Pulmonary Pathophysiology

Pulmonary Pathophysiology

Gerard J. Criner, M.D.

Professor of Medicine
Director, Pulmonary and Critical Care Medicine
Temple University School of Medicine
Philadelphia, Pennsylvania

Gilbert E. D'Alonzo, D.O.

Professor of Medicine
Deputy Director, Pulmonary and Critical Care Medicine
Temple University School of Medicine
Philadelphia, Pennsylvania

Fence Creek
Publishing

Madison,
Connecticut

Typesetter: Pagesetters, Brattleboro, VT
Printer: Port City Press, Baltimore, MD
Illustrations by Visible Productions, Fort Collins, CO
Distributors:

United States
Blackwell Science, Inc.
Commerce Place
350 Main Street
Malden, MA 02148
Telephone orders: 800-215-1000 or 781-388-8250
Fax orders: 781-388-8270

Canada
Login Brothers Book Company
324 Saulteaux Crescent
Winnipeg, Manitoba
Canada, R3J 3T2
Telephone orders: 204-224-4068

Australia
Blackwell Science, Pty Ltd.
54 University Street
Carlton, Victoria 3053
Telephone orders: 03-9347-0300
Fax orders: 03-9349-3016

Outside North America and Australia
Blackwell Science, Ltd.
c/o Marston Book Service, Ltd.
P.O. Box 269
Abingdon Oxon, OX14 4XN England
Telephone orders: 44-01235-465500
Fax orders: 44-01235-465555

2 3 4 5 6 7 8 9 10

TABLE OF CONTENTS

Contributors .... **ix**

Preface .... **xi**

Gerard J. Criner, M.D.

Gilbert E. D'Alonzo, D.O.

Chapter 1 .... **1**

Growth and Development

John M. Travaline, M.D.

Friedrich Kueppers, M.D.

Chapter 2 .... **11**

Normal Lung Structure

Daniel Shade, Jr., M.D.

Francis C. Cordova, M.D.

Chapter 3

Normal Lung Function

Section 3.1: Ventilation 37

Section 3.2: Diffusion Capacity 49

Section 3.3: Lung Circulation 59

Section 3.4: Gas Transport and Acid-Base Status of the Lung 72

Section 3.5: Ventilation-Perfusion Relationships 89

Section 3.6: Normal Exercise Physiology 105

Bernard Borbely, M.D.

Gilbert E. D'Alonzo, D.O.

Chapter 4 .... **115**

Airflow Obstruction

David E. Ciccolella, M.D.

Kathleen J. Brennan, M.D.

Chapter 5 .... **135**

Parenchymal Inflammation and Injury

Clarke U. Piatt, M.D.

Gerald O'Brien, M.D.

Chapter 6 .... **151**

Pulmonary Hypertension

Trudy A. Kantra, D.O.

Gilbert E. D'Alonzo, D.O.

Chapter 7 171

Respiratory Failure

Gerard J. Criner, M.D.

Chapter 8 191

Exercise and Disease

Francis C. Cordova, M.D.

David S. Kukafka, M.D.

Gilbert E. D'Alonzo, D.O.

Chapter 9 211

Asthma

David E. Ciccolella, M.D.

David S. Kukafka, M.D.

Chapter 10 233

Chronic Obstructive Pulmonary Disease

Friedrich Kueppers, M.D.

Chapter 11 243

Sarcoidosis

Daniel Shade, Jr., M.D.

Gerald O'Brien, M.D.

Chapter 12 259

Interstitial Lung Diseases

Yaroslav Lando, M.D.

Gerald O'Brien, M.D.

Chapter 13 285

Pathophysiology of Pulmonary Embolism

Michaela Stanciu, M.D.

Gilbert E. D'Alonzo, D.O.

Chapter 14 301

Lung Cancer

David S. Kukafka, M.D.

John M. Travaline, M.D.

Chapter 15 315

Mycobacterial Diseases

Perwaiz H. Rahim, M.D.

Samuel L. Krachman, D.O.

Chapter 16 .... **331**

    HIV Infection and the Lung

    Ubaldo Martin, M.D.

    Gerard J. Criner, M.D.

Chapter 17 .... **353**

    Sleep Apnea and Sleep-Related Breathing Disorders

    Samuel L. Krachman, D.O.

    Thomas Berger, B.A., R.P.S.G.T.

Chapter 18 .... **367**

    Pleural Disease

    Kathleen J. Brennan, M.D.

Chapter 19 .... **383**

    Occupational Lung Diseases

    Francis C. Cordova, M.D.

    Daniel Shade, Jr., M.D.

Index **405**

CONTRIBUTORS

Thomas Berger, B.A., R.P.S.G.T.
Coordinator, Sleep Disorders Center
Temple University School of Medicine
Philadelphia, Pennsylvania

Bernard Borbely, M.D.
Research Fellow
Temple University School of Medicine
Philadelphia, Pennsylvania

Kathleen J. Brennan, M.D.
Clinical Instructor of Medicine
Temple University School of Medicine
Philadelphia, Pennsylvania

David E. Ciccolella, M.D.
Assistant Professor of Medicine
Director, Inpatient Asthma Center
Temple University School of Medicine
Philadelphia, Pennsylvania

Francis C. Cordova, M.D.
Assistant Professor of Medicine
Temple University School of Medicine
Philadelphia, Pennsylvania

Gerard J. Criner, M.D.
Professor of Medicine
Director, Pulmonary and Critical Care
 Medicine
Temple University School of Medicine
Philadelphia, Pennsylvania

Gilbert E. D'Alonzo, D.O.
Professor of Medicine
Deputy Director, Pulmonary and Critical
 Care Medicine
Temple University School of Medicine
Philadelphia, Pennsylvania

Trudy A. Kantra, D.O.
Fellow
Temple University School of
 Medicine
Philadelphia, Pennsylvania

Samuel L. Krachman, D.O.
Assistant Professor of Medicine
Director, Sleep Disorders Center
Temple University School of Medicine
Philadelphia, Pennsylvania

Friedrich Kueppers, M.D.
Professor of Medicine
Temple University School of Medicine
Philadelphia, Pennsylvania

David S. Kukafka, M.D.
Fellow
Temple University School of Medicine
Philadelphia, Pennsylvania

Yaroslav Lando, M.D.
Fellow
Temple University School of Medicine
Philadelphia, Pennsylvania

Ubaldo Martin, M.D.
Fellow
Temple University School of Medicine
Philadelphia, Pennsylvania

Gerald O'Brien, M.D.
Assistant Professor of Medicine
Medical Director, Lung Transplantation
Temple University School of Medicine
Philadelphia, Pennsylvania

Clarke U. Piatt, M.D.
Fellow
Temple University School of Medicine
Philadelphia, Pennsylvania

Perwaiz H. Rahim, M.D.
Fellow
Temple University School of Medicine
Philadelphia, Pennsylvania

Daniel Shade, Jr., M.D.
Senior Research Fellow
Temple University School of Medicine
Philadelphia, Pennsylvania

Michaela Stanciu, M.D.
Fellow
Temple University School of Medicine
Philadelphia, Pennsylvania

John M. Travaline, M.D.
Assistant Professor of Medicine
Director, Invasive Procedures
Temple University School of Medicine
Philadelphia, Pennsylvania

PREFACE

For the medical student, the transition from classroom and textbook learning to the clinical arena is a difficult and complex one that requires extensive knowledge and clinical acumen and well-honed history-taking and physical examination skills. One of the essential paths for making the transition from the classroom to clinical practice is the pathophysiology course, in which the mechanisms of disease processes are presented in the context of clinical medicine. In this book, we have tried to incorporate in a case presentation format the basic pathophysiologic mechanisms of pulmonary disease states. Moreover, we have made extensive use of illustrations, tables, margin notes, and end-of-chapter review questions in an effort to make the material easier to understand and to foster memory retention.

In this textbook, Chapters 1 through 3 deal with normal lung development and function. Chapters 4 through 8 describe the pathophysiologic changes that occur in specific lung diseases. Chapters 9 through 19 review specific pulmonary diseases and thus reinforce the pathophysiologic principles that are essential to each disorder. In Chapters 5 through 19, one or more clinical case studies are used to highlight important points presented in the chapters, and the text is followed by a series of review questions related to the physiologic principles that need special reinforcement.

We are indebted to the students we have instructed, who have honed our teaching skills; to our contributors, who have devoted much time and effort to the writing of the various chapters; to Darlene Macon for her secretarial support; and to our families for their everlasting support and patience.

Gerard J. Criner, M.D.
Gilbert E. D'Alonzo, D.O.

INTRODUCTION

Pulmonary Pathophysiology is one of six titles in the *Pathophysiology Series* from Fence Creek Publishing. These books have been designed as course supplements and aids for board review for second- and third-year medical students who are studying the pathophysiology of individual organ systems. Each book in the series is an overview of a major organ system with an emphasis on pathophysiology. Diagnosis, treatment, and management of specific diseases are also covered at a level appropriate for preclinical study. Each chapter has one or more clinical cases integrated throughout the text; the resolution of these cases requires mastery of the pathophysiologic concepts presented in the chapter.

Each book in the *Pathophysiology Series* shares common features and formats. Difficult concepts are presented in a brief and focused format to provide a pedagogical aid that facilitates both knowledge acquisition and review. Extensive use of margin notes, figures, tables, and board-review questions illuminates the basic science principles of pathophysiology.

Given the long gestation period necessary to publish a book, it is often impossible for publishers to keep pace with rapid changes and advances. However, the authors and the publisher recognize the need to have access to the most current information and are committed to keeping *Pulmonary Pathophysiology* as up to date as possible between editions. As the field of pulmonology evolves, updates to this text may be posted on our web site periodically at http://www.fencecreek.com.

We hope that students find the format and the text material relevant, interesting, and challenging. The Fence Creek staff and the authors welcome your comments and suggestions for use in future editions.

Chapter 1
GROWTH AND DEVELOPMENT

John M. Travaline, M.D.

Friedrich Kueppers, M.D.

▊ CHAPTER OUTLINE

Learning Objectives
Case Study: Introduction
In Utero Lung Development
Histology of Lung Development
Diaphragm and Pleura Development
Development of the Lung Vasculature
Fetal Circulation
Case Study: Continued
The First Breath
Surfactant
Postnatal, Childhood, and Adult Development
Normal Aging
Abnormalities of Lung Growth and Development
Case Study: Resolution
Review Questions

▊ LEARNING OBJECTIVES

At the completion of this chapter, the reader should:
• Know the important features of lung growth and development.
• Understand fetal circulation and the changes that occur at birth.
• Understand the effects of aging on the lung.
• Appreciate important developmental anomalies that result in lung disease and dysfunction.

Case Study: *Introduction*	E. A. is a 30-year-old woman who recently has discovered that she is pregnant. She sees her obstetrician for her first prenatal visit, at which time the physician examines her and reviews with her recommendations for prenatal health.
	E. A. is elated over her pregnancy and pleased to learn from her physician that everything appears to be fine with her and her baby. She is eager to initiate all of the recommendations that her physician has suggested to ensure the proper and healthy development of her baby.

▊ IN UTERO LUNG DEVELOPMENT

In utero lung development can be broken into four periods: embryonic, pseudoglandular, canalicular, and saccular (Table 1-1).

Table 1-1
Periods of In Utero Lung Development

PERIOD	APPROXIMATE TIME IN GESTATION	MAIN EVENT
Embryonic	26 days to 6 weeks	Major airway development
Pseudoglandular	6–16 weeks	Development of smaller airways (bronchioles)
Canalicular	16–24 weeks	Acinus formation and vascularization of the lung
Saccular	24 weeks to term	Subsaccules form and alveoli begin to appear

EMBRYONIC

The embryonic period begins approximately 26 days after ovulation. The lung develops from a ventral outpouching of the foregut that is lined by endodermal epithelium. This outpouching gives rise to the right and left lung buds, which elongate into the primary lung sacs, and by day 32 to 34 the five lobar bronchi appear as outgrowths of the primary bronchi. In the sixth week of gestation, segmental bronchi form, marking the end of the embryonic period.

PSEUDOGLANDULAR

During the pseudoglandular period, the five lobar bronchi divide, and by the fourteenth week of gestation approximately 75% of all bronchial branching is complete. By the sixteenth week, all conducting airways are present and with time they grow only in size. At this point, the airways are blind tubules lined by cuboidal epithelium and give the lung the histologic appearance of a gland.

By the end of this period, approximately 20 generations of airways have developed. All but the last eight generations of airways will eventually develop cartilage in their walls and be considered bronchi. The last eight generations will not develop cartilage and are termed bronchioles.

CANALICULAR

The canalicular period is characterized by the further development of the peripheral (distal) portion of the bronchial tree, with the lumina of the bronchi and bronchioli becoming larger. The terminal bronchioles are also giving rise to respiratory bronchioles. During this period, the lung is also becoming very vascularized. These events are the basis for the formation of the gas exchange units in the lung. By the twentieth week of gestation, lamellar inclusions that are the sites of surfactant synthesis within granular pneumocytes can be seen.

SACCULAR

The saccular period begins at about the twenty-fourth week of gestation and is marked by the development and proliferation of thin-walled saccules at the ends of the respiratory bronchioles. These saccules are a primitive form of alveoli. During this period the lung increases in volume and surface area.

As early as the thirtieth week, saccules develop into subsaccules that become alveoli. At term, it is estimated that 30 million to 50 million alveoli are present in the lung. Although a relative slowing of alveolar development is thought to occur during the first 3 months after birth, there is a steep increase in the number of alveoli during the first year of life, and by approximately 3 years of age, the number of alveoli reaches an estimated 300 million—the same as in the adult (Table 1-2).

Approximately 10% to 15% of the total number of alveoli in the adult are present at birth.

Table 1-2
Lung Size at Various Ages

AGE	NUMBER OF ALVEOLI ($\times 10^6$)	NUMBER OF AIRWAYS ($\times 10^6$)	SURFACE AREA FOR GAS EXCHANGE (m²)	BSA* (m²)
Birth	24	1.5	2.8	0.21
3 months	77	2.5	7.2	0.29
13 months	129	4.5	12.2	0.45
8 years	280	14	32	0.92
Adult	296	14	75	1.9

* BSA = Body surface area.
Table adapted from Avery ME, Fletcher BD, Williams R: *The Lung and Its Disorders in the Newborn Infant,* 4th ed. Philadelphia: WB Saunders, 1981.

∎ HISTOLOGY OF LUNG DEVELOPMENT

CELL TYPES

During in utero lung development, epithelial thickness of the airways decreases whereas airway diameter increases.

Early in fetal development, the bronchial mucosa consists of a stratified epithelium of vertically oriented cells. By the thirteenth week, ciliated cells begin to appear throughout the bronchial tree. Goblet cells can be seen at the same time; they contain acidic and neutral glycoproteins.

Kulchitsky's cells can be seen in the airway epithelium by gestational week 16. These cells contain characteristic electron-dense granules at their bases and are thought to have an as yet unspecified endocrine function.

Lymphocytes can be found in bronchial epithelium near the basement membrane at about the same time. It is not clear if these cells are related to the so-called bronchial-associated lymphoid tissue that develops after birth.

TRACHEOBRONCHIAL GLANDS

Tracheobronchial glands are found at 10 weeks' gestational age. Initially they are found only in the trachea, but later they also appear more caudally. By the fourth month of gestational age they are present in the bronchial walls. At sites of bifurcations they are present in greater numbers. The ratio of the area occupied by glands as a proportion of the total bronchial wall thickness (Reid index) is similar in adult and late fetal development. In childhood, however, the glandular proportion is greater in the large bronchi. It is estimated that 4000 submucosal glands are present in the human trachea. This number apparently does not change very much in later life. Increased gland area is attributable to greater glandular size and branching.

ALVEOLI

The terminal respiratory bronchiolus divides into several sacs that are lined by cuboidal epithelium; these structures eventually form the alveoli. The cuboidal cells become thin and flat and form the major part of the total alveolar surface (and the lung); these cells are called type I cells. Another type of cell that originates from the primary cuboidal cells is the so-called type II cell, which is present in the alveolar lining. This cell is more cuboidal, has microvilli, and contains surfactant; it is in fact the sole pulmonary source of surfactant.

> Type II pneumocytes are the sole source of surfactant production in the lung.

■ DIAPHRAGM AND PLEURA DEVELOPMENT

The human diaphragm is derived from four embryonic structures: the transverse septum, which is the largest contributor; the pleuroperitoneal membranes; the dorsal mesentery of the esophagus; and the body wall. The dorsal aspect of the transverse septum fuses with the pleuroperitoneal membranes and the dorsal mesentery of the esophagus to form a primitive partition between the pericardial and abdominopelvic cavities. The crura of the diaphragm develop as muscle grows into the dorsal mesentery of the esophagus. By the twelfth week of gestation, lung growth and pleural cavity enlargement appear to burrow into the body wall and separate the body wall into an outer layer, which remains part of the body wall, and an inner layer, which forms the peripheral portions of the diaphragm. Further expansion of the pleural cavities into the body wall results in the formation of the costodiaphragmatic recesses and helps shape the diaphragm into a domelike structure.

The transverse septum lies close to the third, fourth, and fifth cervical spinal nerves. Branches from these nerve roots, along with their associated myoblasts, migrate into the transverse septum and become the primary nerve supply for the diaphragm.

As the lungs grow into the pleural canals, the mesothelium lining the canals becomes the visceral pleura. With time, the pleuropericardial folds wall off the pleural canals, thus creating pleural cavities. The lining of the outer wall of the pleural cavity becomes the parietal pleura.

■ DEVELOPMENT OF THE LUNG VASCULATURE

The pulmonary artery arises from the sixth aortic arch, and the proximal portions on each side form the right and left pulmonary arteries. Whereas the right distal portion loses its connection with the arch, the left distal portion of the arch remains connected with the aorta and forms the ductus arteriosus.

The pulmonary arteries continue to develop during the embryonic and pseudoglandular periods in a fashion similar to that of the airways. By 12 weeks, the preacinar vessels exist in a proportion similar to that in the adult. The remaining time of in utero development is characterized mainly by increases in the diameter and length of the pulmonary arteries.

The pulmonary veins develop from a connection between the common pulmonary vein, which is an outpouching from the sinoatrial region of the heart, and the portion of the splanchnic plexus draining the lungs.

■ FETAL CIRCULATION

Before birth, most of the blood flow from the right ventricle is shunted from the pulmonary artery into the aorta via the ductus arteriosus (Figure 1-1). Approximately 10% of the cardiac output goes to the lungs. Because the right ventricle in the fetus has a greater afterload than the left ventricle, its wall is thicker. In addition to the ductus arteriosus, the fetal circulation uniquely contains two other circulatory channels that help maintain its connection and proper functioning with the placenta.

One of these channels is the foramen ovale. This opening in the atrial septum permits blood to flow from the right atrium into the left atrium. As does the ductus arteriosus, the foramen ovale shunts blood away from the lung. The other channel is the ductus venosus, which shunts blood as it returns to the fetus via the umbilical vein, from the liver into the inferior vena cava.

At delivery, with removal of the placenta from the circulation, there is a marked increase in the systemic vascular resistance and a decrease in the volume of blood returning to the inferior vena cava. As the lung expands with air, pulmonary vascular resistance rapidly falls and the left atrial pressure increases secondary to an increase in

FIGURE 1-1
SCHEMATIC DEPICTION OF FETAL CIRCULATION. This figure is adapted from *The Developing Human*, Keith Moore. Philadelphia: WB Saunders Company, 1982.

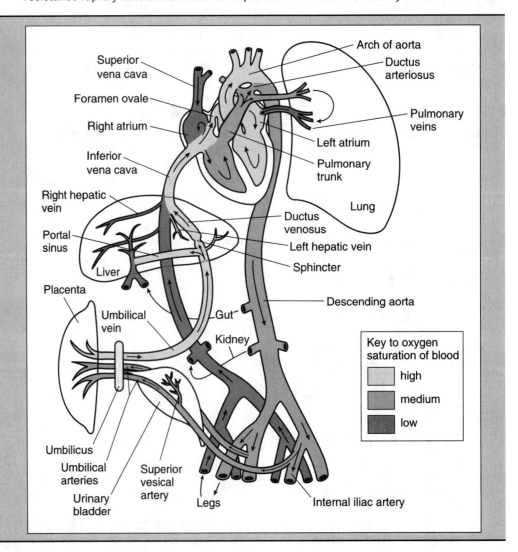

blood flow returning from the lungs and as a result of the increase in systemic vascular resistance. With the drop in pulmonary vascular resistance, the right atrial pressure decreases, and as a result of this decrease, coupled with the increase in left atrial pressure, the foramen ovale functionally closes.

Within hours after birth, the ductus arteriosus is also functionally closed. The trigger is thought to involve the rise in arterial oxygen tension that occurs after birth, but the exact mechanism has not been well elucidated. Following birth, owing to the marked reduction in pulmonary vascular resistance, the wall of the right ventricle becomes thinner in comparison with the thicker wall of the left ventricle. This relationship between the ventricles occurs because of the reduced pulmonary vascular resistance and increased systemic vascular resistance that occur after birth.

E. A. has no complications throughout her pregnancy. Her routine prenatal visits to her obstetrician are characterized by reassurance from the doctor that her baby is developing normally. However, at approximately 32 weeks of gestation, E. A. begins to notice intermittent pelvic and back pain. She sees her obstetrician, who informs her that premature labor has begun. Despite efforts to cease her labor so that her baby can continue to develop in utero, E. A. prematurely delivers a boy.

Case Study:
Continued

■ THE FIRST BREATH

The transition from a fluid-filled lung in utero to an air-filled lung shortly after delivery is a crucial one, and is importantly facilitated by the presence of surfactant. Surfactant is stored in type II pneumocytes and is avidly dispersed into the alveolar space with the first breath.

The transition from fluid-filled to air-filled lungs begins with the first breath. This breath requires the generation of pressure as high as 40 to 100 cm H_2O by the respiratory muscles, predominantly the diaphragm, in order to overcome the elastic and resistive forces of the lung. Surface tension is the force tending to promote alveolar collapse. This force is inversely proportional to the radius of the alveoli, and so smaller alveoli have greater surface tension. Surfactant lines the inner surface of the alveoli and decreases surface tension, and thus the force that must be generated by the inspiratory muscles to inflate the lungs is significantly lower after the first few breaths.

■ SURFACTANT

The single most important biochemical reaction in lung development is the formation of surfactant, which lines the alveolar surface at the air interphase (see Figure 1-2). Pulmonary surfactant is composed of a complex mixture of lipids—particularly phospholipids such as dipalmitylphosphatidylcholine (DPPC). Two distinct proteins of different molecular masses (34 kD and 11 kD) are also intrinsic components of pulmonary surfactant. The detailed structural arrangements of the various components have not as yet been fully elucidated.

> Surfactant reduces surface tension, thereby inhibiting alveolar collapse.

There is a relatively steep increase in surfactant (measured as DPPC) concentration in the lung at about 60% of the gestational period. The material is stored in the alveolar epithelial cells; the concentration within the alveoli is low. At birth, this situation changes rapidly and the intracellular and extracellular (alveolar) pools become approximately equal. If there were no surfactant lining the alveolar surface, there would be a direct fluid-air interface and the surface tension would be approximately ten times as great as it is in the presence of adequate amounts of surfactant. The infant simply does not have enough strength to inflate the lung or sustain even minimal air movement for an extended period of time. The initial breath, which moves approximately 30 mL of air into the lung, requires a negative pressure of 40 to 100 cm H_2O, or approximately 14 times as much as is necessary to move the same volume of air in later, more mature breathing.

> A lack of adequate surfactant in the lung is the primary reason for ventilatory failure in premature infants and is part of the pathophysiology of hyaline membrane disease.

There is considerable variation among individuals in the time of onset of secretion of surfactant into the alveolar space as measured by the amount found in the amniotic fluid. The causes of this variation are not yet understood.

FIGURE 1-2
SCHEMATIC REPRESENTATION OF THE EFFECTS OF SURFACTANT ON THE LUNG. This figure is adapted from *The Ciba Collection*, volume 7, section I plate 41. CIBA Pharmaceutical Company, 1980.

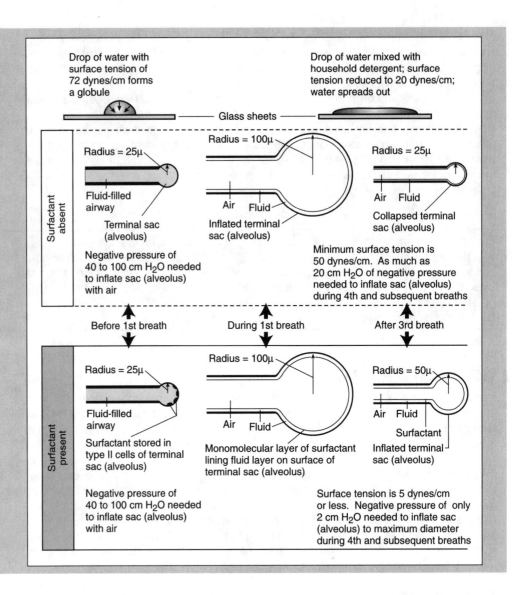

Prematurely born infants can exhibit a condition called hyaline membrane disease—a disorder that results largely from a lack of surfactant in the lung. This disorder is characterized by the failure of the lung to expand fully in the period immediately following birth and for some time thereafter. Thus, there is atelectasis and poor distensibility of the lung. Pulmonary blood flow is impaired, and right-to-left shunting often occurs as a result. The intra-alveolar hyaline membranes that give the disease its name consist of fibrin deposits and cellular debris.

Treatment for this disease includes intratracheal instillation of synthetic surfactant into the lungs. Preventive therapy in situations where premature delivery is anticipated consists of corticosteroid administration to the mother. This therapy may accelerate maturation of the infant's lungs and promote increased surfactant production.

■ POSTNATAL, CHILDHOOD, AND ADULT DEVELOPMENT

Major anatomic changes take place in the thoracic cavity after birth. At birth, the lungs have a greater anterior-posterior diameter in relation to the cranial-caudal dimension. The position of the diaphragm is higher than in later childhood and adulthood. This difference is largely attributable to the relatively greater content of the abdominal cavity, particularly the liver. For adequate gas exchange, rapid, shallow breathing is necessary.

The chest wall of the newborn is more compliant than the chest wall of the adult. It is common, therefore, to see a paradoxical inward movement of the thorax on inspiration in the newborn because of increased chest wall compliance.

Continued growth and development of the lung is characterized by an approximate tenfold increase in the number of alveoli and airways in the lung from birth to adulthood. The surface area for gas exchange is also increased by a factor of approximately 20 (see Table 1-2).

Initially, elastic fibers are found only in the major bronchi and not at the alveolar level. At age 3 months, they can be found at all levels of the lung, including the alveoli.

NORMAL AGING

With advancing age, several changes take place in the respiratory system and the lung (Table 1-3). Some of these alterations are intrinsic to the lung, whereas others occur in response to changes that take place in other organ systems. There is also great variation among individuals in onset and progression of these changes.

FEV$_1$ declines by approximately 10 mL/yr as the lung ages.

EFFECT OF AGING	PATHOPHYSIOLOGIC CORRELATE*
Decreased lung elasticity	Decreased FEV$_1$, increased RV, decreased VC
Increased stiffness of the chest wall	Decreased TLC
Decreased respiratory muscle mass	Decreased MIP
Small airway closure in dependent lung zones	Increased A-a O$_2$ gradient

* FEV$_1$ = forced expiratory volume in 1 second; RV = residual volume; VC = vital capacity; TLC = total lung capacity; MIP = maximal inspiratory pressure; A-a = alveolar-arterial.

Table 1-3
Major Effects of Aging on the Respiratory System

There is a loss of elasticity and hence a decrease in elastic recoil with age. The loss of elastic recoil is greatest at high lung volumes. During conventional pulmonary function measurements, this loss manifests itself by a decrease in the FEV$_1$ (forced expiratory volume in 1 second). The estimated annual decrease in FEV$_1$ varies between 9 and 13 mL depending to some degree on the age range used in the standard reference values and also on whether healthy smokers are included, because smoking independently reduces FEV$_1$ to a greater degree.

A further consequence of the loss of elasticity is the early closure of small airways in dependent lung zones. This results in several consequences: 1) an increased residual volume (RV) and decreased vital capacity, 2) a ventilation/perfusion mismatch and an increased alveolar-arterial (A-a) oxygen gradient, and 3) an increased alveolar duct size.

There are also changes in the chest wall that have consequences for the lung. These changes include: 1) a decrease in chest wall compliance, 2) weakening of the respiratory muscles, and 3) a decrease in muscle mass. These changes also contribute to the loss of vital capacity and the decrease in FEV$_1$.

Chest wall compliance decreases with aging.

ABNORMALITIES OF LUNG GROWTH AND DEVELOPMENT

DEVELOPMENTAL ANOMALIES

These anomalies arise at various stages of lung development, perhaps as a result of somatic mutations of genes that govern differentiation of lung-specific structures. There may be complete bilateral agenesis of the lung, which is of course incompatible with life. There is usually rudimentary development of the trachea or a laryngotracheal bud that ends blindly. There can also be nearly full development of the bronchi but no alveolar differentiation.

Unilateral pulmonary agenesis is a more frequent condition. There can be a total unilateral absence of all lung structures. In other cases there can be a rudimentary bronchus but no lung parenchyma, or there may be bronchial hypoplasia and a reduced amount of lung tissue. Cases of unilateral agenesis are usually discovered early at autopsy, but rare patients have lived to the sixth or seventh decade. The functional states of these conditions depend on various factors such as associated vascular abnormalities and therefore the degree of shunting of blood away from aerated portions of the lung.

Among the minor developmental anomalies that do not always produce clinical symptoms is the complete absence of one or several lobes. In these situations the bronchi either are absent or end in small caps of underdeveloped lung tissue.

Abnormal lobe formation in the lung is relatively common. An azygos lobe, usually in the right lung, is found when a portion of the right upper lobe grows more medially and posteriorly than normal. A cardiac lobe, another rare anomaly, develops when the anterior basal segment of the right lower lobe becomes separated from the lower lobe.

PULMONARY SEQUESTRATION

Lung sequestration refers to lung tissue that is contained within a lobe (usually a lower lobe) but is not connected to the bronchial system. Its blood supply, however, is derived from the systemic circulation.

Sequestrations of the lung are generally separated into two classes: 1) intralobar and 2) extralobar. Intralobar sequestrations are located within the visceral pleura and usually are not associated with other anomalies. Extralobar sequestrations, however, are defined as being separated from the lung and outside of the visceral pleura. Frequently these sequestrations are associated with other anomalies such as diaphragmatic defects.

Sequestrated lung tissue can remain dormant for a long time without producing symptoms. However, infection or cyst formation, or an abnormal chest x-ray, may eventually lead to its detection and possible removal.

> Pulmonary sequestrations are classified as either intralobar or extralobar.

ABNORMALITIES OF THE TRACHEA AND BRONCHI

Major bronchial and tracheal developmental abnormalities can arise at several stages of pulmonary development. The bronchial tree originates from the laryngotracheal bud at about day 24 of gestation. In rare cases, a second respiratory bud develops more caudally from the esophagus or from the poorly differentiated stomach. Accessory bronchi can arise from these structures, or from the primitive trachea.

These bronchi can become part of an otherwise normal lung or they can give rise to an accessory lobe or become atretic. They can also lead to accessory bronchial buds or give rise to esophageal diverticula or cysts depending on the completeness of the development.

CONGENITAL DIAPHRAGMATIC DEFECTS

Failure of the posterior or posterolateral aspect of the diaphragm to close during development may result in herniation of abdominal contents into the thorax. This type of defect occurs in approximately 1 in 2000 births. This defect (Bochdalek's hernia) is usually unilateral and is more commonly present on the left side. Lung development on the affected side is impaired, and hypoplasia of the lung occurs as a result of compression by herniated abdominal contents.

Herniation of abdominal structures through the sternocostal hiatus (Morgagni's foramen) sometimes occurs and is associated with defects in the umbilical region.

Eventration of the diaphragm is produced by failure of muscular tissue to extend into the pleuroperitoneal membrane. This defect in the diaphragm results in an outpouching of the diaphragm in which abdominal contents may be cranially displaced into the saclike structure.

> Diaphragmatic hernias may be posterior (Bochdalek's hernia) or anterior (Morgagni's hernia).

Case Study: *Resolution*

E. A.'s child is placed immediately on a ventilator in order to support his life while exogenous synthetic surfactant is administered and allowed to facilitate his lung function. Time is also afforded to allow continued lung growth and development, so that by 38 weeks of gestation, he is able to sustain sufficient lung function and grow normally into childhood.

▌REVIEW QUESTIONS

1. Match each of the following descriptions with the appropriate period of lung development from the list below.

   (1) During this period, the thin-walled saccules at the ends of the respiratory bronchioles develop into alveoli.
   (2) Lung buds elongate into primary lung sacs.
   (3) Nearly all of the bronchial branching of the lung has been completed.
   (4) During this period, terminal bronchioles give rise to respiratory bronchioles, and the lung becomes more vascularized.

   (A) Embryonic
   (B) Pseudoglandular
   (C) Canalicular
   (D) Saccular

2. Regarding surfactant, all of the following are true except:

   (A) Secreted by type II alveolar cells
   (B) Absence in the newborn impairs lung expansion
   (C) Decreases surface tension in the lung
   (D) Worsens lung compliance

3. Which one of the following is an effect of normal aging on the respiratory system?

   (A) Increase in lung elasticity
   (B) Decrease in A-a oxygen gradient
   (C) Decline in FEV_1
   (D) Increase in vital capacity

4. In fetal circulation, through which structure is blood shunted from the pulmonary artery to the systemic circulatory system?

   (A) Ductus arteriosus
   (B) Foramen ovale
   (C) Ductus venosus
   (D) Bronchial vein

5. A chest radiograph showing an abnormality in the posterior aspect of the thorax could be attributable to any of the following except:

   (A) Eventration of the diaphragm
   (B) Bochdalek's hernia
   (C) Morgagni's hernia
   (D) Pulmonary sequestration

■ ANSWERS AND EXPLANATIONS

1. The answers are 1, D; 2, A; 3, B; 4, C. There are four general stages of human lung development. Each stage is designated by a term related to a major event that occurs during that stage. Thin-walled saccules that form at the ends of respiratory bronchioles become alveoli during the saccular period. Lengthening of lung buds into primary lung sacs occurs during the embryonic stage; this stage is the earliest in lung development. During the pseudoglandular period, nearly all of the lung branching has been completed and the airways are blind tubules lined with cuboidal epithelium that makes them appear as glands. Respiratory bronchiole formation and lung vascularization occur during the canalicular period.

2. The answer is D. Surfactant is composed largely of phospholipids secreted by type II alveolar cells lining the alveoli. The chief function of surfactant is to decrease surface tension in the lung and thereby prevent alveolar collapse. The absence of surfactant would result in decreased lung compliance. This situation is frequently encountered in premature newborns in which a relative lack of surfactant leads to poorly compliant lung function and a condition called hyaline membrane disease.

3. The answer is C. There are several important changes in the respiratory system that normally accompany aging. Loss of elastin in the lung leads to a decrease in lung elasticity. Alterations in gas exchange produce an increase in the alveolar-arterial (A-a) oxygen gradient. FEV_1 declines at a rate of approximately 10 mL/yr with normal aging. Vital capacity also decreases with normal aging.

4. The answer is A. Fetal circulation involves shunting of blood away from the lung into the systemic circulation via the ductus arteriosus. Other important channels that are unique to the fetal circulatory system are the foramen ovale and the ductus venosus. The foramen ovale allows blood to flow from the right atrium into the left atrium and, as does the ductus arteriosus, shunts blood away from the lung. The ductus venosus shunts blood from the liver into the inferior vena cava as it returns to the fetus via the umbilical vein.

5. The answer is C. Structural abnormalities that may exist in the posterior thorax include diaphragm eventration, Bochdalek's hernia, and pulmonary sequestration. Morgagni's hernia is anterior in the thorax (sternocostal hiatus).

■ SUGGESTED READING

Avery ME, Fletcher BD, Williams R: *The Lung and Its Disorders in the Newborn Infant*, 4th ed. Philadelphia: WB Saunders, 1981.

Hislop A, Reid L: Growth and development of the respiratory system—anatomical development. In Davis JA, Dobbing J, eds: *Scientific Foundations of Paediatrics*. Philadelphia: WB Saunders, 1974, pp 214–253.

O'Rahilly R, Muller F: *Human Embryology and Teratology*, 2nd ed. New York: Wiley-Liss, 1996, pp 259–271.

Verhagen AR: Respiratory system. In Rubin A, ed: *Handbook of Congenital Malformations*. Philadelphia: WB Saunders, 1967, pp 157–169.

Chapter 2
NORMAL LUNG STRUCTURE

Daniel Shade, Jr., M.D.

Francis C. Cordova, M.D.

■ CHAPTER OUTLINE

Learning Objectives
Introduction
Case Study: Introduction
The Bony Thorax and Chest Wall
Respiratory Muscles
Airways
Alveolar-Capillary Exchange Units
Lung Compliance
Airway Resistance
Circulation
Case Study: Continued
Lymphatics
Nervous System
Case Study: Resolution
Summary
Review Questions

■ LEARNING OBJECTIVES

At the completion of this chapter, the reader should:
• Understand how the bony thorax facilitates the action of the respiratory muscles.
• Know how the respiratory muscles act to pump air into and out of the thorax.
• Understand how derangements in the mechanical properties and orientation of the respiratory muscles affect airflow.
• Appreciate the specialized function and organization of the airways and gas-exchange units.
• Be familiar with the structure and function of the pulmonary circulation and the differences between intra- and extra-alveolar vessels and their adaptation to pressure-volume changes.
• Understand the structure and function of the pulmonary lymphatic and nervous systems.

■ INTRODUCTION

The respiratory system is extraordinarily well equipped to perform many important functions. The bony thorax, chest wall, and respiratory muscles are arranged to provide the impetus for the movement of gases into the airways all the way down to the alveoli. At the alveoli, an intimate association with a vast capillary network allows gas exchange as well as other metabolic functions to occur. Nervous tissue and lymphatic vessels are omnipresent and perform their respective duties. In this chapter, the structure and organization of these components will be described as well as the consequences that arise when these components are damaged or disturbed.

Case Study:
Introduction

K. G., a 56-year-old housewife with a history of adenocarcinoma of the right breast, presents to your office with a 1-day history of progressive shortness of breath and midchest pain that increases with inspiration. She also has noted pain and swelling of her left lower leg during the last week. Her medical history is remarkable for a diagnosis of stable chronic obstructive pulmonary disease (COPD), which is related to a two-pack-per-day cigarette habit. She has increased her use of a beta-agonist bronchodilator over the night, but to no avail.

On examination, K. G. appears mildly frightened and dyspneic, with a respiratory rate of 35 breaths per minute, and a pulse of 110 beats per minute. She exhibits noticeable retractions of her neck accessory muscles of respiration and marked abdominal tensing on expiration. Her lung fields are slightly diminished to auscultation at the left base, with scant wheezing throughout. The rest of the examination is normal except for a swollen and tender left calf. You order a chest radiograph and arterial blood gas.

■ THE BONY THORAX AND CHEST WALL

The bony thorax

• protects vital thoracic structures.
• serves as scaffolding for respiratory muscles.

The bony thorax not only protects vital structures within the chest cavity (heart, major intrathoracic vessels, and lung) from external injury but also serves as the skeletal framework for attachment of the respiratory muscles. The respiratory muscles, through their thoracic attachments, act as a bellows that drives air in and out of the lung. The adult thorax resembles a truncated cone in that its widest transverse diameter is located at the eighth or ninth rib. It is surrounded by a skeletal and chondral framework consisting of the sternum, ribs, costal cartilages, and thoracic vertebrae. The first seven ribs are connected to the sternum by means of the costal cartilages. The costal cartilages of the eighth, ninth, and tenth ribs articulate with the costal cartilages immediately above them. The cartilaginous tips of the lowest two ribs terminate freely in the lower chest wall. These ribs are also called floating ribs.

The movement of the ribs during inspiration serves to increase both the anteroposterior and transverse diameters of the thoracic cage.

During inspiration, the anteroposterior and transverse diameters of the thoracic cage increase as a result of the cumulative movement of the ribs at each costovertebral joint. For example, contraction of the parasternal muscles, which arise from the lateral border of the sternum and insert into the upper border of the second through the sixth ribs, decreases the angle between the lateral border of the sternum and the upper border of the ribs, resulting in the so-called bucket-handle motion of the rib cage. The inspiratory action of the scalene muscles, which originate from the cervical vertebrae and insert into the upper two ribs, lifts the entire rib cage upward and outward in a pump-handle motion. The movement of the upper, middle, and lower ribs is shown graphically in Figure 2-1.

The upper abdomen contributes to respiratory mechanics by acting as a fulcrum for exertion of force by the diaphragm as it descends during inspiration.

The upper abdomen also contributes to chest wall structure and mechanical function. The internal surfaces of the rib cage and the abdominal cavities overlap because the diaphragm is so closely apposed to the inner surface of the rib cage, the so-called zone of apposition (Figure 2-2). The zone of apposition is important in enhancing the mechanical properties of the diaphragm and will be discussed later. Because of the intimate relationship of the lower rib cage and abdomen, the mechanical properties of the chest wall are determined by the elastic properties of both. Because the lung and the chest wall are arranged in series, the total pressure of the respiratory system (P_{RS}) is the algebraic sum of the pressures exerted by the lung (P_L) and chest wall (P_W), as shown by the equation $P_W + P_L = P_{RS}$. Under static conditions, the pressure exerted by the chest wall is the difference between pleural and body surface pressures ($P_W = P_{PL} - P_{BS}$). On the other hand, the pressure exerted by the lung is the difference between alveolar and pleural pressures ($P_L = P_A - P_{PL}$). The static volume-pressure relationship of the relaxed chest wall and the lung is shown in Figure 2-3. At functional residual capacity (FRC), or resting volume of the respiratory system, the outward recoil of the chest wall is balanced by the inward recoil of the lung. At higher lung volumes, both the chest wall and lung recoil inward, whereas at lower lung volumes, the outward recoil pressure of the rib cage increases.

At functional residual capacity (FRC), the outward recoil of the chest wall is balanced by the inward recoil of the lung. This is the equilibrium point of the respiratory system.

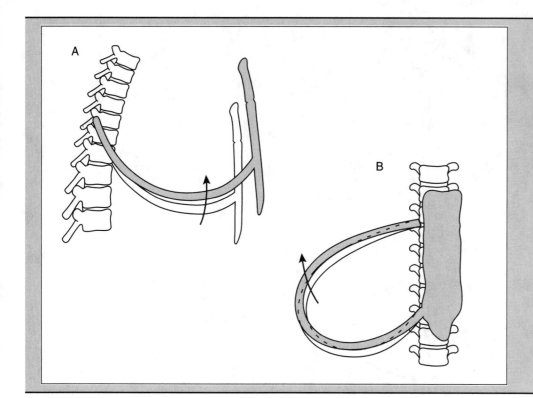

FIGURE 2-1
Diagram illustrating expansion of the ribs with both pump-handle (A) and bucket-handle (B) rotation. The sternum and one rib are shown before and after rib cage expansion (*dark*). Reproduced with permission from de Troyer A, Loring SH: Actions of the respiratory muscles. In Roussos C, ed.: *The Thorax*, 2nd ed. New York: Marcel Dekker, 1995.

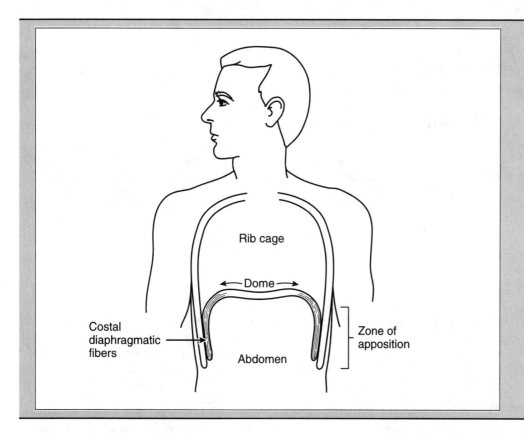

FIGURE 2-2
Diagram demonstrating the relationship of the rib cage, diaphragm, and abdomen, and the zone of apposition (*see text*). Reproduced with permission from de Troyer A, Loring SH: Actions of the respiratory muscles. In Roussos C, ed.: *The Thorax*, 2nd ed. New York: Marcel Dekker, 1995.

FIGURE 2-3
The static volume-pressure curves of the lung (P_L), chest wall (P_W), and total respiratory system (P_{RS}) during relaxation. Adapted from Rahn H, et al.: The pressure-volume diagram of the thorax and lung. *Am J Physiol* 146:161–178, 1946, and Agostoni E, Mead J: Statics of the respiratory system. In Fenn WD and Rahn H. Handbook of Physiology, volume 1, section 3. American Physiological Society, 1964, pp 387–409.

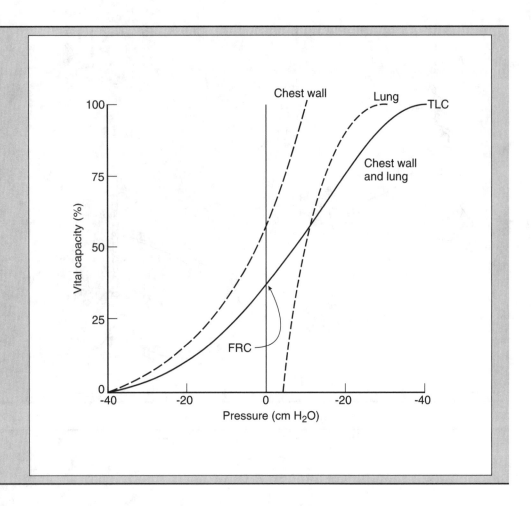

■ RESPIRATORY MUSCLES

The respiratory muscles, in concert with the bony thorax, function as the respiratory pump that drives air in and out of the lung. A good understanding of the functional characteristics of the respiratory muscles and the thorax is important for diagnosis and treatment of the different causes of respiratory failure, such as neuromuscular diseases (i.e., muscular dystrophies, myasthenia gravis, etc.), respiratory muscle fatigue, and deformity of the chest wall (kyphoscoliosis). Moreover, diseases of other organ systems (congestive heart failure, sepsis, systemic lupus erythematosus, hypothyroidism, etc.) can also impair respiratory muscle function and may lead to respiratory muscle dysfunction, hypercapneic respiratory failure, and even failure to wean from the ventilator.

ANATOMY OF THE RESPIRATORY MUSCLES

The diaphragm is the main muscle of respiration. During normal tidal breathing, diaphragmatic contraction results in outward movement of the lower thoracic cage and the anterior abdominal wall. The resulting decrease in pleural pressure causes air to enter the airways and subsequently the alveoli, where gas exchange takes place. During quiet expiration, air is passively expelled from the lung as a result of lung and chest wall recoil. During exercise, when ventilatory demand is increased several fold, accessory muscles such as the external intercostals, scalenes, and sternocleidomastoid muscles exhibit inspiratory action, while the internal intercostal and abdominal muscles exert expiratory action.

Diaphragm. The diaphragm is a musculotendinous skeletal muscle that separates the thoracic from the abdominal cavity (Figure 2-4). Owing to differences in function and attachment to the thorax, the diaphragm is traditionally divided into two separate muscles—namely, the costal and crural components. The costal diaphragm arises from

The diaphragm is the main muscle of respiration.

Normally, in quiet breathing, expiration is passive.

the xiphoid process and from the inner surfaces of the seventh through twelfth ribs while the crural portion arises from the aponeurotic arches on both sides, from the first through third lumbar vertebrae on the right, and from the first and second vertebrae on the left. Both muscles insert into the tendinous portion of the diaphragm, the central tendon. There are three openings (hiatuses) near the central portion of the diaphragm where the aorta, esophagus, and inferior vena cava pass through. The vagus nerve also courses through the esophageal hiatus while both the azygos vein and thoracic duct pass through the aortic hiatus. Because of fiber orientation, a potential cleft may exist posteriorly (foramen of Bochdalek) or anteriorly (foramen of Morgagni), whereby abdominal contents may herniate into the thorax and manifest as respiratory distress during infancy.

The diaphragm is commonly divided into two separate components:

- costal diaphragm
- crural diaphragm

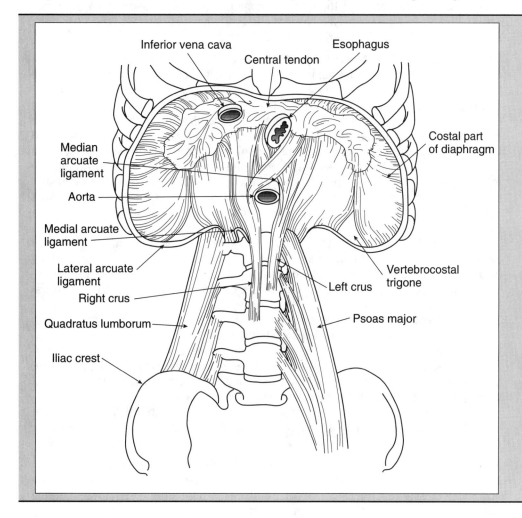

FIGURE 2-4
Schematic coronal section of the human diaphragm, showing its bony attachment. Reproduced with permission from Osmond DG: Functional anatomy of the chest wall. In Roussos C, ed.: *The Thorax*, 2nd ed. New York: Marcel Dekker, 1995, p. 432.

Because of the unique function of the diaphragm in contracting continuously throughout an individual's lifetime, the myofibrils are richly supplied with blood vessels to facilitate transport of nutrients and removal of metabolic waste products. The diaphragm is innervated by the phrenic nerve, a confluence of the fourth, fifth, and sixth cervical roots on each side. On the right side, the phrenic nerve descends into the thorax in close proximity to the superior vena cava, passes in front of the right hilum, and finally passes between the parietal pericardium and the mediastinal pleura before reaching the diaphragm. On the left side, the nerve follows a mid- to lower thoracic course similar to that on the right side after it descends between the left common carotid and subclavian arteries. Sensory innervation to the diaphragm is supplied both by the phrenic nerve and by branches of the sixth to twelfth segmental nerves. The course of the phrenic nerve is important because phrenic nerve injury frequently occurs during cardiac surgery (in 1% to 5% of cases) as a result of the close association of the phrenic nerve with the pericardium.

As the diaphragm contracts, the abdominal contents are pushed downward and the lower rib cage is expanded and elevated. The costal area of the diaphragm where it abuts

The diaphragm is primarily innervated by the phrenic nerve, which courses through the thorax and is vulnerable to various insults, such as tumor encroachment.

The zone of apposition optimizes the mechanical function of the diaphragm by allowing it to use the abdominal contents as a fulcrum.

the rib cage is called the zone of apposition. The zone of apposition optimizes the mechanical action of the diaphragm by allowing it to use the abdominal viscera as a fulcrum to elevate the lower rib cage. During quiet inspiration, the height of this zone decreases by 1.5 cm, whereas the size and shape of the dome of the diaphragm remain constant. Thus, the diaphragm behaves as a piston during much of the inspiration—that is, the radius of curvature is relatively maintained, thereby promoting mechanical coupling between the abdomen and the thorax.

The diaphragm can also function as expiratory muscle in certain circumstances. During total lung capacity maneuvers or hyperinflation as a result of air trapping, as seen in COPD, the diaphragm assumes a more flattened position. Contraction of the diaphragm in this position pulls the lower rib cage inward, thus producing an expiratory action. Paradoxical inward movement of the lower rib cage during inspiration (Hoover's sign) is commonly seen in hyperinflated COPD patients.

Intercostal and Accessory Muscles. There are two groups of intercostal muscles: the external and internal intercostals. The external intercostal muscles extend from the articulations between the ribs and vertebral bodies to the origins of the costal cartilages. Beyond the costal cartilages, the external intercostal muscles become the fibrous aponeurosis called the anterior intercostal membrane. On the other hand, the internal intercostal muscles extend from the sternum to the angles of the ribs dorsally and to the sternocostal junction ventrally. Thus, the only muscles located between the sternum and the chondrocostal junction are the internal intercostal muscles. In this location, the internal intercostal muscles are particularly thick and are sometimes called the parasternal intercostal muscles. Both motor and sensory innervation of the intercostal muscles are derived from the first through twelfth thoracic nerve roots. The lower intercostal nerve contributes to the innervation of the lower abdominal muscles and diaphragm.

Based on their anatomic attachment, the external intercostal muscles and the parasternal portions of the internal intercostal muscles elevate the rib cage during inspiration and thus are considered inspiratory muscles. In contrast, the internal intercostal muscles depress the rib cage during active contraction, thus producing an expiratory action on the chest wall.

The accessory muscles of respiration include the anterior, middle, and posterior scalenus muscles and the sternocleidomastoid muscles. These muscles act as inspiratory muscles, especially during conditions of high ventilatory requirement such as exercise or in the presence of disease states. However, even during normal quiet breathing, the scalenus muscles are invariably active, unlike the sternocleidomastoid muscles, which are recruited only when ventilation increases substantially.

Contraction of both the sternocleidomastoid and scalenus muscles causes cranial displacement of the upper rib cage as well as a significant increase in its anteroposterior diameter.

Abdominal Muscles. The abdominal muscles include the rectus abdominis muscles, the external and internal obliques, and the transversus abdominis muscle. The abdominal muscles are expiratory muscles and are recruited during exercise and during obstruction of airways when exhalation becomes an active process.

Active exhalation is accomplished by the abdominal muscles through two mechanisms. First, contraction of the abdominal muscles results in inward displacement of the abdominal wall and produces an increase in abdominal pressure. As a consequence, the diaphragm is pushed cranially into the thoracic cavity, thereby increasing pleural pressure and emptying the lung. The second action of the abdominal muscles results from their attachment to the lower rib cage. The rectus abdominis muscles originate from the ventral aspect of the sternum and from the fifth to seventh costal cartilages and insert into the pubis bone. The external abdominal oblique originates from the lower eight ribs and inserts into the inguinal ligament and iliac crest. The internal abdominal oblique muscle lies deep to the external abdominal oblique muscle and originates from the iliac crest and inguinal ligament and inserts onto the costal margin. The transversus abdominis muscle is the deepest muscle of the lateral abdominal wall. Its fibers arise from the inner surface of the lower six ribs, lumbar fascia, iliac crest, and inguinal ligament, and it inserts ventrally into the rectus sheath. Contraction of the lower abdominal muscles pulls the lower rib cage caudally, thereby decreasing its anteroposterior dimension.

Intercostal Muscle Groups

- External (primarily inspiratory)
- Internal (primarily expiratory)

Accessory Muscles of Respiration

- Scalenes
- Sternocleidomastoids

The abdominal muscles are expiratory muscles.

FUNCTIONAL CHARACTERISTICS OF THE RESPIRATORY MUSCLES

The respiratory muscles have a biochemical composition similar to that of other skeletal muscles, and thus behave much as do other skeletal muscles in the body. Certain important differences, however, are evident. First, the function of the respiratory muscles is as critical in sustaining life as is the function of the heart. Second, the respiratory muscles are involved in both voluntary and involuntary control. Third, respiratory skeletal muscles must overcome resistive and elastic loads whereas other skeletal muscles must overcome only inertial loads.

Types of Muscle Fibers. Different types of muscle fibers can be identified on the bases of myosin adenosinetriphosphatase (myosin ATPase) content and mitochondrial and glycolytic enzyme activities. There are three main types of muscle fibers. Type I fibers have low myosin ATPase contents, high mitochondrial activities, and low glycolytic enzyme activities. Thus the type I fiber is highly oxidative and fatigue resistant, contracting and dissipating force slowly. In contrast, type II fibers have high myosin ATPase contents and high glycolytic enzyme activities, but lower mitochondrial activities. Type II fibers have a predominantly glycolytic metabolism and can generate higher forces than type I fibers, but are more susceptible to fatigue. Type II fibers are further divided into type IIa and type IIb fibers. Type IIa muscle fibers have higher mitochondrial activities and are more fatigue resistant relative to type IIb fibers.

The respiratory muscles, like skeletal muscles in other parts of the body, are a mixture of slow twitch (type I) and fast twitch (types IIa and IIb) fibers. The mixture of fiber types varies across the respiratory musculature. The diaphragm in adult humans is composed of 55% type I fibers, 21% type IIa fibers, and 24% type IIb fibers. The intercostal muscles contain about 10% more type I fibers than the diaphragm muscle. Abdominal muscle fiber type composition is much more varied compared with the other respiratory muscles.

Muscle Fiber Types
- Type I fibers are oxidative and fatigue resistant.
- Type II fibers are glycolytic and can generate more force than type I fibers, but are more prone to fatigue.

Motor Unit. The muscle fibers are innervated by motoneurons coming out of the neuraxis. A motor unit comprises a single motoneuron and all the muscle fibers it innervates. Within a single muscle, there is a range of motor unit size that depends on the function of the motoneuron. Large, high-threshold motoneurons (not easily excitable) support large motor units, whereas small, low-threshold motoneurons support small units. Moreover, the number of fibers constituting a motor unit varies depending on the size of the muscle itself and its primary function. For example, small muscles in the hand, such as the abductor pollicis, have few motor units compared with large antigravity muscles such as the quadriceps. Muscles requiring fine control of movement have smaller motor units (fewer fibers per motoneuron) than those of muscles that do not require precise muscle coordination.

The pattern of motor unit recruitment also depends on the size of the motor unit—that is, small, slow motor units are recruited during slow contractions (such as quiet breathing) whereas large, fast motor units are recruited only during high-force contraction, such as in hyperventilation during exercise.

A motor unit is a single motoneuron and all the muscle fibers it innervates.

CONTRACTILE PROPERTIES OF THE RESPIRATORY MUSCLES

The function of the respiratory muscles, as for other skeletal muscles, is dependent on their intrinsic contractile characteristics. The force generated during muscle contraction depends on the initial precontraction muscle length (force-length relationship), the velocity of muscle shortening (force-velocity relationship), and the frequency of stimulation (force-frequency relationship). These mechanical properties of the muscle are also dependent on the predominant fiber type found in the muscle and are described below.

Muscle Force-Length Relationship. The active tension developed by the muscle is dependent on the precontractile length of the muscle. The precontractile length at which maximum tension is generated by the muscle is called the optimal muscle length (L_o). The optimal muscle length usually corresponds to the resting length of the muscle. Accordingly, the force generated by the muscle declines on either side of the optimal muscle length, as shown in Figure 2-5.

The tension developed by a muscle is dependent on the precontractile length of the muscle.

FIGURE 2-5
Diagram showing the maximal active tension (% P_O) able to be generated by a muscle (in this example, the diaphragm), and its relationship to optimal length (% L_O). Force generation declines on either side of L_O. Reproduced with permission from Farkas GA: Functional characteristics of the respiratory muscles. *Sem Resp Med* 12(4):251, 1991.

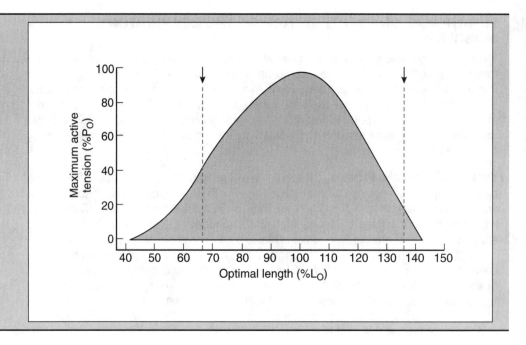

In an intact respiratory system, lung volume becomes the index of muscle length and the pressure generated by the respiratory muscle becomes the index of force. During inspiration, the inspiratory muscles shorten and the expiratory muscles lengthen. Thus the pressure generated by the respiratory muscles is a function of lung volume—that is, as lung volume increases, maximal inspiratory pressure decreases whereas maximum expiratory pressure increases. The converse is true during exhalation.

The force-length relationship for the diaphragm is different from the relationship for other skeletal muscles in that maximal tension occurs at 25% above in situ resting length. In addition, the diaphragm still generates some tension at 40% of in situ resting length, whereas other skeletal muscles develop zero tension at 50% to 60% of in situ resting length.

Muscle Force-Velocity Relationship. Another important intrinsic contractile behavior of the muscle is the relationship between the generated force and the velocity of muscle shortening. As the velocity of muscle shortening increases, the amount of tension the muscle can generate decreases proportionally, as shown in Figure 2-6. In other words, the velocity of muscle shortening is inversely proportional to the force output of the muscle. In an intact respiratory system, a surrogate measure of the velocity of muscle shortening is the rate of airflow. In studies where resistive loading is applied in order to vary airflow, the maximal pressure exerted by the respiratory muscles decreases as the rate of airflow increases.

The force-velocity relationship is an important concept in understanding how the respiratory muscles maintain power output (force multiplied by velocity) during high ventilatory demand. Power output at either extreme of the force-velocity curve is zero. In order to maintain or increase respiratory muscle power output during high ventilatory demand, there is a progressive recruitment of other inspiratory muscles rather than an increase in the force of contraction. Because of this contractile pattern, all of the muscles shorten at a velocity that produces maximum power output.

Muscle Force-Frequency Relationship. The force of muscle contraction is dependent not only on the muscle's initial length and velocity of shortening but also on its stimulation frequency. The force-frequency relationship results from the summation of twitch force during repeated stimulation. The higher the frequency of stimulation, the greater the generated force up to a certain point where generated force plateaus even with further increases in stimulation frequency. The frequency required to achieve this plateau is called the fusion frequency. Fast muscles, such as type IIb fibers, contract and relax more rapidly than slower type I muscle fibers. Thus, at low stimulation frequencies,

The tension developed by a muscle is dependent on the velocity of muscle shortening.

The tension developed by a muscle is dependent on the frequency of stimulation.

slower muscles generate higher forces than faster muscles because relaxation is not completed before the next impulse arrives, which results in a summation of individual twitches (Figure 2-7).

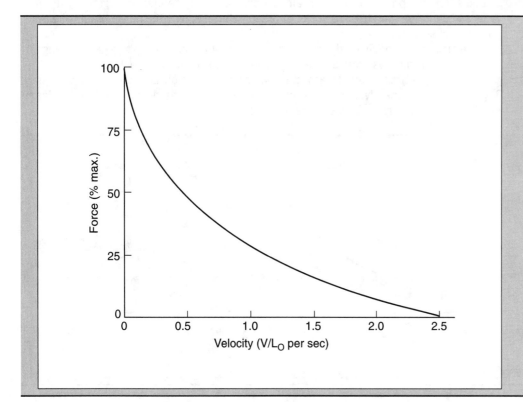

FIGURE 2-6
As the velocity of muscle shortening increases, the amount of force generated by the muscle decreases. Reproduced with permission from Murray J. *The Normal Lung*, 2nd ed. Philadelphia: WB Saunders, 1986, p. 130.

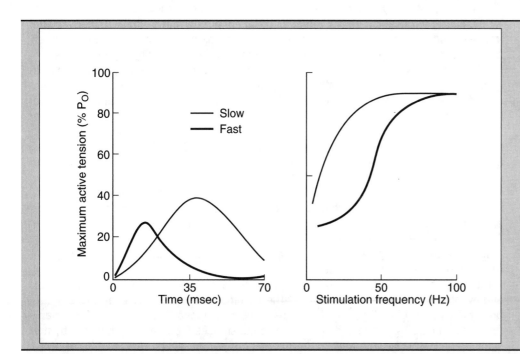

FIGURE 2-7
Isolated properties of fast and slow skeletal muscle. The panel at left shows response to a single twitch. The panel on the right shows response to repeated stimuli. Note that the slow muscle at any level of stimulation is able to generate higher forces than fast muscle. Fast muscle has already fully relaxed by the time slow muscle is achieving peak force in response to a single twitch. (*See text for full explanation.*) Reproduced with permission from Farkas GA: Functional characteristics of the respiratory muscles. *Sem Resp Med* 12(4):250, 1991.

▌AIRWAYS

The primary function of the respiratory system is to provide a conduit for the delivery of oxygen to the alveoli, where gas exchange occurs, and to expel gases and metabolic by-products from the body. Although the airways can be strictly defined as originating at the nares and continuing up to the alveolar-capillary interface, only the intrathoracic airways will be discussed here.

The airways can be divided into two groups depending on their role in gas exchange. The conducting airways start at the trachea and end in the terminal bronchioles. In general, they are thick-walled passages that do not function as gas-exchange units. Beyond this level, the alveolar ducts and alveoli comprise the respiratory bronchioles, which actively participate in gas exchange (Figure 2-8).

The airways may be separated into conducting airways (which do not participate in gas exchange) and respiratory bronchioles (which participate in gas exchange).

FIGURE 2-8
Diagram of the distal airways, showing the terminal bronchioles (TB), respiratory bronchioles (RB), alveolar ducts (AD), and alveolar sacs (AS). The region of the lung distal to the terminal bronchioles is termed an *acinus*.

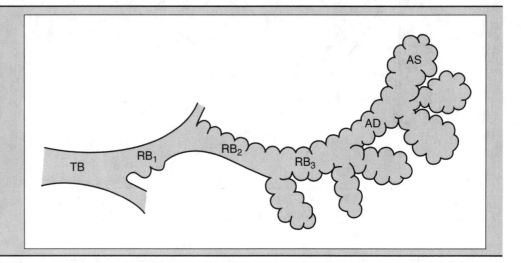

The trachea is supported anteriorly by semicircular cartilaginous rings that provide rigidity, and posteriorly by a thin muscle layer that facilitates removal of airway secretions by decreasing tracheal lumen and inducing turbulent airflow during cough maneuver. The trachea divides at the carina into the left and right main stem bronchi, which further divide into smaller segmental bronchi at irregular intervals for multiple generations.

The walls of the airways contain a myriad of specialized cells that vary in number and composition as one moves distally toward the gas-exchange regions (Figure 2-9). The mucosa is a surface layer of pseudostratified columnar epithelial cells that have cilia on their luminal surfaces. The cilia have a unique arrangement of microtubules (nine peripheral doublets and two central singlets) that is characteristic (Figure 2-10). The rhythmic beating of the cilia creates a mucociliary elevator that transports mucus, cells, and liquid out of the distal airways and into the pharynx. Other cells in the superficial epithelial layer include secretory cells called goblet cells that produce mucus, which is extruded into the lumen; and basal cells, which function as "reserve cells" that are able to differentiate into either goblet or columnar cells, as needed. The basal layer of epithelium may also contain Kulchitsky's cells, or K cells, which are members of the APUD (amine precursor uptake and decarboxylation) system. Their exact role is uncertain, although they may function, in part, as chemical sensors that respond to changes in the compositions of inspired gases.

Kulchitsky's cells are members of the APUD system and may act as chemical sensors.

Distally, the epithelial layer thins into a single layer. Goblet cells decrease in number and eventually disappear at the level of the terminal bronchioles. Also at the terminal bronchioles, nonciliated, cuboidal Clara cells begin to appear. Clara cells perform many functions, including the metabolism of toxic substances (such as carcinogens) by the cytochrome P-450 system, and the formation of important apoproteins and lipids.

The submucosa contains bronchial mucous glands as well as bronchial smooth muscle. The mucous glands produce the majority of the mucus seen in the airways. The number of mucous glands decreases as one approaches the respiratory bronchioles. Smooth muscle exists as a circular band around the epithelium to the level of the respiratory bronchioles, where the overall proportion of smooth muscle is greatest.

Airway smooth muscle tone is determined by:

• the autonomic nervous system
• response to mediators released by inflammatory cells

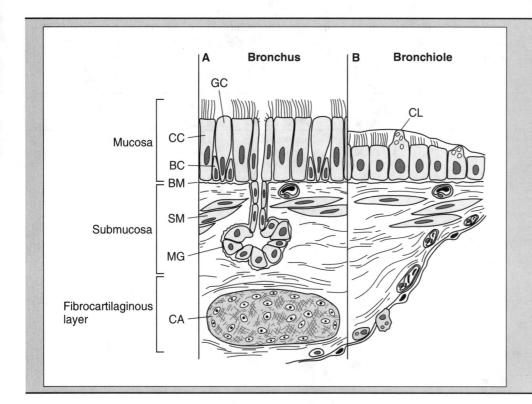

FIGURE 2-9
Cellular components of the airway wall. Panel A depicts cellular composition at the level of the large airways (trachea and bronchi). Panel B shows composition at the smaller airways (bronchioles). CC = ciliated columnar epithelial cell; GC = goblet cell; BM = basement membrane; BC = basal cell; SM = smooth muscle; MG = mucous gland; CA = cartilage; CL = Clara cell.

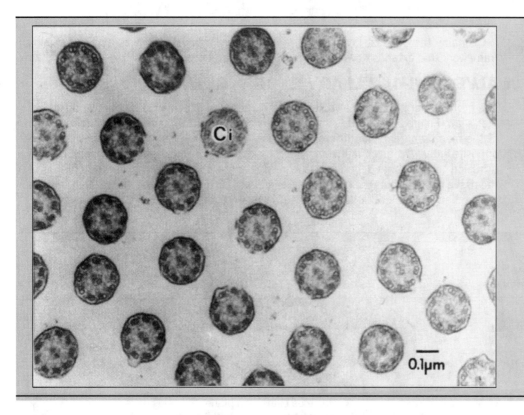

FIGURE 2-10
An electron micrograph of cilia, showing, in cross section, the characteristic arrangement of microtubules (nine peripheral doublets and two central singlets) seen in motile cilia. Reproduced with permission from Staub N, Alkertine KH. Anatomy of the lungs. In Murray J, Nadel J, eds: *Textbook of Respiratory Medicine, 2nd ed.* Philadelphia: WB Saunders, 1994.

Smooth muscle tone is determined by the autonomic nervous system and by mediators released by mast cells and other inflammatory cells. Bronchoconstriction, such as in asthma, can therefore be caused by excessive vagal tone (excess vagal activity can also increase mucus secretion) as well as by the degranulation of inflammatory cells in response to allergens and irritants.

Lymphocytes, individually or in aggregations called BALT (bronchial-associated lymphoid tissue), can be found in the epithelium or in deeper layers of the airway and serve to protect the lung from the potential insult of airborne pathogens and debris. Table 2-1 summarizes the functions of the various respiratory cells.

Table 2-1
Major Airway Cells and their Functions

	PROXIMAL AIRWAYS	CELL FUNCTION	DISTAL AIRWAYS	CELL FUNCTION
Mucosa	pseudostratified columnar	propel mucous and material out of airways	pseudostratified columnar	propel mucous and material out of airways
	goblet cells	secrete mucous	Clara cells	metabolism/ formation of substances
	basal cells	differentiate into goblet or columnar cells	goblet cells*	secrete mucous
	Kulchitsky cells	possible chemical sensors		
Submucosa				
	smooth muscle	bronchial tone	smooth muscle*	bronchial tone
	mucous glands	secrete majority of mucous		
	lymphocytes	defense		
Fibrocartilaginous				
	cartilage	supporting framework		

* Decreased numbers at distal levels

Finally, the deepest layer of the airway is cartilaginous and acts as a supporting framework that extends down to the level of the distal bronchioles.

■ ALVEOLAR-CAPILLARY EXCHANGE UNITS

The exchange of gas at the alveolar-capillary interface is achieved by passive diffusion. Fick's law (Figure 2-11), states that the diffusion of a gas is proportional to the tissue area of the membrane and the difference between the partial pressure of the gases on the opposite sides. Diffusion is inversely proportional to the thickness of the membrane. A diffusion constant that depends on the particular gas studied, as well as on properties of the tissue itself, affects the rate of gas transfer across the membrane. As we shall see, the gas-exchange units of the lung are beautifully arranged to accomplish this task.

FIGURE 2-11
Fick's law.

Fick's Law

V_{gas} (amount of gas transferred) is proportional to:

$$\frac{A}{(T)(D)(P_1 - P_2)}$$

A is the area of the membrane
T is the thickness of the material
D is a diffusion constant
P$_1$ – P$_2$ is the difference in partial pressure of gas

The terminal bronchioles eventually evolve into the respiratory bronchioles, which contain alveoli within their walls and thus are able to participate in gas exchange. A group of three to five terminal bronchioles with its terminal alveolar subdivisions is known as a primary lobule or an acinus. An acinus is the gas-exchange unit of the lung. Proceeding distally, the terminal bronchioles terminate into a rich network of interconnected alveoli. The alveolar walls also contain openings known as alveolar pores of Kohn. Most alveolar pores are covered with surfactant, but large intra-alveolar openings help to ventilate the adjacent alveoli through the process of collateral ventilation. The surface area of the lung available for gas exchange is enormous. It is estimated that the alveolar surface area is 50 to 70 m², or about the size of a tennis court.

The walls of the alveoli are very thin (about 0.5 µm) and are comprised of two major types of cells. Type I pneumocytes are flattened cells with long cytoplasmic extensions that comprise approximately 95% of the alveolar surface. Little metabolic activity occurs in these cells, as evidenced by the relative lack of organelles, but as can be seen in Figure 2-12, the thin cytoplasmic extensions are ideal for gas exchange. In some areas, the adjacent capillary endothelium and the epithelium of the type I cells have a fused basement membrane, thus further decreasing the amount of tissue that the gas has to traverse. Type II pneumocytes are more numerous and contain much more metabolic machinery. The type II cells are capable of differentiating into type I cells and may therefore act as a repair mechanism. In addition, the type II cells produce surfactant, a lipid containing material that acts to reduce alveolar surface tension and thus prevent atelectasis, or collapse, in addition to increasing the compliance (decreasing the stiffness) of the lung. The absence of surfactant is thought to cause the infant respiratory distress syndrome. Type II pneumocytes also remove excess water and material from the alveolar space by actively pumping fluid through sodium-potassium channels located on the basolateral surfaces of their membranes. Lastly, the alveolar spaces contain large numbers of alveolar macrophages that act as an important defense against inhaled pathogens and other materials.

The surface area available for gas exchange is enormous, and approximates the size of a tennis court.

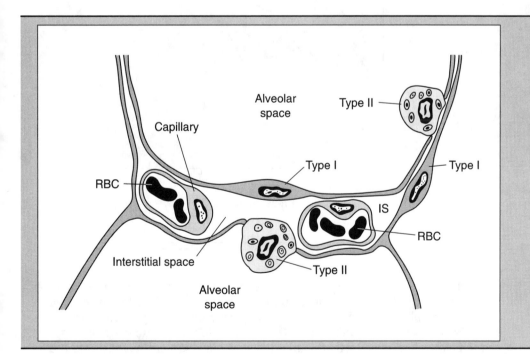

FIGURE 2-12
Diagram of normal alveolar structure showing type I and type II epithelial cells (pneumocytes). Note the thin cytoplasmic processes (which are ideal for gas exchange) in the type I pneumocytes.

■ LUNG COMPLIANCE

Ventilation is the process of moving air from the atmosphere through the upper nasal passages to the conducting airways, and finally to the terminal respiratory units of the lung, where gas exchange occurs. In order for ventilation to proceed, the respiratory muscle has to overcome the mechanical properties of the respiratory system— specifically, the *compliance* (or distensibility) of the lung and chest wall, and the *resistance* of the airways.

Compliance is dictated by the relationship between the change in volume and the change in pressure of a system. Several factors, taken in aggregate, determine the compliance of the lung. The *elastic recoil* of the lung is the force that tends to cause the inflated lung to recoil inward. The primary determinants of lung elastic recoil are the inherent properties of the lung tissue itself—that is, the interrelationship between elastin and collagen fibers within the parenchyma, and the surface forces at the air-liquid interfaces (alveoli), which are largely determined by surfactant. The effect of surface tension on lung compliance is best illustrated by the difference between the volume-pressure curves for a lung filled with saline and a lung filled with air, as shown in Figure 2-13. The saline-filled lung, where surface tension is eliminated, is more compliant than the air-filled lung, which means that less pressure is required to inflate the lung to a given volume. Moreover, the difference in the inflation and deflation limbs of the volume-pressure curve of the lung (hysteresis) is eliminated. In order to decrease the surface tension at the air-liquid interfaces, the alveoli are lined with surfactant. Surfactant is a material composed of lipid (primarily phosphatidylcholine) and protein that is produced by type II alveolar cells and serves to reduce surface tension and thus facilitate inflation. It is responsible for the observed hysteresis loop in an air-filled lung.

$$Compliance = \frac{Change\ in\ volume}{Change\ in\ pressure}$$

FIGURE 2-13
Diagram showing the difference in volume-pressure curves for lungs filled with air and lungs filled with water, based on the elimination of surface tension by saline. The difference between the inspiratory and expiratory curves is called *hysteresis*. Adapted and reproduced with permission from Clements JA, Tierney DF: Alveolar instability associated with altered surface tensions. *In* Fenn WO, Rahn H, eds.: *Handbook of Physiology*, Sec. 3, Respiration, Vol. II. Washington: American Physiological Society, 1964, pp. 1565–1583.

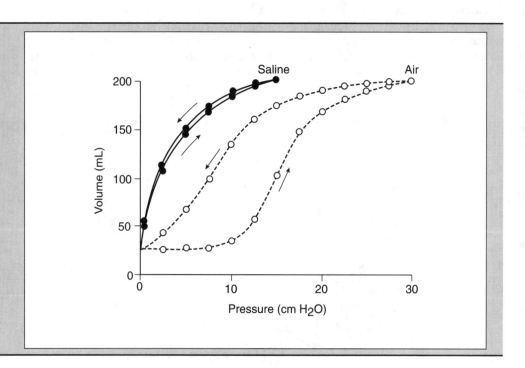

Certain disease states alter the cellular composition of the lung and result in either increased compliance (such as in emphysema, where there is a loss of elastin) or decreased compliance (such as in pulmonary fibrosis), as shown in Figure 2-14. In the adult respiratory distress syndrome (ARDS), damage to the gas-exchange units occurs and initiates a loss of surfactant and an influx of proteinaceous material into the air spaces, resulting in a loss of lung compliance as well as a reduction in the ability to exchange gas.

In addition to the inherent properties of the lung described above, the volume at which compliance is measured also plays a role in lung compliance (specific compliance). At low lung volumes, a small change in pressure produces a large change in lung volume, indicating a high compliance. At high lung volumes, the elastic recoil increases until the limit of distensibility is reached and inspiration cannot continue (Figure 2-15). As previously discussed, the elastic recoil pressure of the total respiratory system is the sum of the pressures generated by the lung and the chest wall.

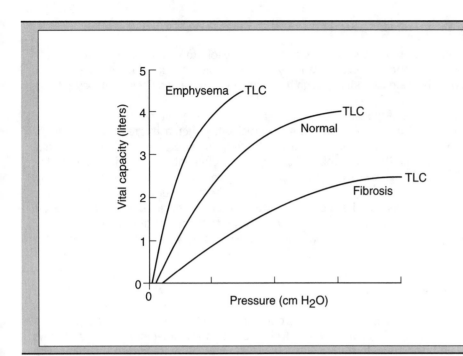

FIGURE 2-14
The compliance of the lung is affected by the intrinsic properties of the parenchyma and airways. The volume-pressure curves depict the very compliant lungs seen in emphysema. In pulmonary fibrosis, the compliance of the lung is low, so that more pressure is needed to inflate the lung. TLC = total lung capacity. Reproduced with permission from Murray JF: *The Normal Lung*, 2nd ed. Philadelphia: WB Saunders, 1986, p. 87.

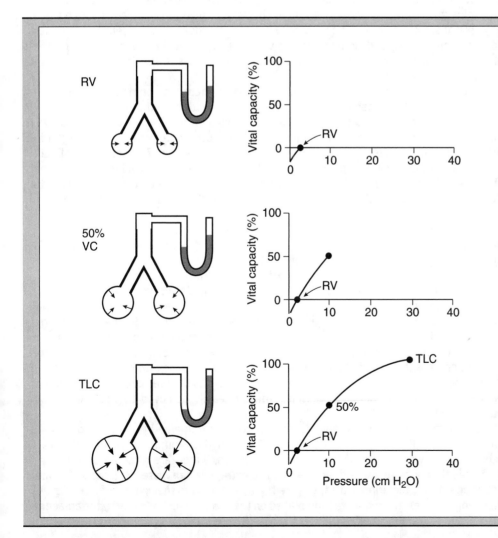

FIGURE 2-15
Schematic representation of the volume-pressure relationships of isolated lungs. As the lungs are inflated from low volume (residual volume, RV) to high volume (total lung capacity, TLC), the recoil pressure is increased. Reproduced with permission from Murray JF: *The Normal Lung*, 2nd ed. Philadelphia: WB Saunders, 1986, p. 86.

■ AIRWAY RESISTANCE

Flow is also determined by the resistance of the respiratory system. For practical purposes, the main source of resistance is the airways (which include the pathway from the nares to the distal airspaces), although the lung parenchyma and chest wall may contribute lesser amounts.

The resistance of the airways is determined by the lung volume, the elastic recoil of the airways, and the airway geometry. Airway resistance increases greatly as the lung is deflated from functional residual capacity (FRC) to residual volume (RV), until a maximal level is reached at RV, where the resistance approaches infinity. At this level, airflow ceases. Elastic recoil provides traction on the airways and thus affects resistance. Lastly, the geometry of the airways, which is determined by the transmural pressure across them as well as by their inherent distensibility related to their composition and smooth muscle tone, is also an important factor that affects airway resistance and airflow. In asthmatics, an inflammatory exudate in the gas-exchange regions as well as increased broncho-constriction lead to marked airflow obstruction and dyspnea.

■ CIRCULATION

The primary function of the pulmonary circulation is to deliver blood to the alveoli in order to participate in gas exchange. As will be seen, this remarkable vascular system is uniquely arranged to perform this duty as well as many other important functions with maximal efficiency.

The pulmonary circulation originates from the right ventricle and includes the pulmonary trunk, the right and left pulmonary arteries, the lobar branches of these arteries, the arterioles, the capillaries, and, on the venous side, the venules and pulmonary veins that empty into the left ventricle. The vessels are thin-walled and contain small amounts of smooth muscle. The pulmonary arteries are located in the centers of lobules and run adjacent to, and branch successively with, bronchi. Pulmonary veins, on the other hand, pass between lobules and run in connective tissue sheaths separated from the arteries and bronchi.

The arterial system extends to the level of the terminal bronchioles and then branches into a dense capillary network that is embedded in the alveolar wall. The alveolar-capillary network has many features that make it very efficient in gas exchange. First, the capillary network is extremely dense. It has been noted that in the congested lung, the blood volume in the alveolar wall may be more than 75% of the total wall volume, a fact that has led some authors to dub this interface a "wall of blood." Next, the alveolar-capillary interface also has an extremely large surface area (estimated at 50 to 70 m²), which aids in diffusion. Lastly, the barrier to diffusion is extremely thin (Figure 2-16).

The pulmonary circulation is unique in that it can adapt to both intra- and extraluminal changes in volume and pressure and still remain a low-pressure system, which is important in preserving the function of the thin-walled right ventricle. The pulmonary arteries receive the entire cardiac output of the right ventricle (6 L/min), but the mean pulmonary arterial pressure is 15 mmHg (normally 25 mmHg in systole and 9 mmHg in diastole), versus a mean systemic arterial pressure of around 100 mmHg. The low pulmonary vascular resistance (Figure 2-17) that is unique to the pulmonary circulation is maintained even in the face of an acute increase in cardiac output to the lung (for example, during exercise) (Figure 2-18). There are two methods by which pulmonary vessels compensate for an increase in pulmonary blood flow: *recruitment* and *distention*. Recruitment is the opening of previously closed vessels as the pressure rises. Distention is an increase in the caliber of vessels, which is easily achieved by the thin-walled pulmonary circuit.

The pulmonary arteries and veins must also adapt to marked pressure and volume changes within the thoracic cavity that may act on their lumina. Physiologists have separated the vasculature into two types of vessels, which are affected by different pressures that occur outside their lumina. The extra-alveolar vessels (Figure 2-19) are not affected by alveolar pressures, but are highly sensitive to the volume of the lung. At high lung volumes, the radial traction placed on the extra-alveolar vessels by the adjacent

---

The alveolar-capillary network is extremely efficient in providing a conduit for gas exchange because:

- the capillary network is very dense.
- the surface area available for gas exchange is quite large.
- the barrier to diffusion is extremely thin.

The pulmonary circulation can adapt to swings in intra- and extraluminal pressure and volume changes and thus preserve the function of the thin-walled right ventricle.

Pulmonary vessels respond to increases in blood flow by recruitment and distention.

There are differences between the manners in which intra- and extra-alveolar vessels respond to changes in lung volume.

lung parenchyma causes dilatation to occur. At low lung volumes, pulmonary vascular resistance within these vessels increases (Figure 2-20). In contrast, the alveolar vessels (in effect, the capillaries that course through the alveolar walls) are exposed to alveolar pressure, and their caliber is determined by the alveolar pressure and the pressure within their lumina. Small vessels in the corners of alveolar walls act in an intermediate fashion between the alveolar and extra-alveolar vessels.

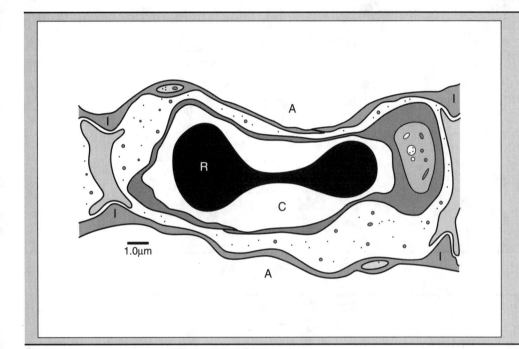

FIGURE 2-16
The thin barrier to diffusion is seen in this cross-sectional diagram of an alveolar wall and adjacent capillary containing a red blood cell. A = alveolus; I = Type I cell; C = capillary; R = red blood cell. Reproduced with permission from Murray JF, Nadel JA, eds.: *Textbook of Respiratory Medicine*, 2nd ed., Vol. 1. Philadelphia: WB Saunders, 1994, p. 25.

Pulmonary Vascular Resistance (PVR)

$$PVR = \frac{PAP - PVP}{Q}$$

PAP = pulmonary arterial pressure
PVP = pulmonary venous pressure
Q = pulmonary blood flow

FIGURE 2-17
Pulmonary vascular resistance.

The behavior of the pulmonary circulation becomes more complex when one considers the effect of gravity on the thin-walled system. Although pressure within the alveoli is roughly uniform in the normal lung, the distribution of pulmonary blood flow in the upright lung is highly dependent on gravity and hydrostatic pressures. Blood flow decreases from the base to the top of the lung. Increasing pulmonary arterial pressure—as a result of exercise, for example—diminishes perfusion differences in the lung by increasing blood flow to both the upper and lower zones.

FIGURE 2-18
Diagram demonstrating the fall in pulmonary vascular resistance that occurs as the pulmonary arterial or venous pressure is raised, an important characteristic that maintains low right ventricular pressure in the face of changing hemodynamic status. Reproduced with permission from West JB: *Respiratory Physiology: The Essentials*, 3rd ed. Baltimore: Williams & Wilkins, 1990, p. 36.

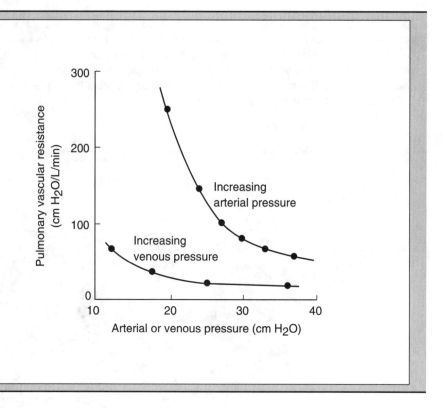

FIGURE 2-19
Diagram showing alveolar and extra-alveolar vessels. Alveolar vessels are exposed to alveolar pressure, whereas the extra-alveolar vessels are sensitive to volume changes within the lung parenchyma. Reproduced with permission from Hughes JMB, Glazier JB, Maloney JE, West JB: Effect of lung volume on the distribution of pulmonary blood flow in man. *Resp Physiol* 4:58–72, 1968.

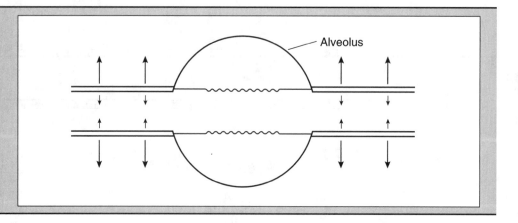

The distribution of pulmonary blood flow in the upright lung is dependent on:

• gravity
• hydrostatic pressure

In order to understand the topographical differences in lung perfusion, the lung has been divided into three zones (Figure 2-21). Zone 1 is a region at the top of the lung where the pulmonary arterial pressure is lower than the alveolar pressure, and the capillaries are closed by the pressure. In normal conditions, true zone 1 conditions (i.e., no blood flow) do not exist, because the pulmonary arterial pressure is sufficient to drive blood to the apex. In addition, the extra-alveolar vessels are still patent, and supply blood to the region. In zone 2, pulmonary arterial pressure is greater than alveolar pressure. Venous pressure here is still lower than alveolar pressure. In this area, flow is dependent on the difference between arterial and alveolar pressures, rather than the difference between arterial and venous pressures. Zone 3 has the usual arrangement in which arterial and venous pressures are higher than alveolar pressure, and the perfusion is driven by the arterial-venous pressure difference. Some authors include a zone 4 at the base of the lung, where lung volumes are low and increased resistance of the extra-alveolar vessels becomes important.

In the discussion above, the passive characteristics of the pulmonary circulation have been explored. There are, however, conditions in which the thin-walled pulmonary

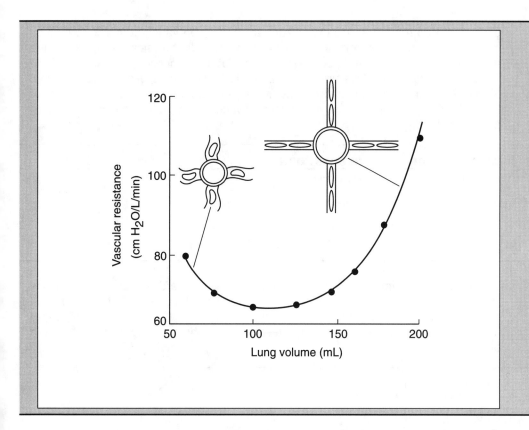

FIGURE 2-20
Diagram demonstrating the effect of lung volume on pulmonary vascular resistance (*see text for explanation*). Reproduced with permission from West JB: *Respiratory Physiology: The Essentials*, 3rd ed. Baltimore: Williams & Wilkins, 1990, p. 62.

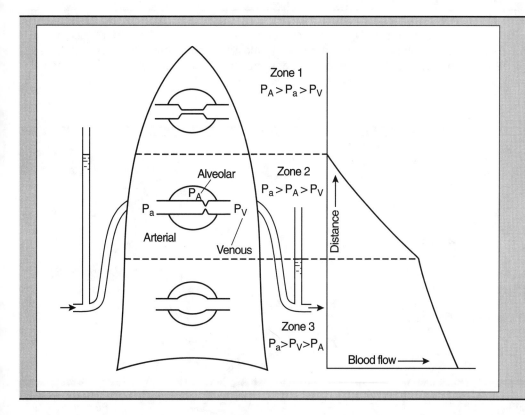

FIGURE 2-21
Diagram showing the topographical differences in lung perfusion, commonly divided into three zones, based on the pressures affecting the capillaries (*see text for explanation*). Reproduced with permission from West JB, Dollery CT, Naimark A: Distribution of blood flow in isolated lung. Relation to vascular and alveolar pressures. *J Appl Physiol* 19:713–724, 1964.

vessels actively vasoconstrict in response to stimuli. Hypoxia is a powerful stimulus for vasoconstriction. The stimulus-response curve for hypoxia in the lung is nonlinear in that PO_2 levels above 100 mmHg do not change vascular resistance, but levels below 70 mmHg cause the circulation to clamp down. The vasoconstriction probably serves to

Hypoxia and acidosis are powerful vasoconstrictors in the pulmonary circulation.

divert blood from areas of low oxygenation and avoid ventilation-perfusion (V/Q) mismatches. Increases in plasma pH augment the vasoconstriction seen in hypoxia. There are many mediators thought to be involved in regulating pulmonary vascular tone (Table 2-2). The autonomic nervous system also plays a small role in regulating vascular tone. Chronic exposure to hypoxia or other vasoconstricting stimuli can lead to thickening of the walls of the pulmonary arteries (pulmonary hypertension) with deleterious effects on the right ventricle.

Table 2-2
Regulators of Pulmonary Vascular Tone

VASODILATATION	VASOCONSTRICTION
acetylcholine	norepinephrine
nitric oxide	angiotensin II
bradykinin	histamine
prostacyclin (PGI$_2$)	serotonin
prostaglandin (PGE$_1$)	thromboxane
	leukotrienes C$_4$, D$_4$
	platelet activating factor

Because the pulmonary vasculature receives the entire cardiac output, it is uniquely suited to act as a filter and to participate in metabolic functions. Certain vasoactive substances are converted or broken down by the circulation (Table 2-3). The lung may also participate in coagulation, act as a reservoir for blood, and filter thrombi from the circulation.

Table 2-3
Some Substances Altered by the Pulmonary Circulation:

serotonin inactivation
bradykinin inactivation
prostaglandin E$_1$, E$_2$, F$_{2a}$ inactivation
IgA secretion
conversion angiotensin I → angiotensin II

A second blood supply, the bronchial circulation, carries 1% to 2% of the cardiac output and supplies blood and nutrients to most intrapulmonary structures, including airways, nerves, and lymph nodes, but does not supply the parenchyma. The bronchial circulation also supplies the visceral pleura (Figure 2-22).

FIGURE 2-22
Schematic diagram of the bronchial circulation. The bronchial circulation contains anastomoses between itself and pulmonary vessels and is thus able to provide some perfusion to alveolar tissues in the event of a blocked pulmonary artery. Reproduced with permission from West JB: *Respiratory Physiology: The Essentials*, 3rd ed. Baltimore: Williams & Wilkins, 1990, p. 1792.

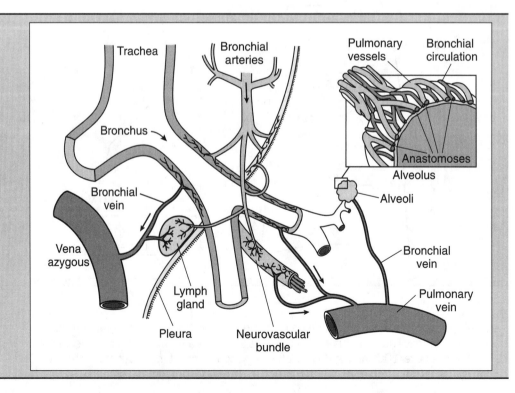

The radiograph reveals a wedge-shaped defect with atelectasis in the left lower lobe, and hyperinflation related to the patient's underlying COPD. The arterial blood gas returns and is significant for an elevated alveolar-arterial (A-a) oxygen gradient. You fear that the patient has suffered a large pulmonary embolism based on the clinical symptoms and history of breast cancer (which is associated with a hypercoagulable state). In addition, the radiograph shows evidence of a wedge-shaped infarct pattern, which is usually present in the distribution of the vessel affected. The atelectasis is caused by impaired surfactant production from type II pneumocytes in response to injury and reduced blood flow. The widened A-a gradient is a result of ventilation-perfusion (V/Q) mismatching in areas of ventilated lung that are deprived of blood flow by the embolus (discussed fully in Chapter 3). You start the patient on anticoagulant therapy and admit her to the hospital. Later that day, her breathing appears more labored and she becomes lethargic. A repeat arterial blood gas shows persistence of the large A-a gradient and marked hypercapnia, with a PCO_2 of 55 (normal, 37 to 43).

■ LYMPHATICS

An extensive lymphatic system exists within the lung and has an important role in fluid homeostasis as well as in defense. Fluid that accumulates from the capillaries in the extra-alveolar interstitium enters the distal ends of lymphatics. The lymphatic vessels contain smooth muscle as well as valves, which facilitate the transport of lymph and fluid from the lung to the hilar and mediastinal lymph nodes. The final destination for lung lymph is either the right lymphatic duct or the thoracic duct. Under certain circumstances, the drainage capability of the lymphatic system can be overwhelmed and can lead to pulmonary edema.

The pulmonary lymphatics act to:

- remove excess fluid from the lung.
- provide defense by removing particulate matter from the lung.

■ NERVOUS SYSTEM

The respiratory system is richly endowed with both sensory (afferent) and motor (efferent) fibers that allow adaptation to a variety of chemical and mechanical changes. Activation and coordination of upper airway receptors is important in the sneeze reflex and the sniff reflex, as well as in coughing and swallowing. The tracheobronchial (afferent) receptors can be separated into myelinated receptors (slowly adapting pulmonary stretch receptors, SARs, or rapidly adapting pulmonary stretch receptors, RARs) and unmyelinated C fibers (Table 2-4). SARs are mechanoreceptors and sense both chemical stimuli (changes in PCO_2) and alterations in lung volume. The precise location of SARs is unknown, but it is thought that they reside in airway smooth muscle cells. RARs also respond to changes in lung volume, but maintain a higher threshold to volume changes than SARs. Chemical stimuli can also discharge RARs. RARs are thought to be housed in airway epithelial cells.

The unmyelinated C fibers are the major sensory fibers in the lung, comprising 75% of fibers that emerge from the lung. Lung volume alterations can discharge C fibers, but endogenous and exogenous chemical agents such as histamine, bradykinin, prostaglandin, serotonin, and cigarette smoke also act as potent stimuli. It is felt that the C fibers may play a role in certain pathologic states that liberate these chemicals, such as pulmonary edema, pulmonary embolism, and asthma. Afferents from SARs, RARs, and C

C fibers are the major sensory fibers found in the lung.

	CELL	LOCATION	MAJOR STIMULI
Myelinated	SAR	?airway smooth muscle cells	chemical, changes in lung volume
	RAR	airway epithelial cells	chemical, changes in lung volume
Unmyelinated	C-fibers (major)	very small airways, alveolar wall, interstitium	many chemicals, changes in lung volume
Other	golgi tendon organs	muscle	changes in muscle tension
	muscle spindle	muscle	changes in muscle stretch

Table 2-4
Major Sensory Afferent Cells

fibers travel back to the central nervous system by way of vagal pathways. Lastly, muscle spindle fibers that detect changes in muscle stretch, and Golgi tendon organs that sense muscle tension, also send impulses from the respiratory muscles back to the central nervous system.

The efferent (motor) nerves have both sympathetic and parasympathetic components. The preganglionic sympathetic nerves originate in the upper four or five thoracic paravertebral ganglia, whereas the preganglionic parasympathetic nerves reside in the vagal brain stem motor nuclei. These fibers then extend from postganglionic nuclei and eventually end near airways, vascular smooth muscle cells, and submucosal glands.

The APUD (amine precursor uptake and decarboxylation) system is also present in the lung, and the characteristic neuroepithelial bodies are usually located at airway bifurcations. It is thought that the APUD system may play a role in peripheral chemoreception, although its exact function is uncertain.

Chemical sensors regulating the control of respiration will be discussed in the next chapter.

Case Study:
Resolution

Your patient has suffered a large pulmonary embolism in the face of underlying lung disease (COPD). As will be discussed in subsequent chapters, COPD results in the loss of elastic recoil in the airways, which leads to air trapping and hyperinflation of the thorax. The hyperinflation changes the orientation of the respiratory muscles, and markedly affects the diaphragm, the major muscle of respiration, by pushing it down or flattening (shortening) it and placing its fibers at a mechanical disadvantage. The respiratory system cannot compensate for the increased work of breathing caused by the loss of pulmonary vasculature by the embolus and increasing V/Q mismatch, and hypercapnia, an ominous sign, ensues.

▮ SUMMARY

The respiratory system is required to perform a myriad of diverse functions including the transport of gases, gas exchange, and immunologic and metabolic activities. The various components of this system are highly specialized and uniquely arranged to accomplish their tasks with utmost efficiency. An understanding of respiratory system structure is of paramount importance if one is to comprehend the consequences of diseases that arise when the framework is deranged.

■ REVIEW QUESTIONS

1. A 64-year-old man with no history of pulmonary disease is admitted to the hospital and undergoes emergent coronary artery bypass graft (CABG) for unstable angina. The patient tolerates the procedure well, is removed from the ventilator without difficulty, and is discharged to home in good condition after 4 days. Three weeks later, the patient is seen in your office and is without complaints. His physical exam is normal except for dullness and decreased breath sounds at the left base. A routine follow-up chest x-ray reveals an elevated left hemidiaphragm. The rest of the film is normal. Decubitus films to detect the presence of pleural effusion are negative. Which one of the following statements is true?

   (A) An ECG and a cardiac enzymes test should be ordered immediately to rule out impending myocardial infarction.
   (B) A chest computed tomography (CT) scan should be ordered.
   (C) The patient should be reassured and released to follow-up.
   (D) The patient should undergo a full oncologic work-up.

2. Which one of the following statements is true about the pulmonary vasculature?

   (A) It receives the entire cardiac output and is a high-pressure system.
   (B) It adapts to changes in volume and pressure by recruitment of closed blood vessels.
   (C) The bronchial circulation receives the majority of the cardiac output.
   (D) Its gas-exchange capabilities are limited by a small capillary bed.

3. A 36-year-old man presents to your office with immotile cilia syndrome. A potential respiratory complication could be

   (A) increased Clara cell mucus production
   (B) decreased epithelial bronchial mucous gland expression
   (C) increased myelinated C fiber discharge
   (D) failure to clear mucus from airways

4. A 39-year-old woman presents to your office with marked elevation in pulmonary arterial pressure. A diagnosis of primary pulmonary hypertension (PPH) is made, and you decide to begin therapy to reduce the pulmonary arterial pressure before irreversible damage is done to the right ventricle. Which agent listed below would be appropriate for reducing the pressure?

   (A) Angiotensin II
   (B) Histamine
   (C) Serotonin
   (D) Nitric oxide

5. Which of the following statements is true concerning the respiratory muscles?

   (A) The major type of fibers present in the diaphragm is type II (fast twitch/glycolytic) fibers.
   (B) The diaphragm is innervated by the vagus nerve.
   (C) The pressure generated by the respiratory muscles is a function of lung volume.
   (D) The amount of tension the respiratory muscles can generate increases with increasing velocity of shortening.

■ ANSWERS AND EXPLANATIONS

1. The answer is C. Phrenic nerve injury following CABG can occur in 2% to 20% of cases owing to the intimate association of the phrenic nerves with intrathoracic structures, most notably the pericardium. The left phrenic nerve is most commonly affected. The injury is usually secondary to damage resulting from the cold cardioplegia solution used for bathing the thoracic structures during cardiopulmonary bypass surgery, although direct mechanical insult may occur also. Unilateral phrenic nerve paralysis is usually well tolerated in patients with no underlying lung disease, and a certain percentage of patients recover full function with time. From the patient's history and exam, there is no evidence of ongoing ischemia. Likewise, there is no evidence of pleural effusion or subphrenic abscess based on the paucity of symptoms and decubitus films. The patient had no evidence of malignancy just 3 weeks prior to his clinic exam.

2. The answer is B. The pulmonary vasculature is a low-pressure system with thin-walled vessels, despite receiving the entire cardiac output per cycle. It accommodates increases in blood flow and pressure by two primary mechanisms: distention and recruitment of blood vessels. Owing to the large number of capillaries and their intimate association with the alveolar walls, the surface area available for gas exchange is enormous. The bronchial circulation receives only about 1% to 2% of the cardiac output.

3. The answer is D. One complication of the immotile cilia syndrome is the inability of pseudostratified columnar cells to clear mucus from the airways as a result of defective cilia motion. This may result in repeated infections and eventual bronchiectatic (dilatated) airways. Clara cells do not produce mucus. The bronchial mucous glands are found in the submucosa. C fibers are unmyelinated fibers and are the major sensory fibers found in the respiratory system.

4. The answer is D. The pulmonary circulation is a low-pressure system that usually adapts well to changes in volume and pressure without marked increases in pulmonary artery resistance. In PPH, pulmonary arterial pressures are quite elevated. The goal of therapy in PPH is to reduce pulmonary arterial pressures and prevent failure of the thin-walled right ventricle (cor pulmonale). Of the agents listed, only nitric oxide is a vasodilator, although its short half-life limits its usefulness in this chronic condition. Prostacyclin and prostaglandins have also been used to treat PPH, but at present the only definitive therapy is lung transplantation.

5. The answer is C. Because the diaphragm, which is innervated by the phrenic nerves, must operate continuously to sustain ventilation, the majority of fibers present are type I (slow twitch/oxidative) fibers, which are relatively fatigue resistant. The amount of pressure that the respiratory muscles can generate is dependent on lung volume. In COPD, as a result of hyperinflation and air trapping, the fibers are shortened and the diaphragm must operate on a less advantageous portion of the length-tension curve, resulting in less force production. With increasing velocity of shortening, the respiratory muscles generate less tension.

■ SUGGESTED READING

Farkas GA: Functional characteristics of the respiratory muscles. *Sem Resp Med* 12(4):247–256, 1991.

Murray JF: *The Normal Lung*, 2nd ed. Philadelphia: WB Saunders, 1986.

Staub NC, Albertine KH: Anatomy of the lungs. In Murray JF, Nadel JA, eds.: *Textbook of Respiratory Medicine*, 3rd ed. Philadelphia: WB Saunders, 1994.

Weinberger SE: *Principles of Pulmonary Medicine*. Philadelphia: WB Saunders, 1996.

West JB: *Respiratory Physiology: The Essentials*, 3rd ed. Baltimore: Williams & Wilkins, 1985.

Chapter 3

NORMAL LUNG FUNCTION

Gilbert E. D'Alonzo, D.O.

Bernard Borbely, M.D.

■ **CHAPTER OUTLINE**

SECTION 3.1   *Ventilation*

SECTION 3.2   *Diffusion Capacity*

SECTION 3.3   *Lung Circulation*

SECTION 3.4   *Gas Transport and Acid-Base Status of the Lung*

SECTION 3.5   *Ventilation-Perfusion Relationships*

SECTION 3.6   *Normal Exercise Physiology*

VENTILATION

Gilbert E. D'Alonzo, D.O.

■ SECTION OUTLINE

Learning Objectives

Introduction

The Simplified Lung

Measurement of Alveolar Dead Space

Regional Differences in Ventilation

Review Questions

■ LEARNING OBJECTIVES

At the completion of this section, the reader should:
- Understand the concepts of minute ventilation, alveolar ventilation, and dead space.
- Be able to measure dead space and describe the differences between anatomic and physiologic dead space.
- Be able to describe the relationship between alveolar ventilation and alveolar PO_2 and PCO_2 and understand the alveolar gas equation.
- Understand the multiple factors affecting the distribution of ventilation that creates regional differences throughout the lungs.
- Be able to describe the concept and measurement of closing volume.

■ INTRODUCTION

Ventilation is the process of air movement into and out of the lung during breathing.

Ventilation consists of the movement of air during inspiration from outside the body through the upper air passages and the divisions and subdivisions of the conducting airways to the terminal respiratory units, and, with expiration, out again. From a functional standpoint, the airways can be divided into conducting and gas-exchange spaces. The upper air passages and the larger airways, including the trachea and major bronchi, are considered conducting airways because they do not participate in gas exchange. The gas-exchange regions of the lung include the respiratory bronchioles, alveolar ducts, alveolar sacs, and alveoli. The amount of inspired air that reaches these sites of gas exchange is determined by many factors, including 1) the way in which air flows through the tracheobronchial tree and 2) lung parenchyma distensibility properties. A pumping action, requiring a neuromusculoskeletal effort, is necessary to expand the lungs and cause air to flow through the respiratory system. These structural and mechanical properties of the lung and chest wall are discussed in Chapter 2.

■ THE SIMPLIFIED LUNG

When air enters the respiratory system, a portion is distributed to the conducting airways and the remainder goes to gas-exchange areas. Figure 3.1-1 is an oversimplified diagram of a lung. The conducting airways are represented by a single tube labeled anatomic dead space. This tube leads into the gas-exchange region of the lung, which involves a blood-gas interface between the alveolar surface and a pulmonary capillary. The alveolar volume

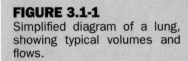

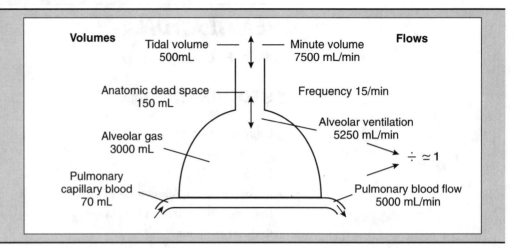

FIGURE 3.1-1
Simplified diagram of a lung, showing typical volumes and flows.

Anatomic dead space in milliliters is approximately equal to the ideal body weight measured in pounds.

is variable, subject to a variety of external forces. With each inspiration, a tidal volume of about 500 mL of air enters the lung. Anatomic dead space accounts for approximately 150 mL. The remainder of each tidal volume makes its way to the alveoli for the exchange of oxygen for carbon dioxide. The gas that resides in the alveolar spaces is generally in excess of 3000 mL, whereas the volume of pulmonary capillary blood is far less, approximately 70 mL. If one were to assume a respiratory rate of 15 breaths per minute, the minute ventilation would be 7500 mL/min and the alveolar ventilation would be more than 5 L. Because heart rate is much higher than respiratory rate, the pulmonary blood flow during each minute of ventilation turns out to be nearly the same as the alveolar ventilation of 5 L/min.

The volume of air entering the lungs each minute is slightly greater than the amount that is expired, because the amount of oxygen taken in is greater than the amount of carbon dioxide released. The volume of air leaving the lung each minute is known as the minute ventilation. In the example presented in Figure 3.1-1, the minute ventilation is 7500 mL/min. Not all the air that passes the lips reaches the alveolar gas compartment, because a portion of the gas remains in the anatomic dead space and does not participate in gas exchange. If the volume of the anatomic dead space is 150 mL, then the amount of air entering this gas-exchange area each minute is less than the minute ventilation. Using our example, the alveolar ventilation would be 350 mL times 15 breaths per minute, or 5250 mL/min. As a rule, anatomic dead space is approximately equal to ideal body weight measured in pounds.

Total dead space includes:

- anatomic dead space
- physiologic dead space

In a variety of diseases, lung tissue may not function as gas-exchange units, and thus such areas contribute to the dead space but would be specifically designated as physiologic dead space. Therefore, in patients with lung disease, one has to consider not only the dead space associated with the conducting airways (anatomic dead space) but also that found in diseased lung areas. These lung areas would be nonperfused alveolar regions (Figure 3.1-2).

We can summarize these concepts conveniently with the mathematical expression

$$\dot{V}_E = V_T \times f,$$

Total minute ventilation equals the volume of air in each breath, or tidal volume, times the number of breaths per minute.

where $\dot{V}_E$ is minute ventilation (4 min), V_T is tidal volume in milliliters, and f is respiratory frequency in breaths per minute.

Substitution of the sum of alveolar volume (V_A) and dead space volume (V_D) for V_T yields the following equation: $\dot{V}_E = (V_A + V_D) \times f$, or $\dot{V}_E = (V_A \times f) + (V_D \times f)$, or $\dot{V}_E = \dot{V}_A + \dot{V}_D$ (where $\dot{V}_A$ is alveolar minute ventilation and $\dot{V}_D$ is dead space minute ventilation), or $\dot{V}_A = \dot{V}_E - \dot{V}_D$.

The alveolar minute ventilation, which discounts dead space effect, is most important for proper gas exchange.

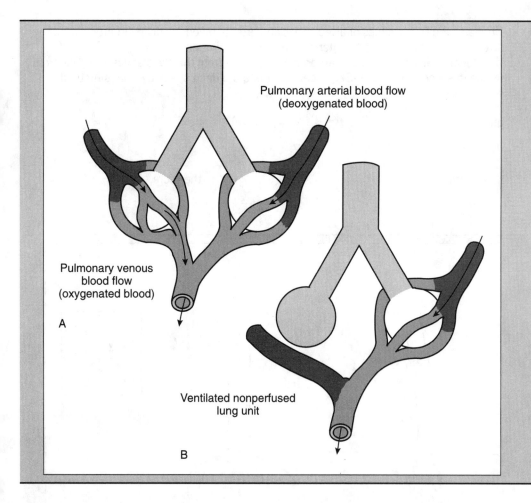

FIGURE 3.1-2
Anatomic and physiologic dead spaces. The light shaded area in panel A shows the anatomic dead space found in the conducting airways of the lung. The light shaded area in panel B shows the anatomic dead space in the alveolus, which is not perfused with blood.

Pulmonary arterial blood flow (deoxygenated blood)

Pulmonary venous blood flow (oxygenated blood)

A

Ventilated nonperfused lung unit

B

■ MEASUREMENT OF ALVEOLAR DEAD SPACE

Although a value for anatomic dead space can be estimated with minimal error, this volume is actually very difficult to measure. Another way of measuring alveolar ventilation is from the concentration of carbon dioxide in the expired gas. Because inspired air contains nearly no carbon dioxide, all of the carbon dioxide in the expired gas comes from the alveoli after it leaves them following gas exchange from the pulmonary circulation. Because no gas exchange occurs in the dead space, there is no carbon dioxide there at the end of inspiration. Therefore, all of the expired carbon dioxide comes from the alveolar gas,

$$\dot{V}CO_2 = \dot{V}_A \times \frac{\%CO_2}{100},$$

where $\dot{V}CO_2$ is the volume of carbon dioxide exhaled per unit of time,

$$\dot{V}_A = \dot{V}CO_2 \times \frac{100}{\%CO_2}.$$

The $\%CO_2/100$ is called the fractional concentration of carbon dioxide and is denoted by FCO_2. Thus the alveolar ventilation can be obtained by dividing the carbon dioxide output by the alveolar concentration of this gas. Using a rapid carbon dioxide analyzer to measure the concentration of carbon dioxide in the final portion of a single prolonged expiration, one can determine the FCO_2. The partial pressure of carbon dioxide (PCO_2) is proportional to the concentration of the gas in the alveoli, or $PCO_2 = FCO_2 \times K$, where K is a constant (equaling 0.863 when V_A is expressed at BTPS and $\dot{V}CO_2$ at STPD),

$$\dot{V}_A = \frac{\dot{V}CO_2}{PCO_2} \times K.$$

Normally, the PCO_2 values of alveolar gas and arterial blood are nearly identical, and the arterial PCO_2 can be used to determine alveolar ventilation.

Because all of the expired carbon dioxide comes from the alveolar gas and none from the dead space (Figure 3.1-3), we can calculate the dead space by Bohr's method,

$$V_T \times F_E = V_A \times F_A$$

and

$$V_T = V_A + V_D$$

therefore,

$$V_A = V_T - V_D$$

substituting

$$V_T \times F_E = (V_T - V_D) \times F_A, \text{ therefore,}$$

$$\frac{V_D}{V_T} = \frac{F_A - F_E}{F_A}.$$

FIGURE 3.1-3

Expired CO_2 comes from alveolar gas, and there is no CO_2 in the dead space, so the tidal volume (V_T) is a mixture of dead space (V_D) gas and alveolar (V_A) gas. The fractional concentrations of CO_2 in the inspired (F_I), expired (F_E), and alveolar (F_A) gas are represented by the dots.

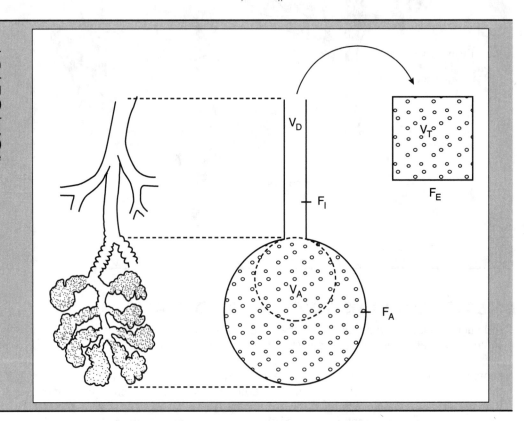

The partial pressure of a gas is proportional to its concentration, and therefore

$$\frac{V_D}{V_T} = \frac{P_ACO_2 - P_ECO_2}{P_ACO_2} \text{ (Bohr's equation),}$$

where A and E refer to alveolar and mixed expired, respectively.

The normal ratio of dead space to tidal volume ranges from 0.20 to 0.35 during rest. Normally, the PCO_2 values of alveolar gas and arterial blood are nearly identical, so the equation is often shown as

$$\frac{V_D}{V_T} = \frac{P_aCO_2 - P_ECO_2}{P_aCO_2}.$$

Therefore, if one measures the end-expiratory gas carbon dioxide concentration and a simultaneous arterial blood-gas value, the ratio of dead space to tidal volume can easily be determined. In a normal subject with a minute ventilation of 6 L/min and a tidal volume of 600 mL, with an arterial blood gas showing an arterial PCO_2 of 40 mmHg and a mixed expiratory gas sample PCO_2 measurement of 28 mmHg,

$$\frac{V_D}{V_T} = \frac{40 - 28}{40} = 0.30.$$

During a constant state of metabolism, alveolar ventilation varies inversely with alveolar PCO_2 and directly with alveolar PO_2.

Therefore, the V_D/V_T ratio is 0.3 and, because the tidal volume is 600 mL, the dead space is 180 mL and the alveolar ventilation is 600 mL − 180 mL, or 420 mL.

The alveolar PCO_2 varies inversely with the alveolar ventilation (Figure 3.1-4) when measured at a constant rate of carbon dioxide production. The magnitude of the change in PCO_2 produced by a change in minute ventilation depends on the relationship between alveolar ventilation and minute ventilation, taking into account the dead space ratio.

Like PCO_2 the alveolar PO_2 is a function of the rate of oxygen uptake across the alveolar-capillary membrane and alveolar ventilation. Because the partial pressures of nitrogen and water vapor are constant within the alveolus, alveolar oxygen and carbon dioxide vary in a reciprocal fashion as the alveolar ventilation is altered (Figure 3.1-5).

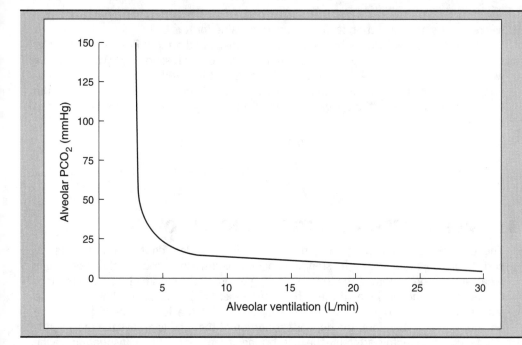

FIGURE 3.1-4
Alveolar PCO_2 initially falls rapidly and then more slowly as alveolar ventilation increases, provided that body metabolism and dead space ventilation remain stable in this normal adult subject. From Grippi MA: *Pulmonary Pathophysiology*. Philadelphia: Lippincott, 1995.

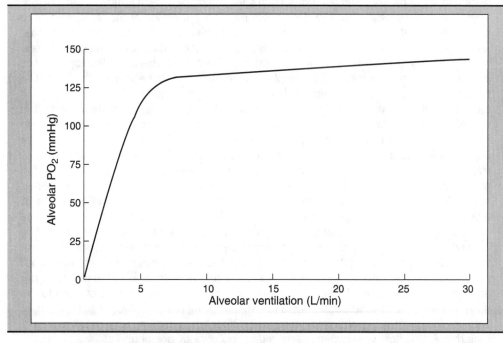

FIGURE 3.1-5
Alveolar PO_2 quickly increases with small initial increases in alveolar ventilation and then rises slowly toward a plateau in the same subject as in Figure 3.1-4 under stable metabolic conditions. From Grippi MA: *Pulmonary Pathophysiology*. Philadelphia: Lippincott, 1995.

This reciprocal relationship between PO_2 and PCO_2 as related to alveolar ventilation can be predicted from the alveolar gas equation, if we know the composition of inspired gas and the respiratory exchange ratio (R). R can be determined from the ratio of carbon dioxide production to oxygen consumption and reflects the metabolism of body tissues at steady state. This R value is known as the respiratory quotient. The sum of the partial pressures of oxygen, carbon dioxide, nitrogen, and water vapor in the alveolus equals

The alveolar gas equation can be used to express the reciprocal relationship between PO_2 and PCO_2 as related to alveolar ventilation.

barometric pressure. Because the nitrogen and water vapor partial pressures are constant, the partial pressure of either alveolar oxygen or carbon dioxide can be calculated if the partial pressure of the other is known:

$$P_AO_2 = (P_IO_2 - P_ACO_2) \times (F_IO_2 + 1 - F_IO_2/R).$$

A simplified form of the alveolar gas equation can be written as

$$P_AO_2 = P_IO_2 - \frac{P_ACO_2}{R} + F,$$

where F is a small correction factor. The normal value for R is 0.8.

A healthy subject who is breathing air has a measured arterial PCO_2 of 40 mmHg, which closely approximates P_ACO_2. Assuming a barometric pressure of 760 mmHg and a water vapor pressure of 47 mmHg, and assuming that inspired air becomes fully saturated with water at normal body temperature, the P_IO_2 is calculated as the product of the total partial pressure of the dry gases in the alveoli and the fractional concentration of oxygen:

$$P_IO_2 = (760 - 47) \times 0.21$$

$$P_AO_2 = P_IO_2 - [40 \times (0.21 + \frac{1 - 0.21}{0.8})] = 149 - 48 = 101 \text{ mmHg.}$$

■ REGIONAL DIFFERENCES IN VENTILATION

Factors Affecting Ventilation Distribution

- Pleural surface pressure
- Lung distensibility
- Resistance to airflow
- Lung volume

The regional distribution of gas in a normal lung is dependent on the pattern of pleural surface pressure change. In the standing position, ventilation per unit volume of lung is greatest near the bottom of the lung and becomes progressively smaller toward the top, but in the supine position, these differences essentially disappear. However, in the supine position, ventilation of the posterior portion of the lung exceeds that of the anterior portion. Therefore, the dependent portion of the lung is always the most ventilated. Additional factors affecting the distribution of ventilation during inspiration are the distensibility of the terminal respiratory units and the resistance to airflow in the airways. Therefore, the regional pleural surface pressure is an expression of the force tending to cause inflation of that part of the lung versus how much inspired air actually reaches that lung region, which is dependent on local lung compliance and airflow resistance factors.

In an upright subject, a pleural pressure gradient exists between the top and the bottom of the lung (Figure 3.1-6). The pleural pressure is most negative at the top of the lung and least negative at the bottom. The gradient is approximately 0.25 cm of water for each centimeter of vertical height. The reason for this is the weight of the lung as it is suspended within the chest. The pressure inside the lung is the same as atmospheric pressure. Because transpulmonary pressure equals the alveolar pressure minus the pleural pressure, the transpulmonary pressure is greater at the apex of the lung than at the base. This larger apical transpulmonary pressure results in greater alveolar distention at the top of the lung than at the base of the lung in the standing position. The basilar resting lung volume is lower than the apical resting volume, so that at the beginning of inspiration any small change in lung volume results in a larger volume change at the base of the lung than at the apex (Figure 3.1-7). Therefore, similar changes in pressure during inspiration result in different alveolar volume and airway caliber changes in one portion of the upright lung than in another portion (Figure 3.1-8). Again, it is important to point out that, although the base of the lung is relatively underexpanded as compared with the apex, it is better ventilated, because more of the overall alveolar ventilation goes to the base. This enhanced ventilation plays a role in improving the efficiency of gas exchange, because the majority of pulmonary blood flow is directed to the lung base or to the area of lung that is the most gravity dependent regardless of body position.

LUNG VOLUME EFFECT ON VENTILATION DISTRIBUTION

Toward the end of a deep inspiration, as lung volume begins to approach total lung capacity, the alveoli at the apices and at the bases of the lungs inflate to nearly the same size (see Figure 3.1-8). This occurs despite the persistent pleural pressure difference,

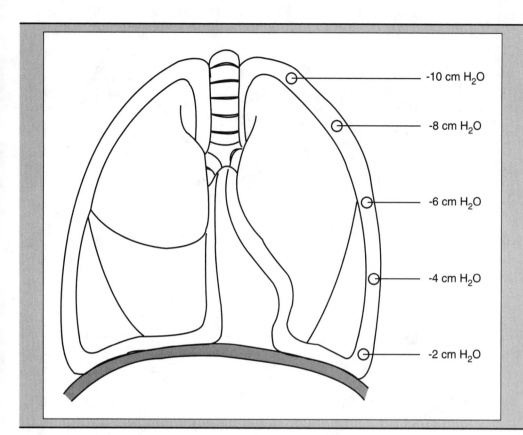

FIGURE 3.1-6
The pleural pressure when measured at end-expiration becomes less negative from the apex to the base of the lung in the standing position.

-10 cm H_2O

-8 cm H_2O

-6 cm H_2O

-4 cm H_2O

-2 cm H_2O

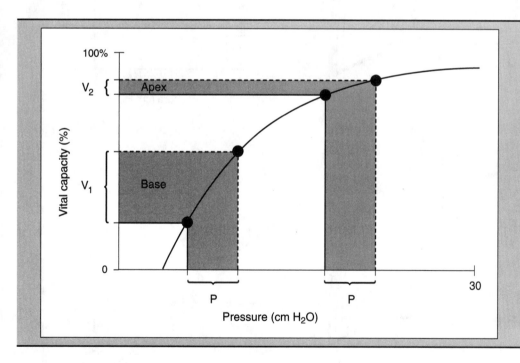

FIGURE 3.1-7
In the standing position, the change in lung volume at the base of the lung (ΔV_1) is larger than the change at its apex (ΔV_2) for a similar degree of inflation pressure (ΔP).

FIGURE 3.1-8

The effects of the pleural pressure gradient on alveolar size and airway caliber at three different lung volumes. The various lung units shown are then plotted on their respected positions on the normal volume-pressure curve. Similar pleural pressure changes during different phases of inspiration result in different alveolar volume and airway caliber changes in one portion of the upright lung as compared with another. From Hinshaw HC, Murray JP: *Diseases of the Chest*. Philadelphia: WB Saunders, 1979.

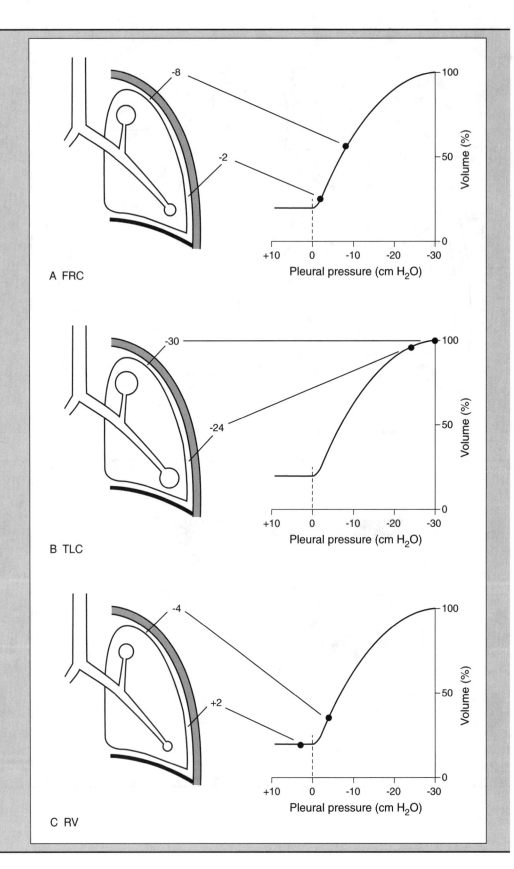

because both regions of the lungs are now functioning on the flat portion of the volume-pressure curve. However, during expiration toward residual volume, when the pleural pressure in the basilar portion of the lung becomes positive and the transpleural pressure actually becomes negative, there is a compressing force that begins to close airways (see Figure 3.1-8). This closure moves progressively up the lungs and involves more and more airways as exhalation continues. Pulmonary blood flow going to these areas of airway closure actually changes, and gas exchange can be disturbed. Airway closure during expiration may occur in dependent lung regions of normal elderly persons breathing at or close to functional residual capacity. Premature airway closure is characteristic of certain diseases, such as obesity, chronic obstructive pulmonary disease, and especially emphysema.

The basilar areas of lung that are being compressed do not have all of their gas squeezed out at the end of a forced expiration. The small airways likely close first, trapping gas in the more distal alveoli. In young, healthy subjects, airway closure occurs at very low lung volumes, but in the elderly, airway closure in the lower portions of the lung occurs at higher volumes and may actually be present at functional residual capacity. The aging lung loses elastic recoil, and intrapleural pressure becomes less negative. Transpulmonary pressure becomes negative and the airways collapse. Therefore, dependent regions of the lung may be only intermittently ventilated, and this can lead to significant problems in gas exchange. Early airway closure occurs in patients with lung disease in which the patency of the peripheral airways is compromised by either reduced elastic recoil, as in emphysema, or by abnormalities of the airways, such as bronchitis and asthma. These diseases are associated with an increase in the closing volume or the closing capacity of the lung.

MEASUREMENT OF CLOSING VOLUME

The single-breath nitrogen washout test can be used to determine ventilation nonuniformity. This test is generally not performed in clinical practice but can be used as a teaching method to help understand the concepts of airway closure (Figure 3.1-9). The

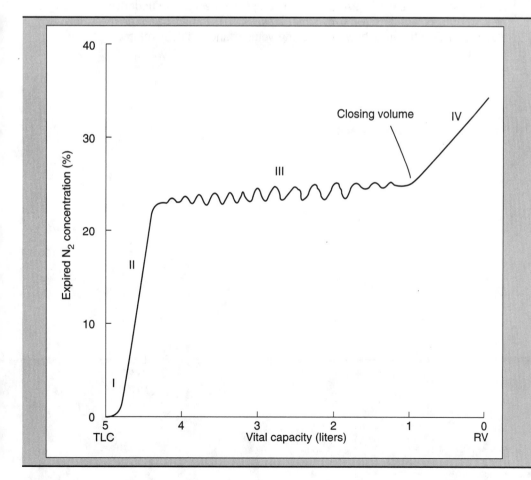

FIGURE 3.1-9
An example of the single-breath nitrogen method of determining airway closing volume. (*See text for details.*) The oscillations found in phase III are cardiac in nature.

subject inhales a single breath of pure oxygen from residual volume to total lung capacity. The subject then exhales slowly back to residual volume and the exhaled gas is measured or quantitated spirographically as the concentration of nitrogen is monitored throughout the exhalation maneuver. When a deep inspiration is taken from residual volume, the usual pattern of ventilatory distribution is reversed. Instead of the gas going to the lower lung regions first, most of the initial inspiration goes to the upper regions of the lung because the lower or more dependent regions are closed and essentially nonventilated.

During slow expiration, emptying normally takes place in a smooth and orderly fashion from the bottom of the lung to the top of the lung when the subject is in the upright position. Because the apices of the lungs were labeled during inspiration, after airway closure begins to occur at the bases late in expiration, the expired gas reflects the high concentration of nitrogen from the slowly emptying lower regions.

The nitrogen washout curve can be subdivided into four phases (see Figure 3.1-9). During the initial part of expiration, gas from the conducting or upper airways (the anatomic dead space) contains only oxygen and no nitrogen. Therefore, this portion of the curve is very brief and nearly flat (phase I). Next, nitrogen-laden gas washes out as alveoli deflate and the nitrogen concentration rises abruptly in phase II. As alveoli empty throughout the lungs, a plateau develops, which represents near homogeneity of ventilation (phase III). In healthy people, this phase of the curve is nearly flat and is known as the alveolar plateau. When phase III is not flat, this indicates the presence of parenchymal and/or airway disease. Phase III provides a measure of ventilation inhomogeneity. Some poorly ventilated lung regions receive little of the inspired oxygen, and therefore these regions have a high nitrogen concentration relative to more normally ventilated areas. Poorly ventilated areas tend to empty later, contributing to a rise in the nitrogen concentration toward the end of phase III, when this portion of the test should be essentially flat. Next, the "plateau" is abruptly terminated by a steep rise in the concentration of nitrogen during phase IV. Closing volume is the junction between phases III and IV and represents the lung volume at which airways in the more dependent regions of the lungs close near the end of expiration. The proposed mechanism underlying phase IV is near closure or actual closure of small airways at the lung bases at these low lung volumes. The difference between closing volume and residual volume is the closing capacity.

■ REVIEW QUESTIONS

1. Concerning ventilation in a healthy subject, which one of the following statements is false?

   (A) Expired carbon dioxide comes from alveolar gas because there is no carbon dioxide in the dead space.
   (B) The tidal volume is a mixture of alveolar gas and dead space gas.
   (C) Alveolar PCO_2 falls slowly and in a linear fashion as minute ventilation increases.
   (D) Alveolar PO_2 quickly increases as minute ventilation increases.
   (E) Dead space is made up of both anatomic and physiologic components of ventilation.

2. Concerning the upright lung, which one of the following statements is false?

   (A) Pleural pressure is most negative at the top of the lung.
   (B) Pressure inside the lung is uniform and the same as atmospheric pressure.
   (C) Alveolar distention is greatest at the apex.
   (D) Ventilation per unit of lung tissue is least near the bottom of the lung.
   (E) For the same inflation pressure, the change in lung volume at the base of the lung is larger than the apical change.

■ ANSWERS AND EXPLANATIONS

1. The answer is C. Because the potential pressures of nitrogen and water vapor are constant within the alveolus, alveolar oxygen and carbon dioxide vary reciprocally as ventilation is increased. With an increase in ventilation, alveolar oxygen rises quickly and alveolar carbon dioxide falls quickly, with smaller and slower changes occurring thereafter.

2. The answer is D. The dependent portion of the lung is always the most ventilated. The distribution of ventilation is also regulated by lung distensibility and resistance to airflow.

■ SUGGESTED READINGS

Anthenisen NR, Fleetham JA: Ventilation: total, alveolar, and dead space. In Farhi IE, Tenney SM (eds). Gas Exchange, Handbook of Physiology, Section 3: the Respiratory System. Bethesda, MD. *Amer Physiol Soc* 1987, Vol IV, pp 113–129.

Bryan AC, Bentivoglio LG, Beeral F, et al: Factors affecting regional distribution of ventilation and perfusion in the lung. *J Appl Physiol* 19:395–402, 1964.

Comroe JH: *Physiology of Respiration*, 2nd ed. Chicago: YearBook 1974, pp 8–21.

Cotes JE: *Lung Function: Assessment and Application in Medicine*, 4th ed. Oxford, England: Blackwell, 1979.

Dubois AB, Botelho SY, Bedell BN, et al: A rapid plethysmographic method for measuring thoracic gas volume: A comparison with a nitrogen washout method for measuring functional residual capacity in normal subjects. *J Clin Invest* 35:322–326, 1956.

Forster RE II, Dubois AB, Briscoe WA, Fisher AB: Pulmonary Ventilation. In *The Lung: Physiologic Basis of Pulmonary Function Tests*, 3rd ed. Chicago: YearBook, 1986, pp 25–64.

DIFFUSION CAPACITY

Gilbert E. D'Alonzo, D.O.

■ SECTION OUTLINE

Learning Objectives

Introduction

Diffusion and Perfusion Limitations

Carbon Monoxide Diffusion Capacity

Measurement of Diffusion Capacity

Carbon Dioxide Diffusion in the Lung

Review Questions

■ LEARNING OBJECTIVES

At the completion of this section, the reader should:
- Understand the concept of lung gas diffusion, including the concept of gas transfer that is diffusion limited, perfusion limited, or a combination of both.
- Be able to explain the importance of measuring carbon monoxide diffusion capacity and how such measurement can be affected.
- Understand the differences between oxygen and carbon dioxide diffusion in the lung.

■ INTRODUCTION

Gas diffusion through a tissue depends on:

- the tissue area and thickness
- the difference in gas partial pressure across the tissue barrier
- the solubility of the gas
- the molecular weight of the gas

The transfer of a gas across the alveolar-capillary membrane occurs by the process of diffusion. Diffusion through such a tissue is described by Fick's law, which states that the rate of gas transfer through a tissue is proportional to the tissue area and the difference in gas partial pressure between its two sides, and inversely proportional to the thickness of the tissue (Figure 3.2-1). The surface area of the alveolar-capillary membrane is between 50 and 100 m^2, and its thickness is less than 1 μm. This thin, massive-surface-area membrane is ideal for gas diffusion. Certain properties of the tissue and the gas are also important to the diffusion process and can be figured into the equation as a constant. The constant is proportional to the solubility of the gas and inversely proportional to the square root of its molecular weight. Taking these factors into consideration, carbon dioxide diffuses through tissue approximately 20 times more rapidly than oxygen, because it has a much higher solubility and a similar molecular weight. The lighter the gas, or the lower the molecular weight, the faster its diffusion.

FIGURE 3.2-1
Diffusion of a gas through tissue is proportional to the area of the tissue, a diffusion constant, and the partial pressure difference of the gas between the two sides, and inversely proportional to the thickness of the tissue (Fick's law). The constant (D) is proportional to the solubility of the gas divided by the square root of its molecular weight.

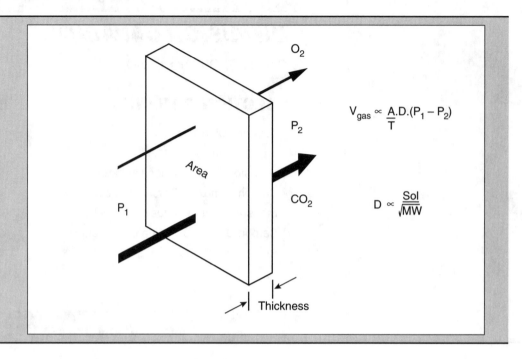

$$V_{gas} \propto \frac{A.D.(P_1 - P_2)}{T}$$

$$D \propto \frac{Sol}{\sqrt{MW}}$$

■ DIFFUSION AND PERFUSION LIMITATIONS

To study diffusion and perfusion limitations, two gases are often used, carbon monoxide and nitrous oxide. Carbon monoxide is used to measure the diffusion capacity of the lung, and nitrous oxide helps measure pulmonary blood flow or perfusion. Both oxygen and carbon monoxide have the ability to combine with hemoglobin, whereas nitrous oxide does not. Nitrous oxide readily diffuses between the gas and blood phases, and a concentration equilibrium between the alveolar gas and blood is reached rapidly. Therefore, the amount of this inert gas that can be taken up or given off by the pulmonary circulation is not limited by lung diffusion properties but is determined by the solubility of the gas and the volume of blood into which it dissolves.

Carbon monoxide is ideally suited for the measurement of lung diffusion capacity ($D_L CO$) because its affinity for hemoglobin is hundreds of times that of oxygen. When carbon monoxide is inhaled in very low concentrations, all the molecules diffuse quickly across the alveolar capillary membrane and move into the red blood cells, where they bind avidly but reversibly to hemoglobin. For practical purposes, the mean capillary partial pressure of carbon monoxide (PCO) is 0. Under these conditions, the amount of carbon monoxide taken up by the pulmonary circulation depends on the diffusion characteristics of the alveolar-capillary membrane and not on the amount of capillary blood. For this reason, uptake of carbon monoxide is "diffusion limited" (Figure 3.2-2).

On the other hand, nitrous oxide does not combine with hemoglobin. This gas moves from the alveoli into the blood and, as the amount of nitrous oxide dissolved in plasma increases, there results a high back pressure whereby further uptake of nitrous oxide into the capillary blood is limited. Therefore, uptake of nitrous oxide is entirely dependent on pulmonary blood flow and volume, not on the diffusion characteristics of the alveolar-capillary membrane, and thus is "perfusion limited" (see Figure 3.2-2).

Oxygen moves across the alveolar-capillary membrane in an intermediate fashion when compared with carbon monoxide and nitrous oxide (see Figure 3.2-2), and its ability to bind to hemoglobin is less than that of carbon monoxide. By the time the red cell traverses approximately one-third of the way through the capillary, the partial pressure of oxygen (PO_2) in the capillary blood is equal to that of the alveolar PO_2 (Figure 3.2-3). It is at this point that further transfer of oxygen is perfusion limited, like that of nitrous oxide. In certain diseases, thickening of the alveolar-capillary membrane occurs and there is the potential for the partial pressure of oxygen in the blood not to reach that of the alveolus by the time the red blood cell reaches the end of the capillary, resulting in some diffusion limitation. With severe exercise, the pulmonary blood flow is greatly increased and the red

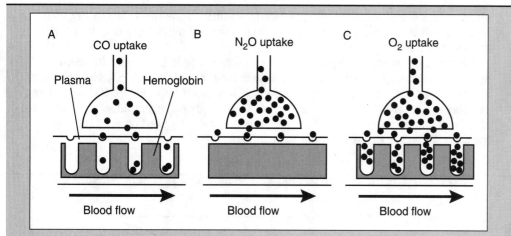

FIGURE 3.2-2
Diffusion-limited and perfusion-limited gas transfer from alveoli to blood. (A) Carbon monoxide transfer is diffusion limited. Because CO is rapidly and avidly bound to hemoglobin, no CO back pressure develops, and the pressure gradient for CO diffusion remains maximal. Gas transfer rate depends on the pressure gradient, membrane characteristics, and physical properties of the gas. (B) Nitrous oxide transfer is perfusion limited. As N_2O builds up in the plasma (N_2O is not bound to hemoglobin), blood becomes saturated with the gas, limiting further transfer. Additional gas transfer depends on continued blood flow to replace saturated plasma. (C) Oxygen transfer is intermediate between transfer of diffusion-limited and perfusion-limited gases.

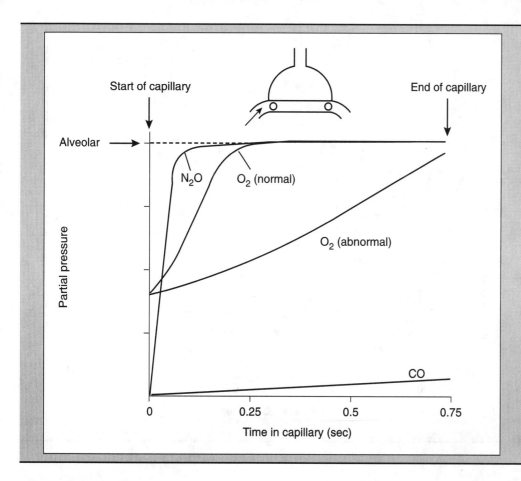

FIGURE 3.2-3
Uptake of carbon monoxide, nitrous oxide, and oxygen along the pulmonary capillary. Note that the blood partial pressure of nitrous oxide virtually reaches that of alveolar gas very early in the capillary so that the transfer of this gas is perfusion limited. By contrast, the partial pressure of carbon monoxide in the blood is almost unchanged so that its transfer is diffusion limited. Oxygen transfer can be perfusion or partly diffusion limited depending on the conditions. From West JB: *Pulm Pathophysiol* 1979.

blood cell capillary transient time is reduced to as little as one-third of its resting value. In patients with thickened alveolar-capillary membranes, limitation of oxygen diffusion is more likely to occur.

If a subject inhales a hypoxic gas mixture or ascends to a high altitude, alveolar hypoxia develops. Alveolar hypoxia generally reduces mixed venous PO_2, and the oxygen diffusion gradient from the alveoli to the capillary blood falls (Figure 3.2-4) and end-capillary PO_2 is far below that of the arterial PO_2. As the cardiac output increases and red blood cell capillary transit time shortens, especially during exertion or at high altitude, the overall effect is worsened, even in fit subjects.

FIGURE 3.2-4
Oxygen time courses in the pulmonary capillary when diffusion is normal and abnormal. Graph A shows time courses when the alveolar PO_2 is normal. Graph B shows slower oxygenation when the alveolar PO_2 is abnormally low. From West JB: *Pulm Pathophysiol* 1979.

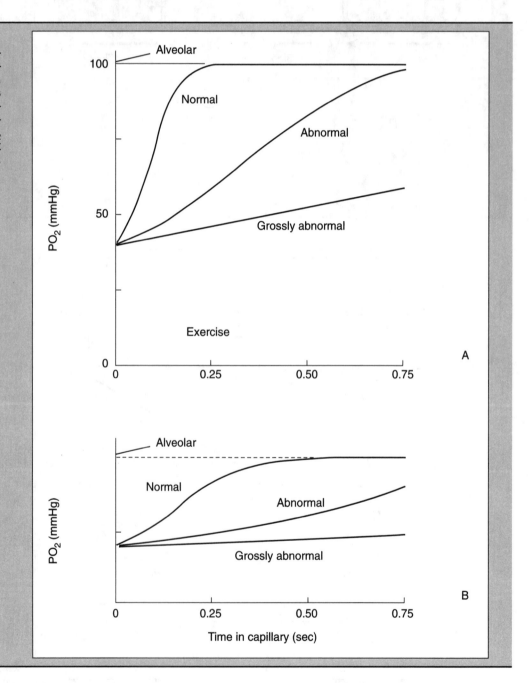

CARBON MONOXIDE DIFFUSION CAPACITY

It has already been pointed out that the lung diffusion capacity (D_L) for a gas such as carbon monoxide is determined by the rate of gas flow (VCO) divided by the pressure gradient of this gas across the membrane (alveolar-capillary),

$$D_L = \frac{VCO}{P_1 - P_2},$$

but the partial pressure of carbon monoxide in capillary blood is zero, so

$$D_L = \frac{VCO}{P_A CO}.$$

The reciprocal of D_L is the resistance to gas flow ($1/D_L$), which includes not only many blood-gas barrier factors (including the alveolar-capillary membrane, plasma, and the red cell membrane), but also the resistance associated with the reaction of binding carbon monoxide (or oxygen) to hemoglobin (Figure 3.2-5). Therefore,

$$\frac{1}{D_L} = \frac{1}{D_M} + \frac{1}{\Theta \times V_c},$$

which represents the overall resistance to diffusion, where D_L is lung diffusion capacity, D_M is the entire surface area of the blood-gas barrier, θ is rate of reaction of CO (or O_2) for hemoglobin, and V_C is capillary blood volume.

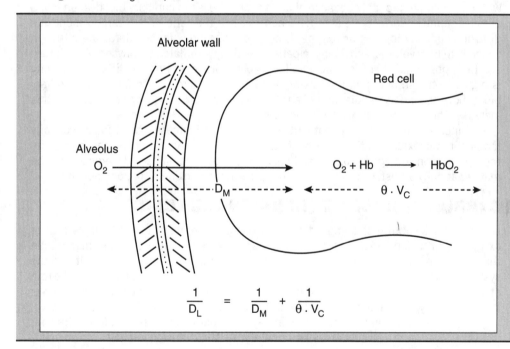

FIGURE 3.2-5
The diffusing capacity of the lung (D_L) is made up of two components, the diffusion process and the time taken for oxygen (or carbon monoxide) to react with hemoglobin.

Therefore, a reduction in lung capillary blood volume reduces the diffusion capacity, whereas an increase in V_C increases the diffusion capacity.

MEASUREMENT OF DIFFUSION CAPACITY

The single-breath method of measuring carbon monoxide diffusion capacity is the most popular way of measuring the diffusion capacity of the lung. With this method the patient inhales a gas mixture containing a low concentration of carbon monoxide and a small amount of helium, which acts as an inert tracer gas. The subject holds the breath for 10 sec at the end of a deep inspiration and, during exhalation, carbon monoxide and helium concentrations are analyzed. It is during the 10-sec breath hold that a fraction of the carbon monoxide diffuses from the alveoli into the blood. This diffusible amount can be calculated from measurements of the carbon monoxide concentration in the gas at the beginning and end of the breath-holding interval. The alveolar concentration of carbon monoxide at the beginning of the breath-holding period is determined from the dilution of inspired helium. Helium is an inert gas, not taken up by lung tissue or blood, so the decrease in helium concentration from its initial value is proportional to the lung value into which the carbon monoxide is distributed, or the alveolar volume. Therefore, by measuring the amount of carbon monoxide transferred into the lung per unit of time, the mean alveolar carbon monoxide concentration, and the mean capillary carbon monoxide concentration (assumed to be 0), the diffusion capacity for carbon monoxide can be calculated. However, in the pulmonary function laboratory, diffusion capacity (D_LCO) is calculated by the equation

$$D_LCO = \frac{V_A \times 60}{(P_B - 47) \times time} \times \ln \frac{F_ACO \text{ (initial)}}{F_ACO \text{ (final)}},$$

where V_A is the alveolar volume, P_B is the measured barometric pressure, and F_ACO is the alveolar CO concentration prior to and after breath holding.

A variety of factors must be considered when measuring the carbon monoxide diffusion capacity. A younger male has a greater carbon monoxide diffusion capacity than an older female. Maximum diffusion capacity occurs in the late teens and early 20s. From the early 20s, diffusion capacity for carbon monoxide declines at the rate of about 2% each year. For any age and height, a woman has approximately a 10% lower diffusion capacity for carbon monoxide than a man. Carbon monoxide diffusion capacity increases with lung volume, probably because of an overall increase in capillary blood volume and alveolar-capillary surface area. Krogh's constant, or the ratio of the carbon monoxide diffusion capacity to alveolar volume, is an important index for standardizing diffusion capacity to lung volume, especially in patients with hyperinflated emphysematous lungs.

Body positional changes affect capillary blood volume, so that the diffusion capacity is higher in the supine than in the standing position. Exercise also increases capillary blood flow secondary to distention and recruitment of pulmonary vessels, and this increases the carbon monoxide diffusion capacity.

An increase in the blood hematocrit or polycythemia increases the diffusion capacity for carbon monoxide. On the other hand, because the hematocrit decreases in anemia, the carbon monoxide diffusion capacity is also reduced. Hematocrit differences can be mathematically adjusted for when measuring carbon monoxide diffusion capacity.

■ CARBON DIOXIDE DIFFUSION IN THE LUNG

Because the solubility of carbon dioxide in tissue is approximately 20 times that of oxygen, its diffusion rate across the alveolar-capillary membrane is 20 times higher than that of oxygen. Therefore, there is a large carbon dioxide diffusion reserve built into the system. However, the reaction of carbon dioxide with hemoglobin is complex, and the rate of diffusion equilibrium of carbon dioxide is nearly the same as or perhaps even lower than that of oxygen, chiefly because of the slope of the carbon dioxide equilibrium curve.

With severe thickening of the alveolar-capillary membrane, carbon dioxide transfer from the blood to the alveolus may be impaired. As the diffusion capacity of the membrane is reduced to one-fourth of its normal value, a small difference between end-capillary blood and the alveolar gas may be found (Figure 3.2-6).

Factors That Enhance CO Diffusion

- Increase in lung capillary blood volume
- Recruitment and distention of pulmonary capillaries
- Supine position
- Müller maneuver

Factors That Decrease CO Diffusion

- Age
- Standing position
- Decrease in lung capillary blood volume
- Loss of pulmonary capillary surface area
- Alveolar disease
- Loss of lung tissue
- Valsalva's maneuver

CO_2 tissue solubility is 20 times greater than O_2 solubility, leading to a 20-fold increase in CO_2 diffusion across the alveolar-capillary membrane.

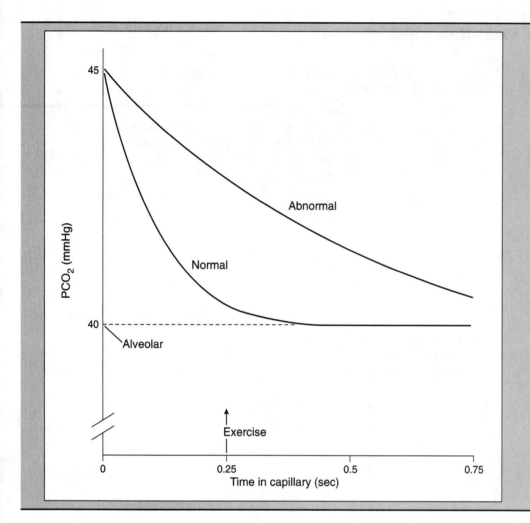

FIGURE 3.2-6
Changes in PCO_2 along the capillary when the diffusion properties are normal and abnormal. From Wagner PD, West JB: *J Appl Physiol* 33:62, 1972.

▌REVIEW QUESTIONS

1. Concerning the transfer of gases across the alveolar capillary membrane, which one of the following statements is false?

   (A) Oxygen diffuses more rapidly than carbon dioxide.
   (B) Gas transfer through tissue is dependent on tissue surface area.
   (C) The thickness of the membrane partially regulates gas transfer.
   (D) Solubility is an important parameter of a transferable gas.
   (E) The lower the molecular weight of the gas, the faster its diffusion.

2. Carbon monoxide diffusion capacity is not directly influenced by

   (A) exercise
   (B) temperature
   (C) blood hematocrit
   (D) lung volume
   (E) position

3. Which one of the following factors does not decrease carbon monoxide diffusion?

   (A) Standing position
   (B) Alveolar disease
   (C) Müller's maneuver
   (D) Age
   (E) Decrease in lung capillary blood volume

■ ANSWERS AND EXPLANATIONS

1. The answer is A. Taking all diffusion factors into consideration as described by Fick's law, carbon dioxide diffuses 20 times more rapidly than oxygen.

2. The answer is B. Exercise, polycythemia, an increase in lung volume, and supine position all increase lung capillary blood volume and carbon monoxide diffusion capacity. The small fluctuations in body temperature do not influence carbon monoxide diffusion capacity.

3. The answer is C. Müller's maneuver is an inspiratory effort against a closed glottis that increases lung blood volume and carbon monoxide diffusion, whereas Valsalva's maneuver is a hard expiratory effort with the glottis closed, a maneuver that decreases lung volume and carbon monoxide diffusion. All other factors are associated with decreases in either lung capillary surface area or lung blood volume.

■ SUGGESTED READINGS

Bates DV, Macklem PT, Christie RV: *Respiratory Function in Disease*, 2nd ed. Philadelphia: WB Saunders, 1971, pp 76–92.

Comroe JH: *Physiology of Respiration*, 2nd ed. Chicago: YearBook, 1974, pp 158–167.

Cotes JE: *Lung Function*, 4th ed. Oxford, England: Blackwell, 1979, pp 203–250.

Filley GF, MacIntosh DJ, Wright GW: Carbon monoxide uptakes and pulmonary diffusion capacity in normal subjects at rest and during exercise. *J Clin Invest* 33:530–539, 1954.

Forster RE II: Diffusion of gases across the alveolar membrane. SM (eds). *Gas Exchange. Handbook of Physiology. Sec 3. The Respiratory System*. Bethesda: Amer Physiol Soc, 1987, Vol 4, pp 71–88.

Krough M: The diffusion of gases through the lungs of man. *J Physiol* 49:271–300, 1915.

Ogilvie CM, Forster RE, Blakemore WS, Morton JW: A standardized breath holding technique for the clinical measurement of the diffusing capacity of the lung for carbon monoxide. *J Clin Invest* 36:1–17, 1957.

Stam H, Krenzer FJA, Versprille A: Effect of lung volume and positional changes on pulmonary diffusing capacity and its components. *J Appl Physiol* 71:1477–1488, 1991.

Roughton FJW, Forster RE: Relative importance of diffusion and chemical reaction rates in determining the rate of exchange of gases in the human lung, with special references to true diffusing capacity if pulmonary membrane and volume of blood in lung capillaries. *J Appl Physiol* 11:290–302, 1957.

West JB: *Respiratory Physiology—the Essentials*, 5th ed, Baltimore: Williams & Wilkins, 1995, pp 21–32.

LUNG CIRCULATION

Gilbert E. D'Alonzo, D.O.

■ SECTION OUTLINE

Learning Objectives
Introduction
Pulmonary Vascular Resistance
Lung Zones
Hemodynamic Monitoring
Review Questions

■ LEARNING OBJECTIVES

At the completion of this section the reader should:
- Be able to describe the process and importance of pulmonary vascular recruitment and distention.
- Be able to discuss the normal pulmonary vascular hemodynamics at rest and during exercise.
- Understand that there is a variety of both active and passive influences on the pulmonary vascular bed and that these factors affect pulmonary vascular resistance.
- Appreciate how the distribution of pulmonary blood flow through any area of lung depends on the interrelationship among pulmonary arterial, venous, and alveolar pressures.
- Be able to describe how the pulmonary artery balloon flotation catheter works and how it can be employed to determine a variety of hemodynamic, gas-exchange, and oxygen transport parameters.

■ INTRODUCTION

Unique Characteristics of the Pulmonary Vascular Bed

- High-capacity system
- Low resistance to blood flow
- Ability to recruit and distend vessels

The pulmonary circulation is a high-capacity, low-resistance vascular circuit that must accommodate the entire cardiac output at rest and during exercise. In order to accomplish this feat, the vascular bed can distend and when necessary recruit a larger vascular surface area with only a slight increase in pulmonary arterial pressure (Figure 3.3-1). From rest to a high level of exercise, the cardiac output of an adult human can go from 5 L/min to as high as 20 L/min (Table 3.3-1). The mean pressure of the pulmonary artery at rest, because this artery is a fairly passive vascular bed, is no more than 18 mmHg. Despite the high cardiac output that occurs during exercise and the large pulmonary vascular volume associated with this change in output, the mean pulmonary arterial pressure generally does not exceed 25 mmHg. In fact, the pulmonary vascular resistance during exercise does not change significantly from values normally found at rest.

Table 3.3-1
Normal Adult Hemodynamics at Rest and During Exercise

	REST	EXERCISE
Cardiac output (L/min)	6	16
Heart rate (beats/min)	80	130
Pulmonary arterial pressures (mmHg):		
Systolic	20–25	30–35
Diastolic	10–12	11–14
Mean	14–18	20–25
Pulmonary arterial occlusion (wedge) pressure (mmHg)	6–9	10–12
Right atrial pressure (mmHg)	4–6	6–8
Systemic arterial pressure (mmHg)	120/80	150/95
Mean	90–100	110–120
Pulmonary vascular resistance (Wood's units)	0.70–0.95	0.60–0.90

FIGURE 3.3-1
The opening of new vessels, or *recruitment*, and the increase in vessel caliber, or *distention*, are the two processes that the lung vasculature undergoes when pulmonary arterial pressure increases in order to minimize pulmonary vascular resistance.

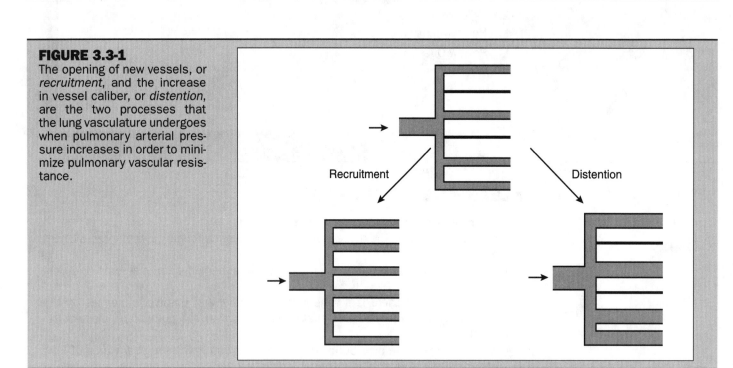

Recruitment   Distention

■ PULMONARY VASCULAR RESISTANCE

Pulmonary vascular resistance (PVR) is a measure of the system's impediment to blood flow, and it is calculated as the driving pressure for blood flow across the circuitry of the lung. This circuitry difference is the difference between mean pulmonary arterial pressure (PAP) and left atrial pressure (LAP), and because blood flow must go through this system, one must consider the cardiac output (CO). Therefore,

$$PVR = PAP - \frac{LAP}{CO}.$$

Left atrial pressure is essentially identical to the pulmonary capillary wedge pressure (PCWP). The PCWP measurement is obtained by occluding blood flow through a branch of the pulmonary artery by either wedging the end of a cardiac catheter or inflating a balloon surrounding the catheter in the vessel. This is generally done during a procedure called Swan-Ganz catheterization (Figure 3.3-2; see Hemodynamic Monitoring, on page 66). Pressures recorded at the tip of the catheter under no-flow conditions reflect pressures downstream within the vascular network such as the reflect left atrial pressure.

Because the pulmonary vascular bed is not equal throughout and it is a dynamic system, numerous factors must be considered when assessing its pressure-flow relationship. As mentioned previously, these vessels are flexible and can change in character with alterations in blood volume and flow. Flow through this system is not laminar but is

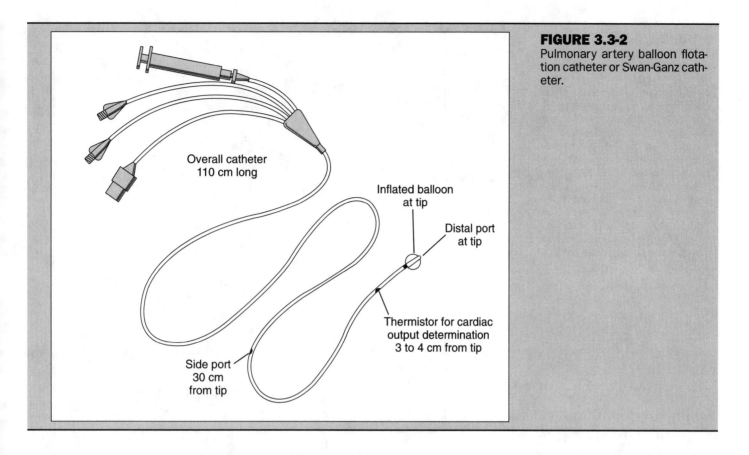

FIGURE 3.3-2
Pulmonary artery balloon flotation catheter or Swan-Ganz catheter.

pulsatile and turbulent, characteristics that create increasing complexities for our understanding of this circulation. The entire system is influenced by body position and changes in transthoracic pressure. Pulmonary vascular resistance is also affected by a variety of passive and active influences on the pulmonary vascular bed.

PASSIVE INFLUENCES ON PULMONARY VASCULAR RESISTANCE

Passive influences relate to mechanical changes within the lungs or hemodynamic changes of the circulation. On the other hand, an active process would imply that the change in pulmonary vascular resistance resulted from a direct effect by the pulmonary vasculature, either humoral or neural in nature. Figure 3.3-3 diagrammatically shows the results of isolated lung perfusion experiments where the effects of changing pulmonary arterial pressure on pulmonary vascular resistance occur at three different ranges of left atrial pressure. As pulmonary arterial pressure increases, pulmonary vascular resistance decreases, but the effect dramatically lessens as left atrial pressure is raised. An increase in pulmonary arterial pressure automatically causes resistance to fall by causing the pulmonary microcirculation either to recruit closed vessels or to further distend open vessels. When left atrial pressure is raised, and pulmonary arterial pressure and lung volume are kept constant, pulmonary vascular resistance decreases (see Figure 3.3-3). The effect of changing left atrial pressure on pulmonary vascular resistance decreases if pulmonary arterial pressure is already elevated.

Lung volumes can influence the pulmonary vascular bed and change vascular resistance. Smaller pulmonary vessels are surrounded by alveolar gas, and changes within the parenchyma of the lung as the lung expands and contracts influence these vessels. When the alveolar pressure rises above the lung capillary pressure, these thin-walled vessels collapse. The pressure difference between the inside and outside of these thin vessel walls is called the transmural pressure. The larger, thick-walled vessels of the lungs, the pulmonary arteries and veins, are also influenced by lung volume. As the lung expands, these vessels are pulled open by the radial traction of the lung parenchyma that surrounds them. Therefore, the vascular behavior of the capillaries and that of the larger blood vessels of the lung are distinctly different. The capillaries, or the so-called "alveolar

Passive Influences on the Pulmonary Vascular Bed

- Left atrial pressure
- Cardiac output
- Changes in lung volume
- Body position
- Alveolar pressure

FIGURE 3.3-3

Effects of changes in pulmonary arterial pressure on pulmonary vascular resistance in three different ranges of left atrial pressure (P_{LA}). As pulmonary arterial pressure increases, pulmonary vascular resistance decreases, but the magnitude of this effect progressively declines as left atrial pressure rises. At a constant pulmonary arterial pressure, a rise in left atrial pressure is accompanied by a decline in pulmonary vascular resistance. From Murray JF: Circulation. *In The Normal Lung*, 2nd ed. Philadelphia: WB Saunders, 1986, p. 156.

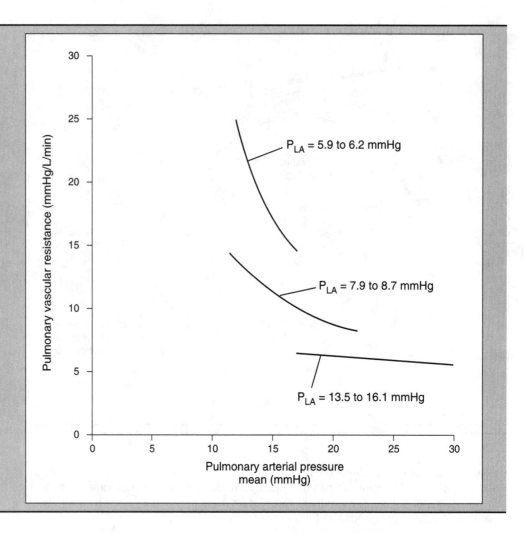

Active Influences on the Pulmonary Vascular Bed

- Neurogenic stimuli
- Humoral and chemical influences
- Alveolar hypoxemia and hypercapnia
- Acidemia

vessels," and the larger blood vessels, or the "extra-alveolar vessels," must be considered both together and separately in order to appreciate how they differ (Figure 3.3-4). Vessels influenced by alveolar pressure, or the so-called alveolar vessels, are the lung capillaries and slightly larger vessels that reside in the corners of the alveolar walls. Their vascular caliber is determined by the alveolar pressure and the vascular pressure that they have. On the other hand, extra-alveolar vessels include all of the arteries and veins that run through the lung parenchyma but are not distinctly influenced by the alveolar pressure. Their caliber is affected by lung volume in that, with expansion, the vessels are pulled open. Finally, the very large vessels that are at the hilar level are actually outside of the lung parenchyma and are influenced by intrapleural pressure. Figure 3.3-4 schematically shows the effects of changing lung volume from residual volume to total lung capacity on pulmonary vascular resistance for the lung vasculature as a whole and then, specifically, for alveolar and extra-alveolar vessels. Pulmonary vascular resistance is lowest at functional residual capacity or at the lung volume at end-expiration during comfortable breathing, and it increases as lung volume decreases toward residual volume or increases as lung volume is maximized at total lung capacity.

ACTIVE INFLUENCES ON PULMONARY VASCULAR RESISTANCE

Certain neurogenic stimuli, including sympathetic and parasympathetic stimuli, and a variety of humoral and chemical influences are responsible for causing active changes in the pulmonary vascular bed. Sympathetic and parasympathetic stimuli can increase or decrease pulmonary vascular resistance, respectively. The influence of the autonomic nervous system on the human lung vasculature remains poorly understood, but it is felt that little effect occurs. A variety of humoral and chemical substances, including catecholamines, prostaglandins, endothelia, and angiotensin, have been shown to increase

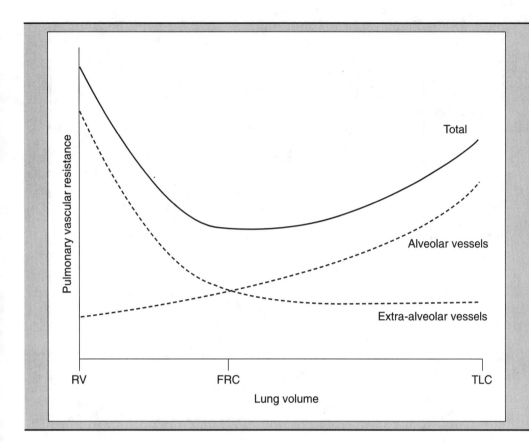

FIGURE 3.3-4
Lung volume and pulmonary vascular resistance. With inflation from residual volume (RV) to total lung capacity (TLC), resistance to flow through alveolar vessels increases, whereas resistance in extra-alveolar vessels decreases. The net result is a U-shaped curve with the nadir at functional residual capacity (FRC). From Murray JF: Circulation. In *The Normal Lung*, 2nd ed. Philadelphia: WB Saunders, 1986, p. 157.

pulmonary vascular resistance. A decrease in pulmonary vascular resistance has been associated with acetylcholine, prostacyclin, and nitric oxide. Alveolar hypoxia and hypercapnia and acidemia have all been shown to increase pulmonary resistance in humans.

Alveolar hypoxia is probably the most potent pulmonary vasoconstrictive influence. Hypoxic pulmonary vasoconstriction is the precapillary muscular pulmonary arterial and arteriolar response to regional alveolar hypoxia. This response appears to be a local humoral-chemical reaction, not at all regulated by the central nervous system. As the alveolar PO_2 falls below 70 mmHg, progressive vasoconstriction occurs and regional blood flow can actually be abolished. This reaction is further modified by changes in blood pH, because acidosis causes a more intense pulmonary hypoxic vasoconstrictive response to occur (Figure 3.3-5).

FIGURE 3.3-5
Diagram of the average results from experiments in newborn calves, showing the effects of changes in inspired PO_2 and pulmonary vascular resistance (PVR) under conditions of different arterial blood pH. As inspired PO_2 is decreased, pulmonary vascular resistance increases; this effect becomes exaggerated and occurs at progressively higher PO_2 values as pH is decreased. From Rudolph AM, Yuan S: Response of the pulmonary vasculature to hypoxia and H^+ ion concentration changes. *J Clin Invest* 45:399–411, 1966.

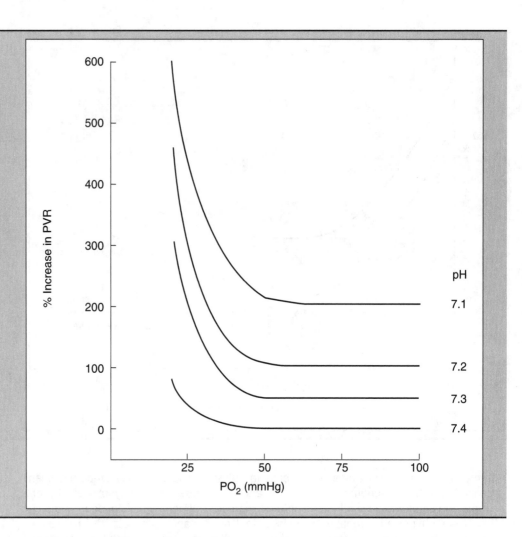

■ LUNG ZONES

So far, we have assumed that all parts of the pulmonary circulation behave identically. However, in the upright position, lung blood flow decreases almost linearly from bottom to top, reaching very low flows at the apex. In the upright position, the uneven distribution of blood flow is explained by hydrostatic pressure differences within the vascular bed. Furthermore, left atrial pressure and the alveolar pressure at different levels within the lung must be considered.

In the standing position, the lung is divided into three or four lung zones (Figure 3.3-6). Each zone is described by how pulmonary arterial, pulmonary venous, and alveolar pressure govern the distribution of blood flow through that portion of lung. The apical portion of the lung is zone 1, where the alveolar pressure exceeds both the pulmonary arterial and venous pressures, and the microvasculature is compressed to closure by this surrounding alveolar pressure. Therefore, blood flow to zone 1 is minimal at best. Because pulmonary arterial blood flow is pulsatile during systole, this transient elevation in pulmonary arterial pressure results in a minimal degree of apical blood flow that is not sustained through diastole. In zone 2, pulmonary arterial pressure exceeds alveolar pressure, but alveolar pressure exceeds pulmonary venous pressure. Therefore, blood flow is not determined by the gradient between the mean pulmonary arterial and left arterial pressures, but the regulatory pressure is alveolar pressure. Therefore, as one moves down the lung from zone 1 through zone 2, there is initially no flow until a point is reached at which alveolar pressure is equal to venous pressure and flow begins.

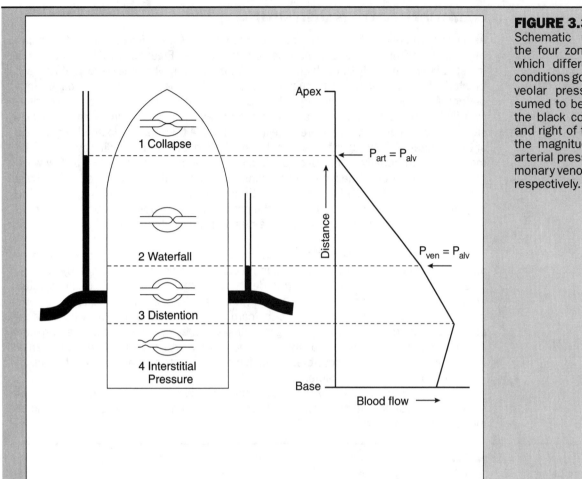

FIGURE 3.3-6
Schematic representation of the four zones of the lung in which different hemodynamic conditions govern blood flow. Alveolar pressure (P_{alv}) is assumed to be 0; the heights of the black columns on the left and right of the lung represent the magnitudes of pulmonary arterial pressure (P_{art}) and pulmonary venous pressure (P_{ven}), respectively.

Alveolar pressure is nearly homogeneous throughout zone 2, but pulmonary arterial pressure increases from the top to the bottom of this zone. Therefore, there is an alternate shifting of alveolar and pulmonary venous pressures that regulates the flow of blood through this zone, acting as a Starling resistor or creating a waterfall effect. Flow through zone 2 is intermittent through vessels that are open when the pulmonary venous pressure exceeds alveolar pressure, and flow stops when alveolar pressure exceeds pulmonary venous pressure.

In zone 3, pulmonary arterial pressure is greater than pulmonary venous pressure, and pulmonary venous pressure is greater than alveolar pressure. Therefore, resistance to blood flow through zone 3 is determined by the pressure gradient from the pulmonary artery to the pulmonary vein.

The final zone, zone 4, is found in the most dependent portion of the erect lung and, despite the fact that hydrostatic pressure is high, pulmonary blood flow actually decreases. This paradox of high vascular pressure resulting from gravitational effects and low blood flow cannot be explained by the same factors that determine vascular flow in the other zones. Other factors cause vessel narrowing and resistance to blood flow. At low lung volumes, the resistance of the extra-alveolar vessels becomes important and a reduction in regional blood flow is seen at the base of the lung where lung parenchyma is least expanded. A reduction in blood flow can be explained by the narrowing of these extra-alveolar vessels. With deep inspiration, vessel distortion, which contributes to blood flow resistance, is relieved, and some flow occurs.

If the supine position is assumed, these zone relationships change. In fact, in the supine position, zone 1 does not exist and the vast majority of the lung is in a zone 3 condition.

■ HEMODYNAMIC MONITORING

As mentioned previously, a balloon flotation catheter called the Swan-Ganz catheter can be used to measure cardiopulmonary hemodynamics (see Figure 3.3-2). The catheter is inserted percutaneously through an introducer needle and, when the balloon at its tip is inflated, the catheter floats through the blood stream until the balloon lodges in a peripheral portion of a pulmonary artery. During flotation, right atrial pressure, right ventricular pressure, pulmonary arterial pressure, and finally pulmonary arterial occlusive pressure or capillary wedge pressure are obtained. A thermistor is located near the tip of the catheter, and through the use of a thermodilution technique, cardiac output can be measured. Additionally, a mixed-venous blood sample can be obtained by a slow withdrawal of blood through the catheter tip channel when the balloon is deflated. Recently, a catheter has been designed to measure continuous mixed-venous oxygen saturation. The placement of this catheter occurs while the patient is in the supine position, and the tip generally floats to a preferred region of the pulmonary vasculature in the lower aspect of the lung, in the zone 3 area.

The thermodilution method for determining cardiac output consists of injecting an aliquot of saline through the catheter and measuring, downstream, the change in temperature of the flowing fluid. The magnitude of the change in temperature of the injected fluid allows calculation of flow or cardiac output. Significant tricuspid regurgitation and intracardiac shunts can falsely reduce the cardiac output measurement with this technique. As pointed out previously, changes in lung volume and intrathoracic pressure can influence cardiopulmonary hemodynamics. Therefore, measurements should be taken at the end of expiration, when possible. Singular measurements are important, but trends in measurements are most valuable.

Using the parameters than can be directly measured (Table 3.3-2), a variety of derived or calculated hemodynamic and gas-exchange and oxygen-transport measurements can be obtained (Table 3.3-3).

Table 3.3-2
Measurements Obtained Using a Pulmonary Artery Catheter

Pressures
Right atrial
Right ventricular
Pulmonary arterial (systolic, diastolic, mean)
Pulmonary arterial occlusion (wedge)

Flow
Cardiac output

Blood Samples
Mixed-venous blood
Pulmonary capillary blood

Oxygen Saturation
Right atrial
Right ventricular
Pulmonary arterial

Cardiac Index (L/min/m²)

$$CI = \frac{\dot{Q}_T}{BSA}$$

where $\dot{Q}_T$ is cardiac output in L/min and BSA is body surface area in m².

Pulmonary Vascular Resistance (dynes • sec • cm⁻⁵)

$$PVR = \frac{\bar{P}_{pa} - \bar{P}_w}{\dot{Q}_T} \times 79.9$$

where $\bar{P}_{pa}$ is mean pulmonary arterial pressure in mmHg, $\bar{P}_w$ is mean pulmonary wedge pressure in mmHg, $\dot{Q}_T$ is cardiac output in L/min, and 79.9 is a conversion factor for adjusting to the unit, dynes • sec • cm⁻⁵.

Systemic Vascular Resistance (dynes • sec • cm⁻⁵)

$$SVR = \frac{\bar{P}_a - \bar{P}_{ra}}{\dot{Q}_T} \times 79.9$$

where $\bar{P}_a$ is mean systemic arterial pressure in mmHg, $\bar{P}_{ra}$ is mean right atrial pressure in mmHg, $\dot{Q}_T$ is cardiac output in L/min, and 79.9 is a conversion factor for adjusting to the unit, dynes • sec • cm⁻⁵.

Stroke Volume Index (mL/beat/m²)

$$SVI = \frac{\dot{Q}_T/HR}{BSA}$$

where $\dot{Q}_T$ is cardiac output in mL/min, HR is heart rate in beats per minute, and BSA is body surface area in m₂.

Right Ventricular Stroke Work Index (g • m/m₂)

$$RVSWI = SVI \times (\bar{P}_{pa} - \bar{P}_w) \times 0.0136$$

where SVI is stroke volume index in mL/beats/m², $\bar{P}_{pa}$ is mean pulmonary arterial pressure in mmHg, $\dot{P}_w$ is mean pulmonary wedge pressure in mmHg, and 0.0136 is a conversion factor for adjusting to the unit, g • m/m².

Left Ventricular Stroke Work Index (g • m/m²)

$$LVSWI = SVI \times (\bar{P}_a - \bar{P}_{ra}) \times 0.0136$$

where SVI is stroke volume index in mL/beat/m², $\bar{P}_a$ is mean systemic arterial pressure in mmHg, $\bar{P}_{ra}$ is mean right atrial pressure in mmHg, and 0.0136 is a conversion factor for adjusting to the unit, g • m/m².

Table 3.3-3
Clinically Useful Calculations Based on Measurements Made Using a Pulmonary Artery Catheter

■ REVIEW QUESTIONS

1. The pulmonary circulation is different from the systemic circulation physiologically. What unique characteristic can be attributed to the pulmonary circulation?

   (A) Low-capacity system
   (B) Low-resistance system
   (C) High-pressure, low-flow system
   (D) Poorly distendable vessel
   (E) Poor vascular recruitment to blood flow

2. Which of the following would not be considered a passive influence on or factor in pulmonary vascular resistance?

   (A) Alveolar hypoxia
   (B) Cardiac output
   (C) Alveolar pressure
   (D) Left atrial pressure
   (E) Body position

■ ANSWERS AND EXPLANATIONS

1. The answer is B. The pulmonary circulation is a high-capacity, low-resistance vascular circuit that accommodates the entire cardiac output not only at rest but also during exercise by the remarkable processes of vascular recruitment and distention.

2. The answer is A. Passive influences relate to lung or hemodynamic mechanical changes, which affect the pulmonary vascular bed, whereas active influences imply that a direct effect is occurring by the pulmonary vasculature itself. Alveolar hypoxia induces precapillary pulmonary vascular constriction by a local humoral or chemical reaction that is not influenced by the central nervous system. All of the other listed factors exert indirect mechanical influences on the pulmonary vascular bed.

■ SUGGESTED READINGS

Borst HG, McGregor M, Wittenberg JL, Berglund E: Influence of pulmonary arterial and left atrial pressure on pulmonary vascular resistance. *Circ Res* 4:393–393, 1956.

Comroe JH: *Physiology of Respiration*, 2nd ed. Chicago: YearBook, 1974, pp 142–157.

Fishman AP (ed): *The Pulmonary Circulation: Normal and Abnormal*. Philadelphia: University of Pennsylvania Press, 1990.

Fishman AP, Fisher AB (eds): *Circulation and nonrespiratory functions. Handbook of Physiology. Sec 3. The Respiratory System*. Bethesda: Amer Physiol Soc, Vol 1, 1985.

Grover RF, Wagner WW, McMurtry IF, Reeves JT: Pulmonary Circulation. In: Shepard JT, Abboud FM (eds). *Handbook of Physiology. Sec 2. The Cardiovascular System, Part I*, Bethesda: Amer Physiol Soc, Vol 3, 1983, pp 103–136.

Harris P, Heath D: *The Human Pulmonary Circulation*, 3rd ed. Edinburgh: Churchill Livingstone, 1986.

Hughes JMB, Glazier JB, Maloney JE, West JB: Effect of lung volume on the distribution of pulmonary blood flow in man. *Respir Physiol* 4:58–72, 1968.

Murray JF: *The Normal Lung*, 2nd ed. Philadelphia: Saunders, 1986, pp 35–43, 139–162.

Voelkel NF: Mechanisms of hypoxic pulmonary vasoconstriction. *Am Rev Respir Dis* 133:1186–1195, 1986.

Weir EK, Reeves JT (eds): *Pulmonary Vascular Physiology and Pathophysiology*. New York: Marcel Dekker, 1989.

West JB: *Ventilation/Blood Flow and Gas Exchange*, 5th ed. Oxford: Blackwell, 1990, pp 15–25.

West JB: *Respiratory Physiology—The Essentials*, 5th ed. Baltimore: Williams & Wilkins, 1995, pp 31–50.

GAS TRANSPORT AND ACID-BASE STATUS OF THE LUNG

Gilbert E. D'Alonzo, D.O.

■ SECTION OUTLINE

Learning Objectives

Introduction

Oxyhemoglobin Dissociation Curve

Oxygen Transport

Carbon Dioxide Transport

Carbon Dioxide–Hemoglobin Dissociation Curve

Acid-Base Status and the Lung

Review Questions

■ LEARNING OBJECTIVES

At the completion of this section, the reader should:
- Understand the concepts of the oxygen capacity and how the affinity of hemoglobin for oxygen changes to meet the demands of the body in order to enhance the oxygen-carrying capacity of the blood.
- Be able to describe the Bohr and Haldane effects and explain why they are so important for oxygen and carbon dioxide transport.
- Be able to explain the concepts and components of oxygen transport and utilization and the relevance of the Fick principle.
- Understand how the lung plays a crucial role in maintaining proper and optimized acid-base balance in the body.
- Be able to describe the differences and interrelationships between respiratory and metabolic pH adjustments that occur in health and in disease states.

■ INTRODUCTION

The amount of oxygen carried in the arterial blood is dependent on the hemoglobin concentration.

As oxygen moves from an alveolus into the plasma, a new concentration gradient is established between oxygen in the plasma and oxygen in the interior of the red blood cell. Oxygen diffuses into the red blood cell and combines chemically with hemoglobin. One gram of hemoglobin can bind to and carry 1.34 mL of oxygen. The oxygen-carrying capacity of blood, therefore, is directly dependent on the hemoglobin concentration: oxygen-carrying capacity (mL/100 mL) equals hemoglobin (gm/100 mL) times 1.34 mL/gm. However, not every oxygen molecule in the blood combines with hemoglobin. A small quantity of oxygen remains dissolved in the plasma. The amount of dissolved oxygen is proportional to the partial pressure of oxygen and its solubility coefficient. The solubility of oxygen in plasma is very low, approximately 0.0031 mL of oxygen in 1 dL of blood per mmHg. Therefore, at an arterial PO_2 of 100, 100 mL of arterial blood contains only 0.31 mL of dissolved oxygen. Dissolved oxygen equals the arterial PO_2 times 0.0031 mL of oxygen/dL mmHg. Therefore, the oxygen content of the blood is the actual amount present in the blood, both combined with hemoglobin and dissolved in plasma.

The maximum amount of oxygen that can be combined with hemoglobin is called the oxygen capacity. If blood is exposed to a very high PO_2 (600 mmHg) and the dissolved oxygen is subtracted, then the oxygen capacity of the blood can be determined. For a subject with a hemoglobin of 15 gm/100 mL, the oxygen capacity is 20.1 mL of oxygen per 100 mL of blood. The relationship between the actual amount of oxygen combined with hemoglobin in a given amount of blood and the oxygen capacity determines the percent saturation of hemoglobin: % SO_2 = (O_2 content − O_2 dissolved in plasma) ÷ (O_2 capacity × 100). Therefore, if the PO_2 is 100, then the oxygen saturation of the arterial blood is 97% and the mixed-venous blood with a PO_2 of 40 mmHg is approximately 75%.

▮ OXYHEMOGLOBIN DISSOCIATION CURVE

Hemoglobin's affinity for oxygen increases as the partial pressure of oxygen in the arterial blood increases. This means that as the molecular concentration of oxygen in the blood increases, hemoglobin becomes increasingly saturated (Figure 3.4-1). This is a reversible chemical reaction and there is a sigmoid shape to the oxyhemoglobin dissociation curve. The shape of this curve has certain advantages. The flat upper portion allows arterial oxygen content to remain high and nearly constant despite fluctuations in arterial PO_2. The steep middle portion of the curve describes how large quantities of oxygen are released at PO_2 values that generally prevail at the capillary level in peripheral tissues. Therefore, peripheral tissues can withdraw large amounts of oxygen for only a small drop in capillary PO_2. The affinity between oxygen and hemoglobin is conventionally expressed as the PO_2 at which the available hemoglobin is half saturated, or the P_{50}, which is measured under standard conditions (temperature, 37°C; blood pH, 7.40). The normal P_{50} of human blood is 26.6 mmHg. A variety of conditions can change the P_{50}, altering the binding affinity of oxygen for hemoglobin. The oxyhemoglobin dissociation curve can be shifted to the right or to the left by changes in pH, PCO_2, and temperature (Figure 3.4-2).

FIGURE 3.4-1
The oxyhemoglobin dissociation curve under the conditions of 37°C, PCO_2 40, and pH 7.40 (solid line). The dissociation O_2 in the plasma and the total blood O_2 content (dashed lines) are shown for a hemoglobin of 15 gm/100 mL of blood. The P_{50} is the arterial PO_2 at which the hemoglobin is 50% saturated (normally 26.6 mmHg), a value used to describe shifts of the curve to the right or the left.

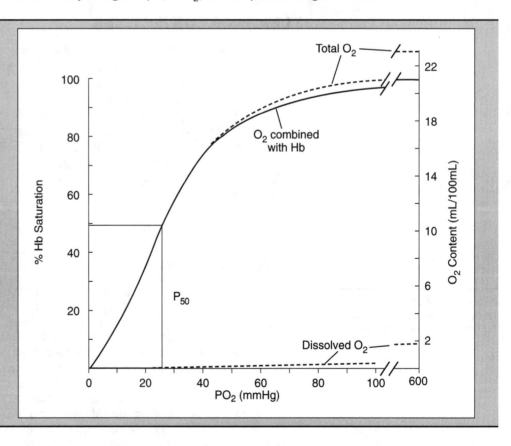

Enhanced affinity of hemoglobin for oxygen is shown by a leftward shift of the oxyhemoglobin curve and a low P_{50}.

- ↓ Temperature
- ↓ PCO_2
- ↑ pH
- ↓ 2,3-DPG

When hemoglobin's affinity for oxygen increases, oxygen is taken up more readily by hemoglobin and released less readily for any PO_2. Enhanced affinity of hemoglobin for oxygen means that the oxyhemoglobin dissociation curve is shifted to the left and the P_{50} is lower than usual (see Figure 3.4-2). A decrease in body temperature, a decrease in PCO_2, and a rise in pH all shift the oxyhemoglobin dissociation curve to the left and are associated with a lower P_{50}. Opposite changes shift the curve to the right, where the affinity of hemoglobin for oxygen decreases and the P_{50} increases.

A rightward shift of the oxyhemoglobin dissociation curve indicates that a higher

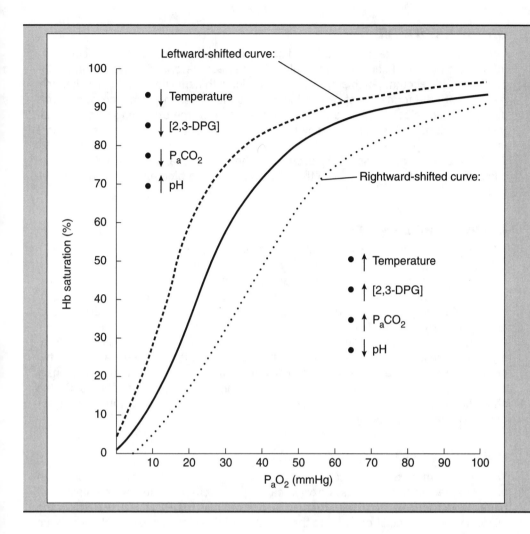

FIGURE 3.4-2
A shift in the oxyhemoglobin curve represents a change in hemoglobin affinity for O_2. A left shift or a fall in the P_{50} means enhanced affinity, whereas a right shift indicates increased P_{50} and reduced affinity.

arterial PO_2 is necessary to maintain a constant oxygen saturation, and therefore the affinity for hemoglobin is decreased. The lower oxygen affinity means enhanced oxygen release to the peripheral tissues. On the other hand, a leftward shift in the curve, with a decreased P_{50}, indicates enhanced hemoglobin affinity for oxygen and less release of oxygen to the peripheral tissues.

The hemoglobin molecule undergoes conformational changes when it reacts with oxygen. When hemoglobin combines with oxygen, its molecular structure seems to contract, and it expands when it releases oxygen. The molecular structure of hemoglobin also changes during reactions with other chemicals, such as carbon dioxide, hydrogen ion, and certain organophosphates such as 2,3-diphosphoglycerate (2,3-DPG). These substances are termed ligands because they can exert effects on the chemical properties of hemoglobin. For this discussion, however, these ligands influence hemoglobin's ability to combine with oxygen, and these relationships are demonstrated by shifts in the oxyhemoglobin association curve.

HYDROGEN ION

Intracellular pH influences the affinity of hemoglobin for oxygen. This is called the *Bohr effect*. The intracellular concentration of carbon dioxide has a direct effect on bicarbonate concentration and an indirect effect on hydrogen ion concentration. During the gas-exchange process at the level of the lungs, hydrogen ion concentration falls as carbon dioxide is eliminated, and the oxyhemoglobin dissociation curve shifts to the left when hemoglobin's affinity for oxygen increases.

On the other hand, in the peripheral tissues, carbon dioxide is added to the blood stream, increasing hydrogen ion concentration, and oxygen's affinity for hemoglobin decreases. These effects are complementary because they provide for enhanced oxygen uptake at the level of the lungs and more efficient oxygen release at the level of the peripheral tissues.

Reduced affinity of hemoglobin for oxygen is represented by a rightward shift of the oxyhemoglobin curve and a high P_{50}.

- ↑ Temperature
- ↑ PCO_2
- ↓ pH
- ↑ 2,3-DPG

CARBON DIOXIDE

One effect of a change in the carbon dioxide concentration in a red blood cell is its influence on intracellular pH, the so-called Bohr effect, described above. Additionally, carbon dioxide accumulation and its binding effect with hemoglobin induce a chemical reaction with the formation of carbamino compounds. A rise in carbamino compounds decreases hemoglobin oxygen affinity, which means that the oxyhemoglobin dissociation curve shifts to the right, thereby releasing oxygen to the peripheral tissues more readily.

On the other hand, as PCO_2 decreases, there is also a decrease in carbamino compounds and the curve shifts to the left, enhancing the binding of oxygen to hemoglobin.

ORGANOPHOSPHATE

2,3-DPG and other organophosphates are metabolized by erythrocytes during glycolysis. These organophosphates are the major energy sources for red blood cells, which do not have mitochondria for oxidative phosphorylation. During anaerobic conditions, usually associated with hypoxia, 2,3-DPG concentration increases. As this organophosphate concentration increases, the P_{50} increases, and there is a decrease in hemoglobin-oxygen affinity and a subsequent burst release of oxygen to the peripheral tissues. Low levels of erythrocyte 2,3-DPG increases oxygen affinity. Low levels of erythrocyte organophosphates are found in a variety of diseases associated with hypoxia, such as anemia, congestive heart failure (CHF), chronic obstructive pulmonary disease (COPD), exposure to high altitude, and a variety of intracardiac shunts. On the other hand, low levels of erythrocyte organophosphates are also found in hypophosphatemia and septic shock.

CARBON MONOXIDE

Carbon monoxide accelerates tissue hypoxia.

- Formation of CO-Hgb decreases O_2 capacity of arterial blood
- ↓ P_{50} by shifting the oxyhemoglobin curve to the right.

The arterial PO_2 can be normal with high levels of carboxyhemoglobin and a low arterial O_2 saturation.

When carbon monoxide binds to hemoglobin, carboxyhemoglobin is formed. Formation of carboxyhemoglobin decreases oxygen-carrying capacity by reducing the amount of hemoglobin available for oxygen binding, and it reduces the P_{50} because it shifts the oxyhemoglobin dissociation curve to the left. Both of these mechanisms enhance tissue hypoxia.

Carboxyhemoglobin anemia is measured by co-oximetry. Even with high levels of carboxyhemoglobin and a low oxygen saturation, the arterial PO_2 can be normal.

Methemoglobin is produced by oxidation of hemoglobin iron from the ferrous to the ferric state. In healthy humans, methemoglobin accounts for less than 3% of the total hemoglobin. When methemoglobin is produced to excess, usually by exposures to certain drugs that accelerate iron oxidation, delivery of oxygen to the peripheral tissues is substantially reduced because it shifts the oxyhemoglobin dissociation curve to the left.

Oxidant drugs include a variety of nitrates, sulfonamides, phenacetin, dapsone, and local anesthetics. In certain patients, there is a congenital defect of the enzyme methemoglobin reductase in red blood cells, and when these patients are exposed to oxidant drugs, this congenital defect expresses itself and serious methemoglobinemia occurs.

There are other abnormal hemoglobins that result from genetic variations. Only a minority of these hemoglobins are associated with a change in oxygen affinity, and most are of little clinical significance. Fetal hemoglobin has a decreased P_{50} that can be attributed to decreased binding of 2,3-DPG to the hemoglobin gamma chains instead of the beta chains in normal fetal hemoglobin. For the fetus, this affinity change has an advantage in that the placental uptake of oxygen is enhanced.

Hemoglobin S, found in sickle cell disease, has a slightly different amino acid sequence in the hemoglobin beta chains. This difference results in a slight rightward shift in the oxyhemoglobin dissociation curve. More importantly, the deoxygenated form of hemoglobin is poorly soluble and crystallizes within the red blood cell, causing it to sickle. The sickle shape actually interferes with capillary transit, and this plays a major role in the cell's ineffectiveness as a transporter of oxygen to peripheral tissues.

■ OXYGEN TRANSPORT

Oxygen transport is the amount of oxygen delivered to the tissues in a unit of time. Oxygen is necessary to maintain aerobic metabolism. Without oxygen, tissues undergo anaerobic metabolism and the formation of certain acid end products, such as lactic acid. After a brief period of time without oxygen, the peripheral tissues begin to undergo irreversible change and eventually cellular death.

Oxygen transport involves transfer of oxygen molecules from the air into the lung and, through the circulation, to the peripheral tissue capillary bed, where the oxygen is eventually released from the red blood cells and used by intracellular mitochondria. The supply of oxygen to the tissues must be plentiful and continuous.

Delivery of oxygen to the peripheral tissues can be calculated by measuring the cardiac output and the arterial oxygen content of the blood. This content is the sum of hemoglobin-bound oxygen and dissolved oxygen in the plasma. Three organ systems are involved in this oxygen delivery process: the circulatory system, which includes cardiac output and arterial blood flow; the erythropoietic system, with its blood volume and red cell mass; and the respiratory system, which optimizes the oxygen saturation of the arterial blood. Disturbances in any of these systems can interfere with appropriate oxygen delivery.

Systemic or total body oxygen delivery (DO_2) can be calculated after cardiac output (CO) and oxygen content of the arterial blood have been determined:

$$DO_2 = CO \text{ (L/min)} \times O_2 \text{ content (MI/L)}.$$

As mentioned previously, the oxygen content is the total amount of oxygen in the blood, including oxygen bound to hemoglobin and oxygen dissolved in plasma. Therefore, the oxygen delivery equation can be shown as

$$DO_2 = CO \times [(Hb \times 1.34 \times \% \text{ saturation}) + (0.0031 \times P_aO_2)].$$

The delivered oxygen is utilized or consumed by the tissue. Some organs receive more blood per unit of tissue than others, and the degree of oxygen consumption may vary. Going from rest to exercise dramatically changes these relationships, as do various disease states. In order to determine the amount of oxygen consumed by an individual organ, one would have to measure that organ's blood flow and the difference between the oxygen contents of its arterial and venous blood, or the arterial-venous oxygen content difference (AVO_2D). However, this type of selective organ measurement is not done in practice. What is done is the measurement of a global or total body oxygen consumption ($\dot{V}O_2$) and the arterial–mixed-venous oxygen content difference by using arterial and Swan-Ganz catheters, as described previously. By measuring DO_2 and VO_2, the oxygen extraction ratio (ER) can be determined:

$$O_2ER = \frac{\dot{V}O_2}{DO_2}.$$

The oxygen ER is normally between 0.25 and 0.35. Body oxygen ER is increased in low-DO_2 states, such as heart failure and anemia, and in hypermetabolic conditions, such as fever and thyroid disease.

FICK PRINCIPLE

The relationship among oxygen consumption, cardiac output, and the arterial and mixed-venous oxygen contents (C_aO_2 and $C_{\bar{v}}O_2$) is the Fick principle:

$$\dot{V}O_2 = CO \times (C_aO_2 - C_{\bar{v}}O_2).$$

$\dot{V}O_2$ can be measured by collecting expired gas spirometrically and measuring oxygen and carbon dioxide concentrations or by determining cardiac output by thermodilution and sampling of the mixed-venous blood with a Swan-Ganz catheter and the arterial blood with a simultaneously puncture-drawn sample.

By the Fick equation, if the cardiac output remains unchanged, an increase in oxygen consumption will increase the AVO_2D. The AVO_2D will decrease if metabolic demand falls and cardiac output has not been permitted to change.

An average-size normal adult can have an oxygen consumption of 250 mL/min and a cardiac output of 5 L/min, and therefore the AVO_2D can be calculated as follows:

$$\dot{V}O_2 = CO \times (C_aO_2 - C_{\bar{v}}O_2)$$

$$(C_aO_2 - C_{\bar{v}}O_2) = \frac{\dot{V}O_2}{CO}$$

$$AVO_2D = 5 \text{ mL/dL.}$$

A normal AVO_2D is approximately 5 mL/dL, the arterial oxygen content is 20 mL/dL at a hemoglobin of 15 g/dL and a normal arterial oxygen saturation, and the mixed-venous oxygen content is normally 15 mL/dL.

■ CARBON DIOXIDE TRANSPORT

Several chemical reactions are important in the transport of carbon dioxide from the tissues to the lungs. As mentioned previously, carbon dioxide is 20 times more diffusible than oxygen. Carbon dioxide is an important end product of aerobic cellular metabolism; therefore, it is continuously produced by body tissues. After carbon dioxide is formed by cells, it diffuses readily into the plasma, where it passes immediately into red blood cells. It then undergoes one of two chemical reactions. However, a small amount is carried in the plasma in solution, or dissolved. The amount of carbon dioxide dissolved in the plasma is determined by its partial pressure and solubility coefficient. Approximately 5% of total carbon dioxide in the arterial blood is in the dissolved form.

Other transport mechanisms involve the bicarbonate ion and carbamino compounds (Figure 3.4-3). Carbon dioxide diffuses into the red blood cell, the greatest portion of

Blood CO$_2$ Transport Mechanisms

- Dissolved in plasma
- Bicarbonate is formal
- Formation of carbamino compounds

FIGURE 3.4-3
Carbon dioxide transport at the level of the capillaries and peripheral tissues, where CO_2 is taken up by the red cell after being released by the tissue and O_2 is released by the red cell for tissue uptake and mitochondrial use. At the level of the lung, the reaction in the pulmonary capillaries is in the opposite direction: O_2 is taken up by the red cell and CO_2 is released to the alveolus. (*See text for a description of the chemical reactions depicted.*)

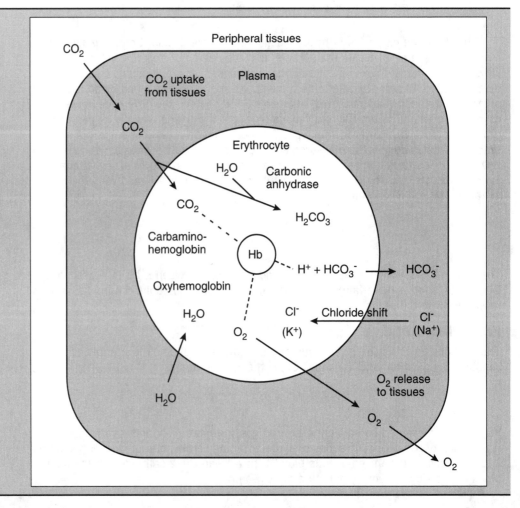

which reacts with water to form carbonic acid (H_2CO_3), which dissociates into hydrogen and bicarbonate ion. This reaction is extremely fast because of the presence of the intracellular enzyme, carbonic anhydrase. Some hydrogen and bicarbonate ions remain in the red blood cell, the hydrogen ion combining with hemoglobin and the bicarbonate ion combining with potassium that has been displaced from hemoglobin during the hydrogen ion reaction (Figure 3.4-4).

Some bicarbonate ion also diffuses out of the red blood cell, not the plasma, because the membrane is more permeable to negatively charged ions than to positively charged ions such as potassium and sodium. With the shift of bicarbonate into the plasma, chloride ions move from the plasma into the erythrocytes (the "chloride shift") in order to maintain electrical neutrality.

Deoxyhemoglobin can handle more H_2CO_3 than oxyhemoglobin, because the deoxy-hemoglobin is a weaker acid, making it a better buffer. This facilitation of hydrogen ion binding by deoxygenated hemoglobin occurs in the peripheral tissues where carbon dioxide concentrations are high. The deoxygenation of arterial blood in peripheral tissues promotes hydrogen ion binding through the generation of reduced hemoglobin. This enhancement of carbon dioxide binding to hemoglobin is known as the *Haldane effect*.

The last form of carbon dioxide transport in the blood is carbamino compounds. A smaller fraction of CO_2 that enters the red blood cell combines, in a reversible fashion, with hemoglobin to form carbamino compounds. The reaction of carbon dioxide to the amino groups of hemoglobin occurs rapidly. This reaction also occurs more readily to deoxyhemoglobin than oxyhemoglobin, again showing that oxygen unloading in the peripheral tissues facilitates the loading of carbon dioxide. Carbamino compounds con-stitute approximately 5% of the carbon dioxide transported in the arterial blood.

The majority of transported carbon dioxide in the blood is in the form of bicarbonate. The amounts found in plasma, in a dissolved form, and in the carbaminohemoglobin form

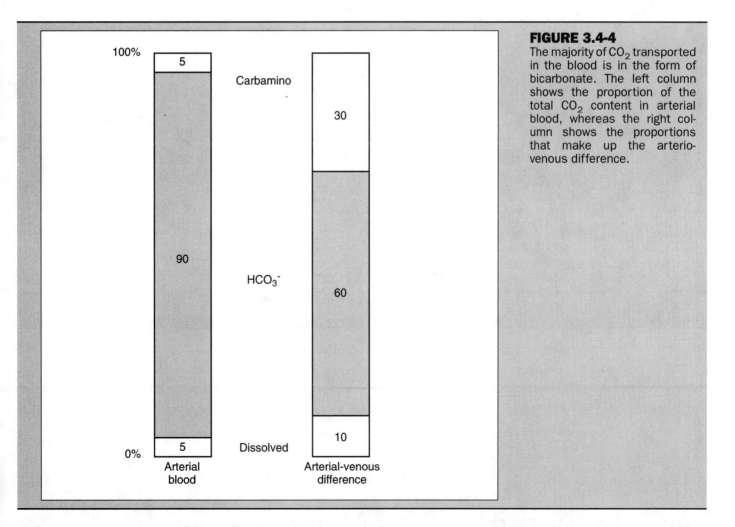

FIGURE 3.4-4
The majority of CO_2 transported in the blood is in the form of bicarbonate. The left column shows the proportion of the total CO_2 content in arterial blood, whereas the right column shows the proportions that make up the arterio-venous difference.

are much smaller. If one looks at the contribution of each of these carbon dioxide transport forms to the arterial-venous difference in carbon dioxide concentration, the bicarbonate form constitutes approximately 60%, the carbamino compounds about 30%, and the dissolved form nearly 10% (see Figure 3.4-4).

CARBON DIOXIDE–HEMOGLOBIN DISSOCIATION CURVE

The relationship between PCO_2 and total carbon dioxide content of the blood is illustrated in Figure 3.4-5. When compared with the oxyhemoglobin dissociation curve, the carbon dioxide–hemoglobin dissociation curve is nearly linear, especially in the physiologic PCO_2 range from 40 to 50 mmHg.

The shift from the lower to the upper curve in Figure 3.4-5 occurs during the deoxygenation of blood as it flows through tissue capillaries. This enhancement of carbon dioxide transport has been explained previously and is called the Haldane effect. Figure 3.4-6 shows that the carbon dioxide–hemoglobin dissociation curve is steeper than the oxyhemoglobin dissociation curve in their normal physiologic ranges. Therefore, there is a greater change in carbon dioxide content than in oxygen content over the range from 40 to 60 mmHg.

FIGURE 3.4-5
The CO_2 dissociation curves for hemoglobin and plasma are shown at different O_2 saturations. Oxygenated blood carries less CO_2 than either venous blood or completely deoxygenated blood (Haldane effect) for the same PCO_2. The inset graph shows what actually occurs to CO_2 content between arterial and mixed-venous blood.

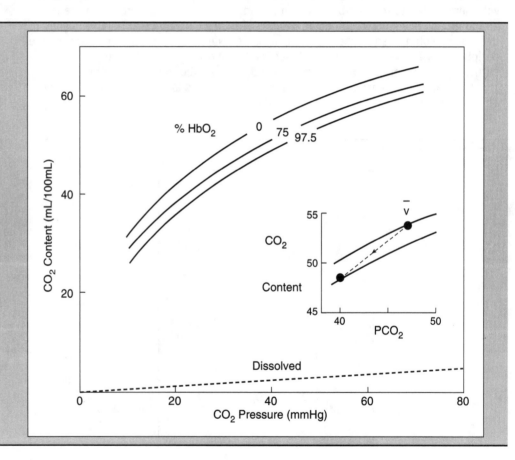

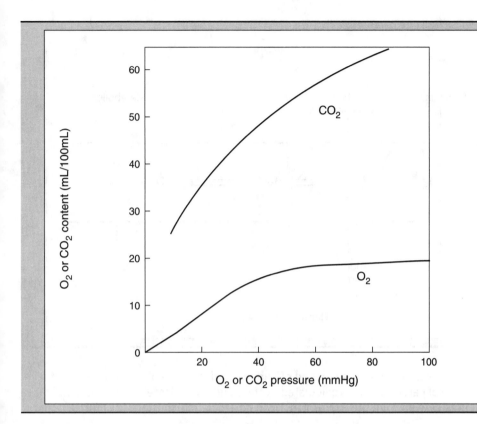

FIGURE 3.4-6
Oxygen and carbon dioxide hemoglobin dissociation curves plotted on the same graph and showing that the CO_2-hemoglobin dissociation is steeper in the normal physiologic range.

ACID-BASE STATUS AND THE LUNG

The elimination of carbon dioxide by changes in minute ventilation allows the lung to play the major role in the minute-to-minute regulation of body acid-base status. Breathing disorders are major causes of acid-base disturbance, and the respiratory system responds to abnormalities in metabolism that alter the body's metabolic status.

The body runs best within a narrow range of pH. Buffering systems play a crucial role in maintaining acid-base equilibrium. There are both extracellular and intracellular buffering systems. The principal buffering system is the carbon dioxide–bicarbonate system, which deals with both extracellular and intracellular disturbances. A few of the other buffering mechanisms include certain blood proteins, hemoglobin, and various constituents of bone.

Nearly all body fluids contain bicarbonate anion in appreciable quantities. This anion is readily available to stabilize changes in pH. There is a huge reservoir of bicarbonate in the body, and it acts as an "alkali reserve" for metabolic disturbances. Bicarbonate reacts with hydrogen ion to form carbonic acid, which exists in equilibrium with carbon dioxide

$$H^+ + HCO_3^- \rightleftharpoons H_2CO_3 \overset{\rightleftharpoons}{CA} H_2O + CO_2$$

and water. Carbonic acid is metabolized rapidly by carbonic anhydrase and the carbon dioxide that is formed, along with water, and rapidly leaves the body through the lungs. The bicarbonate buffering system converts the hydrogen ion, which is formed from the metabolic production of body acids, to carbonic acid. Carbon dioxide is produced during cell metabolism, and the carbonic acid formed is quickly changed to hydrogen ion and bicarbonate. The chief pathways for production and removal of carbon dioxide, hydrogen ion, and bicarbonate are shown in Figure 3.4-7.

FIGURE 3.4-7
Chief pathways for production and removal of bicarbonate, hydrogen ion, and carbon dioxide.

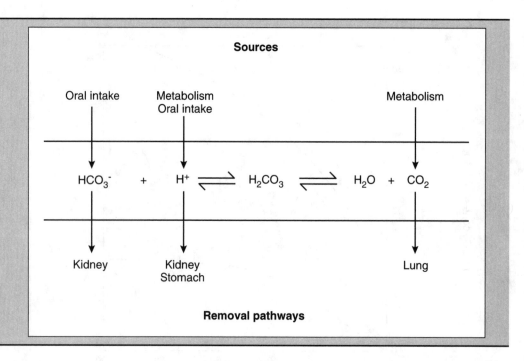

The pH resulting from the solution of carbon dioxide in the blood and the eventual dissociation of carbonic acid is calculated by the Henderson-Hasselbalch equation. This equation is derived from the expression for the dissociation constant (K_A) for carbonic acid:

$$K_A = [H^+] \times \frac{[HCO_3^-]}{[H_2CO_3]}.$$

The logarithmic form of this equation is

$$\log K_A = \log[H^+] + \frac{\log[HCO_3^-]}{[H_2CO_3]}.$$

The concentration of carbonic acid is proportional to the concentration of dissolved carbon dioxide, and we can change the constant and write the pH as the negative logarithm of the hydrogen ion concentration. Then the equation can be written as

$$pH = pK_A + \frac{\log[HCO_3^-]}{[H_2CO_3]}.$$

Because the amount of carbon dioxide is proportional to its solubility coefficient, the carbon dioxide concentration can be replaced by ($PCO_2 \times 0.03$) and the equation becomes

$$pH = pK_A + \frac{\log[HCO_3^-]}{PCO_2 \times 0.03}.$$

The value of pK_A is 6.1, and when the concentration of bicarbonate in the arterial blood is 24 mM/L and PCO_2 is 40 mmHg, then

$$pH = 6.1 + \frac{\log 24}{0.03 \times 40}$$

$$= 6.1 + \log 20$$

$$= 6.1 + 1.3$$

$$= 7.4.$$

If the bicarbonate concentration falls and the arterial PCO_2 remains constant, pH falls. On the other hand, if the bicarbonate concentration rises and PCO_2 remains constant, pH rises. A similar analysis holds for primary changes in arterial PCO_2—a rise or fall in this value, without an accompanying change in bicarbonate concentration, results in a fall or rise in pH, respectively. The bicarbonate concentration is determined chiefly by the kidney, and the PCO_2 concentration is determined by the lung.

The relationships among pH, PCO_2, and plasma bicarbonate (HCO_3) are graphically represented in the Davenport diagram (Figure 3.4-8). Plasma bicarbonate is plotted against blood pH for several levels of arterial PCO_2. Normal values are represented by point A. The line BAC shows the relationship between bicarbonate and pH as carbonic acid is added to or removed from arterial blood ("buffer line"). Going from point A to point B demonstrates the addition of carbonic acid, whereas going from point A to point C represents the removal of carbonic acid from the blood.

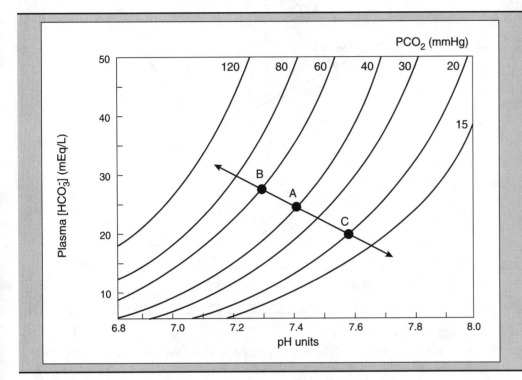

FIGURE 3.4-8
Davenport diagram. Plasma bicarbonate (HCO^-_3) is plotted against blood pH for a variety of arterial PCO_2 values as isobars. Point A is the normal value, and the line represented by BAC is the "buffer line" that is created as carbonic acid is added (AB) or removed (AC).

The Davenport diagram can be used to assist in our understanding of respiratory acidosis and alkalosis and the metabolic compensations associated with these changes (Figure 3.4-9). Normal blood pH is between 7.36 and 7.44. When the pH increases above 7.44, the blood becomes alkalemic. On the other hand, when the pH decreases below 7.36, acidemia is defined. Alkalemia is represented by a shift from point A to point C, and acidemia is represented by a shift from point A to point B. The shifts that occur from A to B and from A to C may be attributable to either changes in arterial PCO_2 or alterations in the plasma bicarbonate concentration. From the diagram it can be seen that a change in pH accompanied by a change in arterial PCO_2 or bicarbonate concentration can be modified by a concomitant alteration in the other variable. A change in the arterial PCO_2 creates a sequence of chemical reactions that causes a change in plasma bicarbonate concentration, or vice versa. These compensatory changes are important homeostatic mechanisms for maintaining proper acid-base balance.

RESPIRATORY ACIDOSIS

Respiratory acidosis is defined as an arterial PCO_2 greater than or equal to 44 mmHg. This increase in arterial PCO_2 reduces the ratio of bicarbonate to PCO_2 and decreases blood pH. After the PCO_2 rises, the bicarbonate must increase because of carbonic acid dissociation. Carbon dioxide retention can be caused by either hypoventilation or ventilation-perfusion inequality.

Using a Davenport diagram (see Figure 3.4-9), the arterial PCO_2 increase that occurs is represented by the line going from point A to point B. If respiratory acidosis persists, the kidney conserves bicarbonate. The increased PCO_2 in the renal tubular cells, which excrete more acid urine by secreting hydrogen ions, allows for the reabsorption of bicarbonate ions. The resultant increase in plasma bicarbonate causes the pH to normalize, as represented on the Davenport diagram by the line going from point B to point D.

For every respiratory change that affects arterial PCO_2, there is a compensatory metabolic adjustment that "normalizes" body pH.

FIGURE 3.4-9
Davenport diagram showing the various changes that occur in respiratory and metabolic acidosis and alkalosis.

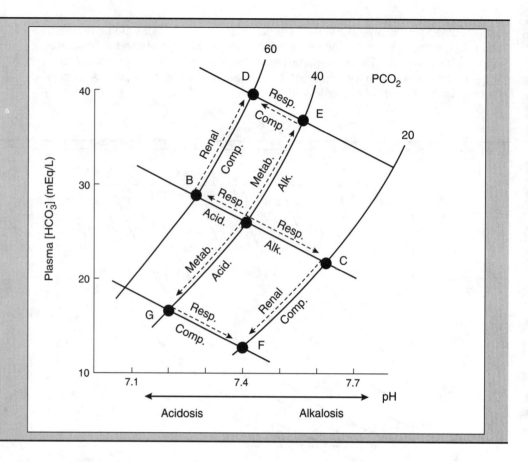

Although the pH often is not completely restored to 7.40, we call this modification a compensated respiratory acidosis. The extent of renal compensation can be determined from the increase in plasma bicarbonate as represented by the difference between points A and D, a value termed the "base excess."

Common causes of carbon dioxide retention and acute and chronic respiratory acidosis are listed in Table 3.4-1. Acute respiratory acidosis can be induced by anesthetics and sedative drugs. Acute brain injury can also cause acute respiratory acidosis. A variety of neuromuscular diseases, such as poliomyelitis, myasthenia gravis, and Guillain-Barré syndrome, have been associated with both acute and chronic respiratory acidosis. The pickwickian or obesity-hypoventilation syndrome is associated with a chronic, partially compensated respiratory acidosis. All of these conditions can occur in individuals with normal lungs. Parenchymal lung diseases, such as severe chronic obstructive pulmonary disease and numerous interstitial lung diseases, are also associated with chronic respiratory acidosis. Patients with kyphoscoliosis have respiratory mechanical problems but also have underlying parenchymal lung disease, generally in the form of atelectasis and fibrosis, and they can also have chronic respiratory acidosis, which is often partially compensated metabolically.

Table 3.4-1
Common Causes of CO$_2$ Retention and Respiratory Acidosis

With Normal Lungs
  Anesthesia
  Sedative drugs
  Neuromuscular disease (poliomyelitis, myasthenia gravis, Guillain-Barré syndrome)
  Obesity (pickwickian syndrome)
  Brain damage

With Abnormal Lungs
  Chronic obstructive pulmonary disease (chronic bronchitis, emphysema)
  Diffuse infiltrative pulmonary disease (advanced)
  Kyphoscoliosis (severe)

RESPIRATORY ALKALOSIS

When the arterial PCO_2 is equal to or less than 36 mmHg, respiratory alkalosis is defined. This condition is generally a result of alveolar hyperventilation. The decrease in arterial PCO_2 increases the bicarbonate-to-PCO_2 ratio and elevates the arterial pH, as represented by a shift from point A to point C on the Davenport diagram (see Figure 3.4-9). Renal compensation occurs by enhancing bicarbonate excretion, thus returning the pH toward normal, as represented by the line going from point C to point F on the Davenport diagram. After a prolonged period of time, renal compensation can be complete, and the plasma bicarbonate is low and there is a negative base excess, or "base deficit."

Patients with normal lungs can hyperventilate and induce an acute respiratory alkalosis. This can occur during periods of anxiety or fever, or in the patient who has a central nervous system lesion, such as a brain tumor or cerebral inflammation. Various drugs, such as aspirin, can also induce hyperventilation. Respiratory alkalosis often occurs in patients with abnormal lungs. Pneumonia, diffuse interstitial lung disease, acute airflow obstruction, heart failure with pulmonary edema, and pulmonary vascular diseases, which are often associated with pulmonary hypertension, are associated with respiratory alkalosis (Table 3.4-2).

Table 3.4-2
Common Causes of Excessive CO_2 Elimination and Respiratory Alkalosis

With Normal Lungs
   Anxiety
   Fever
   Drugs (e.g., aspirin)
   Central nervous system lesions (tumors, inflammation)
   Endotoxemia

With Abnormal Lungs
   Pneumonia
   Diffuse infiltrative pulmonary diseases (early)
   Acute bronchial asthma
   Pulmonary vascular diseases
   Congestive heart failure

METABOLIC ACIDOSIS

The term "metabolic" refers to a primary change in plasma bicarbonate, which often causes a compensatory respiratory response and a change in the arterial PCO_2. The plasma bicarbonate may be reduced secondary to accumulation of acids in the blood or a loss of plasma bicarbonate (Table 3.4-3). The Davenport diagram can be used to explain metabolic acidosis (see Figure 3.4-9). The ingestion of a fixed acid, or an increase in the production of acid or reduced excretion of a fixed acid, lowers the plasma bicarbonate concentration, as represented by a shift from point A to point G on the diagram. The drop in blood pH causes stimulation of body peripheral chemoreceptors, which in turn stimulates the respiratory center and increases minute ventilation, reducing the arterial PCO_2, as reflected on the diagram as a shift from point G to point F. The change in plasma bicarbonate reflects a base deficit, and this is shown as the difference between points A and F.

In metabolic acidosis, one has to determine whether there has been a primary loss of plasma bicarbonate or an accumulation of body acid that lowers plasma bicarbonate.

Table 3.4-3
Common Causes of Metabolic Acidosis

Increased Unmeasured Anions (Excess Nonvolatile Acids)
   Diabetic ketoacidosis
   Alcoholic ketoacidosis
   Lactic acidosis
   Salicylate intoxication
   Renal failure
   Methanol or ethylene glycol poisoning

Normal Unmeasured Anions (Loss of Bicarbonate)
   Diarrhea
   Pancreatic or biliary fistulas
   Renal tubular acidosis
   Chronic pyelonephritis
   Obstructive uropathy

Metabolic alkalosis can be caused by excessive ingestion of an alkali, such as milk, or by a loss of body acid.

METABOLIC ALKALOSIS

An excessive loss of body acid or an accumulation of base produces metabolic alkalosis (Table 3.4-4). The loss of body acid can be responsive or resistant to the administration of chloride. In metabolic alkalosis, there is an increase in plasma bicarbonate, which raises the ratio of bicarbonate to arterial PCO_2 and raises pH. Again, the Davenport diagram can be used to enhance understanding of metabolic alkalosis (see Figure 3.4-9). A shift from point A to point E on this diagram reflects the development of a metabolic alkalosis, and a shift from point E to point D indicates respiratory compensation. This respiratory compensation is actually alveolar hypoventilation, which results in a high arterial PCO_2 or hypercapnia. The plasma bicarbonate is high, and there is a base excess, as represented by the difference between point A and point D.

Table 3.4-4
Common Causes of Metabolic Alkalosis

Alkalosis Secondary to Alkali Administration
  Milk-alkali syndrome
  Ingestion of sodium bicarbonate

Chloride-Responsive Alkalosis
  Gastric fluid losses
  Diuretic therapy

Chloride-Resistant Alkalosis
  Primary aldosteronism
  Bartter's syndrome

MIXED ACID-BASE DISTURBANCES

Mixed respiratory and metabolic disturbances often occur in clinical practice. The sequence of the respiratory and metabolic disturbances is often difficult to unravel unless there is a continuum of data to analyze. A nomogram can be used to evaluate mixed acid-base disturbances. Figure 3.4-10 shows the relationship among arterial pH, arterial PCO_2, and bicarbonate concentration in all types of acid-base disturbances. The clear space in the center (N) of the nomogram represents normal acid-base balance, and any point between the clearly marked bands represents more complex acid-base disturbances. The banded areas represent straightforward acid-base disturbances with or without compensation. At times, even using this nomogram, confusion remains as to the sequence of events that has occurred and that explains a particular acid-base disturbance.

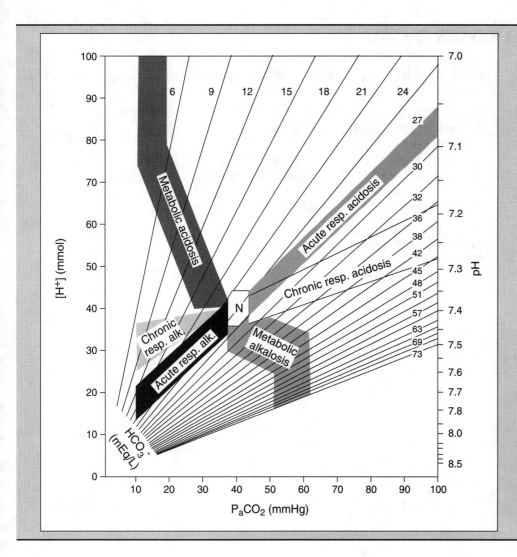

FIGURE 3.4-10
Nomogram for evaluating all types of acid-base disturbances. Each band depicts the relationship among arterial pH, P_aCO_2, and bicarbonate concentration in simple acid-base disturbances. Points falling between bands indicate mixed disturbances. N indicates the normal range. From Goldberg M, Green SB, Moss ML, et al.: Computer-based instruction and diagnosis of acid-base disorders: a systemic approach. *JAMA* 223:269–275, 1973.

▮ REVIEW QUESTIONS

1. Which of the following should not shift the oxyhemoglobin dissociation curve to the right?

   (A) An increase in blood pH
   (B) An increase in body temperature
   (C) Hypercapnia
   (D) An increase in hydrogen ion concentration
   (E) An increase in red cell organophosphate concentration

2. During respiratory acidosis, which one of the following is true?

   (A) Lactic acid is elevated.
   (B) Bicarbonate is decreased.
   (C) Arterial PO_2 is low.
   (D) Arterial PCO_2 is elevated.

▮ ANSWERS AND EXPLANATIONS

1. The answer is A. A rightward shift of the oxyhemoglobin dissociation curve indicates that a higher arterial PO_2 is necessary to maintain a constant oxygen saturation—in other words, red cell affinity for oxygen is decreased. Reduced red cell oxygen affinity means that there is an enhanced release of oxygen for immediate uptake by peripheral tissues. An increase in temperature or any condition that decreases blood pH causes a rightward shift in the oxyhemoglobin dissociation curve.

2. The answer is D. Respiratory acidosis is defined by an arterial PCO_2 that is elevated above a normal acceptable range. Bicarbonate falls over time, and changes in neither arterial PO_2 nor blood lactate value would be indicative of a metabolic component.

▮ SUGGESTED READINGS

Baumann R, Bartels H, Bauer C: Blood oxygen transport. In Farhi LE, Tenney SM (eds). *Gas Exchange. Handbook of Physiology*. Sec 3. The Respiratory System. Bethesda: Amer Physiol Soc, 1987, Vol 4, pp 147–172.

Comroe JH: *Physiology of Respiration*, 2nd ed. Chicago: YearBook, 1974, pp 183–196.

Davenport HW: *The ABC of Acid-Base Chemistry*, 6th ed. Chicago: University of Chicago Press, 1974.

Klocke RA: Carbon Dioxide Transport. In Farhi LE, Tenney SM (eds). *Gas Exchange. Handbook of Physiology*. Sec 3. The Respiratory System. Bethesda: Amer Physiol Soc, 1987, Vol 4, pp 173–197.

Murray JF: *Normal Lung*, 2nd ed. Philadelphia: WB Saunders, 1986, pp 211–231, 183–210.

Nunn JF: *Applied Respiratory Physiology*, 3rd ed. London: Butterworth, 1987, pp 207–219, 256–270.

Rose BD: *Clinical Physiology of Acid-Base and Electrolyte Disorders*, 4th ed. New York: McGraw Hill, 1994.

West JB: Gas transport for the periphery. In *Respiratory Physiology: The Essentials*, 5th ed. Baltimore: Williams & Wilkins, 1995, pp 71–88.

VENTILATION-PERFUSION RELATIONSHIPS

Gilbert E. D'Alonzo, D.O.

■ SECTION OUTLINE

Learning Objectives

Introduction

Determination of Alveolar PO_2 and PCO_2

Alveolar-Arterial Oxygen Difference

Abnormal Gas Exchange

Assessing Lung Gas-Exchange Efficiency

Review Questions

■ LEARNING OBJECTIVES

At the completion of this section, the reader should:

- Understand the principal determinants of alveolar PO_2 and PCO_2 and appreciate the concept of ventilation-perfusion relationships in lung gas exchange.
- Be able to explain the various abnormal gas-exchange mechanisms responsible for the development of arterial hypoxemia.
- Be able to assess lung gas-exchange efficiency.

■ INTRODUCTION

The alveolar gas composition and the ability of the pulmonary capillary blood to reach equilibrium with the alveolar gases are the determinants of the arterial blood-gas composition. Arterial gas concentrations depend on the makeup of the inspired gas, the minute ventilation of the blood delivered to the lungs, and, most importantly, the manner in which ventilation and blood flow are portioned to each alveolus. Important additional determinants of the alveolar and thus the arterial blood-gas composition, especially in the diseased lung, are the partial pressures of oxygen and carbon dioxide in the blood that is returning to the heart and the lung—in other words, the mixed-venous blood.

■ DETERMINATION OF ALVEOLAR PO_2 AND PCO_2

One can measure the inspired concentration of oxygen and the barometric pressure and determine the PO_2 of the inspired air. Normally, the PO_2 of the inspired air is 150 mmHg and the PCO_2 is close to 0. Mixed-venous blood has a PO_2 of 40 mmHg and a PCO_2 of 45 mmHg. The alveolar PO_2 of 100 mmHg is determined by a balance between the inspired oxygen concentration during ventilation and how much is removed via diffusion by the capillary blood flow. The normal alveolar PCO_2 of 40 mmHg is established in the same manner (Figure 3.5-1).

Now let us assume that the ventilation-perfusion ratio of the unit is gradually increased by slowly obstructing and then completely stopping blood flow to that unit (see Figure 3.5-1). Because oxygen is not being pulled from the alveolus into the blood, the alveolar PO_2 rises and the PCO_2 gradually falls as ventilation washes carbon dioxide from the unit. When blood flow to this well-ventilated alveolus totally stops, the ventilation-perfusion ratio is infinity. This unit does not participate in gas exchange and actually becomes part of the dead space ventilation.

FIGURE 3.5-1

Three-compartment model for analysis of effects of differing ventilation-perfusion relationships on alveolar PO_2 (P_AO_2) and CO_2 (P_ACO_2). Assumptions include an inspired PO_2 of 150 mmHg, a mixed-venous PO_2 of 40 mmHg, and a PCO_2 of 45 mmHg. (A) $\dot{V}/\dot{Q}$ = 1.0. Ventilation and perfusion are perfectly matched. P_AO_2 is 100 mmHg and P_ACO_2 is 40 mmHg, as predicted by the alveolar gas equation. (B) $\dot{V}/\dot{Q}$ = 0. The unit is perfused but not ventilated. Alveolar gas tensions equal those of mixed-venous blood. (C) $\dot{V}/\dot{Q}$ = ∞. The unit is ventilated but not perfused. Alveolar gas tensions equal those of inspired gas.

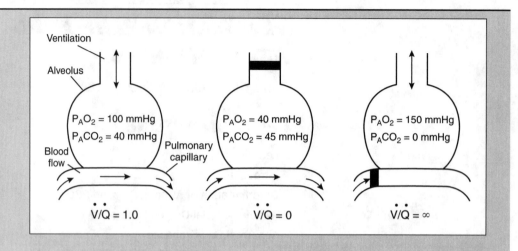

On the other hand, ventilation can be gradually and then completely stopped while alveolar blood flow continues. In this case the alveolar gas composition gradually becomes similar to that of the mixed-venous blood, and the alveolar blood flow relationship contributes to shunted blood flow. The ventilation-perfusion ratio is 0 (see Figure 3.5-1).

A convenient way of demonstrating these changes is to use the blood oxygen–carbon dioxide diagram (Figure 3.5-2). This diagram demonstrates the relationship between varying ventilation-perfusion relationships and their effects on alveolar PO_2 and PCO_2. With lower ventilation-perfusion relationships, there is little effect on the alveolar PCO_2 but a profound effect on the alveolar PO_2. On the other hand, there is a profound effect on the alveolar PCO_2 at ventilation-perfusion ratios greater than 1 but a modest effect on the alveolar PO_2.

FIGURE 3.5-2

Oxygen–carbon dioxide diagram showing a ventilation-perfusion ratio line. The PO_2 and PCO_2 of a lung unit move along this line from the mixed-venous point $\dot{v}$ to the inspired gas point *I* as the ventilation-perfusion ratio is increased. From West JB: *Ventilation/Blood Flow and Gas Exchange.* Oxford: Blackwell, 1977, p. 37.

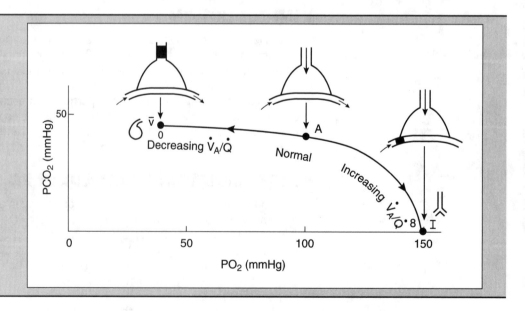

The normal lung does not have homogeneous ventilation-perfusion relationships. Ventilation increases slowly from the top to the bottom of the lung, and blood flow increases more rapidly (Figure 3.5-3). Because there is proportionately more ventilation than perfusion at the apices of the lung, the $\dot{V}/\dot{Q}$ ratios are higher. The opposite occurs at the base of the lung. Therefore, $\dot{V}/\dot{Q}$ ratios decrease from top to bottom (Figure 3.5-4). These differences in ventilation-perfusion ratio affect end-capillary PO_2 and PCO_2 in a profound way, as reflected by the changes in the oxygen and carbon dioxide contents of

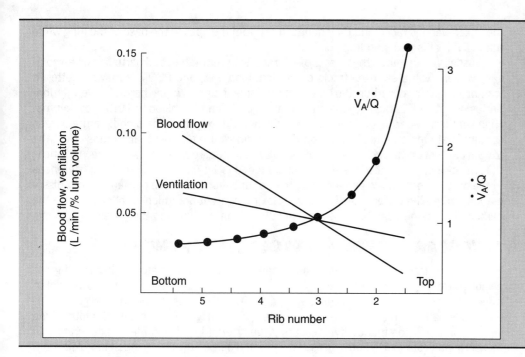

FIGURE 3.5-3
Regional variation of ventilation and perfusion and their relationship to one another ($\dot{V}_A/\dot{Q}$) from the apex to the base of the upright lung. Ventilation and perfusion are greater at the base, and $\dot{V}_A/\dot{Q}$ is lower at the base. From West JB: *Ventilation/ Blood Flow and Gas Exchange.* Oxford: Blackwell, 1977, p. 30.

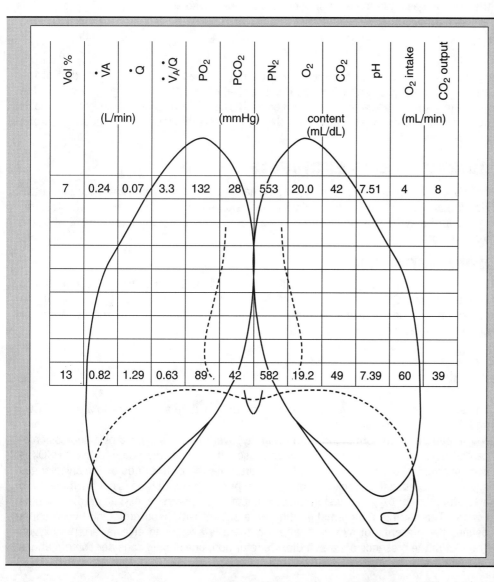

Vol %	$\dot{V}_A$	$\dot{Q}$	$\dot{V}_A/\dot{Q}$	PO_2	PCO_2	PN_2	O_2	CO_2	pH	O_2 intake	CO_2 output
	(L/min)			(mmHg)			content (mL/dL)			(mL/min)	
7	0.24	0.07	3.3	132	28	553	20.0	42	7.51	4	8
13	0.82	1.29	0.63	89	42	582	19.2	49	7.39	60	39

FIGURE 3.5-4
Apical-basal differences in multiple respiratory variables in the healthy, upright lung. The lung is conceptualized as multiple discrete levels from base to apex, each having a certain V_A/P. The V_A/P of each level determines its corresponding alveolar PO_2 and PCO_2, as well as the O_2 and CO_2 contents of blood leaving the level. For purposes of simplification, only values for the top and bottom levels are shown. From West JB: Ventilation-perfusion relationships. In West JB: *Respiratory Physiology: The Essentials,* 4th ed. Baltimore: Williams & Wilkins, 1990, pp. 61, 63.

the mixed-venous blood and the change in pH from the apex to the base of the lung while the individual is in a standing position.

Just as we examined the effects of alterations in ventilation and perfusion on alveolar gas, we can evaluate these effects on end-capillary PO_2 and PCO_2. It may be better to look at oxygen and carbon dioxide contents specifically. When there is a ventilation-perfusion ratio of 1, the oxygen content of the end-capillary blood is 19.5% by volume. High ventilation-perfusion ratios add relatively little oxygen to the blood, so the oxygen content is approximately 20% by volume, but low ventilation-perfusion ratios affect the oxygen content of the end-capillary blood to a greater degree. In fact, when the $\dot{V}/\dot{Q}$ ratio is 0.1, the oxygen content of the end-capillary blood is 14.6% by volume. The differences in the oxygen content are explained by the nonlinear shape of the oxyhemoglobin dissociation curve. The differences in carbon dioxide content are much smaller because the carbon dioxide–hemoglobin dissociation curve is almost linear in the physiologic range.

ALVEOLAR-ARTERIAL OXYGEN DIFFERENCE

The effectiveness of lung gas exchange can be better appreciated by measuring the alveolar-arterial oxygen difference. The carbon dioxide difference can also be determined. In the normal lung, in the standing position, the alveolar-arterial oxygen difference is small in magnitude—approximately 5 mmHg—as a result of global lung ventilation-perfusion inequality. Measuring the arterial PO_2 is simple and accurate, but measuring alveolar partial pressures of oxygen and carbon dioxide is much more difficult. For this reason, it is practical to estimate the mean alveolar gas concentrations by using the alveolar gas equation to approximate the mean alveolar PO_2:

$$P_AO_2 = P_IO_2 - P_ACO_2 (F_IO_2 + 1 - \frac{F_IO_2}{R}),$$

where P_IO_2 is the inspired gas PO_2, P_ACO_2 is the alveolar PCO_2 (close to that of the arterial PCO_2), F_IO_2 is the fractional concentration of inspired oxygen, and R is the respiratory exchange ratio, which is generally 0.8. The respiratory exchange ratio is determined by the current metabolic status, the oxygen consumption, and the carbon dioxide production.

ABNORMAL GAS EXCHANGE

The basic mechanisms of abnormal gas exchange in the lung are hypoventilation, diffusion impairment, shunt, and ventilation-perfusion inequality. The patient with respiratory failure may have abnormal gas exchange as a result of any one or more of these mechanisms.

HYPOVENTILATION

Hypoventilation is defined as a minute ventilation that is insufficient to maintain a normal arterial PCO_2 for a given level of tissue metabolism as defined by the production of carbon dioxide. Considering the lung as a single compartment, the equation for alveolar ventilation adequately describes this relationship:

$$P_ACO_2 = \frac{\dot{V}CO_2}{\dot{V}_A}.$$

> Any decrease in alveolar ventilation will result in an increase in alveolar PCO_2 and therefore in arterial PCO_2.

> A normal alveolar-arterial oxygen gradient in a patient with hypoxemia and hypercapnia defines hypoventilation.

Therefore, any decrease in alveolar ventilation will result in an increase in alveolar PCO_2 and therefore in arterial PCO_2.

In patients with normal lungs, in whom hypoventilation is caused by a depression of central nervous system function or neuromuscular disease, the rise in arterial PCO_2 is accompanied by a corresponding fall in the arterial PO_2 as described by the alveolar gas equation. Because the hypoxemia observed in pure hypoventilation is not attributable to an inefficiency of oxygen transfer, the calculated alveolar-arterial oxygen gradient will be normal. The finding of a normal gradient in a patient with hypoxemia and hypercapnia defines the presence of hypoventilation. If there is a widened alveolar-arterial oxygen gradient in the presence of carbon dioxide retention, one should consider complications such as pneumonia and pulmonary embolism. Other gas-exchange abnormalities can be responsible for the development of a high arterial PCO_2.

DIFFUSION IMPAIRMENT

Impaired diffusion, or the failure of the pulmonary end-capillary blood to equilibrate fully with the alveolar gas, is rarely a significant problem in clinical medicine. The pulmonary capillary blood reaches the alveolar gas tension in approximately one-third the time that it spends in the capillaries, thereby leaving a wide margin for changes in diffusibility before any abnormality would be expected to be seen. In fact, the diffusion capacity for the lung must fall below 20% of normal before any impact on arterial oxygenation occurs.

Theoretically, the gas-exchange system could be stressed sufficiently to permit an alveolar–end-capillary difference for oxygen if red blood cell transient time through the capillaries were markedly shortened, as observed during exercise, or if the driving pressure from the alveolus into the blood were reduced, such as in individuals living at high altitudes. However, even in these situations, the lung can increase its diffusion capacity sufficiently by recruiting additional pulmonary capillary blood volume or by inducing polycythemia to minimize any adverse effect on gas exchange. This would be an appropriate change or physiologically induced polycythemia.

Diffusion impairment may play a role in the hypoxemia observed in both emphysema and the adult respiratory distress syndrome. It may also be part of the gas-exchange abnormality found in patients with advanced lung fibrosis, especially during exertion. It is probably safe to conclude that diffusion impairment is unlikely to be a significant problem in patients with respiratory failure, especially because even small increases in the fractional concentration of the inspired oxygen would abolish any alveolar–end-capillary disequilibrium that might exist.

VENTILATION-PERFUSION INEQUALITY

Recent experimental data have enhanced our understanding of the role of ventilation-perfusion inequality as a mechanism of abnormal gas exchange in the lung. Increasing the mismatch of ventilation and blood flow affects both oxygen uptake and the elimination of carbon dioxide by the lungs.

The normal ventilation-perfusion ratio of a lung unit is nearly 1. If no ventilation is available to a lung unit that is being perfused, the ventilation-perfusion ratio is 0. If there is ventilation going to a lung unit but there is no perfusion, the ratio is infinity and represents physiologic dead space or an alveolus that does not participate in the exchange of oxygen or carbon dioxide. If there is perfusion but no ventilation going to the lung unit, physiologic shunt is indicated. Physiologic dead space and physiologic shunt are the two extremes that must be considered when looking at overall ventilation-perfusion relationships within the lung. In fact, there is the potential for a large number of lung units to have ventilation-perfusion ratios between 1 and 0 and between 1 and infinity. However, it is uncommon for lung units with high ventilation-perfusion relationships to have adverse effects on gas exchange. On the other hand, lung units with ratios of less than 1 often have profound effects on arterial PO_2 and some effects on arterial PCO_2.

A patient who has a large number of ventilation-perfusion lung units, which increases the physiologic dead space, can easily increase the minute ventilation and blow off more carbon dioxide from other lung units that are functioning in gas exchange, thereby compensating for any additional dead space. Hypercapnia develops only when the fraction of alveoli with high ventilation-perfusion ratios is so great that the increase in minute ventilation cannot be sustained. This happens in only very advanced lung disease. Because the carbon dioxide–hemoglobin dissociation curve is linear within its physiologic range, compensatory change occurs with ease.

Although increasing ventilation with ventilation-perfusion inequality is usually effective at reducing the arterial PCO_2, it is much less effective at improving hypoxemia. Again, this is attributable to the differences in the structure of the gas-hemoglobin dissociation curve. The almost flat portion of the oxyhemoglobin dissociation curve means that only units with moderately low ventilation-perfusion ratios benefit appreciably from increases in minute ventilation; units with high ventilation-perfusion ratios benefit very little. Units with very low ventilation-perfusion ratios continue to affect

Impaired diffusion is rarely a significant cause of hypoxemia in disease.

adversely the arterial PO_2 by mixing blood with an oxygen content close to that of mixed-venous blood with better-oxygenated blood coming from units with higher ventilation-perfusion ratios. The overall mixed arterial PO_2 then changes only mildly to moderately, and in some cases hypoxemia remains.

The effects of increasing ventilation-perfusion inequality on arterial PO_2 and PCO_2 can be seen in Figure 3.5-5. This figure represents the mathematical manipulation of a hypothetical lung model that has constant oxygen consumption, carbon dioxide production, hemoglobin concentration, and cardiac output. The solid lines demonstrate the effect of increasing ventilation-perfusion inequality while constraining minute ventilation. As expected, increasing the degree of ventilation-perfusion inequality influences the exchange of both oxygen and carbon dioxide, showing a fall in the arterial PO_2 and a progressive rise in arterial PCO_2. As noted in this example, the minute ventilation is fixed. Normally, when a patient is not ventilation limited or does not have an abnormal chemoresponsiveness to hypercarbia, the rise in arterial PCO_2 results in a progressive increase in minute ventilation in order to maintain a normal PCO_2. If we allow the minute ventilation to increase to a level that maintains the arterial PCO_2 at 40 mmHg, the effect of increasing ventilation-perfusion inequality is shown by the dashed lines. Increases in arterial PCO_2 are prevented by the minute ventilatory response, but this increase in minute ventilation only partially attenuates the fall in arterial PO_2. As mentioned previously, this results from the difference in the shape and position of the oxyhemoglobin and carbon dioxide–hemoglobin dissociation curves. Thus, ventilation-perfusion inequality, not counting the shunt and dead space components of the ventilation-perfusion relationship scheme, is a potent mechanism for both hypoxemia and hypercarbia. An increase in minute ventilation can minimize or completely eliminate hypercarbia, but hypoxemia is only partially affected. Ventilation-perfusion inequality is the major abnormality of gas exchange in patients with all forms of chronic obstructive and interstitial lung disease as well as a variety of other diseases that affect the lung either directly or indirectly.

> Ventilation-perfusion inequality is the major abnormality of gas exchange in patients with chronic lung diseases.

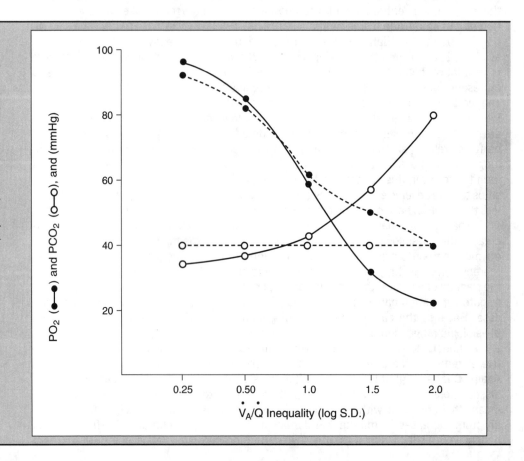

FIGURE 3.5-5
Effects of increasing ventilation-perfusion ($\dot{V}_A/\dot{Q}$) inequality on arterial PO_2 and PCO_2. The solid lines show the changes in gas tensions when cardiac output and minute ventilation are held constant. The changes in gas tensions when ventilation is allowed to increase to maintain arterial PCO_2 at 40 mmHg are shown by the dotted lines. From Dantzker DR: Gas exchange abnormalities. In Montenegro H, ed.: *Chronic Obstructive Pulmonary Disease*. New York: Churchill Livingstone, 1984.

The effect of an increase in the inspired oxygen concentration on the arterial PO_2 in patients with hypoxemia induced by ventilation-perfusion inequality is of major clinical importance. With minor degrees of inequality, there is a rapid rise in arterial PO_2 as the inspired oxygen concentration is increased (Figure 3.5-6). However, as ventilation-perfusion inequality worsens, the rate of increase of the arterial PO_2 decreases and actually becomes curvilinear. Patients with severe ventilation-perfusion inequality may be partially resistant to increasing F_IO_2 until a level of 50% or more is reached. When 100% oxygen is administered, ventilation-perfusion inequality is no longer an obstacle to oxygen exchange, as long as this high concentration of oxygen is breathed for a sufficient period of time to wash out all the nitrogen from those very-low-ventilation-perfusion lung units that are very slowly ventilated. If the patient has been breathing 100% oxygen for a long period of time and there remains an inappropriately low arterial PO_2, a significant amount of shunt must be present.

Figure 3.5-7 demonstrates the patterns of arterial PO_2 increase that occur as the inspired oxygen concentration is increased in lung units that have ventilation-perfusion ratios of less than 1. In this figure, a commonly used and clinically acceptable range of inspired oxygen concentration has been chosen, and, from the line for the lung as a whole as it relates to each of the ventilation-perfusion relationships of that lung, it can be seen that an increase in arterial PO_2 from 52 mmHg while breathing room air to as high as 90 mmHg occurred with only a minor increase in F_IO_2 to 35%. Therefore, if one analyzes the effect of increasing the inspired F_IO_2 on individual lung units found in this patient with severe chronic obstructive lung disease, it can be seen that it varies widely depending on the $\dot{V}/\dot{Q}$ relationship that is being studied. In those lung units in which the ratio is higher, the end-capillary PO_2 leaving that unit is adequate, but at the same time there are still areas of lung with lower ratios where the end-capillary PO_2 is still seriously low. However, in those alveoli that are favorably affected by the higher concentrations of oxygen, the end-capillary PO_2 improves, whereas, in the other units in which the alveolar PO_2 remains low because of severe ventilation-perfusion inequality, the end-capillary PO_2 remains low and the vascular bed is under the influence of hypoxic vasoconstriction. This may have important ramifications for the ability of low-flow oxygen therapy, which generally delivers lower inspired oxygen concentrations, to prevent the development of cor pulmonale, because hypoxic vasoconstriction will not be reversed in the areas of lung with persistent alveolar hypoxia.

SHUNT

Right-to-left shunt of blood in the lung is a major gas-exchange abnormality of cardiogenic and noncardiogenic pulmonary edema, severe pneumonia, and advanced inflammatory lung disease, generally with lung fibrosis. Shunt has also been recognized in the abnormal gas exchange following pulmonary embolism, cardiac bypass surgery, and acute exacerbations of chronic obstructive lung disease. However, for many of these diseases, severe ventilation-perfusion inequality remains the principal cause of the very low arterial PO_2.

The physiologic effect of shunt on gas exchange is different from that of ventilation-perfusion inequality. If there is no ventilation-perfusion inequality present, the effect of increasing shunt in the lung and maintenance of minute ventilation and cardiac output at a constant level can be seen in Figure 3.5-8. The most striking feature is the precipitous fall in the arterial PO_2 with only a small increase in arterial PCO_2 as the percentage of shunt increases to a very high level. The arterial PCO_2 in the diseased patient often does not increase because the minute ventilation increases with the fall in the arterial PO_2. This increase in minute ventilation prevents hypercarbia from developing. In fact, just the opposite generally occurs—that is, the arterial PCO_2 decreases with the increase in minute ventilation. As in severe ventilation-perfusion inequality, an increase in ventilation is unable to alter substantially the hypoxemia that develops. It is unusual for a shunt fraction of more than 50% to 60% to be found in even advanced lung disease.

When oxygen is administered to patients with shunting, it is difficult to increase the arterial PO_2. This makes sense, because the etiology of the hypoxemia in patients with shunting is the admixture of mixed-venous blood that totally bypasses alveoli that are ventilated and directly admixes with arterialized blood. Figure 3.5-9 shows the effect of

FIGURE 3.5-6

V̇/Q̇ and arterial oxygenation. (A) Effects of increasing and decreasing V̇/Q̇ and P_aO_2 as inspired O_2 concentration is increased. A high F_IO_2 is necessary to raise P_aO_2 in regions with low V̇/Q̇. (B) Effects of increasing and decreasing V̇/Q̇ on end-capillary O_2 content as inspired O_2 concentration is increased. For alveoli with very low V̇/Q̇ (e.g., 0.001), F_IO_2 must be increased markedly to raise end-capillary O_2 content. A 10-fold increase in V̇/Q̇ only minimally increases end-capillary O_2 content; however, the presence of low V̇/Q̇ regions results in profound lowering of end-capillary O_2 content. Hence, the presence of alveoli with high V̇/Q̇ cannot compensate for hypoxemia resulting from alveoli with low V̇/Q̇. From West JB: State of the art: ventilation-perfusion relationships. *Am Rev Resp Dis* 116:919–943, 1977.

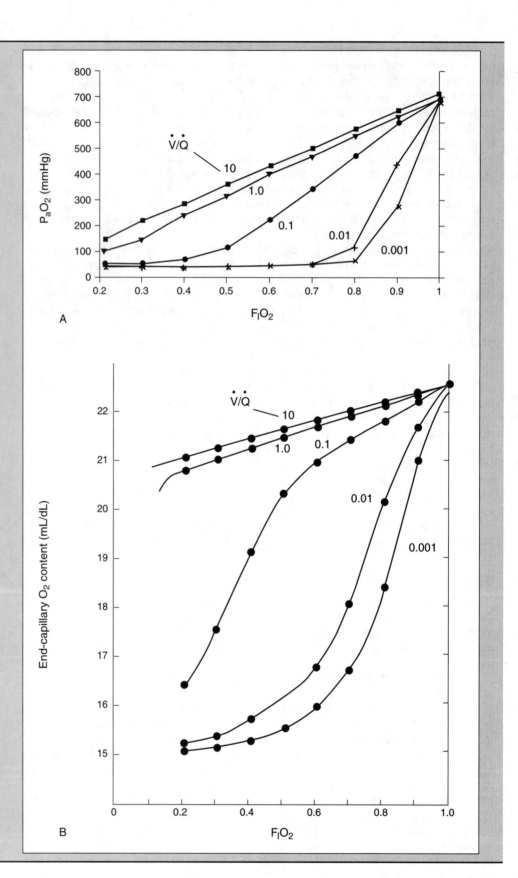

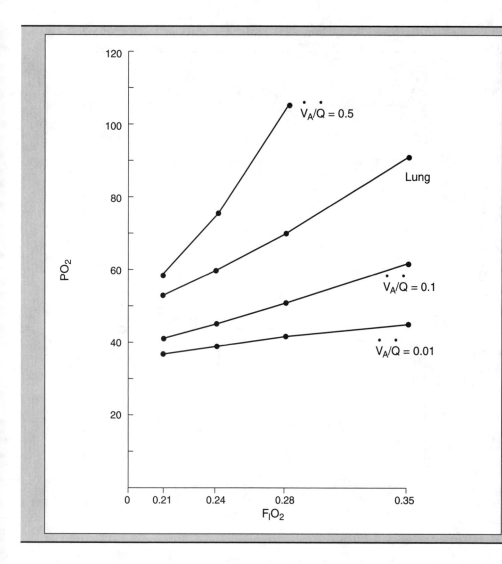

FIGURE 3.5-7
Effects of increasing the inspired oxygen fraction (F_IO_2) on the arterial PO_2 of a patient (lung) with severe $\dot{V}_A/\dot{Q}$ inequality and on the end-capillary blood of individual lung units with varying $\dot{V}_A/\dot{Q}$ ratios. Overall arterial PO_2 promptly rose, but the end-capillary PO_2 from very low $\dot{V}_A/\dot{Q}$ lung units improved only slightly. From Dantzker DR: Gas exchange abnormalities. *In* Montenegro H, ed.: *Chronic Obstructive Pulmonary Disease.* New York: Churchill Livingstone, 1984.

changing the F_IO_2 on the arterial PO_2 and oxygen content in lungs that have shunts ranging from 10% to 50%. At low levels of shunt there is a relatively brisk rise in arterial PO_2 as the F_IO_2 is increased, but as the degree of shunt increases, the change that occurs with increasing F_IO_2 decreases. With small shunts, an increase in inspired oxygen concentration elevates the arterial PO_2 owing to the ability of the higher inspired oxygen concentration to increase alveolar oxygen concentration in areas of the lung where the blood is exposed to those alveoli. As more shunt units develop and less blood is exposed to ventilated alveoli, the effect of increasing the oxygen concentration of the inspired gas becomes less effective. It is clinically relevant to understand that with this severe development of hypoxemia in high shunt states, even small increases in the arterial PO_2 can significantly increase arterial oxygen content and eventually peripheral tissue oxygen delivery, because the change that occurs is along the rapidly increasing portion of the oxyhemoglobin dissociation curve.

NONPULMONARY FACTORS

Nonpulmonary factors may profoundly affect gas exchange, especially in the presence of abnormal lung function. Alterations in the mixed-venous PO_2 may play a role in the eventual arterial PO_2. If one examines the Fick equation, there is a complex relationship that determines the amount of oxygen in the blood returning to the lungs, the mixed-venous oxygen content ($C_{\bar{v}}O_2$):

$$\dot{V}O_2 = CO \times (C_aO_2 - C_{\bar{v}}O_2).$$

FIGURE 3.5-8
Effect of increasing shunt on the arterial PO_2 and PCO_2. From Dantzker DR: Gas exchange abnormalities. In Montenegro H, ed.: *Chronic Obstructive Pulmonary Disease*. New York: Churchill Livingstone, 1984.

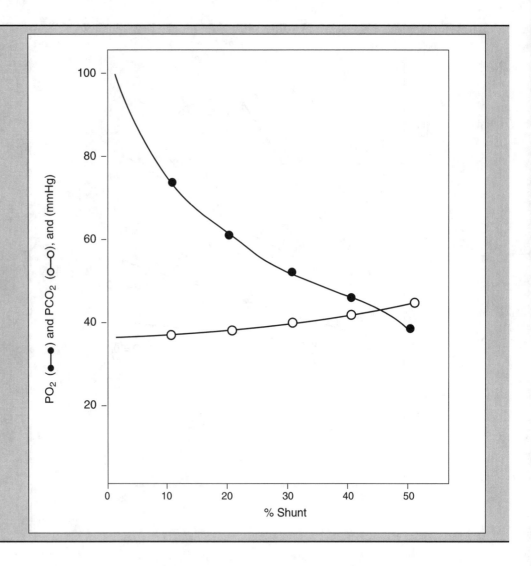

For any lung unit, the end-capillary PO_2 is influenced by the mixed-venous PO_2.

Abnormalities of all these factors—the arterial oxygen content (C_aO_2), oxygen consumption ($\dot{V}O_2$), and cardiac output (CO)—are often found to be present in critically ill patients. The oxygen consumption, a measure of tissue metabolism, is increased in many conditions, including fever, sepsis, burns, trauma, heart failure, and the postoperative state. Cardiac output, an extremely variable factor in critically ill patients, can be severely affected by the underlying disorder or by the therapeutics used in treatment, such as mechanical ventilation, especially when positive end-expiratory pressure is used. Arterial oxygen content varies with changes in the arterial PO_2, oxygen saturation, and hemoglobin concentration. Finally, oxygen saturation can be influenced by the position of the oxyhemoglobin dissociation curve.

For any lung unit, the end-capillary PO_2 is markedly influenced by the mixed-venous PO_2. In the case of shunt, any change in mixed-venous PO_2 affects the arterial PO_2 by direct mixing. For lung units that are ventilated, the magnitude of the effect is greatest for lung units with $\dot{V}/\dot{Q}$ ratios of less than 1, and the influence decreases as this ratio increases above 1. Figure 3.5-10 demonstrates the theoretical effects that an alteration in mixed-venous PO_2 may have on the arterial PO_2 in three settings: a normal lung, a lung with marked ventilation-perfusion inequality, and a lung with a large intrapulmonary shunt. Although many assumptions have been made in relation to these calculations, this figure allows us to visualize the influence that a change in mixed-venous PO_2 might have on the arterial PO_2 in the absence of other alterations. It emphasizes that when the arterial PO_2 in a patient with respiratory failure deteriorates, factors in addition to those directly referable to the underlying lung disease must be considered as possible etiologies of the increased hypoxemia. Furthermore, the degree to which an alteration in any of these nonpulmonary variables will affect gas exchange depends on the ability of the patient to respond by compensatory measures. An increase in oxygen consumption can be offset by an increase in cardiac output, and the effects of a fall in arterial PO_2 can be gradually compensated for by an increase in the hemoglobin concentration of the blood. But it is important to note that patients who are critically ill often lack compensatory reserve.

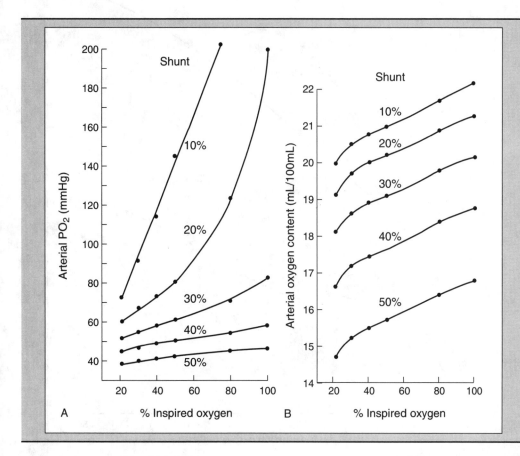

FIGURE 3.5-9
Relationship between inspired oxygen concentration and arterial PO_2. (A) O_2 content. (B) For lungs with various degrees of shunt. From Dantzker DR: Gas exchange in the adult respiratory distress syndrome. *Clin Chest Med* 3:57–67, 1982.

■ ASSESSING LUNG GAS-EXCHANGE EFFICIENCY

Arterial blood gases are the simplest measurements to obtain, but while important in the clinical management of patients, they are relatively insensitive to changes in overall gas-exchange efficiency. The arterial blood gases are influenced by changes in overall minute ventilation and by a variety of nonpulmonary factors that alter the mixed-venous PO_2 and PCO_2. Furthermore, when patients are breathing higher concentrations of inspired oxygen, arterial blood-gas measurement becomes an even more difficult tool to use. In patients with normal lungs or with small shunts or minor degrees of ventilation-perfusion inequality, there is a rapid, almost linear rise in the arterial PO_2 as the F_IO_2 is increased. As the shunt or ventilation-perfusion inequality increases, the response becomes more complex. For example, as the degree of ventilation-perfusion inequality increases, the initial rate of increase of the arterial PO_2 as the F_IO_2 is raised decreases, and the response over the whole range becomes curvilinear (see Figure 3.5-6). A similar but less complex response occurs when shunt is the abnormality.

The alveolar-arterial oxygen gradient is another parameter that is used to assess gas-exchange efficiency. The ideal alveolar PO_2 can be adequately calculated from a simplification of the alveolar gas equation

$$P_AO_2 = P_IO_2 - \frac{P_ACO_2}{R},$$

FIGURE 3.5-10
Effects of changing the mixed-venous PO_2 on the arterial PO_2 in a theoretical lung without $\dot{V}_A/\dot{Q}$ inequality (solid line), with serious $\dot{V}_A/\dot{Q}$ inequality (—), and with a 30% shunt (---). The cardiac output and minute ventilation have been held constant, and the mixed-venous PO_2 has been allowed to fall by increasing the oxygen consumption. From Dantzker DR: Influence of cardiovascular function on gas exchange. *Clin Chest Med* 4: 149–159, 1983.

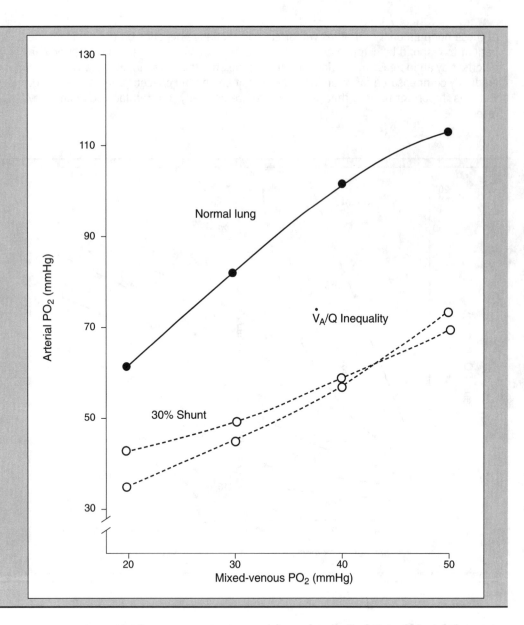

where P_IO_2 is the inspired PO_2 and R is the respiratory exchange ratio. If the lung were perfectly homogeneous, there should be no difference between the calculated alveolar PO_2 and the measured arterial PO_2. Any factor making gas exchange less efficient will lead to a widening of the alveolar-arterial oxygen gradient. This gradient is an index of abnormal gas exchange and has an advantage over routine blood gases in that it is less sensitive to changes in the level of overall ventilation. It does suffer, however, from many of the same problems that are associated with the arterial blood gas, because increasing shunt or ventilation-perfusion inequality leads to a widening of this gradient, but so do changes in the mixed-venous PO_2 by virtue of its tendency to alter the arterial PO_2. Furthermore, changes in the inspired oxygen concentration alter the measured alveolar-to-arterial oxygen gradient in the absence of any changes in the severity of lung disease.

When shunt is the major abnormality, the alveolar-arterial oxygen gradient increases progressively as the inspired concentration of oxygen is increased toward 100%. In patients with ventilation-perfusion inequality, the change in the gradient as the inspired oxygen concentration increases is more complex. In fact, the change is curvilinear, initially increasing and then decreasing as the oxygen concentration that is being inspired is altered (Figure 3.5-11). If this parameter is to be used to follow a patient's

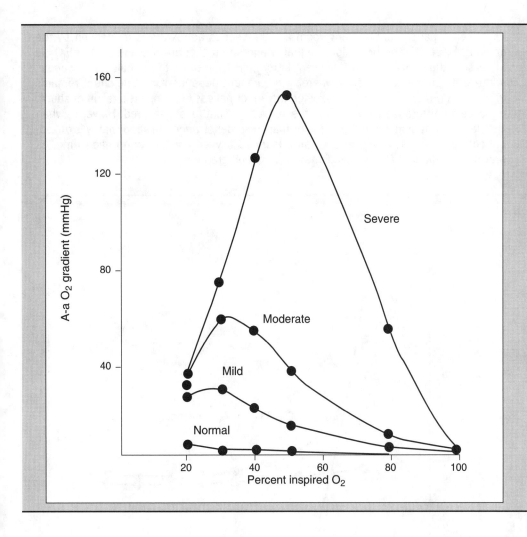

FIGURE 3.5-11
Effects of increasing the percent of inspired oxygen on the
calculated alveolar-arterial gradient for oxygen (A-a O_2) in a
normal lung and in lungs with
mild, moderate, and severe
ventilation-perfusion inequality.
From D'Alonzo GE, Dantzker
DR: Respiratory failure, mechanisms of abnormal gas ex-
change, and oxygen delivery.
Med Clin NA 67:557–571,
1983.

clinical course, the measurement of the alveolar-arterial oxygen gradient must be done at the same inspired oxygen concentration each time.

Another measurement used in clinical practice to assess gas-exchange efficiency is the calculation of the venous admixture ($\dot{Q}_S/\dot{Q}_T$). For the purpose of modeling, this measurement assumes that the lung is composed of two compartments, one that is ventilated and perfused and another that is perfused but not ventilated. Any decrease in the arterial oxygen content is thought to result from the admixture of blood from the unventilated or poorly ventilated compartment. The amount of oxygen in the arterial blood is thus the sum of the oxygen coming from the perfused but nonventilated compart-ment and that coming from the perfused and ventilated compartment. This concept allows for the development of an equation:

$$\dot{Q}_S/\dot{Q}_T = \frac{C_cO_2 - C_aO_2}{C_cO_2 - C_{\bar{v}}O_2}.$$

The arterial oxygen content (C_aO_2) and the mixed-venous oxygen content (C_VO_2) can be calculated from the measured partial pressure and saturation of the arterial and mixed-venous blood. The calculation of the end-capillary oxygen content poses certain problems. Because the blood coming from this compartment is assumed to have the PO_2 of the ideal alveolar value, the end-capillary PO_2 equals the alveolar PO_2 and can be calculated from the alveolar gas equation. If the alveolar PO_2 is greater than 150 mmHg, the saturation of this blood can be assumed to be 100%. If it is less than 150 mmHg, the saturation must be calculated from one of many standard algorithms* for the dissociation curve.

---

* Kelman GR: *J Appl Physiol* 21:1375, 1966.

When a patient is breathing room air, the venous admixture is influenced by the amounts of ventilation-perfusion inequality and shunt that are present. As the F_IO_2 is increased, the contribution of low ventilation-perfusion units to the calculated venous admixture appears to decrease whereas the amount dependent on true shunt remains unchanged (Figure 3.5-12). Thus, when the abnormal gas exchange is a result of shunt, it makes no difference on what F_IO_2 the venous admixture is measured. However, when ventilation-perfusion inequality is the primary disorder or when the abnormality is mixed, patients must be assessed at the same inspired oxygen concentration each time, as previously indicated for the alveolar-arterial oxygen gradient.

FIGURE 3.5-12
Effects of changing the percent of inspired oxygen on the calculated venous admixtures for three clinical situations. From D'Alonzo GE, Dantzker DR: Respiratory failure, mechanisms of abnormal gas exchange, and oxygen delivery. *Med Clin NA* 67:557–571, 1983.

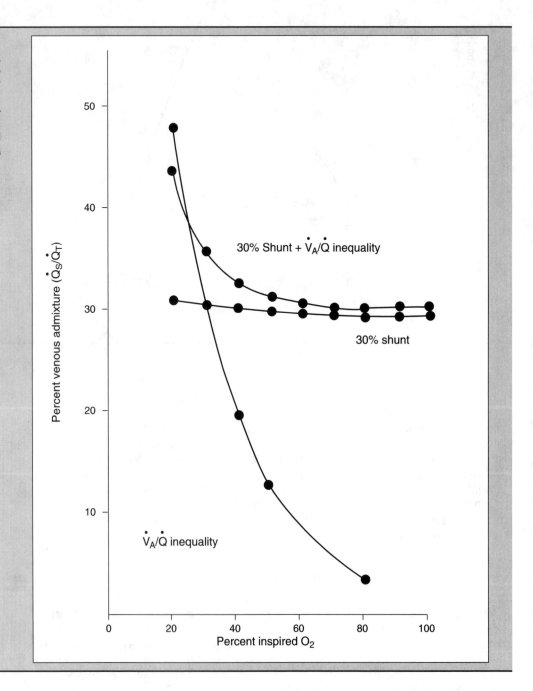

▮ REVIEW QUESTIONS

1. Supplemental oxygen will not correct hypoxemia caused by which of the following?

   (A) Hypoventilation
   (B) Ventilation-perfusion mismatching
   (C) Right-to-left shunting
   (D) Diffusion impairment
   (E) Loss of capillary volume

2. Oxygen delivery to peripheral tissues is least dependent on which of the following?

   (A) Cardiac output
   (B) Arterial oxygen content
   (C) Hemoglobin concentration
   (D) Oxygen bound to hemoglobin
   (E) Oxygen dissolved in plasma

3. A patient's entire left lung is consolidated (unventilated) as a result of a pneumonia process. The arterial PO_2 is 65 mmHg and the arterial PCO_2 is 24 mmHg while the patient is breathing 100% oxygen. The alveolar-arterial oxygen gradient is

   (A) 710
   (B) 689
   (C) 618
   (D) 504

4. Which one of the following does not determine the alveolar PCO_2?

   (A) Carbon dioxide produced by tissues
   (B) Respiratory portion
   (C) Inhaled carbon dioxide concentration
   (D) Alveolar PO_2
   (E) Alveolar ventilation

5. "Pure" alveolar hypoventilation as a cause of hypoxemia, as observed in patients with acute drug overdose and normal lungs, is characterized by

   (A) an increase in the alveolar-arterial oxygen gradient
   (B) a normal A-a DO_2
   (C) a reduced arterial PCO_2
   (D) increased airway secretions
   (E) a reduced alveolar PCO_2

■ ANSWERS AND EXPLANATIONS

1. The answer is C. In order to improve arterial oxygenation with supplemental oxygen, the alveolar concentration of oxygen must increase. Because there is no alveolar ventilation associated with lung units that are participating in right-to-left shunting, supplemental oxygen does not affect the end-capillary oxygen tension.

2. The answer is E. A minor portion of the oxygen delivery scheme is the small amount of oxygen that dissolves in blood plasma ($0.0031 \times$ arterial PO_2).

3. The answer is C. The alveolar PO_2 is determined by subtracting water vapor pressure (47 mmHg) from barometric pressure (760 mmHg), multiplying the result by the inspired oxygen concentration as a ratio, and then subtracting the arterial PCO_2 (as a surrogate value for alveolar PCO_2) after it has been divided by the respiratory exchange ratio, which is generally 0.8.

$$P_AO_2 = (P_B - P_{WV})(F_IO_2) - \frac{P_aCO_2}{0.8}$$

$$= (760 - 47)(1.0) - \frac{24}{0.8}$$

$$= 683$$

Finally, the arterial PO_2 is subtracted from the alveolar PO_2.

$$P_AO_2 - P_aO_2 = \text{A-a } DO_2$$

$$683 - 65 = 618$$

The high A-a DO_2 is a reflection of a serious gas-exchange problem and, in this case, of the presence of a large shunt fraction because the patient's arterial PO_2 did not respond to the 100% oxygen that was administered.

4. The answer is C. The concentration of carbon dioxide in the inspired air is already zero, and therefore it cannot participate as a determinant of alveolar PCO_2.

5. The answer is B. Alveolar hypoventilation results in an increase in alveolar PCO_2 and hence in arterial PCO_2. The rise in the arterial PCO_2 is accompanied by a corresponding fall in arterial PCO_2 as described by the alveolar gas equation. Because this hypoxemia is not attributable to an influence of oxygen transfer, the calculated A_aDO_2 will be normal.

■ SUGGESTED READINGS

Comroe JH: *Physiology of Respiration*, 2nd ed. Chicago, YearBook, 1974, pp 168–182.

D'Alonzo GE, Dantzker DR: Respiratory failure, mechanisms of abnormal gas exchange and oxygen delivery. *Med Clin NA* 67:557–571, 1983.

Dantzker DR: Gas exchange abnormalities. In: Montenegro H (ed). *Chronic Obstructive Pulmonary Disease*, New York: Churchill Livingstone, 1984.

Dantzker DR: The influence of cardiovascular function on gas exchange. *Clinics Chest Med* 4:149–159, 1984.

Farhi LE: Ventilation-Perfusion Relationships. In: Farhi LE, Tenney SM (eds). Gas exchange. Handbook of Physiology, Sec 3. The respiratory system. Bethesda: *Amer Physiol Soc* 1987, Vol 4, pp 199–215.

West JB: *Ventilation/Blood Flow and Gas Exchange*, 5th ed. Oxford: Blackwell 1990, pp 29–49, 80–109.

West JB: *Respiratory Physiology—The Essentials*, 5th ed. Baltimore: Williams & Wilkins 1995, pp 51–69.

West JB: State of the Art: Ventilation-Perfusion Relationships. *Am Rev Respir Dis* 116:919–943, 1977.

NORMAL EXERCISE PHYSIOLOGY

Bernard Borbely, M.D.

Gilbert E. D'Alonzo, D.O.

■ SECTION OUTLINE

Learning Objectives

Energetics

Gas Exchange

Circulation

Effect of Aerobic Training in Healthy Subjects

Review Questions

■ LEARNING OBJECTIVES

At the completion of this section, the reader should:
- Be able to explain how body energy sources are recruited during progressive exercise.
- Understand the interrelationship between ventilation and circulation that allows for a necessary coordinated physiological response during exercise.
- Be able to explain how training affects muscles and the cardiopulmonary system, allowing for more prolonged and higher-intensity exercise to occur.

■ ENERGETICS

Skeletal muscles comprise approximately 45% of the lean body weight and are responsible, in the resting state, for nearly 40% of overall body basal oxygen consumption. During exercise, skeletal muscle metabolism may be responsible for 95% of the total oxygen consumption.

Skeletal muscle uses three energy pools depending on the type of activity being performed (Figure 3.6-1). Adenosine triphosphate (ATP) is stored within the muscle to meet immediate energy demands, but this source is rapidly depleted shortly after the initiation of exercise. Regeneration of ATP allows exercise to continue until anaerobic glycolysis is activated. Continued exercise depends on oxidative phosphorylation. Substrates available for oxidation include carbohydrates and fatty acids. ATP is produced by the intracellular mitochondria and requires oxygen (aerobic exercise) to form intracellular water and carbon dioxide, which is eliminated by the cell.

Circulatory and respiratory mechanisms during exercise have a limited capacity. At higher levels of exercise, as the demand for oxygen outstrips its supply, muscles begin to use local oxygen stores in myoglobin, stores of phosphoryl creatine, and anaerobic glycolysis. These local energy resources can support muscular activity for brief periods of time during progressive exertion. Failure to keep up with ATP requirements creates muscle exhaustion and loss of power output.

Anaerobic glycolysis leads to lactate production. Lactic acid is the end product of this anaerobic metabolism—an acid that must be buffered by bicarbonate. This buffering process produces an excess of hydrogen ions and carbon dioxide that must eventually be removed from the cell. Anaerobic metabolism produces only a small fraction of the ATP that is produced during aerobic carbohydrate-driven metabolism. Accumulation of

FIGURE 3.6-1

Energy sources for muscle as a function of duration of activity. Skeletal muscle has three energy systems. In power events with durations of a few seconds, immediate energy courses are utilized. For rapid, forceful exercises lasting from several seconds to approximately 1 minute, both immediate and nonoxidative energy sources are employed. For activities lasting for more than 1 minute, oxidative mechanisms become increasingly necessary.

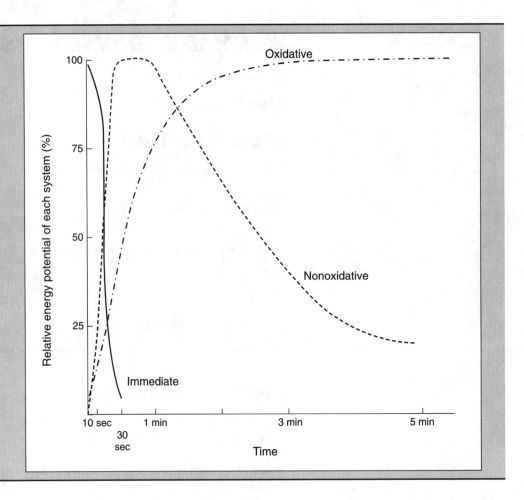

lactate is dependent on the amount produced and its metabolism by the liver. High muscle lactate concentrations are directly related to exhaustion, but there are probably other mechanisms. The way in which the body uses different fuels in aerobic exercise can be evaluated by measuring the respiratory quotient (R). This quotient is determined by looking at the ratio of the carbon dioxide that is produced to the amount of oxygen that is being utilized. For carbohydrates, R equals 1, but for free fatty acids it falls to 0.7. For the body as a whole, at lower levels of work, R equals 0.85, indicating the metabolism of both carbohydrate and fat. During prolonged exercise in the fasting state the R value remains low, but following a meal the R value increases because the continuous availability of carbohydrate inhibits adipose tissue glycolysis. The major carbohydrate fuel is glycogen, which is stored in muscle.

Muscle glycogen concentration is closely related to endurance at high levels of exercise. Furthermore, the amount of glucose released by the liver increases during exercise and is matched by the muscle uptake, with little change in blood glucose concentration. Metabolic needs during exercise are supplied in part by glucose, but the main energy source is muscle glycogen. Following exercise, the depleted muscle glycogen is replenished, but this process can be slow after prolonged high-level exertion.

Fatty acids—mainly triglycerides from adipose tissue and muscle—can be used as an energy source during exercise. Free fatty acids are liberated by the hydrolysis of triglycerides and are transported in a bound form with plasma albumin. The muscles pick up these fatty acids and use them as a fuel source during exercise. The mobilization of fatty acids is part of a complex hormonally controlled process involving catecholamines and insulin.

Amino acids and keto acids can be used as fuel sources by exercising muscle, but their contributions are small. The ability of muscle to use a variety of fuels gives it a flexibility in maintaining energy supply during a wide variety of situations. During low-to-moderate levels of exercise of long duration, the energy supply process is maintained by oxidation of carbohydrates and free fatty acids. In immediate heavy exercise, such as weightlifting, muscle glycogen is mainly used. For short-duration, high-intensity exercise such as dashes, anaerobic glycolysis is important, but if the exertion continues at a lower level, aerobic glycolysis follows. If exercise is prolonged, free fatty acids are used to an ever-increasing degree (Table 3.6-1).

| TYPE OF ACTIVITY | ENERGY SOURCE | EVENT | | **Table 3.6-1** |
		ATHLETIC	DAILY LIFE	Energy Pools Used During Various Types of Activity
Power	Immediate	Shot put	Lift child	
Speed	Nonoxidative	100-yard-dash	Run for bus	
Endurance	Oxidative	Marathon	Deliver mail	

■ GAS EXCHANGE

An essential substrate for ATP production during aerobic metabolism is oxygen, and the source of oxygen is ambient air. Oxygen must be extracted from the air by the lungs, transported to peripheral tissues through the blood stream, and transferred to the intracellar mitochondria for energy production. The entire process is completed by virtue of the availability of an oxygen molecule, which combines with a hydrogen ion to form water at the end of the electron transport chain, where hydrogen ions are shuttled and ATP is produced.

In order to meet the demand for oxygen during exercise, ventilation is regulated. As exercise becomes more strenuous, the oxygen demand increases and minute ventilation must increase. Initially, minute ventilation is increased to a greater extent by larger tidal volumes. Respiratory rate increases, but it is not until later in exercise, when minute ventilation is high and the tidal volume has been maximized, that the breathing process becomes more dependent on respiratory rate (Figure 3.6-2). Overall, minute ventilation increases in a linear fashion through low and moderate levels of exercise, but at higher levels the rate of increase, or slope, of minute ventilation changes (Figure 3.6-3). This change in minute ventilation is a compensatory response to the metabolic acidosis that is occurring, with higher blood lactate levels developing. The point at which the slope in minute ventilation changes is termed the "anaerobic threshold." At that point, the arterial PCO_2, which has remained constant during low and moderate levels of exercise, actually starts to fall and continues to fall at higher levels of exercise as a result of the compensatory hyperventilation (with a dilutional fall in end-expiratory PCO_2) that is occurring in response to the metabolic acidosis that is developing (see Figure 3.6-3).

The important component of the minute ventilation that increases during exercise is the alveolar ventilation. During exercise, anatomic dead space actually increases in proportion to the tidal volume increase, secondary to distention of the large airways that occurs with deep breathing. On the other hand, the ratio of dead space to tidal volume (V_D/V_T) decreases, representing a reduction in wasted ventilation, which is a reflection of more efficient breathing. The resting V_D/V_T ratio of approximately 30% falls to as low as 10% at high levels of exercise (Figure 3.6-4).

As increasing levels of oxygen are transported to the peripheral tissues and ventilation and cardiac output increase, the alveolar and arterial partial pressures of oxygen remain nearly constant. The normal resting alveolar-arterial PO_2 difference (A-a DO_2) is 8 to 12 mmHg. However, there is a slight decrease in this gradient during exercise secondary to more uniformly distributed pulmonary blood flow and a reduction in the small amount of ventilation-perfusion inequality that occurs in a normal subject at rest. At very high levels of exercise, however, A-a DO_2 increases slightly, but the reason for this remains poorly understood. Like the A-a DO_2, the alveolar-arterial PCO_2 difference changes from rest to exercise. At rest, arterial PCO_2 is higher than alveolar PCO_2. With the improvement in ventilation-perfusion matching that occurs during exercise, this difference is minimized.

During high levels of exercise, the minute ventilation increases in a more rapid fashion to compensate for the developing metabolic acidosis and maintain exercise.

FIGURE 3.6-2
Tidal volume (V_T) and respiratory rate (F_B) increase differently during exercise, and minute ventilation increases.

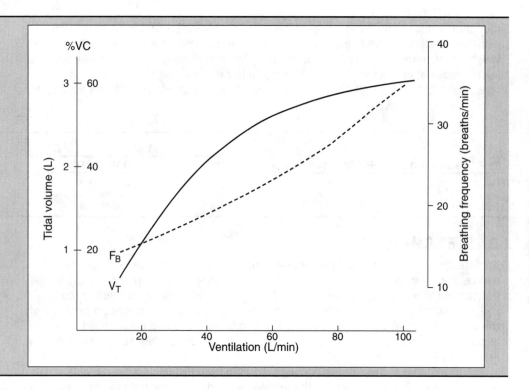

FIGURE 3.6-3
The ventilatory responses (both minute V_E and alveolar ventilation V_A) before and after the anaerobic threshold (AT), with corresponding changes in the arterial PCO_2 (P_aCO_2) and end-expiratory PCO_2 (P_ECO_2).

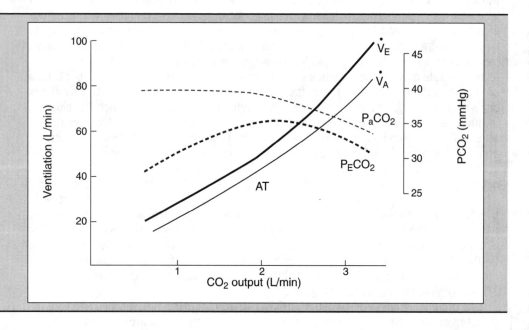

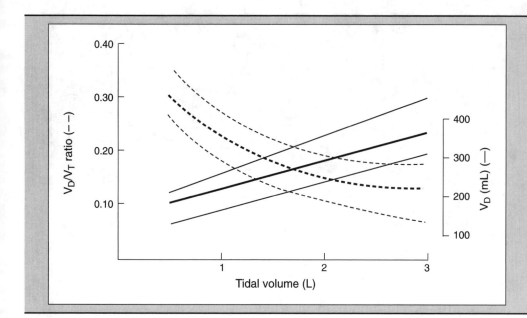

CIRCULATION

Systemic oxygen transport is dependent on blood flow and the oxygen content of the arterial blood. The cardiac output determines the total body blood flow to peripheral tissues. During exercise, oxygen transport is increased mainly through an increase in cardiac output. The relationship between cardiac output and oxygen consumption is linear, until a plateau point known as the aerobic capacity or maximum oxygen consumption (Figure 3.6-5) is reached. The cardiac output is dependent on the heart's stroke volume and rate. Early in exercise, stroke volume increases at a higher rate than the change in heart rate, but at higher levels of exercise, the change in cardiac output becomes more dependent on the linear increase in heart rate (Figure 3.6-6). The maximal heart rate achievable during exercise depends on the patient's age and cardiac status (Figure 3.6-7).

With progressive heart exercise, heart rate increases to the predicted maximum, and at that heart rate, exercise cannot be maintained. Normally, exercise is limited by cardiovascular factors, not ventilatory factors.

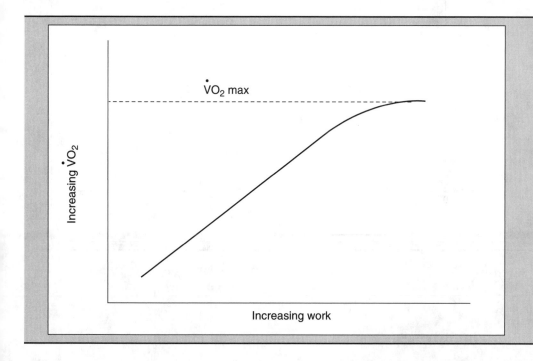

FIGURE 3.6-6

As exercise increases in intensity, O_2 consumption increases and both heart rate (f_c) and stroke volume (V_s) rise. The initial increase in cardiac output is more dependent on V_s, but as a higher cardiac output is needed, the change in f_c predominates. The thick lines represent the effect of training on cardiac performance.

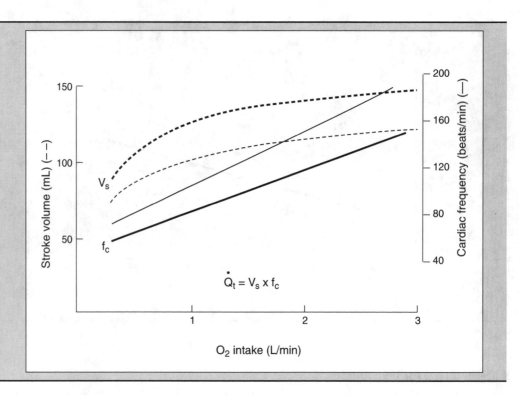

$$\dot{Q}_t = V_s \times f_c$$

FIGURE 3.6-7

Maximum heart rate (f_c) is achievable in a healthy adult during exercise.

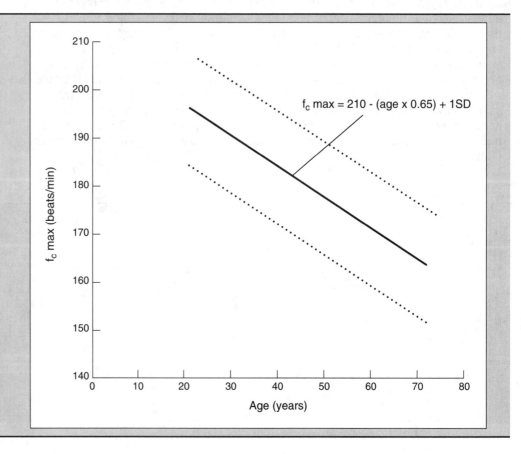

f_c max = 210 - (age x 0.65) + 1SD

During exercise, myocardial contractility increases. Factors that affect contractility during exercise include the increase in heart rate, sympathetic neurologic influences, and the precontractile muscle fiber length of the heart.

At aerobic capacity, maximal cardiac performance is found. That is, the maximum predicted heart rate is achieved and there is no further cardiac reserve. On the other hand, at maximum exercise, there is generally a substantial degree of respiratory reserve. Exercise is not limited by ventilatory factors but by cardiovascular factors in the healthy subject. The ability to achieve higher levels of performance is dependent on the amount of external work that can be performed with the internal work that occurs. Therefore, the more fit an individual is, the higher the degree of external work for the total amount of oxygen that is being consumed.

BLOOD FLOW AND VASCULAR PRESSURES DURING EXERCISE

During mild through moderate levels of exercise, plasma volume remains constant or is slightly decreased. At maximum exercise, plasma volume significantly decreases. In fact, during vigorous exercise, hemolysis may occur. The effects of blood volume and hemoglobin concentration are minimized in well-trained subjects because the baseline circulating blood volume is increased, as is the hemoglobin concentration.

During exercise, peripheral blood flow is regulated by vasodilatation and vasoconstriction at a local tissue level. Vasodilatation occurs in the working muscles and, at the same time, vasoconstriction occurs in nonworking muscles and the abdominal viscera. During maximum exercise, the respiratory muscles may use up to 25% of the oxygen uptake. Because vasodilation in the larger working muscle groups is more pronounced than the vasoconstriction that occurs during exercise in visceral tissue, arterial vascular resistance decreases.

Systolic, mean, and diastolic pressures all tend to increase during exercise. The rate of increase in pressure per change in oxygen consumption is greater for systole than for diastole. In some patients, diastole might decrease slightly.

Heat production that occurs during exercise is proportional to the amount of work that is being performed. The release of heat from the body occurs primarily through the skin, but the increase in minute ventilation also helps dissipate heat. Therefore, skin vascular dilatation occurs to allow for this exchange in heat.

▌EFFECT OF AEROBIC TRAINING IN HEALTHY SUBJECTS

The delivery of oxygen to the tissues requires a coordinated response from the cardiovascular and pulmonary systems in order to sustain aerobic metabolism and remove metabolites. As oxygen consumption increases, there must be an increase in ATP production from aerobic metabolism. If this demand is not met, anaerobic glycolysis is called on, with a resultant increase in lactic acid. The level of work at which the blood lactic acid level begins to rise rapidly is the anaerobic threshold. At this point, the minute ventilation accelerates disproportionately to the rise in carbon dioxide produced chiefly by exercising muscle in order to buffer the added acid load (see Figure 3.6-3). As lactic acid and carbon dioxide continue to accumulate, progressive acidosis occurs and cell function is adversely affected, ultimately causing exercise to stop. The level of work at which no further exercise is possible is called the aerobic capacity or the maximal oxygen consumption (see Figure 3.6-5).

The anaerobic threshold normally occurs at 40% to 80% of the maximal oxygen uptake and represents a barrier above which sustained exercise is not possible, and thus it has a predicted value for determining the level of exercise that an individual can maintain for a prolonged period of time. Limited additional activity is still possible beyond the anaerobic threshold, until maximal oxygen consumption is reached.

The level of fitness required to perform certain activities is determined by an individual's anaerobic threshold and aerobic capacity. A simple way of determining whether a person has sufficient conditioning for a job or an activity is to perform a cardiopulmonary stress test with analysis of oxygen and carbon dioxide concentrations in the expired gas and measurement of minute ventilation to determine oxygen uptake throughout exercise. This study can be performed with a computerized system. The information obtained—anaerobic threshold and maximal aerobic capacity—can be used to determine whether

The level of fitness required to perform an activity is limited by:

- anaerobic threshold
- aerobic capacity

that individual can sustain work or physical activity at a certain level and, when necessary, maximize effort to a level required for performance. Physical training can often result in a physiological adaptation where there is a delay in the development in the anaerobic threshold and an overall increase in aerobic capacity.

Physical training is the regular performance of a work load of sufficient intensity, duration, and frequency to produce a beneficial physiologic change. Training may be directed at increasing muscle strength, which requires brief bursts of muscle activity, or at improving endurance, which requires more prolonged submaximal exertion.

The intensity necessary for training should be greater than that generally encountered during routine activities. As training progresses, the intensity must be increased to achieve further improvement. For the average sedentary adult, exercise at a level greater than 50% of their maximal oxygen consumption is required to improve aerobic capacity by 5% to 10%. The intensity of exercise may be gradually increased to a maximum of 70% to 80% of the maximal oxygen consumption, which often raises the aerobic capacity by as much as 15%. More important than the rather small increase in aerobic capacity is the effect training has on anaerobic threshold. Training can delay the onset of the anaerobic threshold by a substantial amount, thereby allowing the individual to perform at a higher level of sustained work for a longer period of time.

The increase in aerobic capacity and the delay in the development of the anaerobic threshold with training results from a more efficient oxygen transport and utilization process. The cardiovascular changes associated with training include increases in ventricular-diastolic volume, myocardial mass, and plasma volume. The heart rate is lower and the stroke volume higher at rest and at any level of submaximal work (see Figure 3.6-6). At maximal work loads, the increase in cardiac output that occurs is attributable to an increase in stroke volume, because maximal heart rate is not affected by training. At the level of the skeletal muscle, oxygen extraction efficiency increases, possibly as a result of changes in mitochondrial function. Furthermore, muscle hypertrophy and increased vascularity are found.

Another consequence of training is a relative shift in the energy substrate utilization from carbohydrates to fatty acids, which preserves muscle glycogen stores and may enhance exercise performance. Finally, training induces a decrease in ventilation at submaximal exercise loads, and at maximal exercise the ability to ventilate comfortably is increased. The diffusion capacity may also be influenced by training, and there also may be changes in central nervous system respiratory drive.

Training leads to:

- an increase in aerobic capacity
- a delay in the development of the anaerobic threshold
- a lower heart rate and higher stroke volume at any level of work
- a decrease in ventilation throughout exercise

■ REVIEW QUESTIONS

1. Concerning the energetics of exercise, which one of the following statements is correct?

   (A) Anaerobic glycolysis is a major contributor of ATP.
   (B) Skeletal muscle has no energy pools.
   (C) The principal substrates for oxidative phosphorylation are carbohydrates and fatty acids.
   (D) The production of ATP is completely independent of oxygen.
   (E) Amino acids are the major fuels for exercising muscles.

2. Select the one answer that best describes the normal response to increasing levels of exercise in a healthy adult.

   (A) Minute ventilation can increase to as much as 20 times its resting value to prevent hypercapnia at high exercise levels.
   (B) Most of the increase in cardiac output during early exercise is met by an increase in heart rate.
   (C) Most of the increase in minute ventilation during early exercise occurs as a result of an increase in respiratory rate.
   (D) Systolic blood pressure does not increase during exercise.

■ ANSWERS AND EXPLANATIONS

1. The answer is C. Skeletal muscle has substantial energy pools. Adenosine triphosphate (ATP) is stored within muscle, and when ATP is depleted, continued exercise depends on oxidative phosphorylation, a process that uses carbohydrates and fatty acids as major fuels. Amino acids and keto acids are only minor fuel sources. Anaerobic glycolysis produces only a small fraction of the ATP that is produced by anaerobic metabolism.

2. The answer is A. Early in progressive exercise, both cardiac output and minute ventilation increase more in rate than in volume, and the rate of increase in pressure per change in oxygen consumption is greater for systolic than for diastolic pressure. Ventilation increases during progressive exercise in order to meet the demand for oxygen during exercise. Minute ventilation changes early in exercise keep the arterial PCO_2 and pH at resting levels, but later in exercise, at high work rates, changes in minute ventilation are greater in order to compensate for the metabolic acidosis that occurs.

■ SUGGESTED READINGS

Åstarnd P-O, Rodahl K: *Textbook of Work Physiology: Physiological Bases of Exercise*, 3rd ed. New York: McGraw Hill, 1986.

Cerretelli P, DiPrampero PE: Gas exchange in exercise. In: Fahri LE, Tenney SM (eds). *Gas Exchange: Handbook of Physiology*. Sec 3. The Respiratory System. Bethesda: Amer Physiol Soc 1987, Vol 4, pp 297–339.

Jones NL: *Clinical Exercise Testing*, 3rd ed. Philadelphia: WB Saunders, 1988.

Murray JF: *The Normal Lung*, 2nd ed. Philadelphia: WB Saunders 1986, pp 261–282.

Wasserman K, Whipp BJ, Casaburi: Respiratory control during exercise. In: Cherniack NS, Widdicombe JG (eds). *Control of Breathing, Part 2, Handbook of Physiology*, Sec 3 Bethesda: Amer Physiol Soc 1986, pp 595–619.

Wasserman K, Hansen JE, Sue DY, et al: Principles of Exercise Testing and Interpretation. Philadelphia: Lea and Febiger, 1994.

Wasserman K, Whipp BJ, Davis JA: Respiratory physiology of exercise: Metabolism, gas exchange, and ventilatory control. *Int Rev Physiol* 23:149–211, 1981.

Weber KT, Janicki JS (eds): *Cardiopulmonary Exercise Testing*. Philadelphia: WB Saunders, 1986.

Whipp BJ, Pardy RL: Breathing during exercise. In: Macklem PT, Mead J (eds). *Mechanics of Breathing, Part 2. Handbook of Physiology*, Sec 3. Amer Physiol Soc 1986, Vol 3, pp 605–629.

Chapter 4
AIRFLOW OBSTRUCTION

David E. Ciccolella, M.D.

Kathleen J. Brennan, M.D.

▮ CHAPTER OUTLINE

Learning Objectives
Introduction
Anatomical and Physiological Concepts
Regulation of Airway Caliber
Mechanisms of Airflow Obstruction
Pulmonary Function in Obstructive Airway Diseases
Review Questions

▮ LEARNING OBJECTIVES

At the completion of this chapter, the reader should:
- Be able to describe the differences in pathology among the common obstructive lung diseases.
- Be able to describe the mechanisms of airflow obstruction in both asthma and COPD.
- Understand the pathophysiology of airway smooth muscle contraction.
- Understand the physiological consequences of airway narrowing on pulmonary function tests.

▮ INTRODUCTION

Airflow obstruction, which is the impairment of air movement between the alveoli and the mouth, may occur in diseases of the upper and lower airways. The upper airways include the area above the branching of the major bronchi (main stem carina) and the lower airways below the major bronchi. This chapter will examine airflow obstruction resulting from diseases that affect the distal lower airways, including emphysema, chronic bronchitis, asthma, bronchiectasis, cystic fibrosis, and other disorders of the intrathoracic airways (Table 4-1). The exact causes of many of these airway diseases remain unknown. Although all these disorders cause airway narrowing, the site of airflow obstruction varies from those affecting the large airways to those affecting the small airways.

Table 4-1
Obstructive Pulmonary Diseases

Lower Airway Diseases
Asthma
COPD (emphysema, chronic bronchitis)
Bronchiectasis
Cystic fibrosis
Other disorders*

Upper Airway Diseases
Tumor
Vocal cord paralysis
Foreign body

* Includes diffuse diseases of the peripheral airways (e.g., obliterative bronchiolitis) and localized abnormalities of the bronchi (e.g., amyloidosis, tumor compression, broncholithiasis).

All of these diseases, with the exception of emphysema, mainly affect the airways. Emphysema affects the lung parenchyma and is defined pathologically by the presence of alveolar-capillary wall destruction resulting in enlargement of the alveolar spaces. Chronic bronchitis is defined clinically by the daily production of sputum for 3 months over 2 consecutive years. These two diseases have been difficult to differentiate clinically, and patients tend to have varying degrees of both, and therefore these disorders have been classified under the name chronic obstructive pulmonary disease (COPD). Bronchiectasis is a disease characterized by an abnormal dilatation of the bronchi caused by destruction of the elastic and muscular elements of their walls. Cystic fibrosis, the most common genetic disease in Caucasian children, is characterized by abnormalities in airway ion transport, which result in abnormal accumulation of airway secretions and frequent bacterial infections. Asthma is an inflammatory airway disease that results in reversible airflow obstruction resulting from airway smooth muscle contraction.

The mechanisms of airflow obstruction vary in each of these diseases but include effects in the airway lumen, airway wall thickening and compression, and airway smooth muscle contraction. In the following section, we review normal airway anatomy and physiological concepts that are important in understanding airflow obstruction.

■ ANATOMICAL AND PHYSIOLOGICAL CONCEPTS

Normal airway anatomy and lung parenchyma structure and function have been reviewed in Chapters 2 and 3, respectively.

AIRWAY RESISTANCE

Total Pulmonary Resistance to Airflow

- Airway resistance: 80%
- Tissue resistance: 20%

During breathing, greater pressure is required to move air than simply to overcome the elasticity of the lung and the thoracic cage. The additional pressure required is the result of friction between individual air molecules as well as between the air molecules and the airway wall (airway resistance) and of friction between the lung and the thoracic cage (tissue resistance). Airway resistance represents 80%, and tissue resistance represents 20%, of the total pulmonary frictional resistance to airflow. Therefore, airway resistance (R_{aw}) is described as the pressure difference between two points in a tube ($P_{mouth} - P_{alveolus}$) divided by the flow rate,

$$R_{aw} = \frac{P_{mouth} - P_{alveolus}}{airflow\ rate}$$

Airway resistance of a tube is directly proportional to the length of the tube (L) and inversely proportional to the fourth power of its radius (R).

$$R_{aw} \propto \frac{L}{R^4}$$

Therefore, a larger airway (larger lumen) has a lower airway resistance than a smaller airway (smaller lumen). As the airways continue to divide, the airway lumens become smaller, resulting in greater airway resistance in individual airways. However, with increasing airway division, the airways also become shorter and the total cross-sectional airway area increases geometrically, thereby increasing total pulmonary resistance by only a small amount.

Airway Resistance to Airflow

- Central airways: 80–90%
- Peripheral airways: 10–20%

Airway resistance to airflow can be arbitrarily divided into two anatomical areas of the lung: the central airways, which are greater than 2 mm in diameter, and the peripheral airways, which are less than 2 mm in diameter. Airflow resistance in the central airways makes up approximately 80% to 90% of total airway resistance, whereas airflow resistance in the peripheral airways makes up only 10% to 20% of total airway resistance. The high airway resistance in the central airways results from the high gas volumes passing through the relatively small cross-sectional areas of the upper airways (i.e., trachea and bronchi), resulting in high flow velocity and turbulent flow. Turbulent flow is produced by high flow velocity and irregularities in the airway. Contact between gas molecules and the airway wall results in a loss in the energy driving these molecules and therefore requires a higher pressure for air molecule movement. Energy loss is greater with heavier molecules than with lighter ones, making gas density an important factor in the production of turbulent flow. For example, turbulent flow can be reduced by inspiring a lower-density gas such as helium.

In the smaller airways, flow becomes slower because of much larger cross-sectional areas, and this results in the predominance of laminar flow. In laminar flow, air molecule movement is streamlined (i.e., the molecules are moving parallel to each other and to the airway wall). Therefore, in smaller airways, the driving pressure to produce airflow is not dependent on gas density. It is dependent on gas viscosity.

Because a large portion of total airway resistance occurs in the central airways, obstruction in the central airways results in a marked increase in airway resistance and airflow obstruction. Obstructive lesions of the central airways may include foreign bodies, tumors of the large airways, airway strictures, and tracheomalacia. However, in the peripheral airways, because they have a much larger cross-sectional area, significant disease and airflow obstruction are less evident.

Another factor that affects airway resistance is lung volume. At high lung volumes, the airways are larger and resistance to airflow is lower.

FORCED EXPIRATION AND THE EQUAL PRESSURE POINT

During normal breathing, intrapleural pressure is negative in both inspiration and expiration whereas alveolar pressure is negative only in inspiration (Figure 4-1). Intrapleural

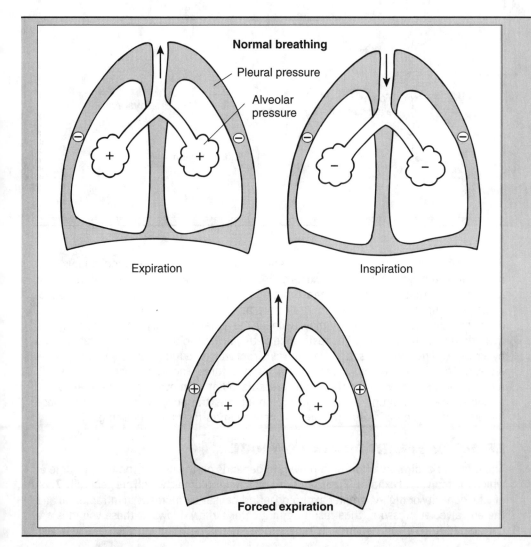

Normal breathing

Pleural pressure

Alveolar pressure

Expiration

Inspiration

Forced expiration

FIGURE 4-1
Alveolar and pleural pressures during normal breathing and forced expiration. In normal breathing, the pleural pressure remains negative during both inspiration and expiration. In forced expiration, alveolar and pleural pressures become positive.

Alveolar pressure, which is equal to airway driving pressure, represents the sum of intrapleural and elastic recoil pressures.

pressure is negative because of the inward retraction of the lungs and the outward retraction of the chest wall at resting lung volume. However, during forced expiration, intrapleural pressure and alveolar pressure are both positive, which may cause airway compression (Figure 4-2). Alveolar pressure, which is equal to the airway driving pressure, represents the sum of intrapleural pressure and elastic recoil pressure. During expiration, this driving pressure is dissipated in the airways as a result of airway resistance. Because the lung elastic recoil pressure, which is transmitted to the lumen of the airway, remains unchanged, there is a point at which airway luminal pressure becomes equal to intrapleural pressure; this point is termed the equal pressure point. Farther upstream from the equal pressure point, airway luminal pressure becomes less than intrapleural pressure, resulting in airway compression and airflow limitation.

FIGURE 4-2

Relationship between pleural pressure and radial traction in normal and emphysematous lungs in the development of the equal pressure point. In the normal lung, the inward-directed pleural pressure is opposed by radial traction on the bronchioles and by the alveolar pressure. Emphysema results in destruction of lung parenchyma and consequently a loss of tethering structures surrounding the bronchioles, causing decreased radial traction. There is also a decrease in elastic recoil owing to decreased lung parenchyma. During expiration, reduction in radial traction results in early airway closure as luminal pressure becomes less than intrapleural pressure, resulting in airway compression and airflow limitation.

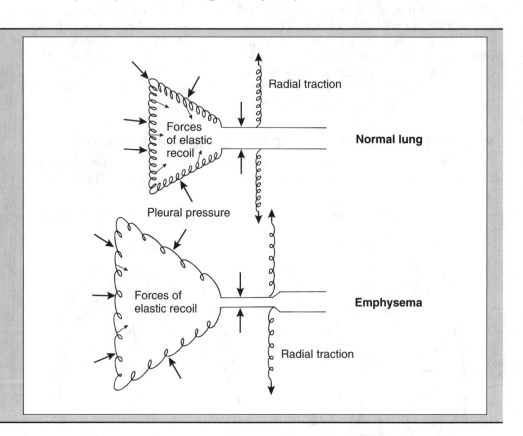

Equal Pressure Point

- Airway luminal pressure equals intrapleural pressure.
- Beyond the equal pressure point, airway compression occurs and airflow is limited.
- Normally, the equal pressure point is not present during quiet breathing.
- In emphysema, the equal pressure point may occur during quiet breathing.

The equal pressure point is not present during quiet breathing in individuals with normal lung function. Normally, it exists only during forced expiration and occurs only at lung volumes that are smaller than functional residual capacity, because the equal pressure point is present in the more flexible peripheral airways. This airway collapse does not occur with high lung volumes, because the equal pressure point is present in the more rigid proximal airways. The resistance of the airways to this collapse is determined by airway wall rigidity, the supporting airway structures, and lung elastic recoil pressure. A weakening of the airway wall or its supporting structures, and a decrease in lung elastic recoil pressures, may cause the equal pressure point to move more proximal to the alveolus, thereby limiting airflow and promoting gas trapping. In emphysema, these factors cause the equal pressure point to occur even during quiet breathing.

EFFECT OF EFFORT ON AIRFLOW RATE

The effect of expiratory effort on airflow rate depends on the size of the lung volume at which the individual exhales (Figure 4-3). At high lung volumes, which are generally 75% of vital capacity or higher, greater expiratory effort causes an increase in intrapleural and thereby alveolar pressure, thus resulting in greater airflow. Flows at these volumes are considered to be effort dependent. However, at lower lung volumes, such as those less

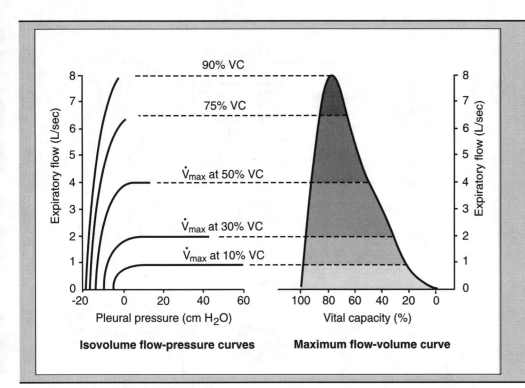

FIGURE 4-3
Isovolume flow-pressure curves during forced expiration. At near total lung capacity (> 75% vital capacity), flow is dependent on amount of effort. However, at lower lung volumes, the flow plateaus and becomes independent of effort, i.e., increasing effort only increases pleural pressure but not flow. Modified from Murray JF. *The Normal Lung* Philadelphia: Saunders, 1986.

than 50% of the vital capacity, the expiratory flow reaches a plateau with increasing intrapleural pressure. At these lung volumes, increasing expiratory effort generates higher pleural pressures, but this does not alter airflow rate. In this case, increased effort does not produce greater airflow because the airways collapse at the same equal pressure point, thereby becoming the limiting factor for airflow. Flows at these lower lung volumes are not affected by effort once airway compression occurs, and are called effort independent.

■ REGULATION OF AIRWAY CALIBER

Airway size normally is regulated by the parasympathetic, sympathetic, and non-adrenergic, noncholinergic (NANC) nervous systems (Figure 4-4). These systems act on airway smooth muscle through receptors for acetylcholine, vasoactive intestinal peptide, peptide histidine methionine, β-adrenergic agonists, and substance P.

CHOLINERGIC NERVOUS SYSTEM

Cholinergic or parasympathetic motoneurons contained within the vagus nerve affect submucosal glands, bronchial smooth muscle, vascular beds, and inflammatory cell function. The cholinergic nervous system is the major neural pathway for bronchoconstriction in the human airways. Cholinergic pathways innervating the respiratory tract originate in the motor nuclei located in the brain stem. Vagal nerve stimulation results in bronchoconstriction whereas cholinergic blockade results in bronchodilation. Cholinergic innervation of the respiratory tract is heterogeneous, with a higher number of cholinergic fibers in the trachea and large airways than in the more peripheral airways. Therefore, stimulation of the vagus nerve or cholinergic blockade results in more prominent central than peripheral effects.

SYMPATHETIC NERVOUS SYSTEM

In contrast, the sympathetic neurons have minimal effects during normal regulation, but the release of epinephrine and in some cases norepinephrine may magnify the effects and result in a more significant indirect effect on the respiratory system. This is supported by the near absence of direct sympathetic innervation in human airways. Thus, sympathetic nervous system control of the human airways occurs largely by modulation of parasympathetic transmission. Locally released and circulating catecholamines may also

Airway size is normally regulated by:

- the parasympathetic nervous system
- the sympathetic nervous system
- the NANC nervous system

The cholinergic nervous system is the major neural pathway for bronchoconstriction.

The sympathetic nervous system plays a minimal role in normal regulation of airway size.

FIGURE 4-4

Neural control of airway caliber. The cholinergic nervous system releases acetylcholine (Ach), producing smooth muscle contraction. In contrast, the nonadrenergic, noncholinergic (NANC) nervous system has both excitatory (E-NANC) and inhibitory (I-NANC) pathways. Vasoactive intestinal peptide (VIP) and nitric oxide (NO) are the primary mediators of I-NANC and result in smooth muscle relaxation and bronchodilation. E-NANC produces bronchocostriction through tachykinins such as substance P, neurokinin A, and neurokinin B. The sympathetic nervous system has no direct innervation of smooth muscle and plays a minimal role in normal airway regulation. However, it may act indirectly through the release of epinephrine or norepinephrine and on parasympathetic ganglion nerve transmission.

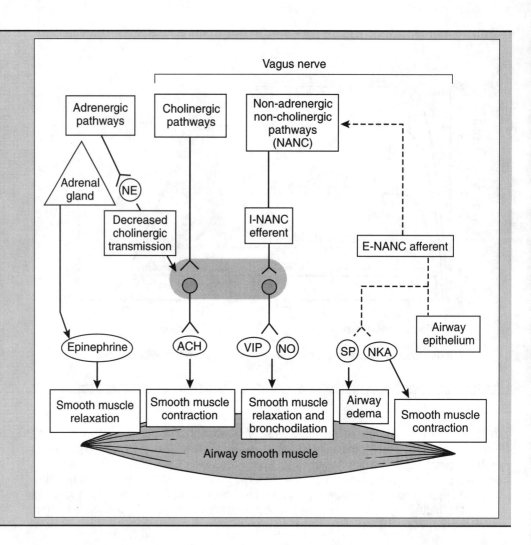

The I-NANC system is the only neural bronchodilator pathway.

modulate airway smooth muscle tone by inhibiting acetylcholine release from postganglionic nerve terminals.

NONADRENERGIC, NONCHOLINERGIC NERVOUS SYSTEM

Neural effects on airways that are not blocked by adrenergic or cholinergic antagonists result from the nonadrenergic, noncholinergic (NANC) nervous system. The NANC nerves have been shown to result in both bronchodilation and bronchoconstriction, vasodilatation and vasoconstriction, and mucus secretion as a result of release of several neurotransmitters. These effects are mediated by the inhibitory (I-NANC) and excitatory (E-NANC) nonadrenergic, noncholinergic nervous system pathways.

The I-NANC nervous system relaxes airway smooth muscle, and because there is no functional sympathetic innervation of the airway smooth muscle, it is the only neural bronchodilator pathway. These responses are probably mediated by both nitric oxide and vasoactive intestinal peptide. Nitric oxide is the major neurotransmitter of I-NANC responses in human airways. It may also be involved in airway and pulmonary blood flow and immune regulation. Vasoactive intestinal peptide is known to be a potent relaxant of airway smooth muscle and dilator of pulmonary vessels, but its effect on mucus secretion is complex.

E-NANC nerves cause bronchoconstriction and may be mediated by the tachykinins. The tachykinins include substance P and neurokinins A and B. Substance P stimulates mucus secretion from submucosal glands in human airways. Substance P has also been shown to contract airway smooth muscle, but neurokinin A is a more potent constrictor.

It has been postulated that the cholinergic nervous system may be involved in airway hyperresponsiveness, but it is not a major cause of airflow limitation in asthma. Bronchodilation of the airways by cholinergic blockade is probably more important in COPD than in asthma. Alterations in the production and degradation of nitric oxide may be important in the pathophysiology of asthma. It is not clear whether neuropeptides contribute to the pathophysiology of asthma.

MECHANISMS OF AIRFLOW OBSTRUCTION

STRUCTURAL ABNORMALITIES

Airflow obstruction may be caused by several mechanisms: luminal obstruction (secretions, debris, foreign bodies, etc), airway wall thickening (edema, inflammatory cell infiltration, scarring, smooth muscle hypertrophy/hyperplasia, mucous gland enlargement, etc.), loss of airway wall supporting structures (loss of connective tissue elastin), and airway smooth muscle contraction (Figure 4-5). These mechanisms vary in their presence and degree depending on the type of obstructive airway disease (Table 4-2). The contribution of each of these mechanisms is also difficult to evaluate. One or more of them may be present in a specific disease.

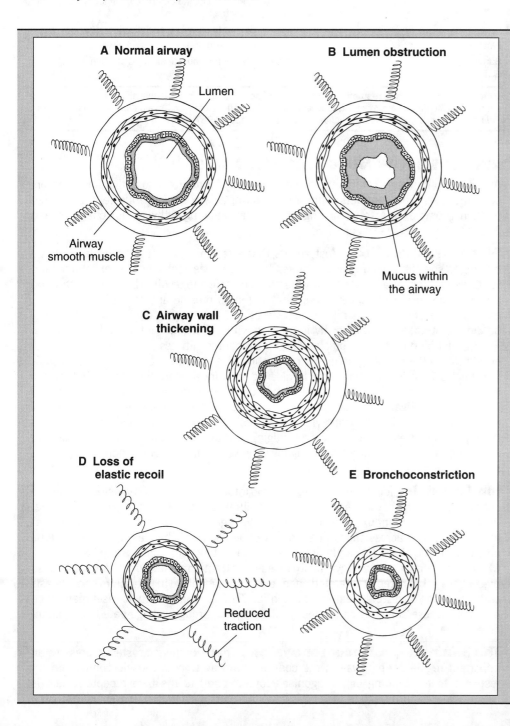

FIGURE 4-5
Mechanisms involved in airflow obstruction. (A) Normal airway. The bronchial walls are composed of an inner layer of columnar epithelial cells. Surrounding the lumen is a ring of smooth muscle. Airway obstruction can be caused by any of the following, alone or in combination. (B) Occlusion of the airway lumen owing to increased secretions or debris. (C) Narrowing of the airway lumen caused by thickening of the wall from edema, smooth muscle hyperplasia/hypertrophy, or mucous gland enlargement. (D) Reduction in luminal diameter caused by decreased elastic recoil from loss of tethering elements that support the bronchial wall. (E) Bronchoconstriction.

Table 4-2
Mechanisms of Airflow Obstruction in Specific Diseases

DISEASE	MECHANISM
Upper Airways (Above the Carina)	
Foreign body	Mechanical
Croup and tracheitis	Mucosal edema of upper airways
Epiglottitis	Swelling of epiglottis
Tumor	Mechanical
Neuromuscular disease	Upper airway muscle weakness
Lower Airways (Below the Carina)	
Asthma	Airway smooth muscle contraction, edema, and secretions
Chronic bronchitis	Airway edema and secretions; airway smooth muscle contraction
Obstructive bronchiectasis*	Partial obstruction of majority of airways; airway secretions and destruction; smooth muscle contraction
Cystic fibrosis	Similar to chronic bronchitis
Emphysema	Decreased elastic recoil and airway wall collapse
Sarcoidosis	Granuloma causing airway distortion
Foreign body	Mechanical

* May also present as a restrictive pulmonary disease if the majority of the airways are completely obstructed. Modified from Martin L: The essentials for patient care and evaluation. *In* Carson D, ed.: *Pulmonary Physiology in Clinical Practice.* St Louis: CV Mosby, 1987, p. 67.

AIRWAY SMOOTH MUSCLE CONTRACTION

Airway smooth muscle contraction and relaxation are controlled through a complex interaction among intracellular signaling pathways, ion channels, and β-adrenergic receptors.

Airway smooth muscle is the final common pathway for neurohumoral and inflammatory cell processes. The contraction and relaxation of airway smooth muscle is controlled through a complex interaction among intracellular signaling pathways, ion channels, and β-adrenergic receptors (Figure 4-6).

Signal Transduction. Most agents that affect airway smooth muscle do so by binding to specific cell surface receptors. Agents such as acetylcholine, histamine, and leukotriene D_4 act as agonists on airway smooth muscle and result in bronchoconstriction through smooth muscle contraction. Airway smooth muscle antagonists such as antiacetylcholine and antihistamine block airway smooth muscle contractions either by binding to surface receptors or by interfering with subsequent intracellular pathways.

Agonist binding to a specific cell surface receptor initiates a series of biochemical events within the cell, beginning with activation of membrane-bound phospholipase C. Phosphatidylinositol bisphosphate is cleaved into inositol triphosphate (IP_3), which releases Ca^{++} from the sarcoplasmic reticulum. The intracellular Ca^{++} binds to calmodulin and activates myosin light chain kinase (MLCK), which subsequently phosphorylates myosin. This phosphorylation of myosin stimulates actin-activated ATPase in the myosin head and results in cross-bridging and airway smooth muscle contraction. Interference in these pathways by antagonists prevents muscle contraction and produces bronchodilation.

Ion Channels. Ion channels also play an important role in airway smooth muscle contraction and regulation. In addition to calcium released from the sarcoplasmic reticulum, there is an influx of calcium through voltage-gated Ca^{++} channels. The movement of calcium across these channels is dependent on changes in the membrane potential. These channels can be inhibited by Ca^{++} blockers such as dihydropyridines, which in turn can inhibit airway smooth muscle contraction. Potassium channels are also present as well as receptor-operated channels that are involved in potassium homeostasis and the setting of resting membrane potential. Through their ability to reset membrane potentials, these channels can influence Ca^{2+} influx through voltage-gated Ca^{2+} channels.

The ß-Adrenergic Receptor System. The β-adrenergic system represents an important regulatory pathway in the control of airway smooth muscle contraction. In response to the binding of a β-agonist (isoproterenol) to the beta receptor, there is

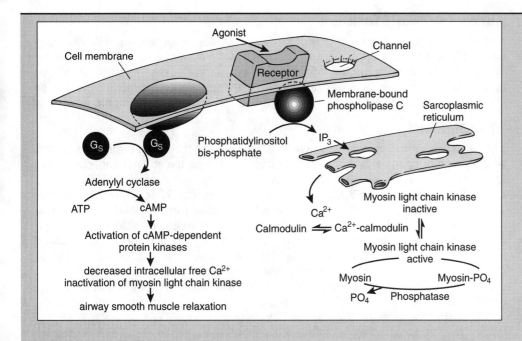

FIGURE 4-6

Signal transduction within the smooth muscle cell. An agonist binding to a cell membrane receptor activates membrane-bound phospholipase C, which converts phosphatidylinositol bisphosphate into inositol triphosphate (IP_3). IP_3 causes the sarcoplasmic reticulum to release Ca^{2+}, which is subsequently bound by calmodulin. The Ca^{2+}-calmodulin compound activates myosin light chain kinase and results in phosphorylation of myosin and subsequent smooth muscle contraction. Smooth muscle contraction can also be affected by the beta-receptor system. Beta-receptor agonist binding stimulates G_s activation of adenylyl cyclase and results in increased cAMP synthesis. Increased cAMP activates various cAMP-dependent protein kinases, which in turn affects a number of intracellular processes, one of which is smooth muscle relaxation. There are also voltage-gated ion channels on the cell membrane that can influence intracellular events.

activation of G_s, a guanosine triphosphate (GTP) binding protein, which results in activation of adenylyl cyclase. Increases in the activity of adenylyl cyclase result in production of cAMP, an important intracellular second messenger, and activation of protein kinase A (PKA). Protein kinase A stimulates phosphorylation of multiple targets within the cell and results in airway smooth muscle relaxation. Phosphodiesterase inhibitors mimic the result of the beta-receptor agonists by preventing the hydrolysis of cyclic adenosine monophosphate (cAMP) and cyclic guanosine monophosphate (cGMP) and increasing intracellular levels with subsequent activation of PKA and thereby relaxing airway smooth muscle. However, recent studies have found that not all effects of beta-receptor agonists occur through PKA activation. Soluble subunits of G_s protein can also act as second messengers through manipulation of the potassium channel.

PULMONARY FUNCTION IN OBSTRUCTIVE AIRWAY DISEASES

AIRWAY RESISTANCE AND EXPIRATORY AIRFLOW RATES

In patients with obstructive lung diseases, there is a reduction in the rate of expiratory airflow. The reduction in expiratory airflow may be a consequence of factors that directly affect the airway, causing a decrease in airway diameter and an increase in airway resistance, or through destruction of lung parenchyma and loss of airway structural support, causing reduced elastic recoil and airway diameter. Airflow resistance is inversely related to the fourth power of the airway radius. Therefore, small changes in radius produce marked increases in airflow resistance. Airway resistance is increased in patients with intrinsic narrowing of the airway lumen owing to airway secretions, smooth muscle contraction, or airway wall thickening, which occurs in asthma and chronic bronchitis. In emphysema, however, intrinsic airway resistance is minimally increased. We can measure alterations in pulmonary function tests caused by obstructive airways diseases using spirometry, lung volumes, diffusion capacity, and arterial blood gases.

AIRWAY CONDUCTANCE

Airway conductance, the reciprocal of airway resistance, is dependent on airway size because it is measured at constant lung volumes while elastic recoil pressure is varied. This minimizes any contribution of reduced elastic recoil as seen in emphysema and isolates the differences in airway resistance. Therefore, airway conductance is usually markedly decreased in asthma and chronic bronchitis compared with emphysema.

SPIROMETRY

Airflow resistance can be indirectly assessed by examining the forced expiratory volumes with the use of spirometry. Important parameters include forced vital capacity (FVC), forced expiratory volume in one second (FEV_1), peak expiratory flow rate (PEFR), and the ratio of FEV_1 to FVC. The FEV_1/FVC ratio normally ranges from 70 to 75, meaning that at least 70% to 75% of the vital capacity should be exhaled in 1 second. The maximal midexpiratory flow ($MMEF_{25\%-75\%}$) is also used but is a less reliable parameter for evaluating lung function. Normal predicted ranges for lung function are commonly based on gender, age, and height. In a large population of individuals, lung function is distributed as a bell-shaped curve. Generally, abnormal values are those outside the 95% confidence interval, which means that 1 in 20 individuals (5%) will be abnormal by convention. Lung function is also expressed as a percent of the normal predicted value.

> The FEV_1/FVC ratio is reduced in obstructive airways disease.

In obstructive airways disease, the FEV_1 and the FEV_1/FVC ratio are typically reduced. The FVC is either normal or reduced depending on the severity of airflow obstruction. Peak expiratory flow rates and the maximal midexpiratory flow ($MMEF_{25\%-75\%}$) are also reduced. The severity of airflow obstruction is gauged by the FEV_1. Generally, the FEV_1/FVC ratio in obstructive lung disease is less than 70 to 75. In contrast, the FEV_1/FVC ratio in restrictive lung diseases (e.g., idiopathic pulmonary fibrosis or asbestosis) tends to be normal or high, with similar reductions for both FVC and FEV_1 (Table 4-3). All lower airway diseases causing airflow obstruction have a similar pattern on spirometry and cannot be differentiated by spirometry alone.

Table 4-3
Obstructive and Restrictive Disease Patterns on Spirometry

	FVC	FEV$_1$	PEFR	FEV$_1$/FVC
Obstructive	↓ or ↔	↓	↓	↓
Restrictive	↓	↓	↓, ↔, or ↑	↔ or ↑

FVC = forced vital capacity, FEV$_1$ = forced expiratory volume in 1 second, PEFR = peak expiratory flow rate; ↓ = decreased, ↔ = normal, ↑ = increased.

> The FVC, FEV_1, and FEV_1/FVC ratio may be normal in small airways disease.

Spirometry is a good technique for evaluating airflow obstruction resulting from disease in the large to medium airways but is less helpful in evaluating airflow obstruction owing to small airways disease (< 2 mm internal diameter). In fact, the spirometric parameters FVC, FEV_1, and FEV_1/FVC may be within the normal range in patients with significant small airways disease. As discussed previously, airflow resistance in the small airways makes up only about 10% to 20% of total lung airflow resistance, and extensive disease of the small airways may not affect FVC or FEV_1. Small airways disease may be evaluated by other, more sensitive tests such as measurement of dynamic compliance, closing volume, and air and helium flow-volume curves. The $MMEF_{25\%-75\%}$, the rate of airflow between 25% and 75% of the vital capacity, is more sensitive to changes in small airways disease but is not specific. These tests may be helpful in evaluation for the presence of early obstructive airways disease in smokers.

FLOW-VOLUME CURVE

The flow-volume curve is the graphic relationship between airflow rate and lung volume. There are two portions of the flow-volume curve—an expiratory portion, where the subject exhales from total lung capacity to residual volume, and an inspiratory portion, where the subject then inhales from residual volume to total lung capacity.

> In diffuse obstructive lower airways disease, the flow-volume curve has a concave expiratory limb.

The expiratory portion of this curve is derived from the graphic relationship between forced expiratory volume and time (Figure 4-7A). The slope of this curve is then determined and plotted against lung volume to obtain the flow-volume curve (Figure 4-7B). The flow-volume curve is helpful in evaluating the presence, type, and location (upper vs.

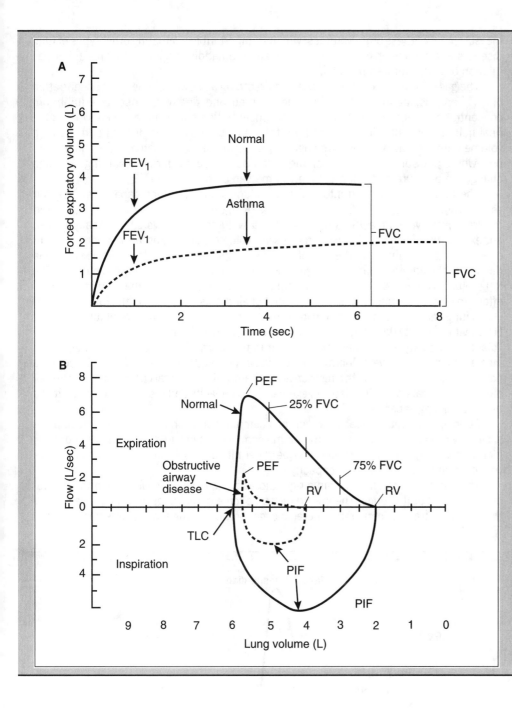

FIGURE 4-7
(A) Forced expiratory volume versus time and (B) flow-volume curve for normal lungs and for obstructive airways disease. (A) Forced expiratory volume is determined by measuring the amount of air forcefully exhaled over time. In obstructive airways disease, FEV_1 and FVC are both reduced from their normal values. The patient with obstructive airways disease exhales at a much slower rate and never attains a plateau after 8 seconds. In contrast, the normal curve shows that the exhaled volume reaches a plateau before 6 seconds. (B) Plot of the slope of the volume-time curve at all lung volumes. In obstructive airways disease, the expiratory curve is concave whereas the normal curve is more linear. In obstructive airways disease, the peak expiratory flow is decreased from its normal value. Note that RV is increased because of air trapping in obstructive airways disease. TLC = total lung capacity, RV = residual volume, PEF = peak expiratory flow, PIF = peak inspiratory flow, FEV_1 = forced expiratory volume in 1 second, FVC = forced vital capacity.

lower airway) of airflow obstruction. In diffuse obstructive lower airways disease, the flow-volume curve has a concave expiratory limb and generally a normal configuration for the inspiratory limb. The flow-volume curve has a different configuration in a patient with airflow obstruction caused by an upper airway lesion (above the main stem carina) than in a patient with lower airways disease. In patients with early lung disease, the flow-volume curve may be concave at the lower lung volumes, indicating small airways disease; the flow rates at 50% and 25% of the vital capacity on the expiratory curve may be reduced. Expiratory time is prolonged in obstructive airways disease as a result of increased airway resistance. The increased airway resistance also hinders emptying of the alveoli, leading to increased lung volumes.

STATIC LUNG VOLUMES AND THEIR MEASUREMENT

Spirometry can measure the volume of air that can be exhaled but cannot measure the remaining volume in the lung, the residual volume, or other volumes and capacities. The measurement of these other volumes, which is important in evaluating other types of lung diseases and airflow obstruction, requires a combination of spirometry and either gas dilution or body plethysmography.

The gas dilution technique is based on breathing a known volume and concentration of an inert gas, helium, which becomes diluted and finally reaches an equilibrium concentration. Because the initial helium concentration and volume are known and the final helium concentration is measured, the final volume can be derived and the lung volume determined. Body plethysmography is performed with the patient in an airtight box, where pressure and volume changes can be measured during breathing. Through changes in pressure and volume, lung volume can be determined.

The lung can be divided into four lung volumes and four lung capacities. The four volumes are tidal volume (TV), residual volume (RV), expiratory reserve volume (ERV), and inspiratory reserve volume (IRV) (Figure 4-8). Tidal volume is the air volume normally inhaled and exhaled with each breath. Inspiratory reserve volume is defined as the additional amount of air that can be inhaled at the end of a normal inspiration. Expiratory reserve volume is defined as the additional amount of air that can be exhaled after a normal expiration. The lung volumes do not overlap. Residual volume is the amount of air remaining in the lungs after a maximal expiration. This is the amount of air that is "trapped" in the lungs.

A lung capacity is made up of two or more component capacities: total lung capacity (TLC), vital capacity (VC), functional residual capacity (FRC), and inspiratory capacity (IC). Total lung capacity is the total amount of air in the lungs after a maximal inspiration. An increase in the TLC above the normal range is usually termed hyperinflation. A TLC below the normal range is consistent with a restrictive respiratory disease. Vital capacity is the maximal amount of air that can be inhaled and exhaled. Vital capacity and the residual volume make up the total lung capacity.

Functional residual capacity, which is a combination of the residual volume and the expiratory reserve volume, is the lung volume commonly measured by gas dilution or body plethysmography. Residual volume can be determined by subtracting expiratory reserve volume from functional residual capacity.

The lungs are contained within a rigid thoracic shell, which is larger than the natural resting volume of the lungs. The inward retractile force of the lungs is counterbalanced by the outward retractile force of the thoracic cage, producing the lung volume known as the

$$TLC = RV + VC$$
$$FRC = ERV + RV$$

FIGURE 4-8

Normal lung volumes and capacities. Lung volumes: IRV = inspiratory reserve volume, TV = tidal volume, ERV = expiratory reserve volume, RV = residual volume. Lung capacities: IC = inspiratory capacity, FRC = functional residual capacity, VC = vital capacity, TLC = total lung capacity. Modified from Warner A and Sackner MA. *Pulmonary Disease*. Boston: Little, Brown, 1983.

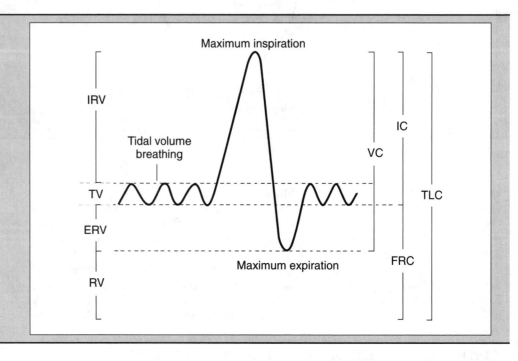

functional residual capacity (FRC), which is the natural resting volume of the lungs. The size of the FRC is determined, in part, by the compliance of the two opposing structures, the lung and the thoracic cage. The higher the lung compliance, the greater the air volume that can be inhaled for a given change in inflation pressure.

LUNG COMPLIANCE

The compliance curves for patients with emphysema, asthma, and fibrosis compared with that of a healthy person are shown in Figure 4-9. The static pressure-volume curve is shifted upward and leftward in asthma and emphysema. The slope is increased in emphysema, indicating a loss of elasticity, but the slope is normal in the asthmatic. In patients with emphysema, elastic recoil is reduced by destruction of alveolar-capillary walls, and the lungs are more easily inflated by a given amount of distending pressure. In patients with pulmonary fibrosis, scar tissue replaces normal lung components, which makes the lungs less compliant and less easily inflated for a change in distending pressure.

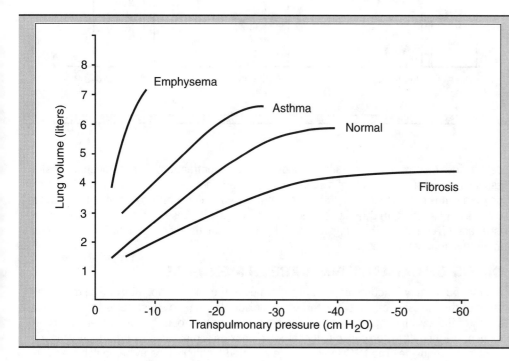

FIGURE 4-9
Compliance curves for subjects with emphysema, asthma, and fibrosis compared with normal lung compliance. In patients with emphysema, elastic recoil is reduced, and the lungs are more easily distended for a given pressure. In asthma, the compliance curve is parallel to the normal curve, but is shifted upward and to the left as a result of alveolar closure. There is no change in lung elasticity. In contrast, the lungs are less distensible in patients with fibrotic lung disease because of scar tissue in the interstitium; the curve is shifted downward and to the right.

LUNG VOLUMES

In general, airflow obstruction causes alterations in lung volumes (Figure 4-10). Increases in RV, FRC, and TLC may occur in obstructive airways diseases. The pattern and degree of alteration in lung volumes vary with the type of disease. The more specific mechanisms and changes in lung volumes will be considered in the respective chapters on the individual diseases.

In an acute exacerbation of asthma, there are typically large elevations in RV and FRC, and modest elevations in TLC. Asthma in complete remission exhibits normal volumes. Some of these volumes may even be increased in the asymptomatic patient. In general, the more severe the airflow obstruction, the more likely these lung volumes will be elevated. In chronic obstructive pulmonary disease (COPD), RV, TLC, and FRC are increased. The increase in TLC is usually greater in COPD—especially in emphysema—than in asthma. It is much more likely to be present during stable periods. In the other obstructive airways diseases (generalized bronchiectasis, cystic fibrosis, etc.), the lung volumes vary in their degree of elevation, both acutely and chronically.

The mechanisms responsible for the changes in lung volumes also vary with the type of obstructive lung disease. Increased lung volumes are due to increased airflow resistance as a result of several mechanisms such as airway wall thickening from inflammation, luminal

Airflow obstruction may result in increases in RV, FRC, and TLC.

FIGURE 4-10

Lung volumes for normal subjects and for those with restrictive and obstructive airways diseases. In restrictive disease, the capacities are reduced. In obstructive airways disease, TLC and FRC are increased whereas VC may be in the normal range or reduced. FRC = functional residual capacity, VC = vital capacity, TLC = total lung capacity.

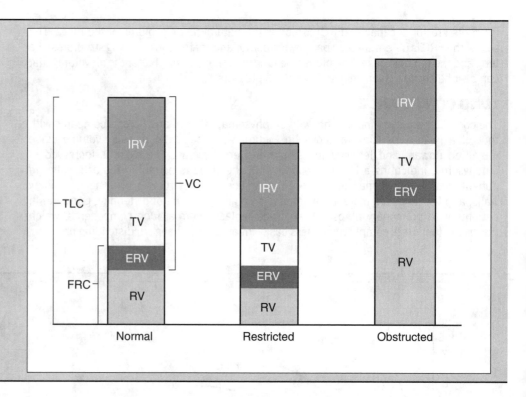

debris and mucus, and reversible smooth muscle contraction. These mechanisms—especially reversible smooth muscle contraction—predominate in asthma. In COPD (emphysema and chronic bronchitis), these mechanisms also contribute to the changes in lung volumes. In addition, in COPD patients—predominantly in those with emphysema—there is a loss of elastin in the lungs, which decreases elastic recoil and further promotes increases in lung volumes.

DIFFUSION CAPACITY FOR CARBON MONOXIDE

Another pulmonary function test that is performed in the clinical laboratory is the measurement of the diffusion capacity for carbon monoxide ($D_L CO$). This test helps to assess the ability of the alveolar-capillary wall to transfer oxygen and carbon dioxide. Instead of using oxygen, the lung diffusion capacity for carbon monoxide is measured using a tracer amount of carbon monoxide. The $D_L CO$ can also be affected by alterations in hemoglobin and in pulmonary-capillary blood volume. However, if these parameters are normal, $D_L CO$ primarily reflects diseases that affect the alveolar-capillary wall. In asthma, the $D_L CO$ is normal or even high, because asthma does not primarily affect the alveoli. Similarly, in predominant chronic bronchitis, the $D_L CO$ is normal or only mildly decreased. However, in predominant emphysema, the $D_L CO$ is reduced by the destruction of alveoli, the gas-exchanging surface. This may help to distinguish emphysema from asthma.

WORK OF BREATHING

The work of breathing is increased in airflow obstruction. The patient must overcome the increased airflow resistance and changes in lung volumes, which also alter the mechanical advantage of the respiratory muscles. Airway obstruction produces hyperinflation through the generation of increased negative intrathoracic pressures needed to overcome increased airflow resistance. This hyperinflation reduces airway resistance but at the expense of an increase in elastic work required for breathing. The static pressure-volume curve, which is shifted upward in patients with airflow obstruction, demonstrates that more work is required to breathe at a higher lung volume. This increase in required work results from the lower compliance and reduced excursion of the lung at the higher lung volumes. This can be experienced by inhaling from a higher-than-normal resting lung volume (i.e., above FRC). It is more difficult and uncomfortable and requires more work by the respiratory muscles to breathe at this higher lung volume.

EFFECT OF AIRFLOW OBSTRUCTION ON CARDIAC FUNCTION

Airflow obstruction, which leads to an increase in intrathoracic pressures, also has effects on cardiac preload and afterload. Higher negative inspiratory pressures in the chest are transmitted to the heart, causing proportional reductions in intracardiac pressures. This results in pulsus paradoxus, which is the transient fall with inspiration and rise with expiration in systemic blood pressure. The severity of the pulsus paradoxus is measured as the difference in systolic blood pressure between expiration and inspiration.

Airflow obstruction may affect cardiac preload and afterload.

GAS-EXCHANGE ABNORMALITIES

Gas-exchange abnormalities observed in acute exacerbation of obstructive lung disease may show a reduction in blood oxygen tension (hypoxemia) with a reduction (hypocapnia) or an increase (hypercapnia) in blood carbon dioxide tension. The mechanisms involved include ventilation-perfusion mismatch, shunt, and hypoventilation (see Chapter 3). In mild asthma exacerbations, ventilation-perfusion mismatch is the predominant cause of hypoxemia. There is some contribution by shunt. In more severe asthma exacerbations, ventilation-perfusion inequality increases further and alveolar hypoventilation becomes more important in the development of hypercapnia (i.e., blood carbon dioxide retention). In emphysema, there is destruction of the alveoli with concomitant airspace enlargement. Ventilation is reduced in proportion to the perfusion, and there is minimal gas-exchange inequality at rest. During exercise, however, gas-exchange abnormalities become more severe. In chronic bronchitis, hypoxemia and hypercapnia are more common and severe than in predominant emphysema. As a group, abnormalities in pulmonary mechanics have a weak correlation with abnormalities in gas exchange.

Patients with obstructive airways disease may exhibit reduced blood oxygen and either decreased or increased blood carbon dioxide.

■ REVIEW QUESTIONS

1. Alterations in expiratory flow in individuals with chronic obstructive pulmonary disease (COPD) are attributable to all of the following except

   (A) increased mucus present in the airway lumen
   (B) a loss of airway tethering forces owing to lung destruction
   (C) inflammation, edema, and smooth muscle contraction of the airways
   (D) an increase in lung elasticity
   (E) decreased elastic recoil

2. In the absence of disease, airway caliber is predominantly under the control of the autonomic nervous system. Which one of the following statements is false regarding neural regulation of the airways?

   (A) The nonadrenergic, noncholinergic (NANC) nervous system has both excitatory and inhibitory effects on airway smooth muscle tone.
   (B) The sympathetic nervous system has a major role in normal regulation.
   (C) Stimulation of the cholinergic system results in release of acetylcholine, a potent bronchoconstrictor.
   (D) Other substances, such as substance P and vasoactive intestinal peptide, participate in local neural arcs to regulate airway smooth muscle tone.

3. In patients with COPD, which of the following changes are likely to be seen on pulmonary function tests?

   (A) $\uparrow$ RV, $\uparrow$ TLC, $\uparrow$ FRC, $\downarrow$ FEV$_1$, $\downarrow$ FVC
   (B) $\downarrow$ RV, $\downarrow$ TLC, $\downarrow$ FRC, $\uparrow$ FEV$_1$, FVC
   (C) $\uparrow$ RV, $\uparrow$ TLC, $\downarrow$ FRC, $\downarrow$ FEV$_1$, $\downarrow$ FVC
   (D) $\uparrow$ RV, $\downarrow$ TLC, $\downarrow$ FRC, $\downarrow$ FEV$_1$, $\downarrow$ FVC

4. For a patient being evaluated for chronic dyspnea, the results of pulmonary function tests were as follows:

TEST	ABSOLUTE VALUE (% OF PREDICTED)
Spirometry	
FVC	2.43 Liters (82%)
FEV$_1$	0.42 Liters (19%)
FEV$_1$/FVC ($\times$ 100)	17
Lung Volumes (Plethysmography)	
Vital capacity (L)	2.43 (82%)
Total lung capacity (L)	7.47 (154%)
Residual volume (L)	5.04 (268%)
Diffusion capacity for carbon monoxide (mL/min/mmHg)	4.7 (27%)

   These results are most consistent with

   (A) emphysema
   (B) idiopathic pulmonary fibrosis
   (C) asthma
   (D) chronic bronchitis
   (E) asbestosis

5. Which one of the following statements is not true of patients with airflow obstruction?

(A) Increases in intrathoracic pressures owing to airflow obstruction can increase ventricular afterload.

(B) The FVC and FEV_1 are reliable tests for the detection of airflow obstruction in small airways obstructive lung disease.

(C) Hypoxemia during COPD exacerbation results predominately from ventilation/perfusion mismatching.

(D) The severity of airflow obstruction is roughly proportional to the severity of pulsus paradoxus.

■ ANSWERS AND EXPLANATIONS

1. The answer is D. In general, there is a reduction in expiratory airflow in patients with COPD compared with normal individuals. This reduction is caused by several factors. For the chronic bronchitis component, there is a partial airway occlusion as a result of increased mucus secretion within the airway caused by an increase in the number of mucous glands. The airway lumen is further compromised because of underlying inflammation and the presence of inflammatory cells and their mediators, which lead to airway edema and smooth muscle contraction. For the emphysema component, there is a decrease in lung elasticity, causing a decreased elastic recoil, and a loss of the tethering forces on the airways as a result of alveolar destruction, causing airway collapse to occur more readily.

2. The answer is B. In normal conditions, the airway smooth muscle is under neural control. Normally, the sympathetic nervous system produces bronchodilation, but the effects are minimal. The cholinergic motoneurons are located in the brain stem and innervate the airways via the vagus nerve. The neurons release acetylcholine, a potent bronchoconstrictor. The NANC nervous system has both excitatory and inhibitory influences on smooth muscle tone. The inhibitory NANC is the primary neural bronchodilator pathway. Peptides such as substance P and vasoactive intestinal peptide are important transmitters released by the NANC system and cause either bronchoconstriction (substance P) or bronchodilation (vasoactive intestinal peptide).

3. The answer is A. In patients with airflow obstruction, several abnormalities can be detected on pulmonary function tests. Because of airflow obstruction from airway wall edema and thickening and smooth muscle contraction, there is an increase in RV as well as increases in FRC and TLC. When there is a loss of elastic recoil, both TLC and FRC are increased. FEV_1 is decreased and FVC is also usually decreased in moderate to severe airflow obstruction. The ratio of FEV_1/FVC is also decreased.

4. The answer is A. The spirometry is consistent with an obstructive process, as indicated by the reduced FEV_1/FVC ratio, which would eliminate the restrictive diseases of idiopathic pulmonary fibrosis and asbestosis. There are diseases with combined defects, but in this case the total lung capacity is increased, which would make the predominant defect obstructive. In emphysema, the lung volumes tend to be increased, and the diffusion capacity for carbon monoxide is reduced as a result of alveolar-capillary wall destruction. In predominantly chronic bronchitis, the diffusion capacity is usually not severely decreased. In asthma, the diffusion capacity is usually normal or high.

5. The answer is B. In airflow obstruction, high negative inspiratory pressures are transmitted to the heart and result in a decrease in intracardiac pressures and an increase in ventricular afterload. On the following beat, the ventricles may not be able to develop enough force to maintain arterial blood pressure, and pulsus paradoxus (a transient decrease in blood pressure with inspiration) develops. The severity of pulsus paradoxus is roughly proportional to the severity of airflow obstruction. The hypoxemia observed in airflow obstruction is thought to be caused by ventilation/perfusion mismatching that occurs in the lung because of: 1) increased ventilation of physiologic dead space, 2) perfusion of low V/Q units, and 3) hypoxic vasoconstriction of pulmonary vasculature. FVC and FEV_1 are reliable tests for detection of airflow obstruction in large airways.

■ SUGGESTED READING

Crapo RO: Pulmonary function testing. *N Engl J Med* 331(1):25–30, 1994.

Ferguson GT, Cherniak RM: Management of chronic obstructive pulmonary disease. *N Engl J Med* 328:1017–1022, 1993.

McFadden ER Jr, Gilbert IA: Asthma. *N Engl J Med* 327(27):1928–1937, 1992.

National Asthma Education Program Expert Panel: Guidelines for the Diagnosis and Management of Asthma (Expert Panel Report 2). Bethesda, MD: National Institutes of Health, 1997, 97–4051:1–86.

Travaline JM, Criner GJ: Pulmonary function testing using a spirometer. *Hosp Pract* 30:57–62, 1994.

Chapter 5

PARENCHYMAL INFLAMMATION AND INJURY

Clarke U. Piatt, M.D.

Gerald O'Brien, M.D.

■ CHAPTER OUTLINE

Learning Objectives
Case Study: Introduction
Pulmonary Parenchymal Structure and Function
Case Study: Continued
Inhalation Injury
Acute Lung Injury
Lung Function
Therapy and Outcome
Case Study: Resolution
Review Questions

■ LEARNING OBJECTIVES

At the completion of this chapter, the reader should:
- Be able to review the normal parenchymal structure of the lung.
- Be able to describe the patho-biological model of acute lung injury (ALI).
- Be able to describe how humoral mediators affect lung repair.
- Understand how parenchymal lung inflammation and fibrosis affect lung function.

Case Study: *Introduction*	*J. S., a 40-year-old firefighter, presents to the emergency room with complaints of progressive shortness of breath that began while he was fighting a house fire. Although he did not enter the structure, he and another firefighter were on the roof of the structure for approximately 2 hours. He initially reported relatively minor symptoms, with a cough and mild dyspnea. However, on arrival at the emergency department, his dyspnea becomes more severe and he is placed on supplemental oxygen delivered by a face mask at 1.0 F_1O_2, which results in some symptomatic improvement.* *The patient denies having other medical problems but admits to smoking one-half pack of cigarettes per day for 10 years. He has been a fireman for 15 years and has had previous smoke inhalation injuries but never as severe as this episode. His review of symptoms is otherwise unremarkable.* *On physical exam, he appears to be in moderate respiratory distress, with a temperature of 99.8°F, a blood pressure of 150/84, and a respiratory rate of 28 breaths per minute. There are no burns, but there is noticeable soot about the nares and his cough is productive of carbonaceous sputum. Initial examination of the nasal mucosa and oropharynx reveals pink mucosa without evidence of burns. No stridor or accessory respiratory muscle use is noted. Auscultation of the chest reveals coarse bilateral wheezes and bibasilar crackles. No clubbing or cyanosis is noted.*

▌PULMONARY PARENCHYMAL STRUCTURE AND ▌FUNCTION

The pulmonary parenchyma is a complex arrangement of tissues and structural elements excluding the larger pulmonary vessels and airways. More specifically, the parenchyma constitutes the terminal respiratory units, which are composed of the alveolar duct together with the accompanying interconnected alveoli (Figure 5-1).

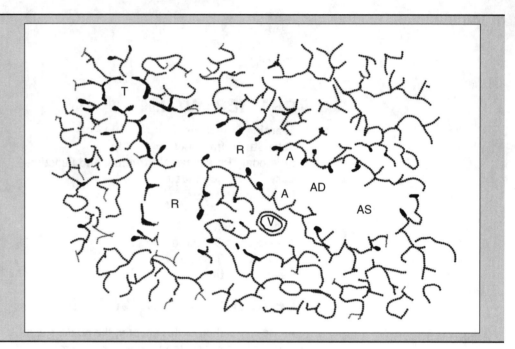

FIGURE 5-1
Terminal respiratory unit. T = terminal bronchiole, R = respiratory bronchiole, A = alveolus, AD = alveolar ducts, AS = alveolar sacs, V = vessel.

The alveolus is a saccular structure composed mostly of capillaries, which form its outer wall. The capillary endothelial cells rest on a basement membrane that appears to be fused with the endothelial basement membrane of the alveolar lumen over half of the capillary perimeter. This thin portion of the alveolar capillary septum allows for optimal gas exchange because of the short distance for gas diffusion. Over the other half of the capillary perimeter, the capillary basement membrane is separated from the alveolar basement membrane, forming an interstitial space (Figure 5-2). The capillaries branch frequently, giving rise to an extensive mesh extending over several alveoli before draining into a pulmonary venule.

The alveolar lumen is lined by type I and type II pneumocytes, which sit on a basement membrane. The type I pneumocyte is a squamous epithelial cell that forms a tight barrier to the passage of both water and solutes into the alveolar space. About 95% of the alveolar lumen consists of type I pneumocytes. The type II pneumocyte is a cuboidal cell with a granular cytoplasm that has several metabolic roles, such as the production of surfactants. Surfactants are lipoproteins that are insoluble and form a thin layer at the air-fluid interface within the alveolar lumen. These molecules serve to reduce surface tension and the elastic forces present within the alveolar wall. Type II cells are also the precursors of the type I cells. The interstitium refers specifically to a potential space interposed between the alveolar epithelial and capillary endothelial basement membranes. This space contains the lung's connective tissue elements consisting primarily of collagen, elastin, and reticulin. These proteins contribute to the lung's normal elastic properties. The bulk of the interstitium, however, is composed of glycosaminoglycosides, which are complex giant polysaccharides that form a gel-like substance. The interstitial space also normally includes a variety of cellular elements such as macrophages, dendritic cells, lymphocytes, and fibroblasts.

The parenchymal interstitium is contiguous with, and extends beyond, the anatomic boundaries of the terminal respiratory unit to include the bronchovascular interstitial space. This space is composed of loose connective tissue that supports the bronchi and the vascular and lymphatic elements of the lung.

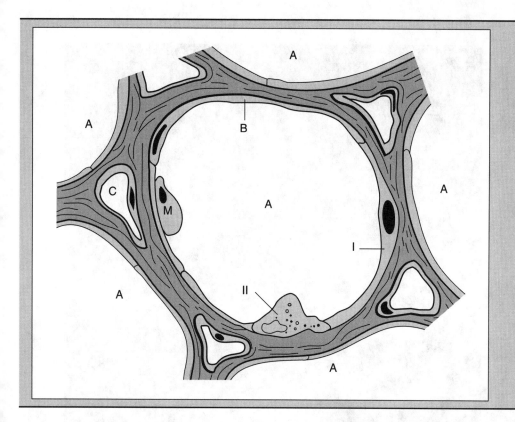

FIGURE 5-2
Interstitial space between alveoli. A = alveolus, C = capillary, I = type I pneumocyte, B = basement membrane, M = monocyte.

Within 6 hours of his presentation to the emergency room, J. S. exhibits progressive symptoms of dyspnea with evidence of respiratory fatigue on physical exam, requiring endotracheal intubation and mechanical ventilation. Inspection of his airway with a bronchoscope does not reveal any evidence of mucosal burns. Frothy, carbonaceous secretions are noted emanating from the lower lobe bronchi. A repeat chest x-ray reveals diffuse bilateral infiltrates consistent with acute lung injury (Figure 5-3).

Case Study:
Continued

■ INHALATION INJURY

Inhalation injury affecting the terminal respiratory unit occurs only through the inhalation of particles or aerosol droplets less than 1 μm in diameter. Chemicals that are water soluble and ionic, such as acids and aldehydes, generally adhere to the mucus lining the respiratory tract and may cause toxic cellular damage to the airway epithelium. However, alveolar injury may occur when these chemicals become adsorbed to small particles of soot that are able to reach the alveoli. Toxic gases that have low water solubility, are nonionic, and are highly lipid soluble, such as phosgene, metal fumes, and ozone, are capable of reaching the alveolar unit in a gaseous phase and can cause direct cellular injury.

The lung must act as a defense barrier against the constant exposure to airborne challenges. Inhaled toxins include gases and vapors of volatile liquids and aerosols. Aerosols consist of suspensions of solid particles and water droplets and may also contain dusts, fumes, and mists. Inhalation of these substances may cause illness through anoxia, direct lung injury, and systemic toxicity. The clinical presentation of this type of injury is dependent on the particular toxin and its kinetics as well as on the length and intensity of exposure. Moreover, pulmonary parenchymal injury may occur if the normal pulmonary defense mechanisms become overwhelmed or if there is ineffective clearing of inhaled debris.

The thermal effects of smoke inhalation are usually isolated to the upper respiratory tract and large airways. The same is true for the water-soluble gaseous by-products of combustion, such as ammonia, chlorine, and sulfur dioxide, which bind to the moist airways and form strong acids. Particles larger than 10 μm are usually trapped by the

Toxic Components of House Fire Smoke

Water-Soluble Components

- Chlorine gas
- Ammonia
- Sulfur dioxide

Lipid-Soluble Components

- Phosgene
- Acrolein
- Nitrous oxide
- Hydrochloric acid

Absorbed Toxins

- Carbon monoxide
- Cyanide

FIGURE 5-3
Chest radiograph of 40-year-old male patient in respiratory distress after inhalation injury.

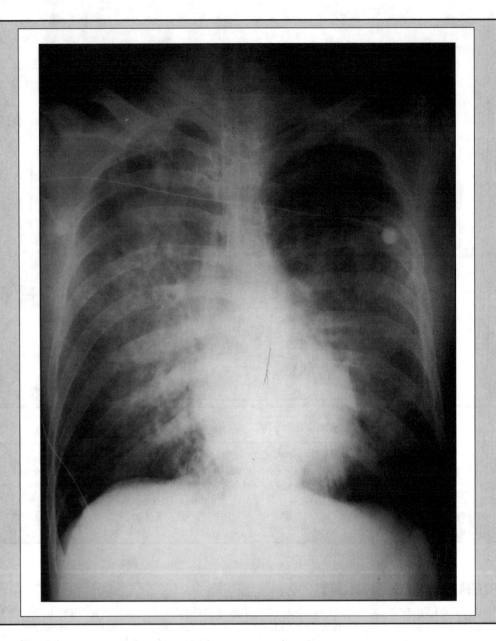

mucociliary defenses of the upper airways and primarily cause mucosal edema, mucus hypersecretion, and airflow obstruction. Direct chemical injury to the epithelium by the toxic by-products of combustion, or by inhaled soot particles, is often the initial step.

ACUTE LUNG INJURY

Definition of Acute Lung Injury (ALI)

ALI is defined as a syndrome of pulmonary inflammation and increased pulmonary capillary permeability that is associated with a constellation of clinical, radiographic, and physiologic abnormalities that cannot be explained by left atrial hypertension.

Patients with significant injury or inflammation of the terminal respiratory units can progress to a syndrome of severe respiratory distress associated with an acute onset of diffuse infiltrates on chest radiograph and with hypoxemia. The diagnosis is usually based on clinical criteria and is termed acute lung injury (ALI).

Respiratory symptoms other than dyspnea are uncommon. Cough, when present, is usually a manifestation of coexisting inflammatory airway injury. On pulmonary examination, crackles can be heard but wheezing and rhonchi usually are not present. The remainder of the physical examination is unremarkable unless an associated comorbid condition exists. Respiratory symptoms often precede the chest x-ray findings, but bilateral alveolar infiltrates usually appear within 24 hours of the inhalational exposure.

Although these infiltrates tend to be bilateral and homogeneous in distribution on chest x-ray, heterogeneous distribution with a predominance in the more dependent lung regions is observed when one performs a more sensitive and specific study, such as a computed tomography (CT) scan.

The acute stage is characterized by an acute and diffuse involvement of the epithelial and endothelial cells, lasts 1 to 3 days, and is commonly referred to as diffuse alveolar damage (DAD). Histologic examination shows epithelial cell necrosis with an intra-alveolar fibrinous exudate dominated by neutrophils and macrophages associated with hyaline membranes, and interstitial edema. This stage is temporally followed by a reparative process and organization dominated by type II cell hyperplasia, fibroblastic infiltration, and resolution of hyaline membranes. A mild degree of interstitial cellular infiltration of lymphocytes and plasma cells is common. The process may resolve or may lead to extensive fibrosis after as little as 7 days. The evolution of acute lung injury can be further defined into three phases: exudative, proliferative, and fibrotic.

EXUDATIVE PHASE

The parenchymal lung inflammation evident during the early phases of ALI is the result of complex cellular and humoral interactions that lead to tissue destruction (Figure 5-4). The type I pneumocytes appear more sensitive to injury than type II pneumocytes. The loss of the tight barrier afforded by the type I epithelial cells results in flooding of the alveolar space with a protein-rich fluid. The delayed clearance of fluid within the alveolar lumen, coupled with epithelial cell death, results in the accumulation of macrophages and debris, causing a characteristic histologic alveolitis. If this exudate is not rapidly cleared from the alveolar airways, it may lead to further epithelial injury and death, producing denudation of the alveolar wall, destruction of the alveolar basement membrane, and humoral amplification of the host immune response. Proliferation and hyperplasia of type II cells, which are the acting precursors for reepithelialization during the normal repair process, are prominent features of the late exudative phase of ALI. These cells are also responsible for the synthesis and secretion of surfactant. However, both secretion and synthesis of surfactant in patients with ALI have been shown to be reduced. Moreover, biophysical studies have demonstrated that the function of surfactant obtained from lungs with ALI is abnormal, presumably as a result of chemical alteration by intra-alveolar fluid.

Acute Lung Injury Criteria

- Identifiable cause or known precipitating condition
- Dyspnea, usually severe hypoxemia
- $P_aO_2/F_IO_2 < 300$ mmHg
- Diffuse radiographic infiltrates
- Reduced compliance
- No evidence for cardiac etiology of pulmonary edema

ALI Pathologic Phases

- Exudative phase
- Proliferative phase
- Fibrotic phase

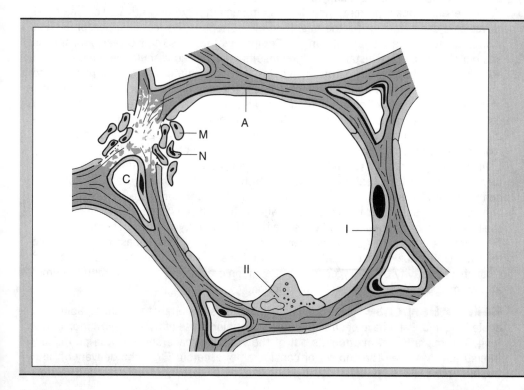

FIGURE 5-4
Exudative phase of ALI: death of type I pneumocyte with damage to underlying alveolar basement membrane (A) and migration of monocytes (M) and neutrophils (N). C = capillary.

Humoral Response. The macrophage is thought to play the central role in the pathogenesis and progression of lung inflammation, because large numbers of macrophages are present within the alveolar space and interstitium in patients with early ALI. Activated macrophages secrete cytokines, which result in the production of secondary mediators and activate other cells that perpetuate the inflammatory reaction (Table 5-1). Cytokines have both systemic and local effects. Systemically, these compounds may

Table 5-1
Cytokines Involved in Acute Lung Injury

CYTOKINE	SOURCES	MAIN EFFECTS
Tumor necrosis factor (TNF)	Macrophages, T cells, mast cells	Fever, leukocytosis, cofactor in macrophage activation, enhances phagocytic immunity
Interleukin-1 (IL-1)	Macrophages, endothelial cells, fibroblasts	Fever, cofactor for proliferation of B, T, endothelial, and stem cells
Interleukin-6 (IL-6)	Macrophages, endothelial cells, T cells	Fever, enhances release of acute phase reactants from liver
Interleukin-8 (IL-8)	Macrophages, endothelial cells	Neutrophil chemotaxis, adherence, and activation
Interferon gamma (IFN-γ)	T cells, null killer (NK) cells	Macrophage activation

Acute Phase Reaction Proteins

- C-reactive proteins (CRPs)
- Proteinase inhibitors (1-AT)
- Coagulation proteins (ferritin)
- Metal-binding proteins (haptoglobin)
- Complement proteins

cause fever and leukocytosis through the accelerated release of white cells from the bone marrow. Locally, they influence tissue repair and regeneration in response to injury and have profound effects on endothelium and fibroblast function. Their effects on endothelium serve to increase neutrophil and lymphocyte adhesion by inducing the synthesis of adhesion molecules. Cytokines can stimulate the synthesis and release of acute phase response proteins. The acute phase response (APR) is the systemic reaction to injury, characterized by abrupt changes in the concentration of certain plasma proteins. The specific function of each these proteins is not fully understood, but they appear to play a role in the maintenance and restoration of systemic homeostasis during and after injury. The production and expression of acute phase proteins are regulated by cytokines and growth factors as well as by glucocorticoids. Initiation of the acute phase response involves several steps that include mediator binding to the appropriate cell receptor, transduction of the signal to the cell nucleus where the acute phase protein gene is either up- or down-regulated, and finally protein synthesis.

Other acute phase proteins include the complement proteins. Activated complement serves as a chemotactant for the migration of neutrophils, eosinophils, basophils, and monocytes to the areas of alveolar injury. Complement may also cause nearby mast cells and platelets to release histamine, which results in increased vascular permeability and edema at the site of injury. Other molecules that participate in systemic response to injury include the arachidonic acid metabolites. These lipid mediators act as regulators of the inflammatory reaction. Arachidonic acid is released from the membrane of injured cells and acts as a substrate for the production of compounds that enhance the inflammatory reaction in the lung. Prostaglandins are generated through the action of cyclooxygenase on arachidonic acid and influence both platelet and neutrophil activation. Leukotrienes generated through the activity of lipoxygenase on arachidonic acid acts as a neutrophil chemoattractant and can induce bronchoconstriction (Figure 5-5). Activated complement also serves to opsonize foreign particles and facilitate phagocytosis. Arachidonic acid is released from the membranes of injured cells and acts as a substrate for the production of compounds that enhance the inflammatory reaction in the lung (Figure 5-5). Prostaglandins are generated through the action of cyclooxygenase on arachidonic acid and influence both platelet and neutrophil activation. Leukotrienes, generated through the activity of lipoxygenase on arachidonic acid, act as a neutrophil chemoattractant and can induce bronchoconstriction.

Leukocyte Retention

Step 1: Rolling
Step 2: Activation
Step 3: Adherence
Step 4: Migration

Cellular Response. Neutrophils are the earliest inflammatory cells to appear in acute lung injury and have been implicated as a major cause of tissue destruction of the lung. The migration of neutrophils out of the vascular space and into the pulmonary interstitium has been the subject of considerable research. First, the delivery of neutrophils into the lung is enhanced by mobilization of demarginated cells and marrow

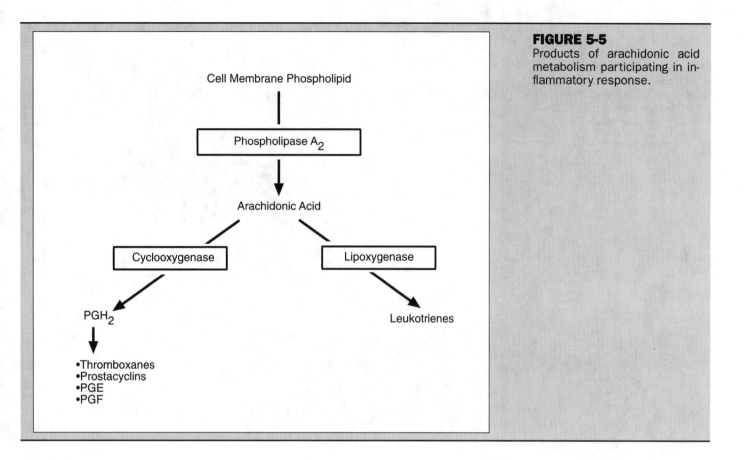

FIGURE 5-5
Products of arachidonic acid metabolism participating in inflammatory response.

reserves. The next phase involves humoral alteration of the normally balanced retentive and dispersive cellular determinants within the pulmonary vasculature, favoring an increase in pulmonary capillary neutrophil retention (Figure 5-6). These determinants include alteration in the neutrophil biophysical properties and increased adhesive properties of both the neutrophil endothelial cells, which promote transmigration of the leukocytes from the intravascular space into the interstitial space, and the alveolar lumen. The neutrophil becomes primed through a complex series of transmembrane signaling events prior to or during migration into the alveolar lumen. This means that when these cells are exposed to an activating stimulus, they become several times more responsive than nonprimed cells. Neutrophil extravasation from the blood is a regulated multi-step process resulting from interactions between the neutrophil and the vascular endothelium. Molecular regulators found on the surface membrane of these cells regulate the process and appear to be the result of cytokine induced expression. The first two steps in this process are called "rolling" followed by "adherence." A family of molecular regulators known as "selectins" facilitates these steps. "Activation" and ultimately "migration" appear to be regulated by another family of molecules known as "integrins." Interleukin-8 has been shown to be the most likely cytokine capable of providing this priming stimulus among patients with ALI.

Neutrophil-mediated alveolar epithelial cell injury may occur through the enhanced release of oxygen metabolites and proteases by the primed neutrophil during particle phagocytosis. Neutrophils contain enzymes that can reduce molecular oxygen into highly reactive free radical species (Figure 5-7). These compounds can cause direct tissue injury through membrane lipid peroxidation. Neutrophil lysosomal proteases are capable of degrading collagen, elastin, proteoglycans, and other structural proteins found within the lung parenchyma. However, proteolytic epithelial injury is normally held in check by antiproteases found within normal lung tissue. Oxidative inactivation of these proteases has been shown to render the epithelium susceptible to proteolytic attack.

Pulmonary Capillary Injury. Pulmonary capillary endothelial integrity is altered early in ALI. Electron micrographic studies have demonstrated cellular edema and

FIGURE 5-6

Interactions of humoral and cellular elements in the inflammatory response. TGF = transforming growth factor, PAF = platelet activating factor, ICAM = intercellular adhesion molecule.

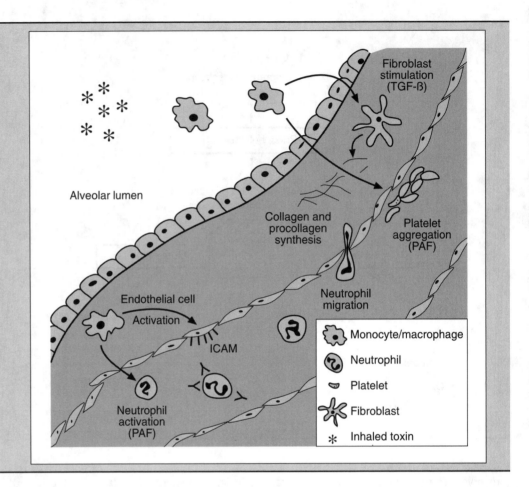

FIGURE 5-7

Free radical production by activated neutrophil. NADH = reduced form of nicotinamide adenine dinucleotide (NAD), NAD$^+$ = oxidized form of NAD.

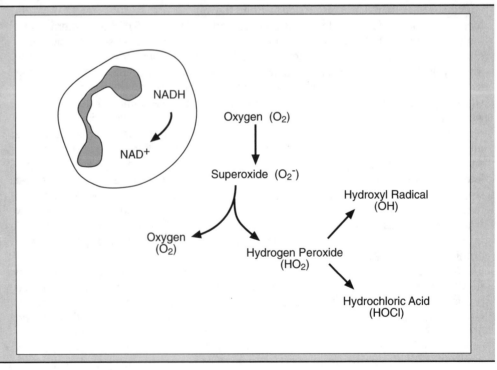

blistering. Injured endothelial cells contract, causing wide intercellular gaps that lead to formation of interstitial edema. The products of arachidonic acid metabolism contribute to the local inflammatory reaction by inducing vasodilation (prostacyclin), vasoconstriction (thromboxane, leukotriene B_4), and increased vascular permeability (prostaglandin E_2, leukotriene B_4). Moreover, vascular occlusion from neutrophil, platelet, and fibrin thrombi are commonly found within pulmonary capillaries. It seems most likely that these lesions develop in situ. This process may result from pulmonary vascular endothelial activation, or from platelet and neutrophil vascular sequestration as a result of humoral mediated enhanced aggregation.

PROLIFERATIVE PHASE

The pathogenic sequence leading to irreversible lung damage has still not been clearly defined, but it is felt that inflammation plays a critical role. If there is resolution of inflammation, lung structure is repaired and pulmonary function returns to a normal or nearly normal state. On the other hand, if inflammation continues, or if the repair process has been affected, severe scarring and fibrosis develop within the lung parenchyma. Fibrin fragments have been shown in vitro to promote fibroblast proliferation, retraction of endothelial cells, and smooth muscle cell proliferation. In this model of lung injury, intra-alveolar macrophages further exacerbate injury by causing alveolar epithelial cell ulceration and migration of fibroblasts into the alveolar space (Figure 5-8).

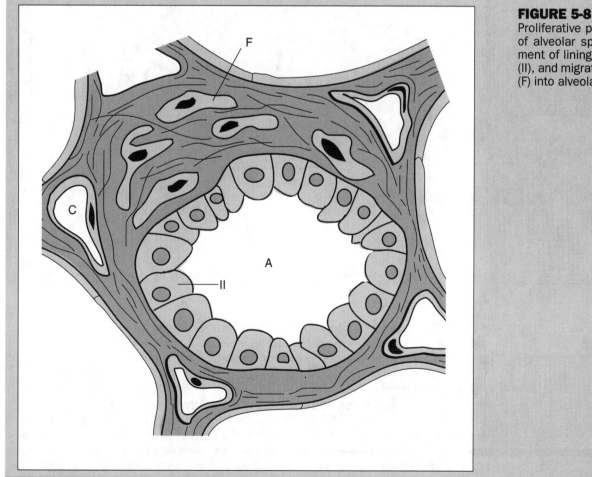

FIGURE 5-8
Proliferative phase of ALI: loss of alveolar space (A), replacement of lining with type II cells (II), and migration of fibroblasts (F) into alveolar space.

Products of Activated Fibroblasts

- Matrix protein elements
  - Collagens, types I and II
  - Fibronectin
  - Elastin
- Arachidonic acid metabolites
- Cytokines

FIBROTIC PHASE

Many pulmonary fibroblasts have distinctive phenotypic markers resembling the myofibroblasts found in skin wound healing and contraction. Ultimately, alveolar fibrosis occurs with fibroblast deposition in a collagen matrix within the air space, leading to alveolar collapse and distortion of normal lung architecture (Figure 5-9).

The rapidity and efficiency with which inflammatory cells and their products are removed from the alveolar space would reasonably be expected to contribute to the balance between resolution and progression of the subsequent fibrotic process. Several theories have been put forth as to why an abnormal repair mechanism may exist in this

FIGURE 5-9

Fibrotic phase of ALI: original architecture of terminal respiratory unit remodeled from collapse and loss of alveolar space (A), forming air cysts (AC) lined with modified epithelium (E) and forming a fibrotic interstitial space (IS).

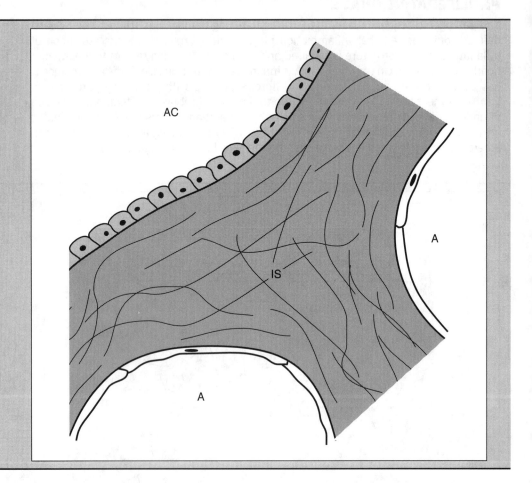

process. One hypothesis suggests that the reparative mechanism is governed by the degree and severity of the initial, or recurrent, alveolar epithelial injury. It has been suggested that disruption of this normal reepithelialization process could set the stage for abnormal alveolar wall repair. For example, if the initial injury is so severe that it results in the destruction of the scaffolding and normal architecture of the lung parenchyma, the reparative process would occur in a disorganized arrangement of connective tissue proteins and scar tissue. The mechanisms by which the immunoeffector cells and cytokines participate in the development of parenchymal lung fibrosis remain undefined.

One of the central questions has been the identification of the cytokines and growth factors driving the fibroproliferative reaction. Attention has been focused on the family of cytokines known as transforming growth factors (TGFs). TGFs are a family of five polypeptide growth factors, produced by macrophages, that stimulate connective tissue growth and collagen formation. Another fibroblast-targeted cytokine is the platelet-derived growth factor (PDGF). PDGF together with insulin-like growth factor (IGF) stimulate fibroblast mitosis and proliferation. Transcription of both fibronectin and procollagen genes has been shown to be increased by TGFs, resulting in increased matrix protein synthesis. Moreover, TGFs inhibit proteolytic degradation of newly formed matrix proteins (Table 5-2).

GROWTH FACTOR(S)	SOURCE(S)	MAIN FUNCTIONS
Transforming growth factors (TFG-α-β)	Macrophages, platelets	Stimulate mesenchymal cell and endothelial cell replication
Platelet-derived growth factor (PDGF)	Platelets, macrophages, endothelial cells, fibroblasts	Stimulate mesenchymal cell migration and replication
Insulin-like growth factor (IGF)	Hepatocytes	Progression signal for fibroblasts that acts on G_1*
Alveolar macrophage growth factor (AMDGF)	Macrophages	Progression signal for fibroblasts that acts on G_1*
Interleukin-1 (IL-1)	Macrophages, lymphocytes	Stimulates synthesis of collagen and collagenase, activates endothelial cells and macrophages

* Cellular growth phase of the cell cycle

Table 5-2
Growth Factors Involved in Lung Repair

■ LUNG FUNCTION

GAS-EXCHANGE ABNORMALITIES IN ACUTE LUNG INJURY

In ALI, it is tempting to assume that the oxygenation abnormality observed is the result of pulmonary edema and thus resembles the hypoxemia seen in congestive heart failure. However, several studies have failed to show a direct correlation between the severity of hypoxemia and the amount of extravascular lung water or lung microvascular permeability. The capillary and the alveolar wall are in direct contact on one side of the capillary with little intervening interstitial matrix. This is where gas exchange occurs. The opposite side of the capillary is the thicker side where extravascular lung water accumulates and where most cases of ALI do not severely affect oxygen diffusion.

The principal cause of hypoxemia is extensive right-to-left intrapulmonary shunting of blood flow. Normally, the regional pulmonary blood flow is reduced in regions of the lung that have become flooded through the mechanism of hypoxic vasoconstriction. In ALI, however, this defense mechanism becomes subverted and the pulmonary circulation does not appear to be capable of directing blood flow distribution away from the injured lung units to optimize ventilation and perfusion. An increase in shunt occurs through the persistent perfusing of atelectatic and fluid-filled alveoli.

Hypoxemia is further worsened by an increase in dead space ventilation. Dead space is the percent of tidal volume (normally less than 30% of total ventilation) that does not participate in gas exchange by ventilating the alveolus but only ventilates the conducting airways. During the fibroproliferative phase of acute lung injury, progressive amounts of the pulmonary capillary bed become obliterated, contributing to the increase in wasted ventilation. During the fibroproliferative phases, dead space increases to as much as 80% of total ventilation. The simplest method of quantifying hypoxemia is simultaneously to measure P_aO_2 and F_IO_2 and express oxygenation as the ratio P_aO_2/F_IO_2. Normal values for this ratio range from 500 to 600. In ALI, this ratio falls below 300.

Physiologic Changes of ALI

- Increased shunt fraction with increased dead space
- Decreased compliance with increased work of breathing
- Compensatory tachypnea

VENTILATION

Ventilation is the process of exchanging oxygen and carbon dioxide between the atmosphere and the individual. This process is achieved through the actions of the muscles of respiration, which include the diaphragm and the accessory respiratory muscles. These muscles must overcome both the frictional resistance to airflow within the tracheobronchial tree and the elastic recoil properties of the chest wall and lung parenchyma. It is possible to assess the elastic properties of the lung during breathing by calculating lung compliance. Lung compliance is a change in lung volume for a given change in intrapulmonary pressure. As the lungs become stiff and compliance becomes reduced, lung elastic recoil pressure varies in a nonlinear fashion that changes with the lung volume. This relationship is known as the volume-pressure curve (Figure 5-10). During the acute phases of ALI, the lungs become stiff as a result of alveolar flooding and edema, and the volume-pressure curve shifts downward and rightward.

FIGURE 5-10
Lung pressure-volume curves: emphysema, normal, and fibrosis. TLC = total lung capacity.

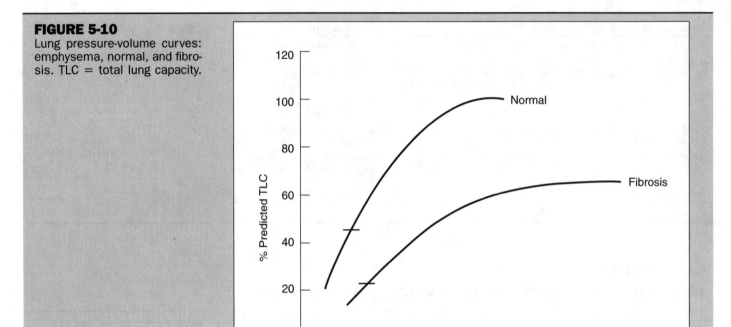

As the lung becomes stiff and more difficult to inflate, the patient is forced to take more shallow breaths. Atelectasis develops, thus further reducing lung compliance. Areas of alveolar flooding adjacent to normal or unaffected lung units result in ineffective ventilation in these regions as well, leading to further problems in oxygenation. To maintain adequate minute ventilation, and to compensate for the increase in physiologic dead space caused by shallow breathing, the patient must breathe faster. A minute ventilation of 30 L/min or more may be necessary to maintain eucapnia. Although the work of breathing may normally account for less than 15% of the total body energy needs, among patients with ALI, this work may exceed more than 50% of total body energy expenditure. This higher elastic work load may ultimately lead to overt ventilatory failure.

PULMONARY HYPERTENSION

Pulmonary hypertension is common in ALI and appears to be related to several factors. Increased pulmonary vascular resistance may result from regional thromboxane-induced vasoconstriction. This process appears to occur early and is usually of only short duration. The most significant cause of pulmonary hypertension appears to result from vascular resistance of neutrophils, platelets, and fibrin thrombi. Sustained elevation in pulmonary artery pressure observed days after the initial injury is more likely a reflection of the degree of lung fibrosis and pulmonary vascular bed obliteration.

■ THERAPY AND OUTCOME

Therapy remains supportive, and includes mechanical ventilation, hemodynamic support, and infection control. Several anti-inflammatory agents have been studied, including corticosteroids, prostaglandin inhibitors, and monoclonal antibodies against tumor necrosis factor (TNF) and interleukin-2 (IL-2). However, none of these therapies has shown significant survival benefit. The use of inhaled nitric oxide has shown promise in improving oxygenation, through its effect as a selective pulmonary vasodilator. Patient outcomes from ALI range from death to complete recovery. Mortality ranges from 40% to 70%. It is impossible to predict clinical course and prognosis in any given patient, but most patients who die do so within the first few days or weeks of ALI. Long-term functional outcome for survivors remains good: patients who survive often regain normal or nearly normal lung function.

Case Study:
Resolution

The patient is transferred to the intensive care unit, and over the next 3 days he requires higher levels of inspired oxygen and becomes increasingly more difficult to ventilate owing to reduced lung compliance. He is given IV sedation, and a pulmonary arterial catheter is inserted and reveals a cardiac output of 8 L/min, a pulmonary arterial pressure of 40/20 mmHg, and a pulmonary capillary wedge pressure of 16 mmHg, consistent with the diagnosis of acute lung injury or noncardiogenic pulmonary edema from smoke inhalation. The chest x-ray shows diffuse alveolar-interstitial infiltrates. He becomes more difficult to oxygenate and eventually requires elective intubation and mechanical ventilation. After several days of supportive care, including ventilation, enteral feeding, and prophylaxis for deep venous thrombosis and stress gastritis, he is successfully weaned and extubated. One year later, he returns to work and has normal lung function and gas exchange.

■ REVIEW QUESTIONS

1. The predominant type of epithelial cell in the normal alveolus is the

   (A) type II cell
   (B) type I cell
   (C) monocyte

2. Smoke inhalation causes acute lung injury at the level of the terminal alveolar unit as a result of

   (A) thermal injury
   (B) carbon monoxide poisoning
   (C) exposure to inhaled irritants
   (D) two of the above

3. Which one of the following is not a condition that may precipitate acute lung injury?

   (A) Asbestos exposure
   (B) Trauma
   (C) Sepsis
   (D) Severe burns
   (E) Drug overdose

4. The phases of acute lung injury are

   (A) proliferation, fibrosis, consolidation
   (B) exudative, proliferative, consolidation
   (C) exudative, fibrotic, consolidation
   (D) exudative, proliferative, fibrotic
   (E) consolidation, exudative, proliferative

5. The predominant inflammatory cells present during the exudative phase are

   (A) neutrophils
   (B) lymphocytes
   (C) macrophages
   (D) A and C
   (E) A, B, and C

6. Which one of the following functions is not performed by cytokines during inflammation and injury?

   (A) Activation of T lymphocytes
   (B) Activation of macrophages
   (C) Inducement of the production of other cytokines
   (D) Activation of clotting factors

7. Fibroblasts are activated by

   (A) the complement system
   (B) interleukins
   (C) TNF
   (D) A and B
   (E) B and C
   (F) none of the above

ANSWERS AND EXPLANATIONS

1. The answer is A. The type II pneumocyte is the most predominant cell in the alveolar epithelium. Type I cells, although they comprise more area of the alveolar epithelium, are fewer in number.

2. The answer is D. Thermal injury and exposure to inhaled irritants toxic to epithelial cells can cause acute lung injury. Although carbon monoxide poisoning causes profound systemic effects with decreased oxygen delivery, carbon monoxide itself does not directly cause epithelial cell injury.

3. The answer is A. Asbestos exposure does not result in acute lung injury but may cause chronic pulmonary fibrosis.

4. The answer is D. The phases of acute lung injury are exudative, proliferative, and fibrotic. The exudative phase follows acute injury and damage to the epithelium and basement membrane with migration of macrophages and neutrophils into the interstitium and alveolar space. The alveolar unit is reorganized, with a change to type II epithelial cells and an influx of lymphocytes and fibroblasts into the interstitium in the proliferative phase. During the fibrotic phase, the collagen is laid down in the interstitium, with overall remodeling of the alveolar unit.

5. The answer is D. The predominant cells of the exudative phase are macrophages and neutrophils, which are recruited after acute lung injury by activation of the complement cascade. These cells in turn release cytokines, which activate other inflammatory cells.

6. The answer is D. Cytokines do not play a direct role in activating the clotting cascade.

7. The answer is E. Both interleukin and tumor necrosis factor activate fibroblasts.

Chapter 6
PULMONARY HYPERTENSION

Trudy A. Kantra, D.O.

Gilbert E. D'Alonzo, D.O.

■ CHAPTER OUTLINE

Learning Objectives
Introduction
Definition and Classification
Case Study: Introduction
History and Physical Examination
Case Study: Continued
Diagnostic Evaluation
Case Study: Continued
Primary Pulmonary Hypertension (PPH)
Case Study: Resolution
Management of Pulmonary Hypertension
Summary
Review Questions

■ LEARNING OBJECTIVES

At the completion of this chapter, the reader should:
- Understand the various causes of pulmonary hypertension (PH) and how its presence can complicate a variety of common diseases.
- Be aware that pulmonary hypertension may substantially change the clinical presentation of the concomitant underlying disease and will worsen the prognosis.
- Be able to appreciate the basic diagnostic process of pulmonary hypertension.
- Appreciate how pulmonary hypertension and its complications can be treated.

■ INTRODUCTION

PH generally remains clinically silent until its pathophysiologic alterations are advanced.

Pulmonary hypertension (PH) may complicate the courses of many pulmonary and cardiac disorders or can develop as a primary disease affecting only the pulmonary vessels. Whether it is primary or secondary, the pathophysiologic alterations caused by PH usually remain clinically silent until the process is far advanced; then the patient often presents with severe exercise limitation, signs of right-sided heart failure, or symptoms suggesting a decrease in left ventricular output. Because a routine screening procedure for this disorder is not available, the physician must have a high index of suspicion when dealing with patients who are at risk for developing PH.

A high index of suspicion is necessary for early diagnosis of PH.

■ DEFINITION AND CLASSIFICATION

PH is defined as a mean pulmonary arterial pressure greater than 25 mmHg at rest or 30 mmHg during exercise.

Pulmonary hypertension is defined as a mean pulmonary arterial pressure greater than 25 mmHg at rest or 30 mmHg during exercise. There are various ways of categorizing etiologies of this disorder. A useful approach, based on the major physiologic mechanism, is shown in Table 6-1. A second classification, organized according to the anatomic site of the underlying disease process, is shown in Table 6-2. In this system, the two major anatomic categories of PH are postcapillary and mixed capillary or precapillary. Postcapillary PH is most commonly associated with the diseases of the left heart that cause the pulmonary venous pressure to be elevated, with a passive increase in pulmo-

Table 6-1
Pathophysiologic Classification of Pulmonary Hypertension

TYPE	MECHANISM	EXAMPLES
Passive	Resistance to pulmonary venous drainage	Mitral stenosis; pulmonary veno-occlusive disease
Hyperkinetic	Increased pulmonary blood flow	Atrial septal defect; ventricular septal defect
Obstructive	Resistance to flow through large pulmonary arteries	Pulmonary thromboembolism; unilateral absence or stenosis of a pulmonary artery
Obliterative	Resistance to flow through small pulmonary blood vessels	Primary pulmonary hypertension; collagen vascular disease
Vasoconstrictive	Resistance to flow from hypoxia-induced vasoconstriction	Chronic mountain sickness; sleep apnea syndrome
Polygenic	Two or more of the mechanisms listed above	Obliterative and vasoconstrictive COPD or interstitial pulmonary fibrosis

nary arterial pressure. Less common diseases that can cause pulmonary venous obstruction, such as pulmonary veno-occlusive disease and constrictive mediastinitis, are also classified as postcapillary. Mixed capillary or precapillary PH is associated with normal left ventricular end-diastolic pressure and is secondary to diseases of the lung parenchyma or pulmonary vessels in which the cross-sectional vascular bed surface area is decreased. Pulmonary hypertension may also occur secondary to left-to-right intracardiac shunts, in which increased pulmonary blood flow is the initial insult, and subsequent anatomic remodeling of the pulmonary vessels accentuates the problem. Extrapulmonary parenchymal diseases, such as severe kyphoscoliosis and fibrothorax, produce distortion of the chest cavity, mechanical compression of the lung parenchyma, and alveolar hypoventilation. This may lead to a substantial degree of PH caused primarily by hypoxic vasoconstriction.

Table 6-2
Classification of Pulmonary Hypertension Based on Anatomic Site of Underlying Disease

ANATOMICAL SITE	UNDERLYING DISEASE
Postcapillary	Left ventricular dysfunction Mitral valve stenosis Atrial myxoma Constrictive pericarditis Constrictive mediastinitis Pulmonary veno-occlusive disease

Mixed capillary and precapillary	Airway and parenchymal diseases
	  COPD
	  Interstitial lung disease
	Pulmonary vascular diseases
	  Pulmonary embolism
	  Congenital heart disease (left-to-right shunt)
	  Vasculitis
	  Primary pulmonary hypertension
	Chest wall diseases
	  Kyphoscoliosis
	  Fibrothorax

Normal or near-normal lungs	High-altitude sickness Chronic alveolar hypoventilation Sleep-disordered breathing Neuromuscular diseases

Patients with normal or near-normal heart, lungs, or thorax may have PH secondary to intermittent alveolar hypoxia. Patients with sleep-related breathing disorders or neuromuscular disease, for example, can have serious hypoxemia during sleep and near-normal arterial blood-gas concentrations while awake.

Primary pulmonary hypertension (PPH), also referred to as unexplained or idiopathic pulmonary hypertension, can be diagnosed only after all other causes have been excluded. Although patients with PPH exhibit a characteristic pulmonary arteriopathy on lung biopsy, none of the pathologic findings is diagnostic of the disease. Pulmonary arteriopathy can also be found in patients with congenital heart disease, PH associated with liver-induced portal hypertension, toxin-induced and drug-induced PH, and human immunodeficiency virus (HIV)-related PH.

T. B. is a 29-year-old, nonsmoking woman who has noticed easy fatigability, light-headedness, and dyspnea on exertion for 3 months. She feels that her symptoms are worsening, and there is concern regarding recent ankle swelling.

On physical examination, the patient's vital signs are normal. Examination of her neck reveals jugular venous distention and a positive hepatojugular reflux (HJR) in the semirecumbent position. While sitting, auscultation of her lungs is normal, but on examination of her heart, there is a loud second heart sound, especially over the pulmonic area (Erb's point), that is barely palpable. The abdominal examination is normal except for mild right upper quadrant tenderness when checking for HJR. There is also mild bilateral ankle edema.

Case Study:
Introduction

■ HISTORY AND PHYSICAL EXAMINATION

The physical examination can be quite helpful in suggesting the presence of pulmonary hypertension (Table 6-3), but the findings are often subtle. The most common physical findings are a loud and occasionally palpable pulmonic valve closing sound and a right ventricular fourth heart sound that waxes and wanes with inspiration and expiration. A sustained left parasternal or epigastric heave or lift may indicate a forcibly contracting hypertrophied right ventricle. A jugular venous giant A wave (Figure 6-1) is an early sign of reduced right ventricular compliance or an elevated right ventricular pressure. With the onset of right ventricular failure, the right ventricle dilates and often produces tricuspid valve regurgitation; in time, regurgitation causes a prominent V wave (see Figure 6-1) in the jugular venous pulse and an inspiration-augmented systolic murmur, heard best with auscultation along the left and right sternal borders. In addition, as the right heart dilates, the pulmonary artery annulus is distorted, and there is regurgitation characterized by a soft-blowing, diastolic murmur that is heard best along the upper left sternal border. The presence of a right ventricular third heart sound is characteristic of right ventricular failure and generally is associated with a poor prognosis. It is frequently accompanied by signs of right-sided heart failure, such as hepatojugular reflux, tender hepatomegaly, ascites, lower-extremity edema, and, eventually, anasarca. Finally, a thorough examination looking for systemic disease, including musculoskeletal and neurologic abnormalities, is essential, with particular attention directed toward the subtle findings often associated with collagen vascular diseases, such as systemic lupus erythematosus.

Early clinical findings related to PH are subtle and include

- loud and sometimes palpable pulmonic valve closing
- a right ventricular fourth heart sound
- sternal lift or heave
- jugular venous A wave

A search for the subtle findings of systemic inflammation in PH patients can help in early diagnosis of collagen vascular diseases.

Collagen Vascular Diseases Associated with Pulmonary Hypertension

- Systemic lupus erythematosus
- Progressive systemic sclerosis
- CREST syndrome
- Mixed connective tissue disease

Loud pulmonic valve closure sound, frequently palpable

Right ventricular third heart sound

Right ventricular fourth heart sound

Sustained left parasternal or epigastric heave or lift (right ventricular heave)

Jugular venous A wave

Prominent jugular V wave

Diminished carotid arterial upstroke

Inspiration-augmented systolic murmur

Soft-blowing diastolic murmur (occasionally harsh)

Signs of right-sided heart failure, such as hepatojugular reflux, tender hepatomegaly (may be pulsatile), ascites, lower-extremity edema, anasarca

Central or peripheral cyanosis

Table 6-3
Physical Findings That Support a Diagnosis of Pulmonary Hypertension

FIGURE 6-1

Waves in the jugular vein. Parts of the heart action are reflected in the jugular venous pulse (JVP). The waves can be compared with the electrocardiogram (ECG), but there is a slight time delay between electrical cardiac events and their neck pulse signs. PH causes great A waves because the right atrium vigorously contracts to fill a poorly compliant right ventricle. Large V waves are transmitted through the neck with tricuspid regurgitation as seen in PH.

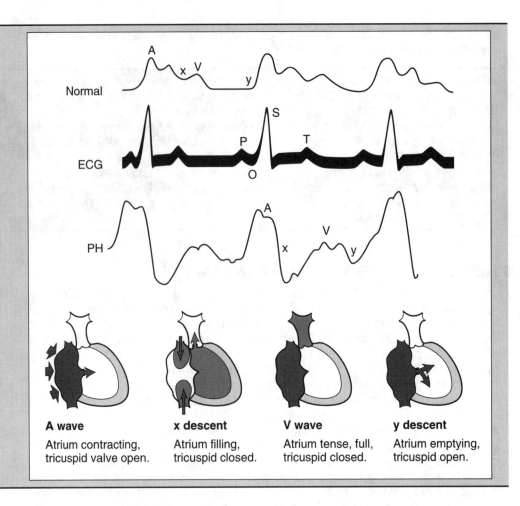

A wave
Atrium contracting, tricuspid valve open.

x descent
Atrium filling, tricuspid closed.

V wave
Atrium tense, full, tricuspid closed.

y descent
Atrium emptying, tricuspid open.

Case Study:
Continued

A series of studies are done on T. B., including a complete battery of blood tests, which are normal. In fact, serology testing for connective tissue diseases is normal. An electrocardiogram suggests PH (Figure 6-2), because there is right ventricular hypertrophy, and a chest x-ray reveals a large heart and prominence of the pulmonary artery (Figure 6-3). A complete pulmonary function test shows a mild restrictive ventilatory defect and a reduction in the single breath carbon monoxide diffusion capacity (Figure 6-4). The arterial blood-gas results also are abnormal: pH, 7.44; PCO_2, 34; PO_2, 64; and oxygen saturation, 93%. Because T. B. has complained of shortness of breath on exertion, she walks on the treadmill, and her arterial oxygen saturation falls to 84% at a low level of exertion.

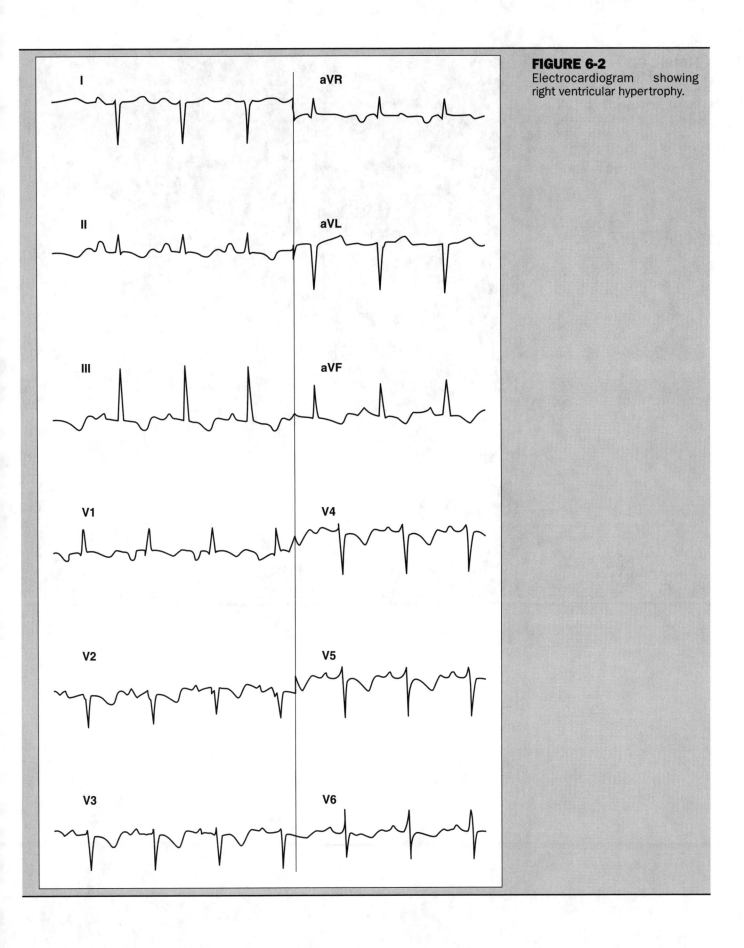

FIGURE 6-2
Electrocardiogram showing right ventricular hypertrophy.

FIGURE 6-3
Chest x-ray revealing cardiomegaly and right pulmonary artery prominence.

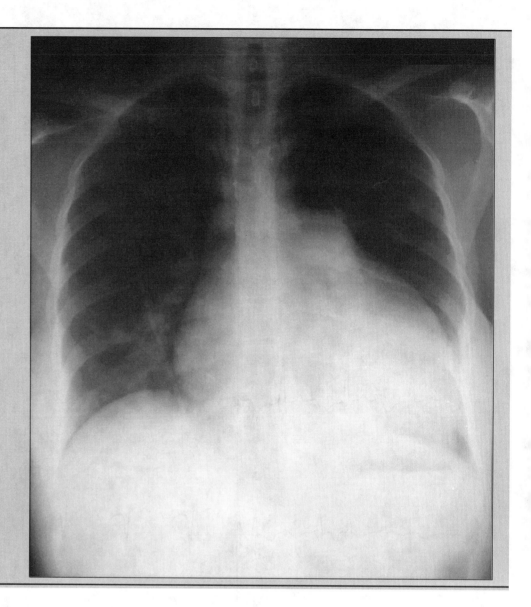

Spirometry (BTPS)		Pred.	Best	%Pred.
FVC	Liters	4.30	2.80	65.00
FEV1	Liters	3.42	2.20	64.00
FEV/FVC	%	79.00	79.00	79.00
Lung Volumes (BTPS)				
TLC	Liters	5.95	5.12	86.00
RV	Liters	1.88	2.20	117.00
RV/TLC	%	29.00	43.00	148.00
FRC PL	Liters	3.35	3.67	109.00
Diffusion Capacity				
DLCO	mL/min/mmHg	24.50	14.60	60.00
DLCO/VA	L/min/mmHg	4.71	3.95	84.00

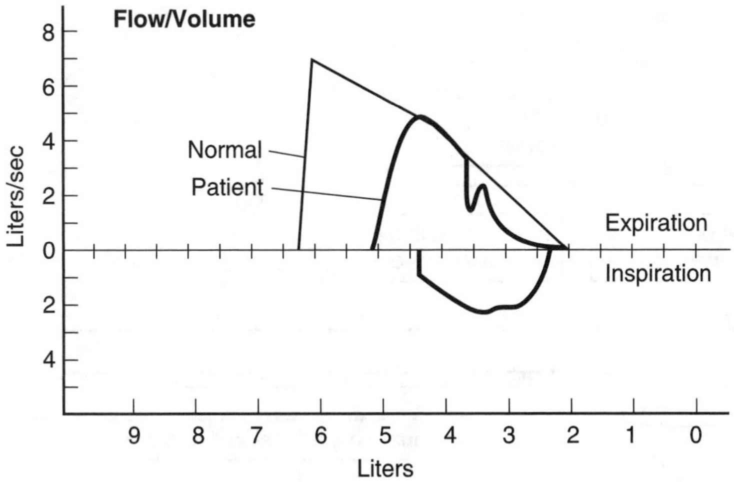

FIGURE 6-4
Pulmonary function tests revealing mild restrictive disease and a decrease in carbon monoxide diffusion capacity.

■ DIAGNOSTIC EVALUATION

The diagnosis of pulmonary hypertension and its causes (Figure 6-5) should follow an orderly and logical progression. An approach to determining the actual cause of PH can be found in Figure 6-6.

FIGURE 6-5
An approach to the diagnosis of PH.

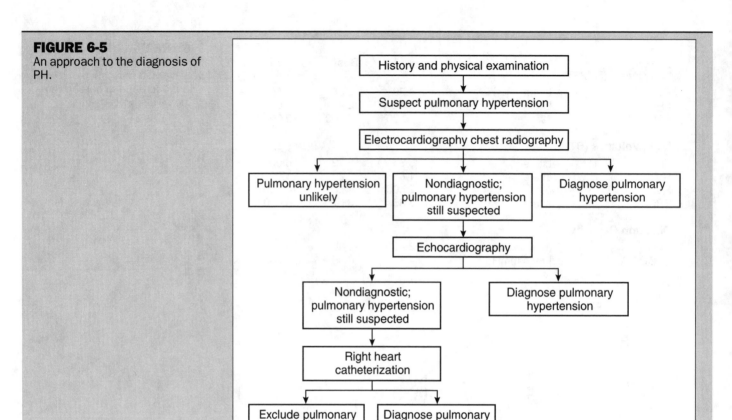

History and physical examination

Suspect pulmonary hypertension

Electrocardiography chest radiography

Pulmonary hypertension unlikely

Nondiagnostic; pulmonary hypertension still suspected

Diagnose pulmonary hypertension

Echocardiography

Nondiagnostic; pulmonary hypertension still suspected

Diagnose pulmonary hypertension

Right heart catheterization

Exclude pulmonary hypertension

Diagnose pulmonary hypertension

FIGURE 6-6
Diagnostic approach to determining the cause of pulmonary hypertension.

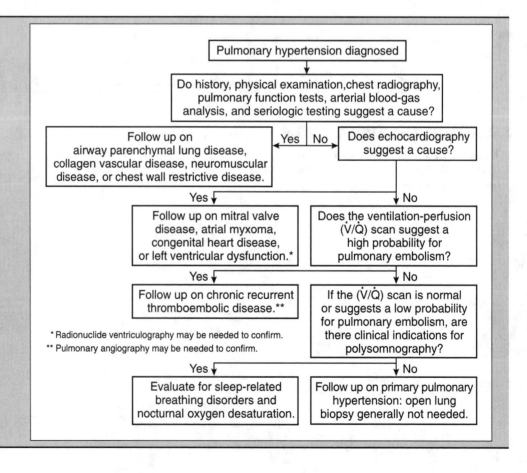

Pulmonary hypertension diagnosed

Do history, physical examination, chest radiography, pulmonary function tests, arterial blood-gas analysis, and seriologic testing suggest a cause?

Follow up on airway parenchymal lung disease, collagen vascular disease, neuromuscular disease, or chest wall restrictive disease.

Yes | No

Does echocardiography suggest a cause?

Yes

Follow up on mitral valve disease, atrial myxoma, congenital heart disease, or left ventricular dysfunction.*

No

Does the ventilation-perfusion (V̇/Q̇) scan suggest a high probability for pulmonary embolism?

Yes

Follow up on chronic recurrent thromboembolic disease.**

No

If the (V̇/Q̇) scan is normal or suggests a low probability for pulmonary embolism, are there clinical indications for polysomnography?

* Radionuclide ventriculography may be needed to confirm.
** Pulmonary angiography may be needed to confirm.

Yes

Evaluate for sleep-related breathing disorders and nocturnal oxygen desaturation.

No

Follow up on primary pulmonary hypertension: open lung biopsy generally not needed.

ELECTROCARDIOGRAPHY

An electrocardiogram that suggests right ventricular hypertrophy is a relatively sensitive test of PH, although the changes do not correlate with the severity of the underlying pressure elevation. Commonly, right-axis deviation and right ventricular hypertrophy with secondary T-wave changes are found.

Unfortunately, mild to moderate PH may exist with no electrocardiographic findings to suggest it, and thus the absence of ECG changes suggestive of right ventricular hypertrophy does not rule out its presence.

Patients with mild to moderate PH may exhibit no ECG anomalies, but often there will be a prominent main pulmonary artery despite the normal ECG.

CHEST RADIOGRAPHY

The chest x-ray can be helpful in identifying the cause of PH; therefore, it is an important part of the evaluation process. Parenchymal abnormalities, redistribution of pulmonary blood flow, general or segmental cardiac enlargement, and chest wall and spinal disorders can provide clues to a specific underlying disorder. The most common finding is prominence of a main pulmonary artery.

PULMONARY FUNCTION AND ARTERIAL BLOOD GAS TESTING

Pulmonary function testing is not directly useful as a diagnostic test for pulmonary hypertension. However, measurements of spirometry, lung volumes, and carbon monoxide diffusion capacity often facilitate the diagnostic evaluation of the specific cause of PH, by demonstrating the presence and degree of obstructive or restrictive pulmonary disease. Pulmonary function studies may disclose certain pathophysiologic abnormalities that are not otherwise clinically apparent.

Hypoxemia is common in disorders associated with PH and should be ruled out as a precipitating or sustaining factor in its development. Clinically significant hypoxic pulmonary vasoconstriction usually does not occur until the arterial oxygen tension falls below 60 mmHg. However, in patients who have sleep-related breathing abnormalities, hypoxemia may occur only during apneic or hypopneic episodes, and blood gases measured while the patient is awake may be only mildly abnormal. Nocturnal episodes of hypoxic vasoconstriction are postulated to be important in the development of PH in patients with chronic obstructive pulmonary disease (COPD) and a variety of restrictive ventilatory diseases as well. Hypercapnia in PH patients implies severe parenchymal lung disease or disordered control of breathing.

A cardiopulmonary exercise test to symptom-limited maximum is useful in the evaluation of patients who complain of dyspnea and in whom no cause is obvious (mystery dyspnea). There is a characteristic pattern of ventilatory and circulatory responses in patients with various forms of cardiac limitations and pulmonary limitations.

T. B. is strongly suspected of having PH, and from the studies performed, her condition does not seem to be attributable to any form of parenchymal lung disease, such as COPD or any restrictive lung disease. At this point, we should be concerned that she may have heart disease (valvular or congenital) or pulmonary vascular disease (primary or secondary). If the patient were older, a sleep-related breathing problem might figure into the differential diagnosis.

An echocardiogram reveals numerous findings consistent with PH, including right ventricular dilatation and hypertrophy, right atrial enlargement, and paradoxical motion at the intraventricular septum (Figure 6-7). The left heart is normal and there is no evidence of congenital heart disease. A ventilation-perfusion lung scan is nearly normal (Figure 6-8). A pulmonary angiogram is not needed.

Case Study:
Continued

ECHOCARDIOGRAPHY

Although the echocardiogram is not specific enough to rule out pulmonary hypertension, several findings are consistent with moderate to severe increases in pulmonary arterial pressure. These findings include the presence of a dilated pulmonary artery, right atrial dilatation, right ventricular dilatation and hypertrophy, paradoxical movement of the intraventricular septum, and abnormal pulmonic valve motion. Of particular diagnostic value are the movement and configuration of the intraventricular septum, as revealed by

FIGURE 6-7
Two-dimensional echocardiogram in a patient with severe PH. There is marked dilatation of the right atrium and ventricle (RA and RV). Normally, the left ventricle (LV) should be larger.

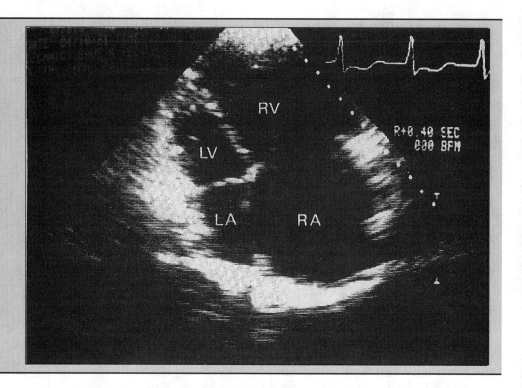

FIGURE 6-8
Perfusion lung scan (two views: left, anterior; right, posterior) in a patient with PH. Low probability for pulmonary embolism with patchy perfusion defects. Ventilation was nearly normal.

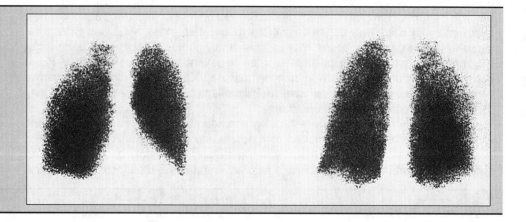

two-dimensional echocardiography. As PH increases, diastolic flattening of the ventricular septum occurs. Eventually, the septum develops a concave configuration relative to the right ventricle.

The echocardiogram can be particularly helpful in establishing if pulmonary hypertension is caused by left ventricular dysfunction, mitral valve disease, or an intracardiac shunt secondary to congenital heart disease.

Exciting developments in Doppler echocardiography make this mode the noninvasive procedure of choice in determining the existence and severity of PH. In certain patients, Doppler echocardiography can estimate pulmonary artery pressure and reduce the need for heart catheterization.

LUNG IMAGING (V/Q SCANNING)

Ventilation-perfusion (V/Q) lung scanning is most useful for distinguishing patients with primary pulmonary hypertension (PPH) from those with major vessel thromboembolic pulmonary hypertension (TPH).

In PPH, the lung scan is either normal (correlating with predominant plexogenic pulmonary arteriopathy) or low-probability, defined as small, patchy perfusion defects (suggesting thrombotic pulmonary arteriopathy) (Figure 6-9). Conversely, in patients with recurrent TPH, the lung scan demonstrates at least one major V/Q mismatch, but more often, two or more are found (Figure 6-10). A high-probability scan for pulmonary embolism may not be of high enough specificity, however, and further evaluation by pulmonary angiography may be required for diagnostic confirmation of chronic embolic disease.

> The V/Q lung scan is either normal or low-probability for pulmonary embolism in patients with PPH.

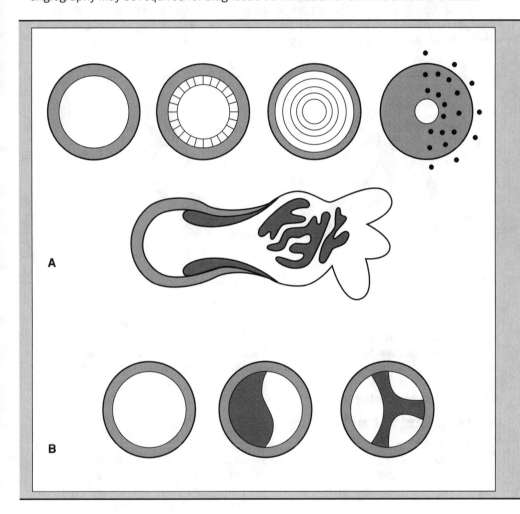

FIGURE 6-9
In patients with PPH who have normal perfusion lung scans, the small pulmonary arteries often show a plexogenic arteriopathy (A). However, in PPH generally a noticeable degree of thrombotic change is found (B). These eccentric vascular changes are attributable to partial resolution of in situ clots.

PULMONARY ANGIOGRAPHY

If the lung scan shows one or more segmental, or greater, V/Q mismatches, a pulmonary angiogram is necessary to rule out thromboembolic disease. In chronic, recurrent TPH, pulmonary angiography shows smooth, convex-bordered occlusions, stenoses, and intravascular webs (Figure 6-11). Signs of large central thrombi, such as filling defects and vessel cutoffs, are found. In TPH, the clots are actually incorporated into the wall of the pulmonary artery and endothelialized so that the angiogram may underestimate the extent of obstruction. By contrast, patients with PPH have proximal and hilar vessel dilatation, which then taper rapidly, with marked bilateral symmetric pruning of the distal vessels.

RIGHT HEART CATHERIZATION

Pulmonary arterial catheterization, using a thermodilution balloon catheter, remains the gold standard for determining the presence and severity of pulmonary hypertension. Unfortunately, at times it can be extremely difficult to pass the catheter into the pulmonary artery in patients with severe PH because of tricuspid valve regurgitation, a dilated right-side chamber, and a low cardiac output. Right heart catheterization may be required to help establish the etiology of the PH; measurement of the pulmonary capillary

Causes of Pulmonary Vessel Obstruction

- Chronic, recurrent pulmonary emboli
- Schistosomiasis
- Filariasis
- Fat emboli (long bone fractures)
- Foreign body emboli (IV drug use; talcosis)
- Tumor emboli
- Multiple thromboses (in situ) of small pulmonary arterioles (sickle cell disease)

> Heart catheterization is often required to diagnose PH resulting from post-capillary causes, such as left ventricular failure and mitral stenosis.

wedge pressure (PCWP) distinguishes postcapillary from mixed capillary-precapillary causes (see Table 6-3). Postcapillary PH is generally identified by a PCWP greater than 15 mmHg, whereas mixed capillary-precapillary PH has a PCWP of less than 15 mmHg. The finding of an elevated PCWP necessitates a further cardiac evaluation to determine whether there is abnormal left ventricular end-diastolic pressure, mitral valve stenosis, or impairment of left atrial filling by stenosis of the pulmonary venous system. Pulmonary veno-occlusive disease can result in a gradient between wedge pressure and left ventricular end-diastolic pressure, although the wedge pressure is usually normal or only mildly elevated. Typical of veno-occlusive disease is the variability in wedge pressure determinations from various sites within the lung.

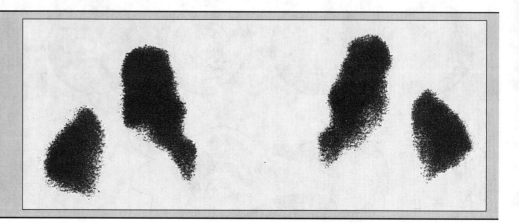

FIGURE 6-10
Perfusion lung scan (left, anterior; right, posterior) in a patient with chronic TPH. Multiple segmental defects are present on perfusion scan. Ventilation scan (not shown) was normal.

Measurements of increased oxygen desaturation in the central veins, right atrium, right ventricle, and pulmonary artery help identify the presence and location of a left-to-right shunt. Congenital heart disease can often be missed (especially in patients with ostium secundum atrial septal defects) if the balloon cathether technique of measuring oxygen saturation is used. There are more sensitive methods of determining the presence of shunt that can be performed in the cardiac catheterization laboratory.

POLYSOMNOGRAPHY

Polysomnography (PSG) is not part of the usual evaluation for pulmonary hypertension; it is used specifically for the diagnosis of sleep-related breathing disorders. Patients with COPD, chronic congestive heart failure, and various neuromuscular diseases are at increased risk for developing sleep-related breathing disorders. Studies performed on unselected sleep apnea syndrome patients have found the frequency of PH to be between 12% and 20%. PH can increase during sleep in COPD patients, exhibiting profound drops in arterial oxygen saturation, particularly during rapid eye movement (REM) sleep. This effect is most noticeable in patients who demonstrate daytime hypoxemia, hypercapnia, and PH, but similar results have been observed in patients with little or no daytime PH. Pulmonary arterial pressures during sleep can exceed daytime values by as much as 25 mmHg.

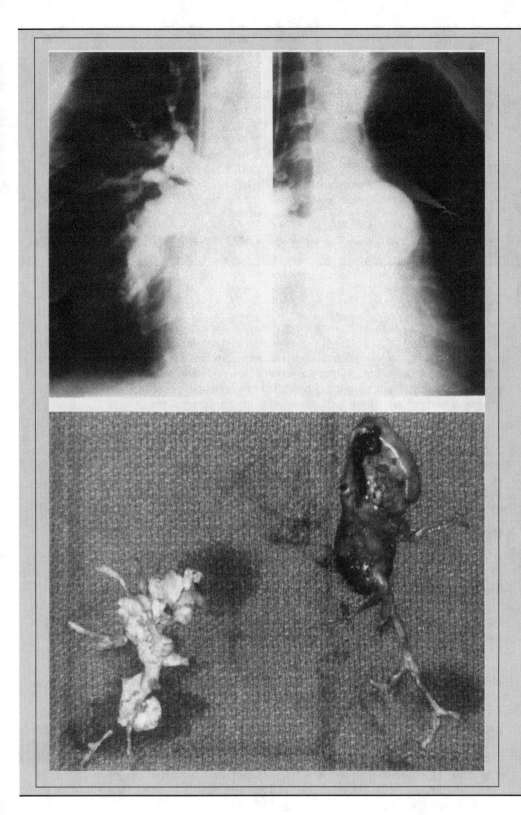

FIGURE 6-11
Chronic TPH. (A) Angiograms demonstrating obstructions, stenoses, and some vessels with poststenotic aneurysmal dilatations. (B) Chronic thrombi removed from pulmonary arteries.

Case Study:
Continued

From our diagnostic evaluation, T. B. has unexplained or primary pulmonary hypertension (PPH). A lung biopsy is not needed. Cardiac catheterization reveals (normal values in parenthesis):

Systemic arterial pressure	*110/86 mmHg (120/80 mmHg)*
Pulmonary arterial pressure	*92/46 mmHg (20/10 mmHg)*
Pulmonary wedge pressure	*10 mmHg (10 mmHg)*
Right atrial pressure	*20/10 mmHg (8/2 mmHg)*
Right ventricular pressure	*90/20 mmHg (20/5 mmHg)*
Cardiac index	*2.4 L/min/m² (3.5 L/min/m²)*
Mixed-venous O_2 saturation	*62% (70%)*
Arterial O_2 saturation	*92% (98%)*

There is no evidence of an oxygen saturation step-up on catheter flotation from the superior vena cava to the pulmonary artery, so an intracardiac left-to-right shunt is not considered.

LUNG BIOPSY

In certain patients with PPH, lung biopsy may be necessary to establish the diagnosis when confounding factors make the diagnosis uncertain. An accurate diagnosis is essential for proper prognosis and management. For example, lung biopsy may distinguish among patients with PPH, pulmonary veno-occlusive disease, and vasculitis.

Transbronchial lung biopsy by fiberoptic bronchoscopy is contraindicated because of the risk of hemorrhage owing to the elevated pulmonary arterial pressure and because the sample is generally small and often does not include blood vessels. Open-lung biopsy, possibly using a thoracoscope, is preferred. This procedure is not without risk, however, particularly in patients with severe PH who cannot tolerate the short period of controlled pneumothorax often necessary to permit sufficient visualization of the lung. It must be stressed that lung biopsy is not considered essential in making an accurate diagnosis of PPH for most patients with this disease process.

■ PRIMARY PULMONARY HYPERTENSION (PPH)

It is important to discuss PPH because it is a disease that principally involves the pulmonary vasculature and can be used to study the clinical presentation of PH and the result of sustained elevated pulmonary vascular resistance on the body.

There is a long asymptomatic period that precedes the diagnosis of PPH because the body, mainly the right heart, compensates for the slow progressive PH that develops. This partially accounts for the advanced manifestations of PH at the time of diagnosis. The mean age at the time of diagnosis is 36 years for both males and females. Although the disease is most common in the third decade for female patients and in the fourth decade for male patients, no age range is immune, and 9% of the patients are older than 60 years of age. The female-male ratio is nearly 2 to 1.

The most commonly reported symptom of PPH is dyspnea, which occurs in 60% of patients as an early symptom, and in all patients as the disease progresses. Atypical angina is also common, as is easy fatigability. Approximately 10% of patients also report symptoms of Raynaud's phenomenon, which occur almost entirely in the female patient population (approximately 95%). The time of onset, from the patient's recognition of first symptoms until eventual diagnosis, is 2 ± 5 years (median 1.3 years), indicating that the diagnosis is often delayed.

The mechanism of dyspnea in patients with PPH is unclear, but it is associated with a characteristic hyperventilation and chronic respiratory alkalosis that is exaggerated during exercise. The near-syncope and syncope are almost always effort related and are believed to result from a limited ability to increase the cardiac output in response to increased metabolic demand. The angina or atypical chest discomfort associated with PPH is also precipitated by stress, suggesting that it may represent right ventricular ischemia.

Syncope is often exercise induced and is likely to be a result of an inadequate cardiac output in response to increased metabolic demand.

Atypical chest pain associated with PPH

- resembles angina.
- is precipitated by dyspnea and stress.
- may represent right ventricular ischemia.

Patients with PPH have physical findings typical of any patient with pulmonary hypertension: an increase in the pulmonic component of the second heart sound is found in 93%, and a right ventricular heave and a right-sided fourth heart sound are found in 38%. More advanced disease is signaled by the presence of a right ventricular third heart sound and tricuspid regurgitation. Patients may also complain of hoarseness. Clubbing is not a feature of PPH and should suggest chronic lung or congenital heart disease.

Patients with PPH have abnormal chest x-rays, with the two most common findings being main pulmonary artery prominence and hilar vessel enlargement with pruning of the more peripheral vessels. As do PH patients in general, PPH patients frequently have right ventricular hypertrophy on ECG.

Patients with PPH generally have abnormal pulmonary function tests. Mild reduction in lung volumes, reduced diffusion capacity for carbon monoxide, and impaired pulmonary gas exchange are typical. The presence of a more than a mild restrictive or obstructive component should suggest another diagnosis. The reduced diffusion capacity for carbon monoxide has been ascribed to obliteration of small pulmonary arteries.

Patients with PPH have mild to moderate abnormalities of pulmonary gas exchange. A respiratory or mixed respiratory-metabolic alkalosis with hypoxemia and a widened alveolar-arterial oxygen gradient are likely to be found in every patient. The hypoxemia that accompanies PPH is attributable to a mild degree of ventilation-perfusion inequality, amplified by the effect of a low mixed-venous PO_2, resulting from an inadequate cardiac output. With exercise, the mixed-venous oxygen saturation falls further and arterial hypoxemia increases. Severe hypoxemia can occasionally occur in PPH, usually caused by intracardiac shunting through a patent foramen ovale or, less commonly, by a markedly depressed cardiac output. The chronic respiratory alkalosis is attributed to increased afferent activity from intrapulmonary stretch receptors or intravascular baroreceptors.

Patients with PPH generally have substantial exercise limitation, with marked fatigue and dyspnea on even mild exertion, as well as excessive ventilation at all exercise levels. These patients usually stop exercising because of dyspnea and lightheadedness. Functional limitation, as determined by the maximal oxygen consumption, is marked in PPH. The heart rate is higher for any submaximal level of work, expressed as a reduction in maximum oxygen pulse. Similar to heart rate, the maximal minute ventilation is higher at any submaximal level in PPH patients than in normal patients. As a consequence, the respiratory alkalosis present at rest in PPH patients is maintained during moderate exercise. The arterial PO_2 falls even further at maximal exercise, and the alveolar-arterial oxygen gradient increases. As noted, the increased hypoxemia with exercise is predominantly a result of inadequate cardiac response to increased metabolic demands and the subsequent exaggerated fall in the mixed-venous PO_2.

M-mode echocardiographic data for PPH patients generally show a normal to small left ventricular end-diastolic internal dimension and right ventricular enlargement. Paradoxical septal motion and partial systolic closure of the pulmonic valve are found. Underfilling of the left ventricle is a reflection of the severity of pulmonary vascular disease, an example of how the left ventricle depends on right ventricular function in patients with pulmonary vascular disease.

Particular attention should be paid to the accurate measurement of right atrial pressure, pulmonary arterial pressure, and cardiac output, because they are important long-term prognostic indicators in patients with PPH. The thermodilution technique seems to be satisfactory for determining cardiac output in most patients with PH. However, the Fick method, with direct measurement of oxygen consumption, is more accurate in patients with low cardiac output states. PPH patients generally have severe PH, with a threefold increase in mean pulmonary arterial pressure, mild to moderate elevation of the mean right atrial pressure with a normal PCWP, and a mildly reduced cardiac index. The correlation between hemodynamic findings and severity of symptoms has been investigated. Patients with more severe symptoms (functional classes III and IV) have higher mean pulmonary arterial pressures, higher right atrial pressures, and lower cardiac indexes than their less symptomatic counterparts.

Hoarseness in PPH patients is attributable to recurrent laryngeal nerve compression by an enlarged left main pulmonary artery.

Cyanosis due to hypoxemia:

- Peripheral cyanosis results from a low cardiac output state.
- Central cyanosis results from a right-to-left shunt (usually with clubbing) or a congenital or patent foramen ovale.

Prostacyclin (prostaglandin I_2, or PGI_2) is a potent vasodilator that reverses the effects of thromboxane (a chemical platelet aggregator).

Case Study:
Resolution

T. B. has severe PPH, and her prognosis is poor. Certain therapeutic issues are entertained, such as the long-term value of vasodilator therapy and lung transplantation. After a vasodilator challenge with intravenous prostacyclin, it is felt that this medication can be constantly infused intravenously while T. B. waits for a lung transplantation. Anticoagulation and the careful use of diuretic therapy are part of the treatment regimen.

Although the condition of T. B. deteriorates slowly over 18 months, a bilateral lung transplantation is performed, and it is anticipated that her functional capacity and prognosis will improve substantially.

■ MANAGEMENT OF PULMONARY HYPERTENSION

Once the cause of PH has been identified, there are several therapeutic options. The management approach depends on the underlying disease and the likelihood that there is a reversible component to the PH.

There is usually considerable reversibility in patients with atrial and ventricular septal defects who have corrective surgery, whereas patients with PPH and PH associated with recurrent emboli have less responsive pulmonary vascular beds. Vasodilators may be administered on a trial basis during hemodynamic monitoring in order to determine the degree of reversibility.

SURGERY

In patients with mitral stenosis, valve replacement usually brings about a dramatic improvement in PH within months. Similarly, significant reduction in PH can occur in patients with cardiac septal defects when surgery is performed before the pulmonary vascular resistance approaches systemic levels and while the net intracardiac shunt is still left to right.

OXYGEN THERAPY

Administration of supplemental oxygen is warranted for the patient who, despite optimal management of an underlying disease, has an arterial oxygen tension (P_aO_2) of less than 55 mmHg while breathing air. Oxygen therapy is also indicated for the patient with signs of cor pulmonale and a P_aO_2 of less than 60 mmHg. Oxygen should be administered as close as possible to 24 hours daily. Continuous use of oxygen is ideal, but may not be practical; thus, the patient with COPD may benefit from oxygen therapy using a low-flow nasal cannula for 18 hours per day. Supplemental oxygen is also used at night for patients with nocturnal desaturation after other correctable causes, such as sleep apnea, have been addressed—even if the daytime P_aO_2 is acceptable.

The goals of oxygen therapy are amelioration of symptoms attributable to systemic hypoxia and alleviation of hypoxic pulmonary vasoconstriction. Oxygen therapy can afford the most dramatic therapeutic effects in patients who have COPD and PH. Improved survival and intellectual function, as well as reduced need for hospitalization, can occur even when pulmonary pressures are only moderately reduced.

BRONCHODILATORS

In patients with COPD and PH, bronchodilators improve ventilatory function and gas exchange, chiefly by decreasing bronchomotor tone. However, these agents also exert other beneficial respiratory and cardiovascular effects. For example, theophylline and β_2-adrenergic agents may cause direct pulmonary vasodilatation. These agents can also enhance mucociliary clearance, improve right ventricular function, and favorably affect diaphragmatic contractility.

DIGITALIS

The role of cardiac glycosides in the management of cor pulmonale is controversial. Digitalis reduces systemic venous congestion in patients with symptoms and signs of overt right heart failure. In patients without heart failure, digitalis enhances the inotropic state of the right ventricle but can also increase pulmonary vascular resistance with an unpredictable effect on cardiac output.

Noninvasive cardiac imaging has demonstrated that patients with pulmonary disease who have compromised left ventricular ejection fractions are likely to respond to digitalis with improved biventricular function. However, one must remember that there is a high incidence of digitalis toxicity in patients with lung disease. Thus, one must weigh the risks of digitalis therapy (an increase in cor pulmonale by hypoxemia; hypokalemia if diuretics are used) with the potential benefits in most patients who do not have left ventricular failure.

DIURETICS

Patients with cor pulmonale often require diuretic therapy. These agents must be used cautiously and sparingly to reduce excessive right ventricular volume preload and to control uncomfortable edema. However, the reduction in right ventricular preload following diuresis may lower cardiac output and cause systemic hypotension and prerenal azotemia. Also, the resultant hypokalemia and metabolic alkalosis may be poorly tolerated by COPD patients who are hypercapnic and hypoxemic.

ANTICOAGULATION

Traditionally, warfarin has been used for long-term anticoagulation therapy in patients who have pulmonary hypertension secondary to chronic pulmonary thromboembolism. This agent has also been used in patients with PPH. Pulmonary thromboendarterectomy has been performed in patients with chronic recurrent thromboembolism who have large proximal pulmonary artery thrombi.

VASODILATOR THERAPY

Numerous systemic vasodilators with different proposed mechanisms of action have been used, chiefly to manage PPH. The rationale for attempting vasodilator therapy in patients with cor pulmonale is based on the concept that right ventricular dysfunction results from an increased afterload, and that pulmonary vasoconstriction constitutes a significant component of the elevation in pulmonary vascular resistance (PVR).

Prolonged vasoconstriction has been suggested as a causative factor for increase in PVR because of the presence of medial hypertrophy on pathologic examination of the pulmonary arteries of patients with PPH. A reduction in vasomotor tone, therefore, should reduce right heart afterload and improve pump function.

A specific vasodilator without systemic effect has not yet been found. However, many nonspecific vasodilators have been tried with limited success.

Calcium channel antagonists (chiefly nifedipine and diltiazem) have become popular for treatment of patients with PPH. Some improvement in exercise tolerance has been demonstrated in these patients, but one must watch for adverse effects, such as systemic hypotension.

Because both the beneficial and adverse effects of vasodilator therapy are unpredictable, certain precautions must be taken when these drugs are used. Catheterization of the right heart is needed to evaluate the patient's acute response to vasodilator therapy.

Acute pulmonary vascular responsiveness to vasodilators can be safely assessed during catheterization. Acute hemodynamic effects are evaluated to determine whether or not patients may benefit from chronic therapy. Prostacyclin is a suitable test drug because of its rapid onset, short duration of action, and potency. Intravenous infusion can be terminated if systemic hypotension, hypoxemia, dyspnea, angina, or other significant effects occur. A 20% reduction in PVR at an infusion rate that does not cause side effects is considered a positive response. Ideally, the fall in PVR should occur with an increase in cardiac output and fall in pulmonary arterial pressure. Consider therapy with oral vasodilators for patients who respond to prostacyclin. Prostacyclin itself can be used chronically by the intravascular constant infusion technique.

A beneficial hemodynamic response to vasodilator therapy is considered to be present when:

- Pulmonary vascular resistance falls by 20% or more.
- Cardiac output remains unchanged or increases.

- The mean difference between pulmonary arterial pressure and pulmonary capillary wedge pressure remains unchanged or decreases.
- Systemic arterial blood pressure remains unchanged or falls only minimally to a level free of side effects.

Ideally, the increase in cardiac output should be the result of an increase in stroke volume—not simply to an increase in heart rate. If a vasodilator is started, the dosage can be gradually increased as tolerated by the patient. Keep in mind that a favorable acute response to a vasodilator may not persist when the drug is administered on a long-term basis. Repeat cardiac catheterizations are necessary for proper assessment of the safety and efficacy of a chronic vasodilator therapy.

TRANSPLANTATION

A small number of patients, usually those with PPH who have met a certain age, psychosocial, and general health criteria, undergo lung transplantation. Tissue rejection has become less of a problem with the use of cyclosporin.

The major drawbacks to lung transplantation include the scarcity of donor organs and institutional availability. Despite these impediments, this surgery is an option worth serious consideration in select patients.

▮ SUMMARY

A high level of suspicion is of paramount importance for the eventual diagnosis of pulmonary hypertension, regardless of the underlying cause. However, once PH is suspected, a methodical work-up using commonly employed diagnostic interventions generally allows rapid confirmation of the presence of the disease, and, usually, a specific diagnosis of its etiology. A proper etiologic evaluation is necessary to ensure that the diagnosis is correct and that the proper therapeutic interventions can be pursued.

■ REVIEW QUESTIONS

1. A 32-year-old woman comes to your office complaining of fatigue, dyspnea on exertion, and near-syncope. She is 5 ft. 4 in. tall and weighs 248 lbs. She admits to taking diet pills for weight reduction and to a 30-pack-year smoking history. Her vital signs are normal. Physical examination reveals neck vein distention, a positive hepatojugular reflux (HJR), and peripheral lower-extremity edema. Her lung sounds are abnormal, revealing a loud pulmonic second sound. Her ECG shows right ventricular hypertrophy. You suspect pulmonary hypertension (PH). Your differential diagnosis includes:

   (A) chronic obstructive pulmonary disease
   (B) congenital heart disease
   (C) vasculitis
   (D) obstructive sleep apnea syndrome
   (E) PH caused by diet pills
   (F) all of the above

2. The initial diagnostic work-up of this patient in Question 1 should include which of the following? (There may be more than one correct answer.)

   (A) Chest x-ray
   (B) Pulmonary arteriogram
   (C) Echocardiogram
   (D) Right heart catheterization
   (E) Polysomnogram (PSG)

3. All of the following may be commonly seen on ECG in patients with PH, except:

   (A) right-axis deviation
   (B) left-axis deviation
   (C) right ventricular hypertrophy
   (D) normal ECG
   (E) atrial fibrillation
   (F) right atrial enlargement

4. The most useful initial treatment for most patients with PH is:

   (A) calcium channel blockers
   (B) oxygen
   (C) prostacyclin
   (D) digitalis
   (E) diuretics

■ ANSWERS AND EXPLANATIONS

1. The answer is F. This patient is a smoker, and thus underlying COPD with possible chronic hypoxemia/hypercapnia causing PH and cor pulmonale must be excluded. Congenital right-to-left shunt, patent foramen ovale, and vasculitis must be ruled out as potential causes. This patient is obese and of short stature, and further delineation of her sleep habits is needed. Finally, weight-reducing drugs have been implicated in PH and in valvular heart disease.

2. The answers are A, C, and D. A chest x-ray will indicate cardiac and pulmonary artery size, will reveal the presence of pleural effusions (at least 200 mL is required for resolution by CXR) or bullous emphysema/hyperinflation, and will show evidence of any existing interstitial lung disease. Echocardiography is the noninvasive procedure of choice for revealing the presence of PH. A pulmonary arteriogram would be indicated only if chronic thromboembolic disease were suspected following an indeterminate or low-probability V/Q scan in the presence of a high clinical suspicion. Right heart catheterization is the gold standard invasive procedure for diagnosing PH and evaluating its extent and severity. Catheterization would also rule out intracardiac shunts and congenital heart disease. Finally, the PSG would be additive in ruling out obstructive sleep apnea as a cause of PH, but it would not be helpful in making a diagnosis of PH.

3. The answer is B. Left-axis deviation is not common in patients with PH. Right-axis deviation, right ventricular hypertrophy, and right atrial enlargement are common, although they are not always evident. The ECG may be normal. Patients with PH and its associated hypoxemia may exhibit atrial fibrillation and other cardiac dysrhythmias.

4. The answer is B. Chronic hypoxemia exacerbates PH. Therefore, the best initial therapy is continuous (24-hr) administration of oxygen. Digitalis and diuretics may help in the treatment of cor pulmonale but must be closely monitored and would not be the initial treatment of choice. Both calcium channel blocker therapy and prostacyclin infusion require cardiac monitoring with a Swan-Ganz catheter prior to initiation of therapy.

■ SUGGESTED READING

D'Alonzo G, Bower JS, Dantzker D: Differentiation of patients with primary and thromboembolic pulmonary hypertension. *Chest* 85:457–462, 1984.

Perkins RC, D'Alonzo G: Pulmonary hypertension: the initial workup. *J Resp Dis* 11(4):11–23, 1990.

Rubin LJ: Pulmonary vasculitis and primary pulmonary hypertension. In Murray JF, Nadel JA, eds.: *Textbook of Respiratory Medicine*, 3rd ed. Philadelphia: WB Saunders, 1994, pp. 1683–1710.

Chapter 7
RESPIRATORY FAILURE

Gerard J. Criner, M.D.

■ CHAPTER OUTLINE

Learning Objectives
Case Study: Introduction
Introduction
Definition of Respiratory Failure
Case Study: Continued
Pathophysiology of Respiratory Failure
Diagnosis of Respiratory Failure
Case Study: Continued
Treatment of Respiratory Failure
Case Study: Resolution
Summary
Review Questions

■ LEARNING OBJECTIVES

At the completion of this chapter, the reader should:
- Be able to define respiratory failure.
- Be able to classify respiratory failure into hypoxemic and hypercapnic subtypes.
- Recognize the signs and symptoms of respiratory failure.
- Know the alveolar gas equation and be able to apply it to the evaluation of respiratory failure.
- Be aware of changes in blood gases that accompany respiratory failure.
- Be aware of the major treatments of respiratory failure.

Case Study:
Introduction

A 43-year-old respiratory therapist with a known history of asthma develops an acute episode of shortness of breath at work. Over the past three days, she has complained of cough and fever following an upper respiratory tract infection. Although her asthma has been well maintained by twice-daily inhalation of corticosteroids and p.r.n. inhalation of beta agonists for symptomatic relief of bronchospasm, her shortness of breath has markedly increased over the past three days.

Today, the patient's breathlessness was more severe on awakening and has increased in severity throughout the day at work. She has failed to respond to multiple inhaled bronchodilator treatments and is found to have a marked increase in respiratory rate, the use of accessory muscles of respiration, and no relief from inhaled bronchodilator therapy. She is evaluated by the medical director of respiratory therapy and is found to be in respiratory distress. She is transported to the emergency room for further evaluation and treatment.

■ INTRODUCTION

Respiratory failure affects patients of all ages and varies markedly in presentation.

Respiratory failure is one of the most serious and life-threatening processes that can affect an individual. It can occur in patients of all ages and can vary markedly in presentation. For example, neonates may quickly develop respiratory failure secondary to meconium aspiration, and older patients with a history of chronic obstructive pulmonary disease (COPD) may exhibit respiratory failure only after developing an acute and superimposed process, such as pulmonary edema or pneumonia. Despite the presentation, the approach to the patient with respiratory failure requires a detailed and consistent exploration of the pathophysiologic mechanisms responsible for its development.

This chapter presents an organized overview of respiratory failure by providing 1) a definition of respiratory failure, 2) a review of the pathophysiologic mechanisms responsible for its development, and 3) insights into its diagnosis and treatment.

■ DEFINITION OF RESPIRATORY FAILURE

The function of the respiratory system is to supply the body with adequate oxygen for aerobic metabolism and to remove its major metabolic waste product—carbon dioxide. This process is achieved through three distinct mechanisms: 1) ventilation, the delivery of ambient air to the alveoli, where it is exposed to blood; 2) diffusion, the movement of oxygen and carbon dioxide across the alveolar air sac and capillary wall barriers; and 3) circulation, the method by which oxygen is carried from the site of gas exchange to the cells of the body, where active metabolism occurs.

To accomplish these processes, the respiratory system functions as a pump for effective ventilation and as an area of gas exchange (Figure 7-1). Failure of the respiratory system to perform optimally in either of these two roles will result in an elevation of PCO_2 (i.e., hypercapnia) and/or a reduction of oxygen in the blood (i.e., hypoxemia), both of which can be considered parameters of respiratory system failure. Hence, respiratory failure is defined as impaired gas exchange—that is, hypoxemia with or without hypercapnia.

> The function of the respiratory system is to supply the body with adequate oxygen and to remove CO_2.

> Respiration is accomplished by means of ventilation, diffusion, and circulation.

> The respiratory system functions as a pump and as an area of gas exchange.

> Respiratory failure is impaired gas exchange: hypoxemia with or without hypercapnia.

FIGURE 7-1
Breakdown of respiratory failure into its two major components: pump failure and lung failure. The end result of pump failure is hypercapnia, and the end result of lung failure is hypoxemia. (Adapted from Bone RC: Acute respiratory failure: definition and overview. *In* Bone R, ed: *Pulmonary and Critical Care Medicine*. St. Louis: Mosby, 1997.)

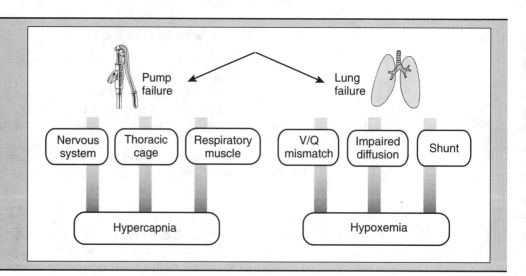

> Respiration is dependent on vital links of anatomic subcomponents.

Although the respiratory system can easily be subdivided into its pump and gas-exchange functional components, the anatomic components that constitute the respiratory system are greater in number and more diverse in nature. Overall, the respiratory system can be physiologically divided into seven anatomic components: 1) the central nervous system; 2) the peripheral nervous system (including the spinal cord and peripheral nerves); 3) the neuromuscular system (including the myoneural junction and respiratory muscles); 4) the thorax and pleura; 5) the upper airways; 6) the cardiovascular system (including the red blood cells, which bind hemoglobin and carbon dioxide); and finally 7) the lower airways, including the alveoli. This classification system, whereby optimum function depends on normal operation of all vital links, highlights the fact that failure of any one of these links may have serious implications and lead to respiratory failure (Figure 7-2).

A helpful way to characterize the many different disease processes that lead to respiratory failure is to separate them into disorders that primarily precipitate pump failure and those that primarily precipitate lung failure. Table 7-1 lists the major pathophysiologic processes that lead primarily to pump failure and to lung failure.

PUMP FAILURE	LUNG FAILURE
Brain Drug overdose Cerebrovascular accident Head trauma	**Lower Airways and Lung** Asthma Bronchitis Chronic obstructive pulmonary disease Pulmonary embolism Acute respiratory distress syndrome Pneumonia Alveolar hemorrhage
Spinal Cord, Neuromuscular Myasthenia gravis Polio Guillain-Barré Spinal cord trauma or tumors	
	Heart Congestive heart failure Valvular abnormalities
Chest Wall Flail chest Kyphoscoliosis Burn eschar	
Upper Airways Vocal cord paralysis or paradoxical motion Tracheal stenosis Laryngospasm	

Table 7-1
Examples of Diseases That Cause Respiratory Failure

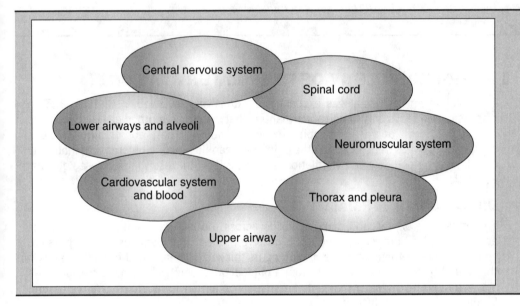

FIGURE 7-2
Seven anatomic subcomponents whose functions are vital to the maintenance of normal respiration. Interruption in the function of any of the links has serious implications for the functioning of the system as a whole. (Adapted from Bone RC: Acute respiratory failure: definition and overview. *In* Bone R, ed.: *Pulmonary and Critical Care Medicine.* St. Louis: Mosby, 1997.)

Besides classifying respiratory failure into pump failure and lung failure subtypes it can be further subdivided into acute and chronic presentations (Table 7-2). In acute presentations of either hypoxemic or hypercapnic respiratory failure, the disease process occurs in minutes to hours, whereas in chronic conditions, gas-exchange disturbances develop over several days or longer. Measurement of blood pH can be an additional aid to further characterization of acute or chronic presentations of hypercapnic respiratory failure. In acute presentations, an inadequate reabsorption of bicarbo-

Respiratory failure can be subclassified into acute and chronic presentations.

PREDOMINANT TYPE	HYPERCAPNIC[a]	HYPOXEMIC[b]
Acute	Minutes to hours; no compensatory changes	Minutes to hours; no compensatory changes
Chronic	Days to months; compensatory mechanisms present are $\uparrow$pH and $\uparrow$ HCO$_3$	Days to months; compensatory mechanism present is $\uparrow$hemoglobin

Table 7-2
Acute Versus Chronic Presentations of Respiratory Failure

[a] $P_aCO_2 > 45$ mmHg
[b] $P_aO_2 < 55$ mmHg while inspiring supplemental O_2 ($F_iO_2 > 40\%$)

nate occurs; in chronic disorders, pH is higher and closer to normal levels as a result of renal conservation of bicarbonate, which buffers chronic elevations in carbon dioxide levels.

Case Study: *Continued*	*Following presentation to the emergency room, the patient is found to be in severe respiratory distress. She cannot speak in one sentence, and she fails to follow simple commands. On physical examination, her respiratory rate is 40 breaths per minute, and she is observed to have paradoxical inward motion of the upper abdomen along with marked use of the accessory inspiratory muscles of the neck and chest wall with flaring of the ala nasi. The patient is promptly intubated with an endotracheal tube, sedated, and placed on mechanical ventilation. While she inspires 100% oxygen on mechanical ventilation with a respiratory rate of 12 breaths per minute and a tidal volume of 600 mL, an arterial blood gas shows a P_aO_2 of 114, a P_aCO_2 of 32, and a pH of 7.47. A chest x-ray shows diffuse alveolar infiltrates.* *Physical examination after intubation reveals a temperature of 101°F, a respiratory rate of 12 breaths per minute, a blood pressure of 120/60 mmHg, and a heart rate of 110 beats per minute. A chest exam shows diffuse end-expiratory wheezes with a 1:4 inspiratory-expiratory ratio. End-inspiratory crackles are also heard at both bases with bronchial breath sounds. Cardiac, abdominal, and extremity examinations are unremarkable.*

PATHOPHYSIOLOGY OF RESPIRATORY FAILURE

Pathophysiologic mechanisms include problems in gas transfer, mismatched perfusion and ventilation, and alveolar hypoventilation.

The mechanism of normal gas exchange is extensively reviewed in Chapter 2. This discussion will focus only on the abnormalities that result in disturbed gas exchange and lead to hypoxemic and/or hypercapnic respiratory failure. These abnormalities include disturbances in gas transfer across the pulmonary capillary bed, problems with matching of pulmonary blood flow and ventilation, and disorders that result in decreased alveolar ventilation.

DIFFUSION ABNORMALITY

Diffusion abnormalities are rarely the sole cause of respiratory failure.

The transfer of oxygen and carbon dioxide across the alveolar capillary membrane is accomplished by diffusion, which is a passive process that depends on the physical characteristics of the membrane, including its thickness, area, and diffusibility, and on the solubility of the gas. However, from a clinical standpoint, abnormal diffusion plays only a minor role in gas-exchange imbalance in patients with acute respiratory failure. Further discussion of diffusion is provided in Chapter 2.

VENTILATION-PERFUSION INEQUALITY

Ideally, each of the lung's alveolar capillary exchange units would have perfect matching of ventilation and perfusion such that optimum gas transfer would occur across each alveolar unit. Realistically, however, this does not occur even in a normal individual, where there is a spectrum of ventilation-perfusion (V_A/Q) ratios varying from those of lung units that are relatively underventilated to those of lung units that are ventilated but not perfused. In normal lungs, V_A/Q may range anywhere from 0.6 to 3.0, with a mean of 1.0. Despite this range of ventilation-perfusion imbalance in a normal lung, however, ventilation-perfusion balance on the whole remains fairly tightly controlled. In the setting of disease, however, considerable mismatching of ventilation and perfusion may occur and may contribute to the development of respiratory failure.

In patients with obstructive or restrictive lung diseases, decreased ventilation resulting from structural or functional abnormalities of the airways can lead to decreased V_A/Q units (Figure 7-3B). Conversely, lung units with high ventilation-perfusion ratios can develop in disorders that lead to overventilation of lung units, such as in emphysematous patients with development of air space enlargement, or to development of underperfusion, as in pulmonary embolism or pulmonary vasospasm (Figure 7-3C).

The development of ventilation-perfusion abnormalities can have a dramatic effect on gas exchange and result in the development of hypoxemia with or without hypercap-

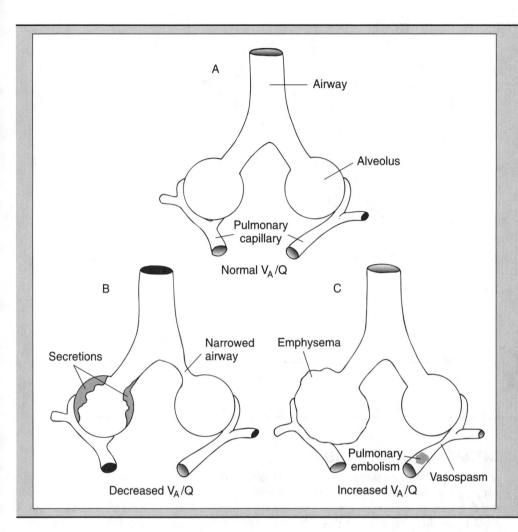

A

Airway

Alveolus

Pulmonary
capillary

Normal V$_A$/Q

B

Secretions

Narrowed
airway

Decreased V$_A$/Q

C

Emphysema

Pulmonary
embolism

Vasospasm

Increased V$_A$/Q

FIGURE 7-3
Examples of ventilation-perfusion inequality. (A) Normal idealized alveolar capillary unit. (B) Examples of decreased ventilation-perfusion units as a result of alveolar secretions or airway obstruction. (C) Examples of increased ventilation-perfusion units owing to the presence of emphysema or problems in the pulmonary vascular bed, such as pulmonary embolism or pulmonary vasospasm.

nia. In a practical sense, however, most of the clinical derangement that is observed following ventilation-perfusion inequality is attributable to the development of profound hypoxemia rather than to the development of hypercapnia. In fact, in most cases, patients with substantial ventilation-perfusion inequality have normal P$_a$CO$_2$ levels or are hypocapnic. This appears to be explained by the differences in the shapes of the oxyhemoglobin and carboxyhemoglobin dissociation curves (Figure 7-4). An increase in P$_a$CO$_2$ sensed by chemoreceptors leads to an increase in minute ventilation, which results in an increase in ventilation of the already well-ventilated lung units. This causes an increase in ventilation-perfusion ratio and an increase in the PO$_2$ of end-capillary blood. However, because of the nonlinear portion of the oxyhemoglobin curve, an increase in PO$_2$ does not result in an increase in the oxygen content of the blood. By contrast, however, a decrease in end-capillary PCO$_2$, because of the linear relationship of carbon dioxide content with the partial pressure of carbon dioxide, most likely results in normocapnia or hypocapnia.

Ventilation-perfusion imbalances also respond in a variable way to increasing concentrations of supplemental oxygen. This fact helps to distinguish ventilation-perfusion imbalance from intrapulmonary shunt as the cause of hypoxemia. As shown in Figure 7-5(A), when disease results in a mild ventilation-perfusion imbalance, the response in arterial PO$_2$ to increased concentrations of supplemental oxygen is relatively linear and approximates the normal condition. With moderate and more severe ventilation-perfusion imbalances, however, higher concentrations of supplemental oxygen are required to demonstrate an increase in arterial PO$_2$. Even with severe ventilation-perfusion imbalances, high concentrations of supplemental oxygen may result in substantial increases in arterial PO$_2$.

Even with substantial V$_A$/Q mismatch, P$_a$CO$_2$ remains low or normal.

V$_A$/Q inequality causing hypoxemia is relatively responsive to inspiration of supplemental oxygen.

FIGURE 7-4

Carboxyhemoglobin and oxyhemoglobin dissociation curves. An increase in the partial pressure of oxygen above a certain level (60 mmHg) does not result in a greater increase in the oxygen content of the blood. However, a linear relationship is seen between the partial pressure of carbon dioxide and carbon dioxide blood content. (Adapted from Dantzker MD, David R: Pulmonary gas exchange. *In* Bone R, ed.: *Pulmonary and Critical Care Medicine*. St. Louis: Mosby, 1997.)

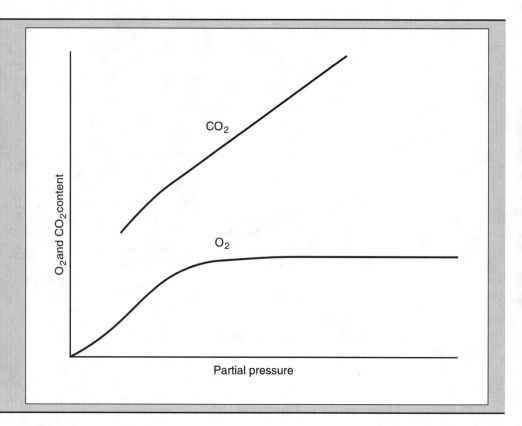

INTRAPULMONARY SHUNT

Intrapulmonary shunt represents mixed-venous blood that is not exposed to the alveolus. Although shunt can be considered an extreme case of V_A/Q inequality, it requires different therapeutic approaches, which makes it uniquely distinct from disorders that cause V_A/Q inequality. Because of this, shunt should be considered as a discrete entity. In normal conditions, 1% to 3% of mixed-venous blood flows directly into the systemic circulation through bronchial and thebesian blood vessels. Clinical disorders resulting in hypoxemic respiratory failure occur in diseases associated with intracardiac or intrapulmonary shunt.

Examples of intracardiac shunt include atrial and ventricular septal defects in which pulmonary hypertension exists. When pressure becomes high enough in the pulmonary vascular bed, right-to-left intracardiac shunt occurs and results in profound hypoxemia. In cases of intrapulmonary shunt, mixed-venous blood passes through pulmonary capillaries into alveoli that are collapsed (atelectatic) or filled with pulmonary edema fluid or inflammatory debris (Figure 7-5A). This is the condition that leads to hypoxemia in patients who present with congestive heart failure, acute respiratory distress syndrome, or severe pneumonia.

> Intrapulmonary shunt greater than 30% causing hypoxemia is relatively refractory to inspiration of supplemental oxygen.

As shown in Figure 7-6(B), intrapulmonary shunts of 30% or greater are relatively refractory to inspiration of higher concentrations of supplemental oxygen. Breathing even 100% oxygen has a minimum impact on increasing arterial PO_2 in patients with severe shunts. This fact can be used as a clinical tool to help identify intrapulmonary shunt rather than V_A/Q inequality as the underlying pathophysiologic mechanism in patients who present with hypoxemia and elevated A-a gradients. In contrast to patients with severe shunts, patients with elevated A-a gradients resulting from V_A/Q inequality exhibit substantial increases in PO_2 while breathing supplemental oxygen.

> Treatment of intrapulmonary shunt includes supplemental oxygen with treatment of the underlying process and attempts to recruit lung volume with CPAP, PEEP, or mechanical ventilation.

Because of the relative refractoriness of moderate to severe shunts to supplemental oxygen, the underlying pathophysiologic process must be treated by recruiting lung units by the application of positive pressure to the alveolus.

HYPOVENTILATION

To prevent the development of respiratory acidosis, the carbon dioxide produced each day as an end product of metabolism (approximately 17,000 mEq of acid) must be exhaled

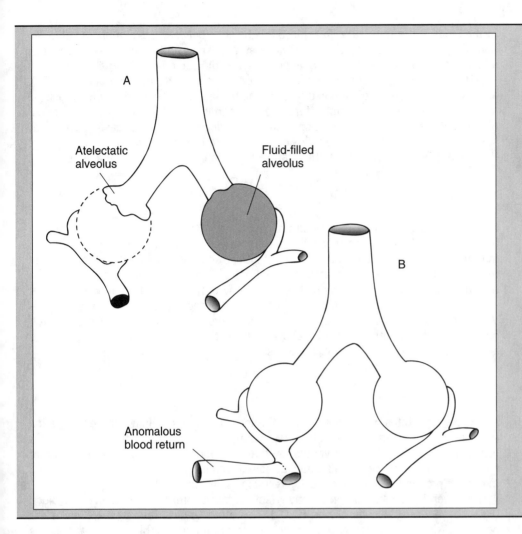

FIGURE 7-5
Examples of intrapulmonary shunt. (A) Collapsed alveolus and fluid-filled alveolus as examples of intrapulmonary shunt. (B) Effect of anomalous blood return of mixed-venous blood bypassing the alveolus and contributing to intrapulmonary shunt.

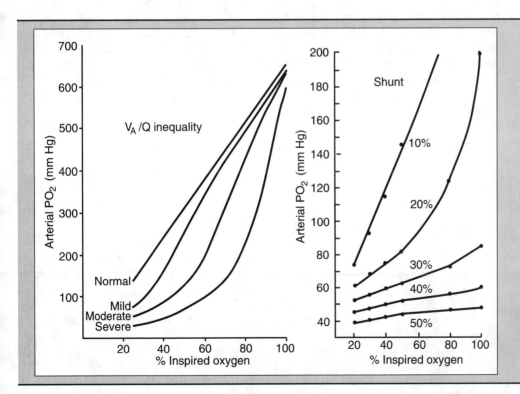

FIGURE 7-6
Response of ventilation-perfusion inequality or intrapulmonary shunt to supplemental oxygen. (A) Ventilation-perfusion inequality under mild to severe circumstances. Even with the presence of severe V_A/Q inequality, high levels of supplemental oxygen have a profound impact on increasing arterial PO_2. (B) By contrast, intrapulmonary shunts of 30% or greater are relatively refractory to supplemental oxygen increasing arterial P_aO_2. (Adapted from Dantzker MD, David R: Pulmonary gas exchange. *In* Bone R, ed.: *Pulmonary and Critical Care Medicine.* St. Louis: Mosby, 1997.)

by the lungs at the same rate. To achieve this balance between production and elimination of carbon dioxide, the central nervous system and carotid body chemoreceptors adjust ventilation over a fairly wide range of carbon dioxide production.

The relationship among alveolar ventilation (V_A), carbon dioxide production (VCO_2), and the partial pressure of carbon dioxide in the blood (P_aCO_2) can be described using a modification of the Fick principle of mass balance that quantitates VCO_2 as the product of V_A and the fractional concentration of carbon dioxide in the alveolar gas. Under steady state conditions, in which carbon dioxide is eliminated from the body at a rate equal to the rate at which it is produced, the relationship among P_aCO_2, VCO_2, and V_A is

_P_aCO_2 is inversely related to alveolar ventilation (V_A)._

$$P_aCO_2 = \frac{K(VCO_2)}{V_A},$$

where K is a constant and R (the respiratory quotient, VCO_2/VO_2) = 0.863. In the normal lung, V_A generally is a fixed proportion of minute ventilation (V_E), the total ventilation measured over a collection period of 1 minute. Dead space ventilation (V_D), the portion of minute ventilation that insufflates the conducting airways and does not participate directly in gas exchange, approximates the volume of the conducting airways. Alveolar ventilation then is the total minute ventilation minus dead space ventilation ($V_A = V_E - V_D$). Thus one can consider V_E and P_aCO_2 to be inversely proportional to one another. If one rewrites the equation for P_aCO_2 above and substitutes $V_E - V_D$ for V_A, the relationship among P_aCO_2, VCO_2, and V_A becomes

$$P_aCO_2 = \frac{K(VCO_2)}{V_E - V_D}.$$

Therefore, states of alveolar hypoventilation are those in which minute ventilation (V_E) is reduced or dead space ventilation (V_D) is high. Either or both of these mechanisms result in a decrease in alveolar ventilation that is abnormally low for a given amount of carbon dioxide production. Inadequate alveolar ventilation to compensate for increased metabolic production of carbon dioxide results in a rise in P_aCO_2.

Hypoventilation may also indirectly affect the partial pressure of oxygen in the blood (P_aO_2) by reducing alveolar oxygen (P_AO_2). This effect is described by the alveolar gas equation, which is discussed later in the subsection on arterial blood-gas analysis. As shown in Figure 7-7, a fall in alveolar ventilation or a rise in carbon dioxide production greater than an increase in alveolar ventilation will result in an increase in P_aCO_2 and a decrease in alveolar PO_2 with a consequent decrease in P_aO_2. In this case, because all of the parameters used in calculating alveolar PO_2 change together, the alveolar-arterial oxygen gradient remains normal. It is important to differentiate hypoxemia caused by alveolar hypoventilation from hypoxemia caused by ventilation-perfusion inequality because these disease processes and their treatments differ markedly. Although hypoxemia in both cases may be treated by inspiration of supplemental oxygen, in most cases hypoventilation must be treated with an augmentation of ventilation to avoid the progressive development of respiratory acidosis.

Hypoventilation reduces P_aO_2 indirectly by increasing P_aCO_2 and reducing P_AO_2.

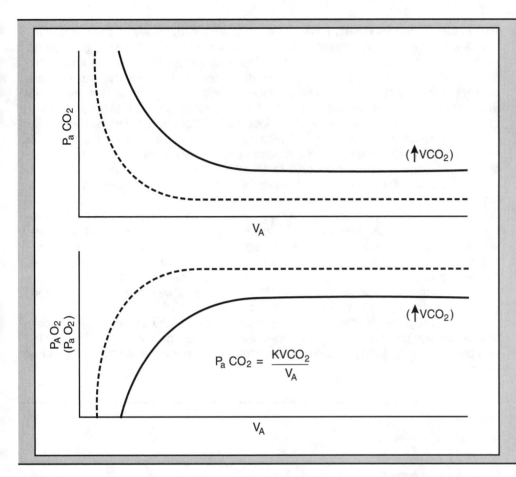

FIGURE 7-7
The relationship of P_aCO_2, P_AO_2, and P_aO_2 to alveolar ventilation. As alveolar ventilation (V_A) increases, P_aCO_2 decreases. As the amount of CO_2 production (VCO_2) increases, this relationship is shifted upward and to the right. Conversely, with an increase in alveolar ventilation (V_A), alveolar oxygen (P_AO_2) and consequently arterial oxygen (P_aO_2), increase. (Adapted from Dantzker MD, David R: Pulmonary gas exchange. *In* Bone R, ed: *Pulmonary and Critical Care Medicine.* St. Louis: Mosby, 1997.)

$$P_aCO_2 = \frac{KVCO_2}{V_A}$$

■ DIAGNOSIS OF RESPIRATORY FAILURE
HISTORY AND PHYSICAL EXAMINATION

Patient Symptoms. The clinical manifestations and symptoms in patients with respiratory failure may vary in accordance with the severity and acuity of the inciting event and with the patient's underlying condition. In patients with catastrophic disorders, and in those with severe underlying diseases who have limited ventilatory reserve, respiratory failure presents acutely. Examples include, respectively, patients who suffer major acute intracranial bleeding and pneumothorax in severe COPD. In other cases, respiratory failure may present insidiously over weeks to months after mechanisms compensating for the gradual development of hypoxemia and/or hypercapnia have failed. Examples include respiratory failure developing in patients with slowly progressive neurologic disorders, such as Duchenne's muscular dystrophy.

In patients who present with respiratory failure, the earliest respiratory complaint is dyspnea, which occurs first with exertion and later, with progression of the disease, at rest. Cough, sputum production, and chest pain may also indicate a primary pulmonary process that triggers the development of respiratory failure. As respiratory failure progresses and precipitates substantial gas-exchange imbalances (i.e., hypoxemia with or without hypercapnia), mental function may also be affected and the patient may complain of headache, visual disturbances, confusion, memory loss, or, in extreme cases, loss of consciousness (Table 7-3).

Dyspnea is the earliest symptom of respiratory failure.

Mental function: headache, visual disturbances, confusion, memory loss, hallucinations, loss of consciousness

Dyspnea (resting vs. exertional)

Cough, sputum production, chest pain

Table 7-3
Patient Symptoms in Respiratory Failure

Physical examination begins with a quick overview of the patient's condition.

Physical Examination. Physical examination in patients with respiratory failure begins with a general assessment. A quick overview of the patient's vital signs, mental alertness, and ability to speak can rapidly triage patients into those who have more severe and those who have less severe manifestations of respiratory failure. In those patients who present with a significant decrease in mental alertness, a more severe manifestation of respiratory failure exists. Moreover, patients unable to speak in complete sentences usually have an FEV_1 of less than 1 liter and similarly suffer from a severe manifestation of a disease precipitating respiratory failure. Other helpful clues are a respiratory rate greater than 35, a heart rate 20 to 30 beats greater than normal, and the presence of pulsus paradoxus (a 15 to 20 mmHg decrease in systolic blood pressure during inspiration). These findings all signify an increased respiratory work load. Similarly, an elevated work of breathing can be assumed when patients use the accessory muscles of ventilation or, in some cases, by the pattern of breathing, especially when paradoxical movements of the rib cage or abdominal compartments are present during inspiration. Paradoxical rib cage or abdominal movements during inspiration (i.e., rib cage and abdominal movements in opposite directions rather than similar outward movements) signify either the development of respiratory muscle dysfunction (respiratory muscle fatigue or respiratory muscle weakness) or a ventilatory work load that is higher than the ventilatory capacity.

Finally, the presence of abnormal auscultatory sounds of the upper airways (stridor) or lower airways (wheezes, rhonchi, or rales) may indicate a primary underlying pulmonary process (e.g., asthma, pneumonia, or sarcoidosis) that is contributing to respiratory failure (Table 7-4).

Table 7-4
Physical Examination in Respiratory Failure

Mental alertness
Ability to speak in sentences
Respiratory rate, heart rate
Pulsus paradoxus present?
Work of breathing (use of accessory muscles)
Pattern of breathing (paradoxical movements of rib cage or abdominal compartments)

Abnormal auscultatory sounds:
   Stridor
   Wheezes
   Rhonchi
   Rales

Findings on history and physical examination must be complemented by laboratory evaluation.

Although the above mentioned findings may indicate the severity, or even in some cases the etiology, of respiratory failure, in most cases the clinical history and physical examination of patients with respiratory failure are relatively nondescript and must be complemented by results from laboratory evaluation.

LABORATORY DIAGNOSIS OF RESPIRATORY FAILURE

The laboratory diagnosis of respiratory failure involves four major categories of testing: arterial blood-gas analysis, measurements of respiratory mechanics, chest imaging, and results of general laboratory testing (Table 7-5). The following is a description of the important features of each of these tests.

Arterial blood-gas analysis is the most important laboratory test in the diagnosis of respiratory failure.

Arterial Blood-Gas Analysis. Arterial blood-gas analysis is the single most important laboratory test used to subclassify the type of respiratory failure. It also provides an indication of the duration and the severity of the episode of respiratory failure. Arterial blood-gas analysis provides information on the presence of three major abnormalities: hypoxemia (reduction of partial pressure of oxygen in the blood), hypercapnia ($P_aCO_2 > 45$ mmHg), and the arterial pH.

Hypoxemia is a reduction of the partial pressure of oxygen in the blood.

Hypoxemia. Hypoxemia is a reduction of the partial pressure of oxygen in the blood. Although normal resting P_aO_2 ranges from 75 to 80 mmHg, a P_aO_2 of less than 60 mmHg is considered to be a lower limit of safety, because lower values represent displacement to

Table 7-5
Laboratory Diagnosis of Respiratory Failure

Arterial Blood-Gas Analysis
P_aO_2
P_aCO_2
pH

Measurements of Respiratory Mechanics
Spirometry (FVC, FEV_1, peak flow)
Respiratory muscle pressures

Chest Imaging
Chest x-ray
CT scan
Ventilation-perfusion scan

Other Tests
Hemoglobin/hematocrit
Electrolytes, bun, creatinine
Creatinine phosphokinase, aldolase

the steep slope of the oxyhemoglobin dissociation curve. In cases of respiratory failure, oxygenation failure is defined as a P_aO_2 of 60 mmHg or less on F_IO_2 of 40% or less.

The mechanisms by which clinically significant reductions in P_aO_2 are produced include right-to-left intrapulmonary or intracardiac shunting of blood, mismatching of ventilation and perfusion, and alveolar hypoventilation, as previously discussed. Hypoxemia caused by alveolar hypoventilation is characterized by a normal alveolar-arterial oxygen difference ($P_AO_2 - P_aO_2$). This difference can be calculated by using the alveolar gas equation to estimate alveolar oxygen (P_AO_2) and measuring the arterial oxygen level of blood during arterial blood-gas analysis (P_aO_2).

As fresh gas is breathed at atmospheric pressure, it is warmed and humidified. The inspired oxygen (P_IO_2) depends on the barometric pressure (P_B). P_B at sea level is 760 mmHg or 1 atm. $P_IO_2 = F_IO_2 (P_B - \text{water vapor pressure})$, where P_IO_2 is the partial pressure of oxygen in the central airways, F_IO_2 is the fraction of oxygen in inspired gas, and P_B is barometric pressure at sea level (760 mmHg). The water vapor pressure exerted at 100% saturation is 47 mmHg, which is the condition in the lower airways.

Measurement of alveolar gas exchange is important because the difference between P_AO_2 and measured P_aO_2 (i.e., the alveolar-arterial oxygen gradient) represents the efficiency of gas exchange between the alveolus and the pulmonary capillary bed. The amount of oxygen at the alveolar level (P_AO_2) can be calculated by the simplified alveolar gas equation:

$$P_AO_2 = P_IO_2 - \frac{P_aCO_2}{R}.$$

The alveolar-arterial oxygen gradient is normally 10 to 20 mmHg but varies with age, body posture, and percentage of the inspired oxygen concentration.

An example calculation of the alveolar-arterial oxygen gradient in a representative patient is as follows:

$$\text{Alveolar-arterial oxygen gradient} = P_IO_2 - \frac{P_aCO_2}{R} - P_aO_2,$$

where $R - 0.8$ (respiratory quotient, VCO_2/VO_2), $P_IO_2 = F_IO_2 (P_B - 47 \text{ mmHg})$, and P_aO_2 and P_aCO_2 are measured by arterial blood-gas measurement.

If a patient breathes room-air oxygen ($F_IO_2 = 0.21$) at sea level ($P_B = 1 \text{ atm} = 760$ mmHg), water vapor pressure is 47 mmHg and P_IO_2 becomes 150:

$$P_IO_2 = F_IO_2 (760 - \text{water vapor})$$

$$= 0.21 (760 - 47)$$

$$= 150$$

If an arterial blood gas measures a P_aCO_2 of 80 mmHg and a P_aO_2 of 40 mmHg, the alveolar oxygen gradient becomes 10. Severe hypoxemia in this case is the result of hypoventilation, not intrapulmonary shunting or ventilation-perfusion imbalance.

Calculation of the alveolar-arterial (A-a) gradient enables one to differentiate hypoxemia caused hypoventilation from hypoxemia resulting from other causes.

$$\text{Alveolar-arterial oxygen gradient} = P_IO_2 - \frac{P_aCO_2}{R} - P_aO_2$$

$$= 150 - \frac{80}{0.8} - 40 = 10$$

Hypercapnia is defined as a P_aCO_2 greater than 45 mmHg.

Hypercapnia. Hypercapnia is an elevation in arterial carbon dioxide tension (P_aCO_2) above the upper limit of normal (45 mmHg). Hypercapnia is more commonly present in chronic cases of respiratory failure resulting from neuromuscular diseases, impaired sensorium, thoracic cage abnormalities, or chronic obstructive pulmonary disease (COPD). Hypercapnia that exists in acute conditions (such as asthma or pulmonary embolism) most likely represents acute severe respiratory failure and has more ominous implications. In all cases, the only mechanism by which hypercapnia occurs is alveolar hypoventilation.

Changes in pH can help differentiate acute from chronic elevations in P_aCO_2.

Arterial pH. The relationship between P_aCO_2 and plasma bicarbonate as described by the Henderson-Hasselbalch equation dictates arterial pH (Table 7-6). This relationship, however, varies according to the duration over which P_aCO_2 has increased. By using the arterial blood gas to measure arterial pH and P_aCO_2, the Henderson-Hasselbalch equation can be used to calculate the bicarbonate level. Only small increases in plasma bicarbonate accompany acute increases in P_aCO_2 over minutes to hours. Over a period of several days, renal conservation of bicarbonate causes bicarbonate levels to increase and buffers pH changes that would otherwise result from a rise in the partial pressure of carbon dioxide. Therefore, changes in pH are much less severe in situations where carbon dioxide retention has been present for longer periods of time. Examples of the effects of acute and chronic variations in P_aCO_2 and plasma bicarbonate on pH levels are shown in Figure 7-8.

Table 7-6
Henderson-Hasselbalch Equation

$$pH = pK_A + \log \frac{[HCO_3^-]}{[H_2CO_3]}$$

$[CO_2]$ can be substituted for $[H_2CO_3]$ and expressed as the product of PCO_2 and 0.03 mL/dL/mmHg, the CO_2 solubility coefficient.

FIGURE 7-8
Effects of acute and chronic variations in P_aCO_2 on plasma bicarbonate and pH. The line connecting points A and C represents the effect of an acute change in P_aCO_2 to a value above or below 40 mmHg. More chronic rise in P_aCO_2 that allows for the effect of renal compensation shows a shift in this relationship to the curve connecting points D and B. In the latter circumstance, renal conservation of bicarbonate attenuates the decline in pH by a rise in arterial P_aCO_2. Reproduced with permission from Murray JF: *The Normal Lung.* Philadelphia: WB Saunders, 1976, p. 224.

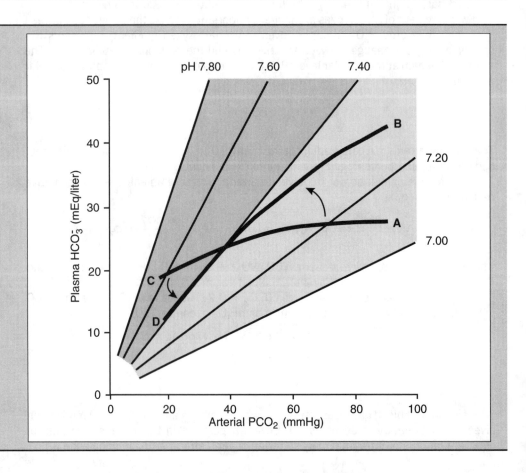

Measurements of Respiratory Mechanics.

Although measurements of lung function are somewhat limited in critically ill patients, in certain circumstances, measurements of respiratory mechanics may help to grade the severity of the abnormality causing respiratory failure and provide insight into the causative mechanism.

In most cases, measurements of spirometry or respiratory muscle pressures are the only respiratory mechanics tests that are applicable in the patient presenting in respiratory failure. Measurements of vital capacity (VC), forced expiratory volume in 1 second (FEV$_1$), and peak expiratory flow rate (PEFR) are the most common parameters used in assessment.

VC is the maximum volume of air that can be exhaled after a maximal inspiration and provides an indication of the patient's maximum ventilatory capability. VC is influenced by the functioning of the central and peripheral nervous systems, the elastic properties of the lung and chest wall, and airway caliber. It cannot be used to assess specific abnormalities of the individual components of the respiratory system but helps to provide a simple, useful measurement of its aggregate function. In most cases, the minimal acceptable VC before respiratory failure ensues is approximately 10 to 15 ml per kilogram of body weight. Lower values usually signify significant impairment of the respiratory system as a pump and predict imminent need for ventilatory assistance. However, as for any laboratory tool used in the diagnosis of respiratory failure, the results of the test must be used only in light of an individual's particular clinical circumstance.

FEV$_1$ is that portion of forced VC measured over the first 1 second of expiration and is used to measure the severity of airflow obstruction. FEV$_1$ values less than 25% of the predicted value are usually associated with increases in P$_a$CO$_2$. The FEV$_1$ test can also be used serially to assess the patient's response to therapy. Measurement of the peak expiratory flow rate (PEFR), the maximum point on the forced expiratory limbs of the flow volume curve, provides information similar to the FEV$_1$.

Measurements of respiratory muscle pressures can also be useful in identifying the cause and also the severity of respiratory muscle weakness contributing to respiratory failure. Maximum inspiratory pressure is a global measurement of inspiratory muscle strength performed under conditions of maximum effort at a known lung volume. Because lung volume affects the precontraction length of the respiratory muscles, maximum inspiratory pressure should be recorded at or near residual volume in order to measure inspiratory muscle pressures under the most optimum condition. Conversely, measurements of expiratory muscle strength (maximum expiratory pressure) should be conducted at or near total lung capacity in order to place the expiratory muscles on the optimum portion of the length-tension curve. As with other measurements of respiratory mechanics, full patient cooperation is required to ensure maximum contraction such that submaximal effort is not a factor limiting the interpretation of values that are lower than normal.

Chest Imaging.

In selected patients, imaging of the chest can provide important information as to the cause of respiratory failure. The test imaging techniques most commonly used in the assessment of the patient who presents in respiratory failure include the chest x-ray, computed tomography (CT) scanning of the thorax, and ventilation-perfusion lung scanning.

The chest x-ray may be important in demonstrating the severity of the chest wall abnormality causing respiratory failure, which is found in cases of severe kyphoscoliosis or flail chest. In patients with abnormalities of the bony thorax who present with respiratory failure, predominantly hypercapnic respiratory failure owing to pump dysfunction, the amount of deviation of the thoracic spine on chest x-ray can be quantitated and used to predict the onset of respiratory failure. Moreover, other patterns on chest x-ray that indicate the presence of severe COPD, pneumonia, or diffuse lung infiltrates, as seen in cases of diffuse interstitial lung disease or the acute respiratory distress syndrome, provide insight into the cause and magnitude of the primary pulmonary process that leads to respiratory failure. The chest x-ray in selected respiratory diseases is important not only in identifying the cause of respiratory failure, but also in assessing the patient's response to therapy.

Although the chest x-ray is the most important initial tool used in the radiologic assessment of the thorax in patients with respiratory failure, the chest CT scan is a more

Measurements of respiratory mechanics may be helpful in identifying the cause of respiratory failure in some patients.

FEV$_1$ and PEFR are used to measure the degree of airflow obstruction.

Respiratory muscle pressures can be helpful in identifying the cause and severity of respiratory muscle weakness.

Chest imaging in respiratory failure includes the chest x-ray (CXR), chest computed tomography (chest CT), and ventilation-perfusion (V/Q) lung scanning.

The chest x-ray is the simplest and most common chest imaging test used in the assessment of respiratory failure.

The chest CT scan is sensitive and specific in delineating pleural from parenchymal processes.

Ventilation-perfusion lung scanning is helpful in the diagnosis of massive and submassive pulmonary thromboembolism as causes of respiratory failure.

General laboratory tests can aid in diagnosing the chronicity of respiratory failure and the contributions of metabolic factors to its precipitation.

sensitive and specific imaging modality. Chest CT is the best imaging test for differentiating pleural from parenchymal abnormalities and characterizing their distribution. The use of an intravenous contrast medium may also help to identify pulmonary vascular abnormalities and their roles in the pathogenesis of respiratory failure.

In selected patients who suffer predominantly from unexplained hypoxemic respiratory failure, ventilation-perfusion scanning of the lung may be helpful. This test allows one to assess how individual regions of the lung participate in ventilation and perfusion. Specific patterns of ventilation-perfusion imbalance can be considered as diagnostic of pulmonary thromboembolism and can help to diagnose pulmonary embolism as a cause of respiratory failure. In cases where ventilation-perfusion scanning is nondiagnostic, performance of a pulmonary angiogram helps to rule in or rule out pulmonary embolism as an etiologic possibility.

Other Tests. In selected patients, results of routine tests performed to assess the patient's general condition may help to provide clues to the cause or chronicity of the problem causing respiratory failure. For example, the presence of secondary polycythemia indicates the presence of chronic hypoxemia, a fact that may be important in constructing the differential diagnosis. Electrolyte imbalances may indicate not only the reason for respiratory pump dysfunction (hypocalcemia, hypomagnesemia, hypokalemia, and hypophosphatemia all impair skeletal muscle contractility) but also the presence of other related metabolic abnormalities; for instance, metabolic acidosis or metabolic alkalosis indicates the presence of a systemic problem that has major implications for respiratory work load and cardiopulmonary function. In selected patients, measurements of creatinine phosphokinase or aldolase may be important in determining the presence of a systemic neuromuscular disease as a cause of hypercapnic respiratory pump failure.

Case Study:
Continued

The patient is admitted to the intensive care unit and is maintained on mechanical ventilation in an assist control mode. She is placed on 100% oxygen with increasing levels of positive end-expiratory pressure (PEEP) to decrease intrapulmonary shunting and improve oxygenation. With 10 cm H_2O PEEP applied with an F_IO_2 of 100%, her P_aO_2 is 70 mmHg.

The patient continues to receive aggressive use of bronchodilators to alleviate bronchospasm and is given parenteral sedation and neuromuscular blocking agents to facilitate ventilation, decrease patient effort, and improve patient comfort.

A Gram stain of the sputum shows a marked increase in white blood cells and gram-positive diplococci. The patient is placed on cefotaxime, at a dosage of 1 gram three times a day, and on prophylactic therapy for GI bleed and deep venous thrombosis. She is fed enterally through a nasoduodenal feeding tube.

■ TREATMENT OF RESPIRATORY FAILURE

Treatment of respiratory failure is based on characterizing the underlying process as to whether it impairs the respiratory system primarily as a pump (hypercapnia) or as an area of gas exchange (hypoxemia). Therefore, treatment for respiratory failure is best done after it has been characterized as hypoxemic, hypercapnic respiratory failure or as hypoxemic, nonhypercapnic respiratory failure. Figure 7-9 outlines an approach to the treatment of respiratory failure based on pump or lung failure as the predominant cause.

OXYGEN

Oxygen should always be used to treat hypoxemic respiratory failure.

The most important initial approach to the treatment of a patient with respiratory failure is to identify the need for supplemental oxygen. Oxygen is frequently necessary for patients who present with hypoxemia or with conditions known to predispose the patient to hypoxemia. Various types of external oxygen delivery devices are available to provide supplemental oxygen. The choice of a particular device depends on 1) the magnitude of supplemental oxygen required by the patient, 2) the need for precise control of supplemental oxygen to avoid excessive oxygenation and hypercapnia, 3) the need for airway control and suctioning for excessive secretions, and 4) the need to increase lung volume

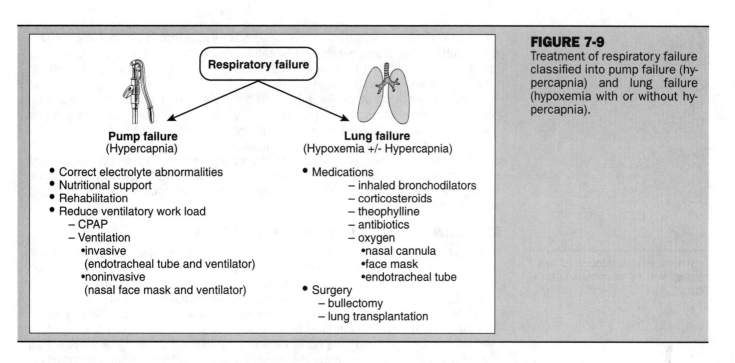

FIGURE 7-9
Treatment of respiratory failure classified into pump failure (hypercapnia) and lung failure (hypoxemia with or without hypercapnia).

by externally applied tidal volumes or the use of positive end-expiratory pressure (PEEP) to improve oxygenation.

Delivering supplemental oxygen by the use of nasal prongs is the simplest and most comfortable method for patients, but this type of apparatus, despite its comfort, cannot be used to provide high levels of oxygen or provide them in an extremely precise manner because of the entrainment of room air with mouth breathing or during high levels of ventilation. Face mask devices that fit more tightly and have nonrebreathing valves and reservoir bags provide higher and more precise concentrations of supplemental oxygen even up to oxygen concentration levels of 80% to 90%. In addition, these devices can also accommodate the use of one-way valves that may allow one to provide external PEEP in order to increase end-expiratory lung volume and thereby decrease intrapulmonary shunting in an attempt to improve oxygenation. Delivery of oxygen by means of a face mask with a Venturi device, a calibrated in-line device, provides high flows of oxygen in more precise increments.

Many devices are used to deliver supplemental oxygen to patients in respiratory failure. Nasal prongs are the easiest but are inefficient, whereas masks are cumbersome but more efficient. Venturi delivery devices allow oxygen prescription to be more precise.

MEDICATIONS

The use of selected medications for the treatment of respiratory failure depends on the underlying disorder. In patients who present with exacerbation of airway obstruction, aggressive inhaled bronchodilator therapy may lessen airway obstruction, improve secretion elimination, and decrease patient ventilatory work load. Inhaled beta agonists, anticholinergics, and, on occasion, systemic theophylline preparations may lessen airway obstruction and help treat the primary disturbance leading to respiratory failure. For patients who have asthma as the primary cause of airway obstruction, systemic corticosteroid therapy has been repeatedly demonstrated to be the cornerstone of medical therapy. Currently in patients who present with primary pulmonary infection as the cause of respiratory failure, the use of antibiotics based on Gram stain and culture of respiratory secretions is mandatory.

SUPPORTIVE THERAPY

Electrolyte or acid-base disturbances known to compromise respiratory pump failure or add to ventilatory work load should be identified and corrected. Hypocalcemia, hypokalemia, hypomagnesemia, and hypophosphatemia all should be identified and corrected if present. Moreover, the presence of a metabolic acidosis should be confirmed and its etiologic event identified so that proper treatment can be instituted. For example, the presence of diabetes ketoacidosis in a patient with underlying pulmonary disease may be the metabolic abnormality that provokes respiratory failure as a result of the effects of metabolic acidosis on increasing ventilatory work load in an otherwise compromised patient. Therefore, direction of attention toward treatment of the metabolic acidosis secondary to diabetic ketoacidosis should be the focus of therapy in such a patient who presents with respiratory failure.

Besides identification of electrolyte and metabolic abnormalities, nutritional support and in some cases reconditioning are important in restoring respiratory pump function and reversing the presence of respiratory failure. Poor nutrition complicates the course of the disorder in the majority of hospitalized patients and even in outpatients with underlying respiratory diseases and is commonly encountered in patients hospitalized with severe systemic diseases. Therefore, ensuring adequate nutrition in order to restore respiratory muscle mass and normal respiratory fiber type composition are important adjuncts to therapy.

REDUCING VENTILATORY WORK LOAD

In some patients, however, because ventilatory work load far exceeds ventilatory capabilities, the measures described above are inadequate for reducing ventilatory work load so as to permit spontaneous ventilation. In these cases, augmentation of the patient's spontaneous ventilation by the use of mechanical ventilation is required.

Augmentation of the patient's spontaneous ventilation can be achieved by either invasive or noninvasive techniques. Invasive forms of ventilation require the use of an artificial conduit inserted in the patient's airway—either a translaryngeal endotracheal tube or a subglottic tracheostomy tube. In noninvasive ventilation, a nasal or nasal-oral face mask is used to augment the patient's spontaneous efforts without the use of an artificial airway.

Invasive ventilation is the most frequently used method of augmenting the patient's spontaneous respiratory effort. In this case, airway intubation is considered to be requisite for the patient's therapy so as to 1) protect the airway, if the patient's consciousness is impaired; 2) suction secretions for patients with excessive mouth or lower respiratory tract secretions; 3) achieve higher oxygen concentrations than are possible with a face mask; and 4) facilitate the use of mechanical ventilation to increase lung volume or to stabilize gas-exchange imbalance.

Endotracheal intubation may be accomplished by means of either nasal or oral translaryngeal intubation. Oral intubation allows a larger tube to be used and is easier to perform under emergent conditions when the vocal cords are visualized by the use of a fiberoptic endoscope or laryngoscope. However, in the long term, oral intubation is uncomfortable for the patient, is less stable, and presents more difficulties in terms of nursing care and oral hygiene. The nasal tube is more comfortable for the patient, is easier to place in a spontaneously breathing patient, and remains stable for longer periods of time, although it can be complicated by the development of sinusitis. In addition, because of its smaller size, the nasally placed endotracheal tube has a higher resistance than the larger, orally placed tube. This latter factor may be important in patients with respiratory failure resulting primarily from an increase in airway resistance, such as in asthma or COPD, and may hinder the weaning process.

Mechanical ventilators are intended to stabilize gas-exchange imbalances until the primary process resolves, not necessarily to achieve normal gas-exchange parameters of pH, PCO_2, or P_aO_2. In some patients, normal values cannot be easily attained without significant complications. For example, if maintaining a normal pH or PCO_2 value predisposes the patient to unacceptably high airway pressures and results in hypotension or lung injury, the goal of ventilation must be refocused to one of stabilizing the patient without subjecting him or her to undue risk for complications from the therapy.

Mechanical ventilators, although variable in size, shape, flow pattern, and other characteristics, must share certain essential features, including delivery of a wide range of tidal volumes (from 100 to 2000 mL), adjustment of respiratory rates from 2 to 60 breaths per minute, and accurate adjustment of inspired oxygen concentrations from 21% to 100%. The ability to adjust inspiratory and expiratory flows, and safety alarms for low and high airway pressures, are also mandatory. Finally, the device must be able to support the patient completely or to assist patient-initiated breaths in patients capable of

Mechanical ventilation is used to augment spontaneous ventilation.

The goal of mechanical ventilation is to stabilize gas exchange, but normal values of pH, P_aCO_2, and P_aO_2 are not paramount.

assisting the machine to ensure their comfort and facilitate their weaning from mechanical ventilation as the primary process resolves.

In general, tidal volumes of 6 to 10 mL/kg are used to augment the patient's spontaneous ventilation, with a backup respiratory rate of approximately 80% of the patient's spontaneous rate. Patients who, because of sedation or severe weakness, are incapable of triggering the ventilator are maintained on controlled forms of ventilation that require frequent assessment of tidal volume and respiratory rate and arterial blood-gas analysis to maintain satisfactory gas exchange.

Although not essential, the capability of providing continuous airway pressure at controlled levels throughout the respiratory cycle (continuous positive airway pressure, or CPAP) or at end-expiration (positive end-expiratory pressure, or PEEP) has been shown to be a helpful tool in oxygenating the patient or transitioning the patient from full ventilatory support to spontaneous breathing (i.e., weaning from mechanical ventilation).

Although mechanical ventilation has been demonstrated to be effective in stabilizing patients with severe life-threatening medical or surgical processes, it is not without complications. Mechanical ventilation has been reported to be associated with about a 60% incidence of lower respiratory tract infection and a 10% to 24% incidence of barotrauma, and most patients who have undergone mechanical ventilation report it to have been an unpleasant experience because of patient-ventilator dyssynchrony and the inability to communicate. In addition, once patients require invasive mechanical ventilation for treatment of respiratory failure, hospital stays are lengthened and mortality increases. Because of these factors, physicians are resorting to noninvasive forms of ventilatory assistance to stabilize patients presenting with respiratory failure so as to avoid the need for invasive ventilation.

The most recent form of noninvasive ventilation employs a nasal or nasal-oral mask with a preset pressure that allows the patient to initiate a breath and receive ventilatory support to the preset pressure in order to augment the patient's own tidal volume and decrease the work of breathing. In several recent prospective, randomized, controlled trials conducted in patients presenting with acute respiratory failure, the use of this form of therapy, in contrast to standard medical therapy, has resulted in a reduced need for invasive ventilation, more rapid stabilization of gas exchange and vital signs, and a decrease in hospital mortality. Characterization of the patients who may best benefit from noninvasive forms of ventilation and those who are not appropriate candidates awaits further study. However, those patients who have rapidly progressive disease, cannot control their airways, are hemodynamically unstable, or do not benefit immediately from the various forms of noninvasive ventilation should be stabilized with endotracheal intubation and mechanical ventilation (i.e., invasive ventilation).

OTHER THERAPY

Selected patients with severe, advanced, end-stage lung disease may be candidates for surgical treatment of respiratory failure. In selected cases, this may include biopsy of lung tissue to determine the cause of respiratory failure, a procedure that almost always is used in patients with unidentified processes involving the pulmonary parenchyma. In selected cases, stabilization of the chest wall in patients who suffer from flail chest, decortication of fibrotic pleura trapping the lung after a significant pleural space infection, and resection of a large bulla that compresses viable lung tissue in patients with advanced COPD are indications for surgical treatment of respiratory failure.

In the last 10 years, however, single-lung, double-lung, and heart-lung transplantation has been used to treat patients with advanced lung diseases causing respiratory failure. In these cases, respiratory failure is most likely a result of end-stage COPD, pulmonary hypertension, cystic fibrosis, interstitial lung disease, or some other disorder wherein the lung is severely and irreversibly incapable of effective gas exchange in spite of maximal medical therapy.

Surgery has a limited but occasionally important role in the treatment of respiratory failure.

Case Study:
Resolution

The patient's clinical condition continues to improve with the use of antibiotics, bronchodilators, and supportive care measures. Subsequent chest x-rays show significant clearing of parenchymal infiltrates, and the patient is eventually able to be titrated to an F_IO_2 of 40% with gradual removal of PEEP. While breathing 40% oxygen through a T-piece, the patient is comfortable, exhibits satisfactory hemodynamics and respiratory variables, and is extubated. Following extubation, the patient suffers from weakness of the lower extremities secondary to high-dosage steroids and neuromuscular blocking agents. Following extubation and transfer to a Step Down Unit, the patient receives extensive whole-body rehabilitation and is discharged from the hospital to home.

The final diagnosis for this patient is pneumococcal pneumonia, status asthmaticus, and the development of the acute respiratory distress syndrome. She continues to do well 2 years later in follow-up in the outpatient clinic, where she is treated for asthma.

∎ SUMMARY

The approach to the patient who presents with respiratory failure should include a systematic investigation to identify the cause of the respiratory failure and to subcharacterize it into a disorder that primarily impairs the respiratory system as a pump or as an area of gas exchange. A combination of medical history, physical examination, and selected laboratory tests enables one to make the correct diagnosis of the cause of the respiratory failure and to direct treatment in the majority of causes. Treatment options include oxygen, medical therapy, the selected use of artificial ventilation, and, in certain instances, surgical treatment.

■ REVIEW QUESTIONS

1. An example of a disease that primarily causes respiratory system pump failure is congestive heart failure. This statement is

   (A) true
   (B) false

2. A 28-year-old woman presents to the emergency room 30 minutes after injecting heroin and is found to have an oxygen saturation of 70% by pulse oximetry. An arterial blood-gas analysis taken while the patient is breathing room air oxygen shows a P_aO_2 of 40 mmHg, a PCO_2 of 80 mmHg, and a pH of 7.15. The most likely cause of hypoxemia in this patient is

   (A) ventilation-perfusion mismatch
   (B) intracardiac shunting
   (C) intrapulmonary shunting
   (D) alveolar hypoventilation

3. The most important laboratory test to perform in the assessment of respiratory failure is

   (A) chest x-ray
   (B) hemoglobin level
   (C) arterial blood-gas analysis
   (D) serum phosphorus
   (E) ventilation-perfusion lung scan

4. A 44-year-old man complains of fever with cough productive of yellow mucus for 3 days. Today, on presentation to the emergency room, he complains of progressively severe breathlessness. After evaluation, an arterial blood gas is drawn and shows a P_aO_2 of 40 mmHg, a P_aCO_2 of 30 mmHg, and a pH of 7.48. After the patient is placed on 100% oxygen by face mask, a repeat arterial blood gas shows a P_aO_2 of 60 mmHg. The pathophysiologic disorder most likely to be causing hypoxemia in this patient is

   (A) ventilation-perfusion mismatch
   (B) intracardiac shunting
   (C) intrapulmonary shunting
   (D) alveolar hypoventilation

5. The first therapy to consider as a treatment for a patient presenting in respiratory failure is

   (A) bronchodilators
   (B) antibiotics
   (C) surgical treatment
   (D) mechanical ventilation
   (E) oxygen

■ ANSWERS AND EXPLANATIONS

1. The answer is B. Congestive heart failure is an example of lung failure wherein hypoxemia results from the alveolus becoming filled with fluid. Examples of diseases in which respiratory failure is caused by pump failure include central and peripheral nervous system disorders and disorders that affect the chest wall or the upper airways.

2. The answer is D. In a person breathing room air at sea level, the P_IO_2 is 150. Subtracting from this value the PCO_2 divided by R (assuming R = 0.8) and then subtracting the patient's P_aO_2 of 40 mmHg yields an alveolar-arterial (A-a) oxygen gradient of 10 mmHg. An A-a oxygen gradient of 10 mmHg is normal, which suggests that the lung is normal and that pump failure or alveolar hypoventilation is the cause of this patient's hypoxemia.

3. The answer is C. The arterial blood gas allows one to measure the P_aO_2, the PCO_2, and the pH. One can also derive the alveolar-arterial oxygen gradient to determine whether reduction in P_aO_2 is secondary to hypoventilation, pulmonary shunt, or ventilation-perfusion inequality.

4. The answer is C. Calculation of the alveolar-arterial oxygen gradient in this patient yields a value of approximately 75 mmHg, which is markedly greater than the normal value of 10 to 20 mmHg. Following inspiration of 100% supplemental oxygen by face mask, there is only a mild increase in arterial oxygen, which is consistent with an intrapulmonary shunt of at least 30%.

5. The answer is E. In most cases, patients who present with respiratory failure have either hypoxemia or a respiratory-failure-causing disorder that is known to cause hypoxemia. Of all the disorders, hypoxemia is the most important one that can result in progression of the patient's respiratory distress or lead to further complications, such as stroke, myocardial infarction, or some other end-organ dysfunction. Therefore, oxygen (E) is the first theory to consider in a patient who presents in respiratory failure. In some patients who present primarily with pure pump failure, mechanical ventilation is warranted (D), but these patients represent a smaller percentage of those who present with respiratory failure and is not considered first line theory. Bronchodilators (A) and antibiotics (B) are used as adjunctive therapies for patients who present with bronchospasm or infection as the major cause of respiratory failure. Similar surgical treatment (i.e., pullectomy or transplantation) is only considered in extreme cases as a matter of last resort.

■ SUGGESTED READING

Bone RC: Acute respiratory failure: definition and overview. In Bone R, ed.: *Pulmonary and Critical Care Medicine*. St. Louis: Mosby, 1997.

Dantzker MD, David R: Pulmonary gas exchange. In Bone R, ed.: *Pulmonary and Critical Care Medicine*. St. Louis: Mosby, 1997.

Roussos C: Ventilatory failure. In Bone R, ed.: *Pulmonary and Critical Care Medicine*. St. Louis: Mosby, 1997.

Chapter 8

EXERCISE AND DISEASE

Francis C. Cordova, M.D.

David S. Kukafka, M.D.

Gilbert E. D'Alonzo, D.O.

▌CHAPTER OUTLINE

Learning Objectives
Introduction
Review of Normal Exercise Physiology
Clinical Exercise Testing
Clinical Signs of Exercise Limitation
Measurements During Exercise Testing
Physiologic Parameters in Respiratory Exercise Limitation
Physiologic Parameters in Cardiac Exercise Limitation
Case Study 1: Introduction
Obstructive Lung Diseases
Exercise Physiology in Obstructive Lung Diseases
Case Study 1: Continued
Case Study 2: Introduction
Restrictive Lung Diseases and Infiltrative Lung Diseases
Case Study 2: Continued
Exercise Physiology in Restrictive Lung Diseases
Case Study 3: Introduction
Exercise Physiology in Pulmonary Vascular Diseases
Summary
Review Questions

▌LEARNING OBJECTIVES

At the completion of this chapter, the reader should:
- Understand the basic ventilatory and circulatory responses to exercise.
- Know the clinical indications for performing cardiopulmonary exercise testing.
- Understand the terminology of exercise physiology and be able to use a variety of exercise parameters in the interpretation of exercise studies.
- Recognize and be able to differentiate the typical exercise physiology patterns in patients with obstructive, restrictive, and pulmonary vascular diseases.

▌INTRODUCTION

Normal exercise physiology is reviewed extensively in Chapter 3. In this chapter, we will explore the usefulness of clinical exercise testing in the diagnosis and treatment of patients with cardiopulmonary disorders. Specific clinical vignettes will be provided to facilitate understanding of the key concepts in exercise pathophysiology.

As discussed in Chapter 3, the increased metabolic demand of exercising muscles can severely stress both the cardiovascular and respiratory systems, especially in the presence of diseases that impair lung function and tissue gas exchange. Because of close coupling of respiratory, circulatory, and intracellular aerobic metabolism (Figure 8-1), a wide variety of diseases, as listed in Table 8-1, may present as exercise limitation early in disease evolution.

Table 8-1
Diseases Commonly Associated with Exercise Limitation

Heart Diseases
Coronary artery disease
Cardiomyopathies
Valvular heart disease
Congenital heart disease

Pulmonary Vascular Diseases
Primary pulmonary hypertension
Cor pulmonale

Ventilatory Disorders
Obstructive lung diseases
  Emphysema
  Chronic bronchitis
  Asthma
Restrictive lung diseases
  Pulmonary fibrosis
  Sarcoidosis
  Hypersensitivity pneumonitis
Chest wall defects
  Kyphoscoliosis
  Pectus excavatum

Blood Disorders
Hemoglobinopathies
Anemia
Carboxyhemoglobinemia

Muscle Disorders
McArdle's syndrome (myophosphorylase deficiency)

Anxiety and Malingering

FIGURE 8-1
Exercise requires intact pulmonary, cardiovascular, and skeletal muscle systems for the performance of efficient muscular work. There is very close coupling among the three systems such that any deficiency in one system results in exercise limitation. Adapted from Wasserman K et al, *Exercise Testing and Interpretation*: an overview. In *Principles of Exercise Testing and Interpretation*. Malvern, PA: Lea & Febiger, 1994.

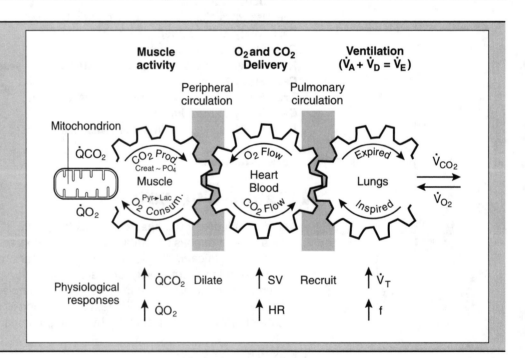

Early Symptoms of Exercise Limitation

• Dyspnea on exertion
• Easy fatigability
• Muscle pain

Early indication of exercise limitation is typically manifested by dyspnea on moderate exertion, easy fatigability with unclear etiology, and leg or chest pain—as in patients with ischemic vascular disease. Exercise limitation can be quantified from the clinical history using the New York Heart Association Functional Classification, as shown in Table 8-2. Simple but objective assessment of exercise endurance can be done using a timed distance test (6- or 12-minute walk). This test measures the distance covered during a defined period of time. However, the "gold standard" for evaluating exercise performance is the symptom-limited integrated cardiopulmonary exercise test. This test is an objective and accurate assessment of exercise limitation. In addition, the etiology of the functional impairment can be diagnosed accurately, and response to treatment can be assessed objectively.

Class 1	No symptoms with ordinary physical activity
Class 2	Symptoms with ordinary activity; slight limitation of activity
Class 3	Symptoms with less than ordinary activity; marked limitation of activity
Class 4	Symptoms with any physical activity or even at rest

Table 8-2
New York Heart Association Functional Classification

Adapted from The Criteria Committee of the New York Heart Association: *Diseases of the Heart and Blood Vessels: Nomenclature and Criteria for Diagnosis*, 6th ed. New York: New York Heart Association/Little, Brown, 1964.

■ REVIEW OF NORMAL EXERCISE PHYSIOLOGY

In order to meet the increased metabolic requirement during exercise, both the cardiovascular and respiratory systems must be able to respond so as to increase oxygen delivery to the skeletal muscle in order to fuel aerobic cellular respiration and maintain tissue homeostasis. Muscle contraction is an energy-requiring process, and the chemical energy stored in the terminal phosphate bond of adenosine triphosphate (ATP) and creatine phosphate provides this energy. Energy is derived from the oxidation of ingested food (carbohydrate and fat) by a series of chemical reactions that lead to oxidative phosphorylation in the mitochondria. Proteins may be used as fuel sources as well, but their principal function is to maintain the structural and functional integrity of the body.

> Chemical energy derived mainly from aerobic metabolism of carbohydrate and fat is required for sustained muscular work.

An individual's exercise performance depends on the capacity of the cardiovascular and respiratory systems to cope with the increased metabolic stress and energy demand that occur during exercise. Optimal oxygen delivery to the exercising muscles should be maintained for ATP production if sustained and efficient muscular work is to be performed. At the cellular level, the most efficient metabolic pathway for the production of ATP is the complete oxidation of the glucose by means of aerobic metabolism. In the presence of oxygen, glucose completely metabolizes to water and carbon dioxide during a series of biochemical reactions involving glycolysis, the cytoplasmic Krebs cycle, and mitochondrial oxidative phosphorylation. Through this pathway, there is a total gain of 36 moles of ATP from complete oxidation of 1 mole of glucose. In contrast, during anaerobic metabolism, the oxidation of glucose stops at the glycolytic pathway, and the net gain in ATP production is only 3 moles. Moreover, two molecules of lactic acid are formed from each mole of glucose, which eventually leads to intracellular and systemic acidosis. Thus it is clear that aerobic respiration is more efficient in maintaining optimal cellular energetics than anaerobic metabolism.

The role of the respiratory system in exercise is to maintain adequate lung gas exchange by 1) ensuring oxygen absorption for eventual delivery to the working muscle and 2) maintaining elimination of carbon dioxide and thus preventing acidosis. A detailed normal ventilatory response has been discussed previously, but to summarize, the normal ventilatory response to exercise is to increase the ventilatory capacity or minute ventilation (V_E) by means of an initial increase in tidal volume (V_T) followed by an increase in respiratory frequency (f_b). In addition, because of improved ventilation/perfusion (V/Q) matching in the lung during exercise, dead space ventilation (V_D/V_T) decreases whereas the diffusion capacity for carbon monoxide (DL_{CO}) increases, causing an overall improvement in pulmonary gas exchange. The respiratory system is closely linked with, and dependent on, the circulatory system to maintain oxygen delivery to peripheral tissues. Normal circulatory responses to exercise include a fivefold increase in the cardiac output (CO) through an initial increase in stroke volume closely followed by a gradual, then progressively more rapid, increase in heart rate. The increase in inotropic and chronotropic stimulation of the heart during exercise is mediated by the release of catecholamines during exercise. Increased sympathetic activity results in venoconstriction and increased venous return to the heart. Whereas only 15% to 20% of cardiac output goes to the muscle when the body is at rest, as much as 80% of the cardiac output during exercise is delivered to the exercising muscle. This is accomplished by selective vasoconstriction of the visceral vascular beds and vasodilatation in actively contracting muscles. As a result of regional vasodilatation, systemic vascular resistance decreases. Despite these impressive cardiovascular responses, the inability to sustain exercise above a certain level, called the anaerobic threshold, results mainly from the inability of cardiac output to meet the oxygen demand of exercising muscle.

Normal Ventilatory Responses to Exercise

- Increase in minute ventilation
- Increase in tidal volume followed by increase in respiratory rate
- Improvement in V/Q matching
- Decrease in dead space ventilation
- Increase in diffusion capacity

Normal Cardiovascular Responses to Exercise

- Fivefold increase in cardiac output
- Increase in stroke volume followed by increase in heart rate
- Decrease in systemic vascular resistance
- Increase in venous return as a result of venoconstriction

Any disease that disrupts the close relationship between the cardiopulmonary system and cellular respiration eventually leads to exercise limitation. Such diseases include disorders of the lungs, the chest wall, central respiratory control, the heart, the peripheral circulation, and the blood.

CLINICAL EXERCISE TESTING

Integrative cardiopulmonary exercise testing permits simultaneous evaluation of the abilities of both the cardiovascular and pulmonary systems to support exercising muscles. Traditional exercise stress testing is limited in scope and primarily addresses the issue of myocardial ischemia. In reality, it is not possible to stress the cardiovascular and pulmonary systems in isolation because of their highly coordinated and interdependent functions. Abnormal cardiac function can adversely affect breathing pattern and eventually gas exchange in the lung. Similarly, pulmonary disorders can have a negative impact on cardiac function. Integrative cardiopulmonary exercise testing not only detects problems in oxygen delivery (as in patients with heart disease, peripheral and pulmonary vascular abnormalities, anemia, hypoxemia, and elevated carboxyhemoglobin level) but also objectively measures exercise capacity. In addition, impaired work efficiency, reduced ventilatory capacity, abnormal ventilation-perfusion matching, and even poor exercise effort can be detected during symptom-limited cardiopulmonary exercise testing.

The indications for exercise testing include 1) dyspnea of uncertain etiology so a more direct diagnostic work-up can be pursued further, 2) objective measurement of exercise capacity for purposes of impairment evaluation, 3) assessment of the effects of therapy and rehabilitation, and 4) preoperative evaluation in high-risk surgical patients undergoing thoracic surgery. Contraindications to exercise testing are presented in Table 8-3. Indications for stopping an exercise test are listed in Table 8-4. Complications that arise in exercise testing are usually the results of life-threatening cardiovascular events such as cardiac ischemia, cardiac arrhythmias (ventricular tachycardia, second- or third-degree atrioventricular block, or atrial fibrillation), and hypotension. Respiratory decompensation during exercise is seldom life-threatening except in cases of serious arterial oxygen desaturation.

Indications for Exercise Testing

- Evaluation of unexplained dyspnea
- Disability evaluation
- Assessment after therapeutic intervention
- Preoperative evaluation of surgical risk

Complications of Exercise Testing

- Cardiac ischemia
- Cardiac arrhythmias
- Hypotension
- Hypoxemia
- Wheezing

Table 8-3
Contraindications to Exercise Testing

Acute Febrile Illness
Acute Cardiovascular Events
  Acute myocardial infarction
  Unstable angina
  Malignant cardiac arrhythmias
    Uncontrolled atrial and ventricular arrhythmias
    Third-degree AV block
  Decompensated congestive heart failure
  Suspected dissecting aortic aneurysm
  Recent systemic and pulmonary embolism
  Acute myocarditis or pericarditis
  Uncontrolled hypertension
  Severe aortic stenosis

Pulmonary Disorders
  Uncontrolled asthma
  Respiratory failure
  Hypoxemia

Severe Electrolyte Abnormalities
  Hypokalemia
  Hypomagnesemia

Onset of symptoms and signs suggestive of coronary artery disease
Chest pain
Ischemic changes on 12 lead EKG
Hypotension
Malignant cardiac arrhythmias (multiforms premature ventricular contraction, R on T wave, Ventricular tachycarida)
Second and third degree heart block
Appearance of left bundle branch block pattern

Onset of symptoms and signs of low cardiac output state
Pallor and sweating
Mental confusion
Dizziness
Hypotension (fall in systolic BP > 20 mmHg with exercise)

Onset of symptoms and signs of impaired pulmonary gas exchange
Severe dyspnea
Cyanosis

Claudication

Subjects requests to stop

Table 8-4
Indications for Stopping an Exercise Test

Exercise-limiting claudication
Exercise-limiting angina
Sick sinus syndrome
Beta-adrenergic blockade
Lung disease
Poor effort

Table 8-5
Clinical Conditions Associated with High Heart Rate Reserve

CLINICAL SIGNS OF EXERCISE LIMITATION

Clinically, the most common factors that stop an individual from exercising are dyspnea, pain, and fatigue. Dyspnea is a perception of shortness of breath or uncomfortable breathing that is disproportionate to the stimulus. As mentioned, the role of the ventilatory system is to regulate the acid-base (pH) status of the body by means of elimination of carbon dioxide and absorption of oxygen. Carbon dioxide and water are the final by-products of substrate oxidation. When the aerobic system is overwhelmed, anaerobic metabolism becomes an important source of energy, and carbon dioxide is produced by the breakdown of lactic acid. V_E is driven by the arterial pH, so that when H^+ increases as a result of increased carbon dioxide, V_E increases. If the ventilatory system is unable to keep up with increased H^+ production, dyspnea develops.

Fatigue occurs when a contracting muscle can no longer generate enough force to maintain a certain level of muscular work. Physiologically, fatigue occurs when the energy requirement of the contracting muscles is not met and there is biochemical deterioration of the intracellular milieu. Some of the proposed mediators of fatigue are lactic acidosis, increased amount of inorganic phosphates, impaired calcium release from the sarcoplasmic reticulum, and decreased ATP production. However, the exact pathophysiologic mechanism of fatigue remains to be elucidated.

Muscle pain, in the form of either angina or claudication, can limit exercise. Angina is caused by a relative decrease in coronary blood flow in response to increased myocardial demand during exercise. Claudication reflects a relative decrease in flow to exercising skeletal muscles in response to increased demand.

Clinical Signs of Exercise Limitation

• Dyspnea
• Fatigue
• Muscle pain

MEASUREMENTS DURING EXERCISE TESTING

MAXIMAL OXYGEN UPTAKE

Because external respiration (i.e., gas exchange at the level of the lung) and internal respiration (i.e., tissue gas exchange) are closely linked, measurement of expired gases (oxygen and carbon dioxide) from the mouth can closely reflect cellular metabolism at steady state. Oxygen uptake (VO_2) represents the amount of oxygen absorbed from the lung. VO_2 is calculated as the product of V_E and the difference between measured oxygen in inspired and expired air: $VO_2 = V_E \times [0.254 (1 - F_EO_2 - F_ECO_2) - F_EO_2]$. In contrast, oxygen consumption (QO_2) reflects cellular oxygen utilization. Similarly, carbon

The most important measure of exercise capacity is the maximal oxygen uptake, VO_{2max}. During steady state, oxygen uptake from the lung equals oxygen consumption.

dioxide output (VCO_2) measures release of carbon dioxide from the lung to differentiate it from production of carbon dioxide by the cells (QCO_2). Assuming steady state conditions (when both O_2 and CO_2 stores are constant), the ratio of VCO_2 to VO_2 (the gas-exchange ratio, R) reflects QCO_2/QO_2, the metabolic respiratory quotient (RQ). During acute hyperventilation, when more carbon dioxide is unloaded from the lung, or in the presence of acute metabolic acidosis, when carbon dioxide production evolves from bicarbonate buffer, R exceeds RQ.

During exercise, VO_2 depends primarily on the amount and efficiency of the work performed by the exercising muscles. Clearly, the body has an upper limit of oxygen consumption as determined by cardiovascular fitness, ventilatory capacity, and the capacity of the exercising muscles to extract oxygen. During symptom-limited cardio-pulmonary stress testing, maximal oxygen consumption (VO_{2max}) is identified when there is no further increase in VO_2 with progressive increases in external work (Figure 8-2). In contrast, maximal VO_2, or peak VO_2, indicates the highest VO_2 achieved for a certain symptom-limited maximal effort. VO_{2max} is the point at which the aerobic capacity of the system is outstripped and anaerobic metabolism becomes an increasingly necessary source of energy. Typically, VO_{2max} occurs after 4 to 10 minutes of incremental exercise. An individual normally can reach up to 80% of the VO_{2max} predicted by age, gender, and height during testing. Thus, any process that impairs the respiratory, circulatory, or muscular system can be seen physiologically as a decrease in exercise capacity. During interpretation of the different exercise parameters, VO_{2max} should be examined first because it indicates the patient's capacity for maximal aerobic function.

TOTAL EXERCISE TIME

If a standardized cardiopulmonary exercise protocol is utilized, the exercise duration is a useful marker of exercise capacity—especially in severely debilitated patients who may be able to exercise for only a few minutes or when serial testing is obtained after an intervention.

FIGURE 8-2
Maximum oxygen uptake (maximum VO_2) is the highest oxygen uptake attained during symptom-limited exercise testing. Maximal oxygen uptake (VO_{2max}) is the maximum aerobic capacity of an individual. It can be identified during exercise testing as a VO_2 plateau despite increasing work load. Adapted from Wasserman K et al. Measurements during integrative cardiopulmonary exercise testing. In *Principles of Exercise Testing and Interpretation.* Malvern, PA: Lea & Febiger, 1994.

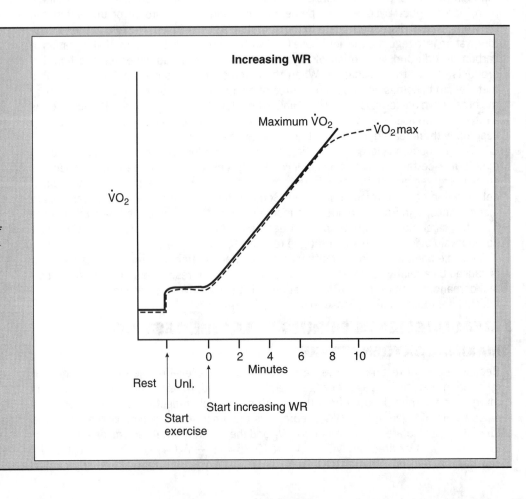

ANAEROBIC THRESHOLD

Anaerobic threshold (AT) is the VO_2 during exercise at which anaerobic metabolism supplements aerobic high-energy phosphate production, resulting in a net increase in intracellular lactate production. During progressive exercise, oxygen demand outstrips delivery of oxygen to muscle, resulting in a lower cytosolic redux state owing to the inability of the mitochondrial membrane proton shuttle to accept extra reduced nicotinamide adenine dinucleotide ($NADH + H^+$) produced in the cytoplasm for oxidative phosphorylation. In order for glycolysis to continue, pyruvate reacts with extra reduced $NADH + H^+$ to regenerate oxidized nicotinamide adenine dinucleotide (NAD^+). In the process, pyruvate is converted to lactate, lowering the lactate-pyruvate ratio. The resulting lactic acidosis then is buffered by sodium bicarbonate to maintain intracellular pH. Exercise duration below AT can be sustained for prolonged periods of time and is limited by skeletal muscle injury and the availability of substrate for continued energy production. In contrast, exercise duration above AT is reduced and is limited by fatigue and dyspnea. Thus it would appear that muscle fatigue is partly attributable to intracellular acidosis as a result of lactic acid production. However, research in exercise physiology has also shown that intracellular lactic acidosis can in fact improve oxygen unloading at the tissue through facilitation of oxygen-hemoglobin dissociation (Bohr effect) (Figure 8-3). In addition, accumulation of lactate causes local vascular bed vasodilatation, further improving oxygen delivery.

The anaerobic threshold generally occurs between 40% and 60% of VO_{2max} and can be determined by the rate at which VO_2 and VCO_2 increase during incremental exercise. At the start of exercise, V_E, VO_2, and VCO_2 increase linearly until lactic acidosis develops. Above AT, the rate of rise of VCO_2 increases more rapidly than that of VO_2 because of the extra carbon dioxide produced by bicarbonate buffering of lactic acid. The abrupt change in the slope of the rise in VCO_2 compared with the slope of the rise in VO_2 (Figure 8-4A) identifies AT during exercise testing (V slope method).

An alternative method of identifying AT is the ventilatory equivalence method. This method is based on identification of the isocapneic buffering period—that is, the period during which metabolic acidosis is buffered by bicarbonate instead of hyperventilation. The linear increases in minute ventilation and VCO_2 at low levels of work change to a curvilinear pattern at higher work rates while the VO_2 continues to increase linearly. Thus, this brief period when the rate of rise of the ventilatory equivalence of VO_2 (V_E/VO_2) increases faster than the ventilatory equivalence of VCO_2 (V_E/VCO_2) indicates that AT has been exceeded (Figure 8-4B).

Anaerobic threshold (AT) is identified when the following metabolic changes occur:

- increase in anaerobic metabolism
- increase in lactate production
- intracellular and systemic acidosis

AT during exercise can be identified noninvasively by either the V slope method or the ventilatory equivalence method.

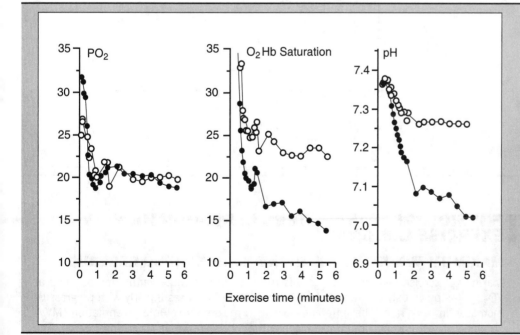

FIGURE 8-3
Femoral venous P_aO_2, oxyhemoglobin saturation, and pH at two constant work rates, one below (open circles) and one above (closed circles) the anaerobic threshold. During exercise above the AT, oxygen saturation is lower despite similar P_aO_2 compared with exercise below the AT, because of the rightward shift in the oxyhemoglobin curve to the right as a result of progressive intracellular acidosis secondary to lactic acidosis. Wasserman K, et al. Interaction of physiological mechanisms during exercise. *J Appl Physiol* 22:71–85, 1967.

FIGURE 8-4

The anaerobic threshold can be determined noninvasively by measuring expired oxygen and carbon dioxide at the mouth during progressive exercise. The V slope method, as depicted in (A), looks at the rate of rise of VO_2 compared with VCO_2. At low work rates, the increase in VO_2 is matched by a similar increase in VCO_2. AT is identified when VCO_2 increases faster than VO_2 owing to an increase in carbon dioxide production. Alternatively, AT can be determined by the ventilator equivalence method, as shown in (B). AT is identified when isocapneic buffering has occurred—that is, when the rate of rise of the ventilatory equivalence of VO_2 (V_E/VO_2) is faster than that of the ventilatory equivalence of VCO_2 (V_E/VCO_2). Adapted from Wasserman K, et al. Measurements during integrative cardiopulmonary exercise testing. In *Principles of Exercise Testing and Interpretation*. Malvern, PA: Lea & Febiger, 1994.

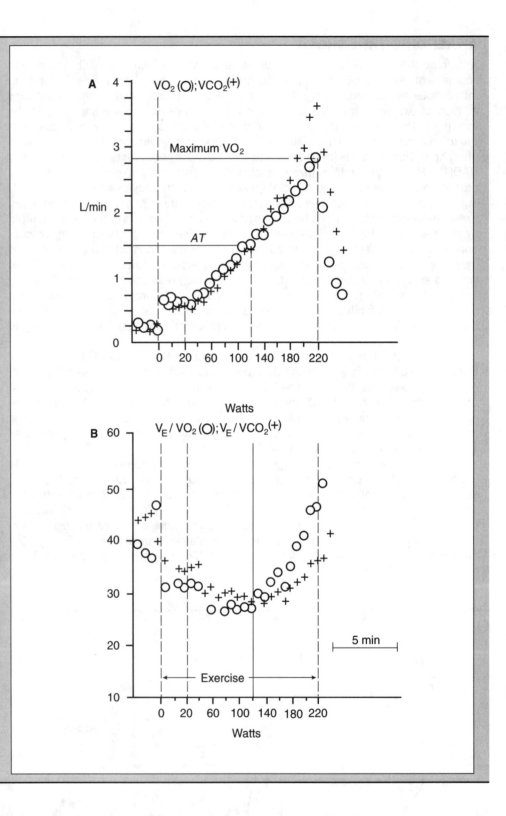

PHYSIOLOGIC PARAMETERS IN RESPIRATORY EXERCISE LIMITATION

MAXIMUM MINUTE VENTILATION AND BREATHING RESERVE

Maximum exercise ventilation (V_{Emax}) is the maximum minute ventilation attained at VO_{2max}. As previously discussed, minute ventilation increases linearly with progressive increases in work rate. The difference between maximum voluntary ventilation (MVV) obtained at rest and maximum exercise ventilation is known as breathing reserve. The

Low breathing reserve is typically seen in patients with chronic airflow obstruction.

normal breathing reserve is usually 10% to 40% of the MVV or at least 15 L/min. A low breathing reserve during exercise usually indicates ventilatory limitation to exercise unless it is found in an extremely fit individual who can attain very high minute ventilation. Patients with moderate to severe chronic airflow obstruction typically have low or no breathing reserve at the end of incremental exercise.

BREATHING PATTERN DURING EXERCISE

Increases in minute ventilation during progressive exercise can be achieved by increasing either tidal volume or respiratory rate. During early exercise, tidal volume increases first, followed by increases in respiratory rate, as discussed in Chapter 3 (Section 3.6). This pattern of breathing ensures an effective increase in alveolar ventilation. In patients with airflow obstruction, the increase in minute ventilation is attained mainly during early low-work-rate exercise by an increase in respiratory rate. In patients with advanced restrictive lung disease, the capacity to increase tidal volume as minute ventilation increases during exercise is limited by a small inspiratory capacity. Thus, the ratio of tidal volume to inspiratory capacity (V_T/IC) increases at high work rate and approaches 1, as shown in Figure 8-5. Moreover, in order to meet an increased minute ventilation requirement, respiratory rate at peak exercise often exceeds 50 breaths per minute.

A rapid and shallow breathing pattern during exercise is usually observed in patients with limited ventilatory capacity. A high ratio of tidal volume to inspiratory capacity and a respiratory rate higher than 50 during peak exercise suggest restrictive lung disease.

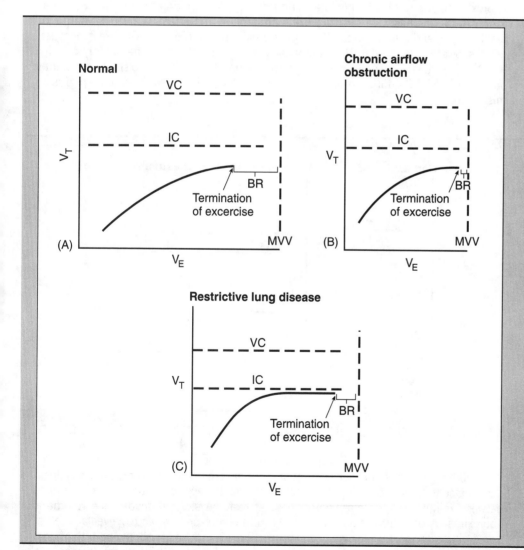

FIGURE 8-5
(A) Normal increase in tidal volume (V_T) as minute ventilation requirement increases during exercise. At maximum oxygen uptake (depicted here as termination of exercise testing), the increase in V_T approaches 80% of the inspiratory capacity. Moreover, at the end of exercise, the maximum minute ventilation approaches only 60% to 80% of resting maximum minute ventilation (MVV) giving a normal breathing reserve (BR) of at least 15 liters or 20% to 40% of MVV. (B) In patients with chronic airflow obstruction, the breathing reserve is severely reduced. (C) In patients with severe restrictive lung disease, the increase in V_T approaches inspiratory capacity in early exercise as a result of small volumes. As in patients with chronic airflow obstruction, the BR is also reduced.

Causes of Hypoxemia During Exercise

- Ventilation/perfusion abnormality
- Right-to-left shunt
- Diffusion limitation

OXYGENATION

Several exercise parameters can be monitored during integrative pulmonary exercise to detect exercise-induced hypoxemia. Hypoxemia can be detected by continuous monitoring of oxyhemoglobin saturation by pulse oximetry or by serial determinations of arterial blood gas. In normal individuals, arterial oxygen tension does not decrease and alveolar-arterial oxygen difference remains normal during exercise. In patients with obstructive airway disease, further hypoxemia may result from a worsening ventilation-perfusion (V/Q) relationship or the development of right-to-left shunting caused by a patent foramen ovale. Pulmonary vascular diseases such as primary pulmonary hypertension and chronic thromboembolic disease may develop, worsening pulmonary hypertension during exercise as a result of an inability of the pulmonary vascular bed to accept an increased cardiac output. The resultant high right atrial pressure may open a previously closed but potentially patent foramen ovale, causing right-to-left shunting and worsening hypoxemia that is refractory to supplemental oxygen.

MEASUREMENT OF VENTILATION-PERFUSION MISMATCH

Ventilation/perfusion mismatch during exercise is suggested by:

- a persistent positive arterial and end-tidal P_aCO_2 difference
- a persistent elevated dead space–tidal volume ratio
- an elevated ventilatory equivalence at AT

A useful measure of the gas-exchange function of the lung is the difference between arterial and end-tidal carbon dioxide pressures. In normal individuals at rest, P_aCO_2 is approximately 2 mmHg higher than end-tidal $P_{ET}CO_2$. During progressive work-load exercise, the increases in carbon dioxide production and effective alveolar ventilation result in a faster rise in end-tidal CO_2 compared with P_aCO_2 (Figure 8-6). Direct measurement shows that end-tidal CO_2 approaches venous blood. Thus, the slightly positive $(P_a-P_{ET})CO_2$ at rest becomes negative (4 mmHg on average) on exercise. A persistently positive $(P_a-ET)CO_2$ during exercise is an indication of impaired ventilation-perfusion mismatch.

FIGURE 8-6
At rest, P_aCO_2 is slightly higher than $P_{ET}CO_2$. Because of increases in effective alveolar ventilation during exercise, $P_{ET}CO_2$ becomes higher than P_aCO_2 by 4 mmHg on average. A persistently positive difference in P_aCO_2 and $P_{ET}CO_2$ is seen in patients with limited ventilatory capacity (B, obstructive disease and C, restrictive disease). Reproduced with permission from Wasserman K, et al. Measurements during integrative cardiopulmonary exercise testing. In *Principles of Exercise Testing and Interpretation*. Malvern, PA: Lea & Febiger, 1994.

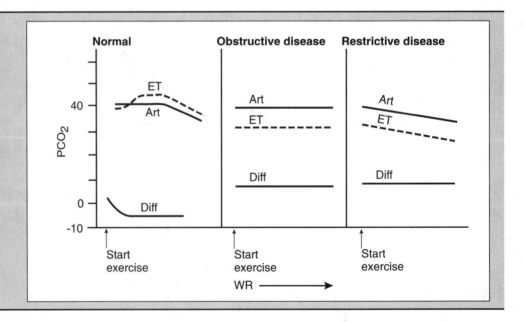

Another measure of uneven ventilation-perfusion matching is the ratio of physiologic dead space to tidal volume (V_D/V_T). Physiologic dead space ventilation is the difference between minute and alveolar ventilations. At rest, physiologic dead space volume is approximately one-third of tidal volume. With the increase in effective alveolar ventilation during exercise, physiologic dead space volume is reduced to about one-fifth of tidal volume. In other words, the physiologic dead space of 0.40 to 0.30 at rest decreases to 0.20 to 0.19 during exercise. In patients with primary pulmonary vascular disease or secondary pulmonary vascular disease, V_D/V_T is elevated at rest and remains elevated during exercise. Physiologic ventilation can be measured noninvasively using the $P_{ET}CO_2$. Because of the inconsistent relationship of P_aCO_2 and $P_{ET}CO_2$ in patients with lung disease, a more accurate method of estimating physiologic dead space volume requires arterial blood-gas sampling and the equation $V_D/V_T = (P_aCO_2 - P_{ET}CO_2)/P_aCO_2$.

Alternatively, ventilatory equivalence for VO_2 (V_E/VO_2) and VCO_2 (V_E/VCO_2) can be used to detect the presence of abnormal V/Q. Normally the nadir of V_E/VO_2 corresponds to the beginning of AT whereas the nadir of V_E/VCO_2 indicates the start of compensation of metabolic acidosis. Normal V_E/VO_2 at the nadir is between 22 and 27 and V_E/VCO_2 is between 26 and 30. An elevated ventilatory equivalence at the anaerobic threshold could be attributable to acute hyperventilation, increased V_D/V_T, or uneven V/Q. However, acute hyperventilation is easily discounted by an R value greater than 1.

PHYSIOLOGIC PARAMETERS IN CARDIAC EXERCISE LIMITATION

OXYGEN PULSE

Oxygen pulse (O_2P) is a calculated value and is derived by dividing oxygen uptake by heart rate. It is the amount of oxygen extracted by the peripheral tissues with each heartbeat and is dependent on stroke volume and the difference between arterial and mixed-venous oxygen. O_2P progressively increases during exercise until it plateaus, as shown in Figure 8-7. The initial increase in O_2P during early exercise results primarily from an increase in stroke volume. Thus, a low O_2P, or an early plateau of the O_2P curve, may indicate low stroke volume and a possible cardiac limitation of exercise. It is important to remember, however, that a low O_2P could be attributable to impaired exercise capacity from respiratory limitations. The predicted O_2P can be calculated by dividing predicted VO_{2max} by predicted maximum heart rate. Other factors that may result in low O_2P are anemia, high carboxyhemoglobin levels, and severe hypoxemia.

A low oxygen pulse suggests cardiac limitation of exercise.

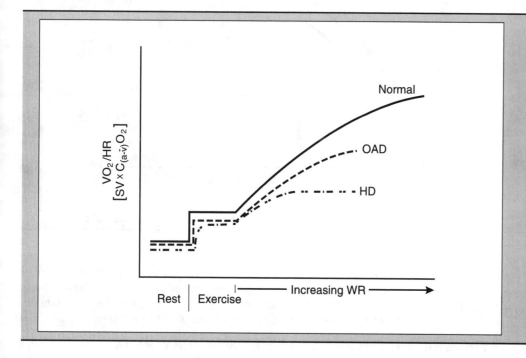

FIGURE 8-7
Oxygen pulse, mathematically represented by VO_2/HR, increases linearly with progressive increase in work load until it plateaus at maximum exercise. An early plateau in oxygen pulse during exercise suggests the presence of heart disease. In patients with obstructive airway disease (OAD), the maximum oxygen pulse may be low as a result of limited ventilatory capacity and early termination of exercise. Reproduced with permission from Wasserman K, et al. Measurements during integrative cardiopulmonary exercise testing. In *Principles of Exercise Testing and Interpretation*. Malvern PA: Lea & Febiger, 1994.

BLOOD PRESSURE AND HEART RATE RESPONSES

The normal blood pressure response to exercise is an incremental increase in blood pressure, although systolic blood pressure increases more than diastolic blood pressure. An increase in systolic blood pressure results mainly from augmented stroke volume with the release of catecholamines during exercise, whereas diastolic blood pressure increases only modestly because of the decrease in systemic vascular resistance resulting from vasodilatation in peripheral muscles. In patients with cardiomyopathy, hypotension

Hypotension during exercise and a steep increase in heart rate at low work rate both suggest cardiac limitation of exercise.

may develop during exercise. Some patients may have an abnormal hypertensive response to exercise characterized by an excessive increase in diastolic blood pressure.

As mentioned earlier, the increase in minute ventilation in response to a higher metabolic demand with exercise is matched by a similar increase in cardiac output. The relationship between the increase in heart rate and VO_2 may be a marker of cardiac dysfunction (O_2P). A steeper increase in heart rate as VO_2 increases, as shown in Figure 8-8, suggests a low stroke volume or cardiac dysfunction. In patients with coronary artery disease, the increase in VO_2 is slow despite a rapid increase in heart rate for a given work load. This implies that stroke volume is low and that the increase in cardiac output cannot keep pace with the increase in oxygen consumption. Similarly, the presence of pulmonary vascular disease also causes an inappropriate heart rate response owing to inadequate left ventricular preload in the presence of right ventricular failure.

FIGURE 8-8
The heart rate increases linearly during exercise. The increase in cardiac output in early exercise results primarily from an increase in stroke volume. An early increase in heart rate at a relatively low work load suggests cardiac limitation of exercise. Reproduced with permission from Wasserman K, et al. Measurements during integrative cardiopulmonary exercise testing. In *Principles of Exercise Testing and Interpretation*. Malvern, PA: Lea & Febiger, 1994.

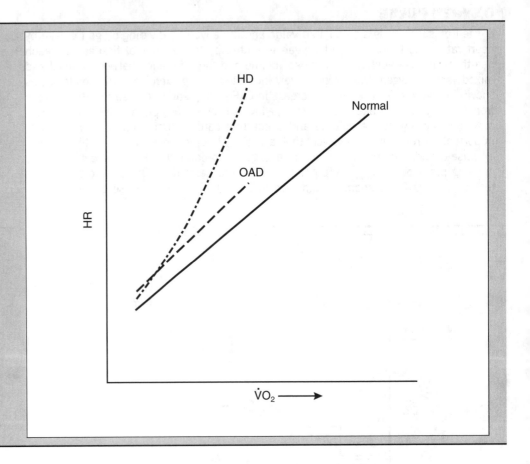

Maximum heart rate during exercise is usually within 90% of predicted maximum heart rate. Heart rate reserve is the difference between the actual maximum heart rate achieved and the predicted maximum heart rate. In certain disease states (see Table 8-5), premature termination of exercise may lead to a high heart rate reserve.

MYOCARDIAL ISCHEMIA AND CARDIAC ARRHYTHMIA

Electrocardiographic monitoring was used in cardiac stress testing to detect myocardial ischemia and the presence of serious cardiac arrhythmias even before the widespread use of clinical integrative cardiopulmonary exercise stress testing. The onset of myocardial ischemia during exercise is usually heralded by the complaint of chest pain and ST segment depression in two or more contiguous leads on the electrocardiogram. In patients with coronary vasospasm, ST segment elevation may be noted instead of depression. Depending on the presence of coronary artery disease, the symptoms and signs of ischemia may occur during moderate to severe exercise and may persist during the recovery phase of the exercise testing.

The presence of myocardial ischemia is suggested by:

- chest pain
- ST segment depression in two contiguous chest leads
- ST segment elevation
- cardiac arrhythmias

The presence of a malignant cardiac arrhythmia, such as multifocal premature ventricular beats, new-onset atrial fibrillation with a rapid ventricular response, or ventricular tachycardia/fibrillation, indicates cardiac dysfunction.

A.V., a 52-year-old postal worker presents with a history of worsening shortness of breath. He admits to having smoked 1 to 2 packs of cigarettes daily since he was in the army at age 18. At the urging of his family, he was able to quit smoking 2 months prior to presentation. He says that he feels well at rest but is bothered by increasing shortness of breath when he tries to exert himself. His dyspnea has increased to the point where he fatigues after walking three city blocks or climbing one or two flights of stairs. He denies having chest pain or weight loss. He has had yellow sputum production every morning for the past 10 years, which he attributes to a "smoker's cough" that has improved since he discontinued tobacco use.

On physical exam, he is comfortable at rest. He is 5 ft 6 in. tall and weighs 156 lb, and his blood pressure is mildly elevated at 150/95. His physical examination is remarkable for an increased anteroposterior diameter of the chest and a marked decrease in breath sounds bilaterally. His cardiac examination is unremarkable. He has no cyanosis, clubbing, or peripheral edema.

A chest x-ray reveals marked hyperinflation without evidence of pulmonary infiltrates or cardiac enlargement. Pulmonary function studies are as follows: forced expiratory volume in 1 second (FEV_1), 0.92 liter (29% of predicted); forced vital capacity (FVC), 3.12 liters (74% of predicted); FEV_1/FVC, 29%; total lung capacity (TLC), 7.10 liters (122% of predicted); residual volume (RV), 3.98 liters (203% of predicted); and DL_{CO}, 13.4 mL/min/mmHg (59% of predicted). A resting arterial blood gas with the patient breathing air reveals a pH of 7.44 (normal, 7.37 to 7.43); a PCO_2 of 38 mmHg (normal, 35 to 45 mmHg); and a PO_2 of 76 mmHg (normal, 76 to 96 mmHg), with an S_aO_2 saturation of 94%.

Case Study 1:
Introduction

OBSTRUCTIVE LUNG DISEASES

The etiologies and pathophysiologies of the obstructive lung diseases are discussed in depth in Chapters 4, 9, and 10. From an exercise standpoint, a variety of different processes can lead to exercise limitations as a result of airflow obstruction. The most common include COPD (emphysema and chronic bronchitis) and asthma. Other diseases that can cause airflow obstruction and affect exercise performance in a similar pattern include bronchiectasis, cystic fibrosis, and disorders of the larynx and trachea.

EXERCISE PHYSIOLOGY IN OBSTRUCTIVE LUNG DISEASES

The most common symptom that limits patients with airflow obstruction is dyspnea, which subsequently leads to exercise limitation. The patient with airflow obstruction may have an impairment in either ventilatory capacity (decreased) or ventilatory requirement (increased). COPD with an emphysematous component (such as that illustrated by Case Study 1) exhibits a functional decrease in useful lung parenchyma that causes a decrease in elastic recoil as well as distal gas trapping and airflow obstruction, both of which lead to a decrease in ventilatory capacity. Disorders with superimposed inflammation and plugging of the airways by mucus, such as asthma, chronic bronchitis, and bronchiectasis, exhibit regional areas of inhomogeneous ventilation with an intact circulation, thus leading to an increase in V/Q mismatch. Overall, V_D/V_T in the lung, which normally decreases during exercise, may not change or may increase because of high-V/Q areas in the lung. As a consequence of V/Q mismatch, P_aO_2 commonly decreases, as manifested by exercise-induced oxyhemoglobin desaturation on continuous pulse oximetry. These events lead to an increased ventilatory requirement (increased ventilation needed to oxygenate and eliminate CO_2) and exercise limitation with dyspnea. The breathing reserve is low, which suggests respiratory limitation.

Patients with serious obstructive lung disease, such as the patient in Case Study 1, typically demonstrate a reduced VO_{2max}. The AT is usually not reached, but when it is

Exercise Abnormalities in Patients with Chronic Airflow Obstruction

- Low VO_{2max}
- Low breathing reserve
- High V_D/V_T
- Hypoxemia

reached, it develops at the lower end of normal as lactic acidosis develops earlier in less conditioned muscle (often the patient cannot exercise to the point of AT).

Case Study 1: *Continued*	*A.V. has a substantial tobacco use history, severe airflow obstruction with signs of hyperinflation and gas trapping, and a reduced diffusion capacity, and is diagnosed with COPD with a significant emphysematous component. He is able to walk 1289 ft (393 m) at a moderate pace while breathing air. His initial oxygen saturation is 97%, and his minimum oxygen saturation is 93%. As a further work-up, a complete exercise study is performed using incremental increases in exercise on a treadmill. The results are as follows: VO_{2max}, 20.16 mL/kg ideal body weight (IBW) (65% of predicted); AT, 15.2 (normal, 12.4 to 24.8); maximum ventilation/MVV, 97% (normal, 60% to 80%); S_aO_2, 97% at rest and 88% at maximum exercise; V_D/V_T, 32% at rest and 31% during exercise; maximum heart rate, 126 beats per minute (72% of predicted); and total exercise time, 6 minutes. The test is stopped because of severe dyspnea.*

Case Study 2: *Introduction*	*A.Z. is a 55-year-old man who has had several months of increasing dyspnea on exertion. Otherwise, he has felt well and denies chest pain, weight loss, and sputum production. He admits to having smoked ½ pack of cigarettes per day for approximately 5 years in the early 1960s. He has been employed for the past 20 years as a machinist. On further questioning, he notes that he worked for 7 years as a pipe fitter in the early 1960s.* *On physical examination, the patient is found to be overweight (5 ft 8 in. tall, 245 lb). His resting respiratory rate is 30 breaths per minute, and examination of his lungs reveals decreased breath sounds with fine "velcro"-like bibasilar crackles. No digital clubbing is noted, and the remainder of his exam is unremarkable.* *A chest x-ray reveals increased interstitial basilar densities with bilateral pleural thickening and areas of pleural calcification. A CT scan of the chest reveals diffuse interstitial disease at the lung bases with bilateral pleural plaques. Pulmonary function studies are as follows: FVC, 1.79 liters (43% of predicted); FEV_1, 1.30 liters (43% of predicted); FEV_1/FVC, 73% (normal, above 70%); TLC, 3.23 liters (56% of predicted); DL_{CO}, 11.5 mL/min/mmHg (43% of predicted); and DL_{CO} corrected for alveolar volume, 103% predicted. An arterial blood gas on room air demonstrates a pH of 7.41, a PCO_2 of 46 mmHg (normal, 35 to 45 mmHg), a PO_2 of 66 mmHg (normal, 76 to 96 mmHg); and an S_aO_2 of 93%.*

RESTRICTIVE LUNG DISEASES AND INFILTRATIVE LUNG DISEASES

Restrictive lung diseases encompass a wide variety of disorders. The common functional finding is that some pulmonary processes have decreased the total amount of functioning lung tissue available for gas exchange. This leads to a smaller, noncompliant lung. The altered chest anatomy is manifested in the pulmonary function test as a decrease in TLC or FVC. There is a large variety of disorders that can have restrictive defects as major components of the pathologic process. These disorders include 1) processes with unknown causes, such as idiopathic pulmonary fibrosis, sarcoidosis, idiopathic hemosiderosis, alveolar proteinosis, amyloidosis, and eosinophilic granuloma, and 2) processes with known causes or precipitants, such as infections, occupational disorders (asbestosis and silicosis), physical irritants (radiation and oxygen toxicity), acute respiratory distress syndrome (ARDS), and neoplasms (bronchogenic and metastatic). These diseases are discussed in detail in Chapters 11, 12, and 19.

A.Z. presents with a severe restrictive ventilatory defect on pulmonary function testing, a reduced P_aO_2 on arterial blood-gas examination, and a clinical and radiographic history consistent with asbestos-related restrictive lung disease. To better assess the extent of his limitations, simple exercise ambulation with S_aO_2 monitoring is done and demonstrates rapid desaturation from 93% S_aO_2 at rest to 76% S_aO_2 after 1 minute of walking.

A complete exercise protocol is done with supplemental oxygen (F_iO_2 of 43%). The results are as follows: VO_{2max}, 20.7 ml/kg IBW (74% of predicted); AT 11.5 (normal 11.2-22.4); maximum ventilation/MVV, 62% (normal, 60% to 80%); S_aO_2 at rest, 99%, which drops to 91% with maximal exercise; V_D/V_T at rest, 29%, which decreases to 24% during exercise; maximum heart rate, 138 beats per minute (80% of predicted); and total exercise time, 7 minutes. The maximum respiratory rate during exercise is 54 breaths per minute. The test is terminated because of severe dyspnea.

Case Study 2:
Continued

EXERCISE PHYSIOLOGY IN RESTRICTIVE LUNG DISEASES

In patients with restrictive lung disease, the abnormal exercise physiology is highlighted by worsening hypoxemia, an inefficient rapid-shallow breathing pattern, and severe dyspnea at low work load. As with the obstructive lung diseases, there is a marked increase in the ventilatory requirement at rest and even more so during exercise, which generally leads to dyspnea with mild exertion. This condition is a result of altered gas exchange reflected by an increased V_D/V_T. Because anatomic and physiologic dead space ventilation occupies a fraction of the inspired tidal volume, alveolar ventilation with each tidal breath is smaller when the patient's breathing is rapid and shallow. Both V/Q mismatch and diffusion impairment may contribute to exercise-induced hypoxemia. The combination of increased distance for diffusion from capillaries to alveoli (owing to alveolar or interstitial fluid and fibrosis) and an increased rate of blood flow through the reduced capillary bed during exercise results in relative decreases in oxygen diffusion and absorption.

Breathing pattern during exercise is an important diagnostic discriminant factor in determining whether exercise limitation is attributable primarily to restrictive or to obstructive lung disease conditions. Because of reduced lung compliance in restrictive lung diseases, all lung volumes (total lung capacity, residual volume, inspiratory capacity) are reduced. Normally, the increase in tidal volume during high work levels of exercise approaches 80% of the inspiratory capacity. In contrast, the V_T/IC ratio approaches 1 in patients with restrictive lung disease. Because of the limited capacity to increase minute volume, their respiratory rate is often higher than 50 breaths per minute at peak exercise.

In summary, the patient with restrictive lung dysfunction typically exhibits the following pattern during exercise: decreased VO_{2max}, low breathing reserve (maximum ventilation/MVV ratio), high V_T/IC ratio, high breathing frequency, and exercise-induced oxygen desaturation.

Exercise Abnormalities in Patients with Restrictive Lung Disease

- Low VO_{2max}
- High V_T/IC ratio
- Low breathing reserve
- Breathing frequency greater than 50 at peak exercise
- High V_D/V_T
- Hypoxemia

A.B., a 53-year-old woman, presents to the pulmonary clinic with a 1-year history of progressive dyspnea with exertion to the point where she experiences severe shortness of breath, chest discomfort, and lightheadedness after walking 50 ft. She notes a 7-pack-year smoking history but quit in 1965. Her medical history is significant for insulin-dependent diabetes mellitus (IDDM) and hypertension. There is no significant occupational history. She denies any dermatologic or rheumatologic complaints.

Physical examination shows a comfortable-appearing woman with a respiratory rate of 16 breaths per minute. Her lung examination is normal, but her cardiac examination is significant for a prominent pulmonic component to the second heart sound. No other abnormalities are found.

The chest x-ray is normal except for the suggestion of prominent central pulmonary vasculature. Pulmonary function studies are normal, but the echocardiogram reveals abnormal left ventricular function. A room air blood gas is significant for mild respiratory alkalosis (PCO_2, 34 mmHg). A right heart catheterization reveals pulmonary artery pressure of 77/22 mmHg with a mean of 44 mmHg (normal, 25/10 with a mean of 15). A work-up for secondary causes of pulmonary hypertension is done, but the patient is diagnosed with primary pulmonary hypertension.

Case Study 3:
Introduction

Case Study 3:
Continued

As part of her continued evaluation and consideration for lung transplantation, an ambulation study with S_aO_2 monitoring is done and reveals an initial S_aO_2 of 97% on room air at rest, which slightly decreases to 92% after walking 1327 ft (404 m). An incremental exercise study on a treadmill is performed with the following results: VO_{2max}, 17 mL/kg IBW (61% of predicted); AT, 9.1 (normal, 11.2 to 22.4); maximum ventilation/ MVV, 102% (normal, 60% to 80%); S_aO_2 at rest, 98%, which drops to 92% with maximal exercise; V_D/V_T at rest, 11%, which increases to 17% with exercise; maximum heart rate, 138 beats per minute (79% of predicted); and total exercise time, 7 minutes 40 seconds. The maximum respiratory rate during exercise is 47 breaths per minute. The test is terminated because of severe dyspnea.

Exercise Abnormalities in Patients with Pulmonary Vascular Disease

- Low O_2 pulse
- Hypoxemia
- Low AT
- High V_D/V_T

EXERCISE PHYSIOLOGY IN PULMONARY VASCULAR DISEASES

The pathophysiology of the pulmonary vascular diseases is discussed in Chapter 6. Briefly, the pulmonary vascular diseases comprise a spectrum of disorders that cause elevation of pressures in the pulmonary vascular circuit, resulting in limitations in cardiac function. The elevated pressures may be caused by primary disorders of the pulmonary circulation (primary pulmonary hypertension, pulmonary thromboembolic disease) or may be secondary to disorders that involve other parts of the body (collagen vascular disease, drug-induced vasculopathy).

Regardless of the cause, elevation of pulmonary pressures has a pronounced effect on the respiratory system. At rest, early in the disease, there may be a mild respiratory alkalosis. A reduction in exercise tolerance is invariably one of the earliest manifestations of pulmonary vascular disease. This reduction in exercise tolerance is typically exhibited by arterial oxygen desaturation with exercise and dyspnea. The oxygen desaturation results from V/Q mismatching caused by reduced perfusion through partially occluded capillaries to ventilated areas of the lung. The high pulmonary pressures favor right-to-left shunting if there are any anatomic openings (patent foramen ovale or ventricular septal defect). During exercise, the pulmonary pressures increase even further, and thus may worsen the degree of either functional or anatomic shunting.

Another manifestation of pulmonary vascular disease is an abnormally high V_E relative to the amount of exercise or VO_2 (see Figure 8-3). The degree of V/Q mismatch, although possibly accounting for the decreased oxygen saturation, is probably not enough to account for the marked ventilatory response. For unclear reasons, patients with pulmonary hypertension have resting respiratory alkalosis (as did our patient in Case Study 3). It is thought that this may be attributable to increased afferent nerve input from baroreceptors in the lung or the heart. The markedly increased V_E noted during exercise may be a further reflection of this altered physiology.

Finally, pulmonary hypertension is a disorder of circulation that has direct cardiac effects. There is a decrease in right heart function, which can affect the left ventricle, resulting in a lower cardiac output (CO) than is required during exercise. Thus, a portion of the limitation on exercise is attributable to reduced cardiac reserve, as demonstrated by a low stroke volume and oxygen pulse. This decreased cardiac reserve results in premature lactic acid buildup and an early AT.

In summary, the following factors contribute to the decreased VO_{2max} typically seen in patients with pulmonary vascular disease: oxygen desaturation with exercise, higher-than-expected V_E, lower cardiac reserve (low oxygen pulse), low AT, and high V_D/V_T.

SUMMARY

Symptom-limited integrative cardiopulmonary exercise testing is a useful clinical tool in the evaluation of patients with limited exercise capacity. Abnormal cardiopulmonary response to exercise may lead to earlier diagnosis of certain diseases even when routine resting examination is normal. Proper interpretation of cardiopulmonary stress testing requires not only a knowledge of normal exercise physiology but also the ability to recognize an abnormal pattern of physiologic response to exercise in certain disease states. Moreover, the interpretation of the exercise test should be done in light of the clinical history and physical examination.

∎ REVIEW QUESTIONS

1. A 45-year-old bank executive complains of dyspnea with moderate exertion. He has occasional episodes of chest pain while playing golf but dismisses them as heartburn. Other than the patient being 20 lb above his ideal body weight, a routine physical examination by a company physician is normal. The patient has a history of 15 pack-years of smoking and a father who died of myocardial infarction at age 55. His serum cholesterol level 1 month ago was 220 mg/dL. Which one of the following is not an expected cardiopulmonary stress test finding in a patient with coronary artery disease?

   (A) Low maximum VO_2
   (B) Low maximum oxygen pulse
   (C) Low breathing reserve
   (D) High heart rate reserve
   (E) A high heart rate at any level of work

2. A 65-year-old retired welder complains of dry coughing and exertional dyspnea with walking for 6 months. He has a 25-year history of smoking, but stopped smoking nearly 2 years ago. Physical examination is remarkable for a respiratory rate of 25 breaths per minute and bibasilar crackles without wheezing on auscultation of the chest. He has significant digital clubbing. Pulmonary function testing reveals: FVC, 2.0 liters (65% of predicted); FEV_1, 1.4 liters (55% of predicted); and FEV_1/FVC, 70%. Lung volume testing reveals: TLC, 4 liters (60% of predicted); and RV, 2.0 liters (64% of predicted). Arterial blood-gas examination shows a pH of 7.45, a PCO_2 of 35 mmHg, and a PO_2 of 65 mmHg. Using this clinical data, which one of the following is not an expected finding during a symptom-limited cardiopulmonary stress test?

   (A) Low maximum VO_2
   (B) High V_T/IC
   (C) Low breathing reserve
   (D) Worsening hypoxemia
   (E) Low respiratory rate

3. Which one of the following statements regarding anaerobic threshold is not correct?

   (A) A low anaerobic threshold on exercise usually indicates either cardiac or circulatory limitation of exercise.
   (B) The anaerobic threshold usually occurs between 40% and 60% of the maximum oxygen consumption.
   (C) Above the anaerobic threshold, lactic acid rapidly accumulates in the blood and within tissues, resulting in acidosis with impaired cellular function.
   (D) During exercise testing, the anaerobic threshold can be determined noninvasively by either a V slope or a ventilatory equivalent technique.
   (E) In a trained athlete, sustained progressive exercise above the anaerobic threshold is possible because of efficient muscular work and energy utilization.

4. Which one of the following is not a physiologic finding in patients with pulmonary vascular disease?

   (A) High minute ventilation at submaximal work rates
   (B) High V_D/V_T
   (C) Low maximum VO_2
   (D) Low oxygen pulse
   (E) Low breathing reserve

5. Match each of the following disorders with the corresponding pathophysiologic mechanism of exercise limitation from the list below.

(1) Obesity
(2) Metabolic acidosis
(3) Malingering
(4) Chest wall disease
(5) Peripheral vascular disease

(A) Irregular breathing, respiratory alkalosis; little or no metabolic acidosis
(B) Increased metabolic requirements; cardiorespiratory restriction
(C) Prevents normal vasodilatation
(D) Reduced buffering capacity; low P_aCO_2 set point
(E) Decreased chest wall compliance; respiratory muscle weakness

■ ANSWERS AND EXPLANATIONS

1. The answer is C. Several points in the patient's clinical history, including angina, excessive weight, a high serum cholesterol, a positive smoking history, and a family history of coronary artery disease (CAD), are worrisome and suggestive of CAD as the cause of his dyspnea. All except (C) the answer options for this question are usually found during progressive exercise to symptom-limited in patients with CAD. Because of the disparity between myocardial oxygen demand and supply during exercise in patients with CAD, several signs and symptoms, such as angina, hypotension, and arrhythmias, may develop during exercise and cause premature termination of exercise. As a result, VO_{2max} and AT are typically low, whereas heart rate reserve is elevated. In addition, depending on the extent of impaired left ventricular function, a low oxygen pulse or an inappropriately high heart rate at lower levels of exercise can be indicative of a low stroke volume state.

2. The answer is E. The clinical history and pulmonary function data are the classic indications of restrictive ventilatory disturbance as the cause of this patient's exercise limitation. A variety of occupational lung diseases (asbestosis, silicosis, hypersensitivity pneumonitis, etc.) can lead to pulmonary fibrosis and restrictive lung disease. In this patient, prolonged and chronic exposure to welding is the cause of the restrictive defect. Typical findings during exercise in restrictive lung disease include a low VO_{2max} as a result of limited ventilatory capacity. Specifically, the small lung volume of patients with restrictive pulmonary disease results in a low breathing reserve and a high V_T/IC ratio. Because of reduced lung compliance, the high minute ventilation during exercise can be achieved only by a progressive increase in respiratory rate, instead of an increase in tidal volume. Often, the respiratory rate at peak exercise is greater than 50 breaths per minute, and exercise-induced hypoxemia occurs because of worsening V/Q mismatch.

3. The answer is F. The anaerobic threshold occurs when the metabolic demand during exercise exceeds the capacity of the circulatory system to deliver nutrients to cardiac and skeletal muscles. Biochemically, glycolysis becomes an important source of ATP above the anaerobic threshold, resulting in lactic acidosis and progressive intracellular metabolic acidosis. Because of these changes, prolonged and sustained exercise above the anaerobic threshold is not possible even in well-trained athletes.

4. The answer is E. The hemodynamic alterations associated with pulmonary vascular disease are pulmonary hypertension and right heart failure. Thus, the low cardiac output state results in a low maximal VO_2 and a low oxygen pulse. The V/E inequality owing to decreased pulmonary capillary blood volume results in a high minute ventilation requirement at submaximal work rates and high V_D/V_T. Because patients with pulmonary vascular disease have normal respiratory mechanics, they have normal breathing reserve not a reduced reserve. In fact, breathing reserve is generally attributable to premature termination of exercise as a result of cardiac limitation.

5. The answers are 1, B; 2, D; 3, A; 4, E; 5, C. Although fatty tissue is metabolically inert compared with skeletal muscle, the added weight of the fatty tissue increases the energy required to accomplish a given level of exercise. In addition, excess fatty tissue located in the chest wall and abdomen impairs the pump function of the respiratory muscles and thus limits overall exercise performance. A narrow physiologic pH range, from 7.35 to 7.45, is vigorously defended during stress by the body's buffer systems so as to maintain an optimal cellular milieu. Exercise worsens an already existing metabolic acidosis at rest, resulting in further disruption of function. In addition, metabolic acidosis increases the minute ventilation requirements both at rest and during exercise. Malingering occurs when an individual tries to fake exercise limitation in order to obtain disability benefits. The normal physiologic responses to exercise as discussed in this chapter are usually absent. Thus, instead of the usual incremental increase in tidal volume followed by a progressive increase in respiratory rate at high work loads, malingering individuals exhibit irregular breathing patterns. Respiratory alkalosis may occur early despite a low work load, and AT is usually not achieved. Chest wall diseases such as scoliosis or kyphoscoliosis decrease chest wall compliance and increase the work of breathing. In addition, distortion of chest wall configuration impairs respiratory muscle force generation by shortening the resting lengths of the respiratory muscles. Peripheral vascular diseases such as atherosclerosis prevent the occurrence of physiologic peripheral vasodilatation during exercise. As a result, the delivery of nutrients and removal of metabolic waste products in exercising skeletal muscles are impaired.

■ SUGGESTED READING

Gallagher CG: Exercise limitation and clinical exercise testing in chronic obstructive pulmonary disease. *Clin Chest Med* 15(2):305–323, 1994.

Marciniuk DD, Gallagher CG: Clinical exercise testing in interstitial lung disease. *Clin Chest Med* 15(2):287–301, 1994.

Murray JF: Chapter 11 (Exercise) In Murray JF, ed.: *The Normal Lung*. Philadelphia: WB Saunders, 1986.

Murray JF: Chapters 5, 41, 54, and 59 In Murray JF, Nadel JA, eds.: *Textbook of Respiratory Medicine*. Philadelphia: WB Saunders, 1988.

Tjahja IE, Reddy HK, Janicki JS, et al: Evolving role of cardiopulmonary exercise testing in cardiovascular disease. *Clin Chest Med* 15(2):271–285, 1994.

Wasserman K: Chapters 1, 3, and 4 In Wasserman K, ed.: *Principles of Exercise Testing and Interpretation*. Malvern, PA: Lea & Febiger, 1994.

Weisman IM, Zeballos RJ: An integrated approach to the interpretation of cardiopulmonary exercise testing. *Clin Chest Med* 15(2):421–445, 1994.

Chapter 9

ASTHMA

David E. Ciccolella, M.D.

David S. Kukafka, M.D.

∎ CHAPTER OUTLINE

Learning Objectives
Case Study: Introduction
Introduction
Clinical Features
Pathology
Airway Inflammation and Inflammatory Mediators
Airway Hyperresponsiveness
Case Study: Continued
Diagnosis and Laboratory Evaluation of Asthma
Pulmonary Function Changes in Asthma
Effects of Airflow Obstruction on Cardiac Function
Gas-Exchange Abnormalities
Special Categories of Asthma
Case Study: Resolution
Assessment of Severity
Therapy for Acute and Chronic Asthma
Complications of Asthma
Review Questions

∎ LEARNING OBJECTIVES

At the completion of this chapter, the reader should:
- Understand and be able to describe the clinical effects of airway narrowing and pulmonary function tests in asthma.
- Be able to describe the cells and mediators involved in the airway inflammation of asthma.
- Know the criteria for the diagnosis of asthma and how to clinically stage or classify this disease.
- Be able to describe the treatment of acute and chronic asthma, stressing the importance of both environmental control measures and pharmacologic therapy.
- Be able to identify the acute and chronic complications of asthma.

Case Study:
Introduction

J. L. is a 24-year-old graduate student who presents to the emergency department because of increased shortness of breath, associated with cough and minimal sputum production, over the last 4 days. He previously noted an intermittent cough, particularly worse at night, over the last 6 months, which he never had evaluated because of a "lack of time." The patient also had a recent "cold" associated with sneezing, nasal congestion, and sore throat. He denies any prior illnesses or medication use. His family history is significant for his father having asthma and rhinitis. His social history shows that he lives alone in an apartment, which has no carpets. He also acquired a cat 18 months ago.

On physical examination, the patient appears moderately short of breath. His blood pressure is 160/80, his pulse rate is 115, and his weight is 150 lb. His chest exam is significant for bilateral expiratory wheezes. He has sternoclavicular retractions, and he appears very uncomfortable.

■ INTRODUCTION

The definition of asthma has remained elusive. Most recently, asthma has been defined as a chronic inflammatory disorder characterized by intermittent symptoms, which include wheezing, chest tightness, and cough associated with airway hyperresponsiveness and variable airflow obstruction.

Asthma can occur at any age but most frequently develops in childhood or young adulthood. The prevalence of asthma in the general population is approximately 5% to 7%, which represents approximately 12 to 17 million Americans. Over the last decade, there has been a rising hospitalization rate for asthma; the hospitalization rate for females is approximately 2.5 times that for males. Asthma has also been a frequent cause of absenteeism from both school and work. In 1990, the total cost (direct and indirect) of asthma care in the United States was estimated to be $6.21 billion. Moreover, there was a 30% increase in mortality from 1980 to 1987, and in 1992 there were approximately 6000 deaths from asthma in the United States.

■ CLINICAL FEATURES

The usual clinical symptoms of an asthma exacerbation are dyspnea, cough, chest tightness, and wheezing. However, these symptoms have variable severity and may not be present simultaneously. In milder cases, some patients may have only a persistent cough, which is worse nocturnally, or dyspnea, especially with exertion. Frequently, in more severe attacks, some or all of these symptoms occur over several days or longer before the patient seeks medical help; a minority of patients may have a rapid onset of severe symptoms over a few minutes or hours. If the patient does not seek medical help early in the asthma exacerbation, she or he may present with a very severe attack resulting in respiratory failure, requiring tracheal intubation and mechanical ventilation, or even death.

The patient may be able to identify a trigger of the attack, such as exercise, pets, dust, smoke, or strong smells. Some patients may have attacks following the ingestion of aspirin or other nonsteroidal anti-inflammatory medications such as ibuprofen, probably as a result of alterations in arachidonic acid metabolism leading to increases in leukotriene production.

In patients who present with asthma attacks, physical examination commonly reveals tachypnea (increased breathing rate), use of accessory muscles of ventilation in more severe cases, an increased expiratory time, and wheezing. In severe attacks, patients may be diaphoretic and may not be able to speak in complete sentences as a result of their dyspnea. Wheezing is a nonspecific sign, indicating only airflow through narrowed airways, and may be present in other disease states. The degree of wheezing is not a good indicator of the severity of the attack. Moreover, in a very severe asthma attack, wheezing may not be present because of severely reduced airflow.

Arterial blood gases may show decreased arterial oxygen (hypoxemia) and decreased carbon dioxide (hypocapnia), but in severe cases the arterial carbon dioxide level may be elevated (see Chapter 4). Expiratory airflow, which usually is reduced, is a much better indicator of the severity of the attack.

■ PATHOLOGY

Airway narrowing leading to increased airway resistance and airflow obstruction in asthma can occur through three main mechanisms: 1) airway smooth muscle contraction, 2) airway wall thickening, and 3) airway lumen debris (Table 9-1).

The airway narrowing and resulting airflow obstruction can be understood by examining the pathology of the airway (Figure 9-1). In asthma, epithelial cell damage with

---

Definition of Asthma

- Airway inflammation
- Airway hyperresponsiveness
- Variable airflow obstruction

Symptoms of Asthma Exacerbation

- Dyspnea
- Cough
- Audible wheezing
- Chest tightness

Signs of Acute Severe Asthma Exacerbation

- Tachypnea
- Diaphoresis
- Wheezing
- Speaks in incomplete sentences
- Use of accessory muscles of ventilation

Table 9-1
Mechanisms of Airway Narrowing in Asthma

Airway smooth muscle contraction

Airway wall thickening:
    Cellular infiltration/edema
    Smooth muscle hyperplasia/hypertrophy (chronic effect)

Airway secretions and cellular debris

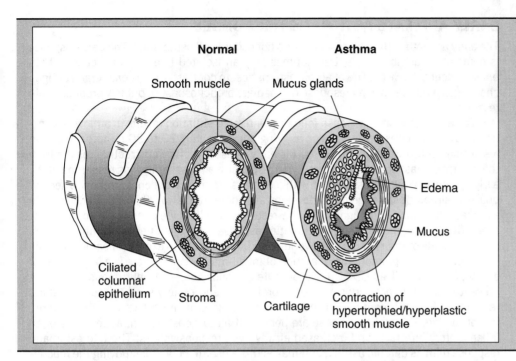

FIGURE 9-1
Morphologic changes in asthma producing airway obstruction.

detachment of the surface epithelial cells is present. Airway wall thickening or narrowing can occur by means of the chronic effects of smooth muscle hypertrophy and hyperplasia, as well as by epithelial basement membrane thickening and hypertrophy of the mucus-secreting glands. In addition, inflammatory cell infiltrates and edema also narrow the airway, causing airflow obstruction. The third component is smooth muscle contraction, which leads to acute symptoms of airflow obstruction in asthma.

AIRWAY INFLAMMATION AND INFLAMMATORY MEDIATORS

The inflammatory cell infiltrate in asthma is consistently characterized by an increase in mast cells, eosinophils, and activated T lymphocytes. These cells and mediators are thought to be major contributors to the pathophysiology of asthma.

The mechanisms for the development of airway inflammation in asthma involve the release of mediators through IgE-dependent and IgE-independent T-lymphocyte processes. The immune system can be divided into antibody-mediated and cell-mediated processes. The antibody-mediated processes involve production and secretion of antibodies by B lymphocytes. The B lymphocytes mature into plasma cells that synthesize and secrete the specific immunoglobulin antibodies. The production of IgE antibodies to allergens is important in allergic asthma. The cell-mediated processes involve T-lymphocyte regulation of B-lymphocyte function—especially IgE synthesis—and the development of a variety of inflammatory effects through the production and release of cytokines. Subpopulations of T lymphocytes called CD4+ helper cells and CD8+ suppressor cells play a significant role in airway inflammation. The normal function of CD8+ T lymphocytes is down-regulation of immunoglobulin synthesis to prevent excessive immunoglobulin levels.

The cellular components of inflammation may release preformed granules and rapidly generated mediators. Cytokines, histamine, leukotrienes, and proteases are among the mediators released into the extracellular milieu. The leukotrienes are derived from arachidonic metabolism and play a role in asthma inflammation.

Airway inflammation has been investigated experimentally by bronchoscopic instillation of an antigen into a bronchial airway of a sensitive asthmatic. In the asthmatic, instillation of the antigen may produce an early phase of airflow obstruction—the early asthmatic response—and a late phase of airflow obstruction—the late asthmatic response.

EARLY AND LATE ASTHMATIC RESPONSES

The early and late asthmatic responses do not occur in all asthmatics. The early response is common in asthmatics, but sometimes only an isolated late response occurs; both phases occur in 30% to 50% of atopic asthmatics. In contrast, many nonallergen antigen challenges produce an early response (immediate bronchospasm), but few produce a late response.

The early asthmatic response following antigen instillation results in airflow obstruction in a few minutes, with a peak occurring approximately 20 to 30 minutes later and resolution occurring within an hour. This early phase of airflow obstruction results from the release of mast cell mediators on hyperresponsive airways. Following resolution of the early response, which is associated with a decrease in mediator concentration, a second phase of airflow obstruction often develops anywhere from 4 to 10 hours later. This late asthmatic response is thought to be the result of specific cytokines released during or soon after initiation of the early asthmatic response. The cytokines elicit inflammatory cells to the site of injury and induce venular endothelial cells to express specific adhesion molecules so as to promote the migration of inflammatory cells. There is a large influx of eosinophils, as well as CD4+ T lymphocytes, monocytes, and neutrophils. The cells present in the inflammatory site release preformed and rapidly synthesized mediators, resulting in further inflammation and the manifestations of clinical asthma. Characteristics of the late asthmatic response are persistent airflow obstruction, appearance of an inflammatory infiltrate, and increased airway hyperresponsiveness. The late asthmatic response mimics chronic asthma and makes this a useful model for studying the mechanisms of airway inflammation.

MAST CELLS

Mast cells play a major role in asthma. These cells can be found in the bronchial epithelium, in the submucosa, and near blood vessels. Mast cells or peripheral blood basophils are passively sensitized by IgE antibodies. Mast cells bind IgE through Fc receptors on the cell surface. On encountering an antigen, the IgE becomes crosslinked, inducing degranulation and release of mediators within minutes. The release of products by these cells is important in the development of the early asthmatic response following an allergen challenge.

The mast cell can release preformed mediators present in granules and also rapidly formed mediators. Preformed mediators include histamine, peroxidase, chemotactic factors, and neutral proteases. These mediators have been shown to cause airway smooth muscle contraction, vasodilation, increased vascular permeability, and glandular secretion. Rapidly formed mediators, which include superoxide anion, cytokines, platelet activating factor, and arachidonic metabolites, have similar effects. Some of these rapidly formed mediators, which include the cytokines IL-3, IL-4, and IL-5, the tumor necrosis factor (TNF), and interferon-γ (IFN-γ), also help to establish the late asthmatic response phase.

LYMPHOCYTES AND CYTOKINES

The lymphocyte has been recently postulated to play a major role in the regulation of airway inflammation and asthma through the production of a large array of cytokines and other modulating mediators. There are increased numbers of lymphocytes, predominantly T cells, in the airways or airway walls. They consist mainly of CD4+ helper cells with no evidence of activated CD8+ suppressor cells. It is generally agreed that the airway T lymphocytes are necessary for the development of the late asthmatic response, especially leukocyte transmigration. The lymphocytes signal other cells in the airway using specific cytokines to develop the inflammatory response.

In the mouse, the CD4+ helper T-cell populations have been found to be of two different subsets, T_H1 and T_H2, based on their pattern of cytokine production (Table 9-2). Similar T-helper cell subsets have been found in humans, but they are not as well defined. The T_H1 cells, which are involved primarily in "classical" cell-mediated immunity against intracellular pathogens and in delayed hypersensitivity reactions (type 4), preferentially secrete IL-2, TNF-β, and IFN-γ. IL-2 stimulates T-lymphocyte proliferation and IFN-γ inhibits B-lymphocyte activation and IgE synthesis by B lymphocytes. The principal effector cell of the T_H1 group is the macrophage. The T_H2 cells, which are involved in IgE-mediated allergic reactions (type 1) and phagocyte-independent host defense, preferentially secrete IL-4, IL-5, IL-10, and IL-13. Both T-helper cell subsets also produce granulocyte-macrophage colony stimulating factor (GM-CSF) and IL-3. The T_H2 cytokines affect B-lymphocyte IgE synthesis; mast cell growth and development; and eosinophil production, survival, and activation. Different T-helper cell subsets may be important in different disease states, such as atopic and nonatopic asthma. These cytokines can also induce adhesion molecules and migration of inflammatory cells into the lungs.

CYTOKINE	T_H1 SUBSET	T_H2 SUBSET
IL-2	+	−
IL-3	+	+
IL-4	−	+
IL-5	−	+
IL-10	−	+
IL-13		+
IFN-γ	+	−
GM-CSF	+	+
TNF-β	+	−

Table 9-2
Cytokines Produced from
T-Lymphocyte Subsets

Modified from Horwitz RJ and Busse WW: *Clinics in Chest Medicine*, 1995.

EOSINOPHILS

The eosinophil is present in the blood, sputum, and airway submucosa of the asthmatic and is probably the predominant effector cell in asthma inflammation. The significant relationship between the number of eosinophils in blood and lung lavage and the severity of asthma, along with the presence of eosinophil granular proteins in the airway submucosa, supports the prominent role of the eosinophil. Furthermore, blocking of eosinophil infiltration by a monoclonal antibody against a specific adhesion molecule prevents the development of allergen-induced airway hyperresponsiveness.

The eosinophil is capable of releasing various mediators that can contribute to airway inflammation. The processes of eosinophil differentiation, migration, and activation are mediated mostly by the actions of IL-3 and IL-5, GM-CSF, and RANTES. RANTES is a chemoattractant for CD4+ T lymphocytes and monocytes to inflammatory sites. The CD4+ T lymphocytes are the most important sources of these molecules.

Eosinophils may cause tissue damage through the release of stored granular compounds and bioactive mediators. The major stored granular compounds in eosinophils are major basic protein, eosinophil cationic protein, eosinophil-derived neurotoxin, and eosinophil peroxidase. In an asthma exacerbation, eosinophil granular proteins are present in high concentrations in the sputum. Major basic protein can increase airway contractility and damage respiratory epithelial cells, and is associated with enhanced airway responsiveness. The bioactive mediators include platelet activating factor (PAF); arachidonic acid metabolites such as leukotriene C4; and cytokines IL-3, IL-5, and GM-CSF. These mediators may be responsible for several effects in asthma, including airway smooth muscle contraction, increased mucus secretion, and vascular permeability. Moreover, the resulting epithelial cell damage may expose sensory nerve endings, thus increasing airway wall edema and smooth muscle responsiveness.

ADHESION MOLECULES AND MIGRATION OF LEUKOCYTES

The migration of leukocytes from the blood stream to sites of tissue inflammation are partially dependent on adhesion molecules. Adhesion molecules are necessary for mounting an inflammatory response. The process of leukocyte migration mediated by cellular adhesion appears to occur in stages. These include random contact and rolling of the leukocyte on the postcapillary venular endothelium near the inflammatory focus, activation and firm adhesion of selected cell populations, and diapedesis and migration into the subendothelial tissue.

The adhesion molecules can be divided into three groups: the selectins, the integrins, and the immunoglobulin gene superfamily of receptors. The adhesion molecules from each group are found on leukocytes, on venular endothelial cells (epithelial cells and fibroblasts), or on both.

Adhesion molecules are regulated by a wide variety of mediators released during the inflammatory cascade. Inflammatory cell recruitment in asthma is associated with an increased expression of specific adhesion molecules on postcapillary venular endothelial cells and the activation of complementary ligands on leukocytes. In summary, adhesion molecules, which promote leukocyte migration to the inflammatory site, are necessary for the development and control of the inflammatory response.

CONSTITUTIVE CELLS

Lung constitutive cells—namely, epithelial cells, endothelial cells, and fibroblasts—may contribute to chronic airway inflammation in asthma through the release and production of cytokines. The epithelial cells can release the cytokines IL-6, IL-8, GM-CSF, IL-1 β, and TNF-α. Endothelial cells can produce IL-1 β, IL-5, and GM-CSF, whereas fibroblasts produce mast cell growth factor, GM-CSF, and IL-8. The cytokines from these resident cells may serve as a mechanism for maintenance and enhancement of the inflammatory response.

■ AIRWAY HYPERRESPONSIVENESS

Two main features of asthma are airway inflammation and hyperresponsiveness. The precise features have not been defined for the airway inflammation, which also occurs in very mild conditions. The secondary effects of airway inflammation are airway hyperresponsiveness and obstruction as well as many of the symptoms and signs of asthma.

Airway hyperresponsiveness, which is defined by the ease with which the airways narrow in response to various nonsensitizing physical and chemical stimuli, is a hallmark of asthma. Hyperresponsive airways in asthma may be thought of as being more *twitchy*. Airway hyperresponsiveness can be assessed by measuring lung function before and after the inhalation of increasing doses of either methacholine or histamine. The hyperresponsive airways develop obstruction at lower cumulative doses than those required for obstruction of normal airways. Physiologically, hyperresponsiveness may help to protect the lung from the detrimental effects of irritating inhalants.

The magnitude of airway hyperresponsiveness seems to be correlated with the degree of airway inflammation. It is also correlated with the numbers of lymphocytes and eosinophils, the amounts of eosinophil major basic and cationic proteins, and the degree of epithelial damage found on bronchial biopsy. Airway hyperresponsiveness in the asthmatic correlates with the clinical symptoms and status of the asthma and with the diurnal variation in airflow obstruction measured by the peak expiratory flow rate. It is not correlated with the severity of airflow obstruction.

The finding of airway hyperresponsiveness is characteristic of asthma but is not unique to its diagnosis, because it is present in some healthy people and in a significant portion of patients with only hay fever. It may also be found in patients with other inflammatory conditions, such as chronic obstructive pulmonary disease (COPD), sarcoidosis, tuberculosis, silicosis, adult respiratory distress syndrome (ARDS), and cystic fibrosis.

Factors that can produce or increase airway hyperresponsiveness include allergen inhalation associated with the late asthmatic response, viral and chlamydial respiratory infections, and some occupational inhalants. Conditions that may increase airflow obstruction but not produce or increase airway hyperresponsiveness in asthmatics are exercise, inhalation of cold dry air, hyperventilation, cigarette smoking, inhalation of irritants, and methacholine or histamine challenge.

The mechanisms underlying airway hyperresponsiveness in asthma are obscure and somewhat controversial. The possible mechanisms are many and various, but there is strong support for the theory that airway hyperresponsiveness is caused by airway inflammation. Other possible mechanisms are physical or structural abnormalities of the airway; autonomic nervous system abnormalities such as increased α-adrenergic responsiveness, cholinergic overactivity, alterations in the nonadrenergic, noncholinergic

(NANC) nervous system, and changes in local axon reflexes; humoral mediators; airway smooth muscle abnormalities; and loss of certain inhibitory mechanisms.

Case Study:
Continued

The patient's laboratory data reveal a peak expiratory flow (PEF) of 180 L/min, a blood gas that showed a pH of 7.49, a PCO_2 of 32 mmHg, a PO_2 of 74 mmHg, and a calculated bicarbonate of 23. His chest x-ray shows mild hyperinflation with no infiltrates. Wright's stain reveals many eosinophils in the sputum. Spirometry shows a mildly reduced forced vital capacity (4.0 liters) but a reduced forced expiratory volume in 1 second (2.4 liters) and an FEV_1/FVC ratio of 60. The patient is treated with aerosolized albuterol by a hand-held nebulizer with marked improvement in his symptoms; peak expiratory flow is 300. Repeat spirometry shows an FVC of 4.5 liters, an FEV_1 of 3.0 liters, and an FEV_1/FVC ratio of 66.

DIAGNOSIS AND LABORATORY EVALUATION OF ASTHMA

The diagnosis of asthma is based on clinical impression, including a consistent history and objective evidence of reversible airflow obstruction. The classic symptoms of asthma—wheezing, cough, chest tightness, dyspnea, and production of sputum containing eosinophils—are nonspecific. Moreover, these symptoms may not be present simultaneously, and some patients may present with cough only—a condition known as cough-variant asthma. In an asthmatic, these symptoms tend to wax and wane and often occur nocturnally.

The prominent nocturnal symptoms of an asthmatic are associated with an exaggerated circadian (day-to-night) rhythm in the peak expiratory airflow (PEF), as compared with that of normals. A normal subject generally has a day-to-night PEF variation of less than 8%. Usually peak expiratory airflow tends to be higher in the late afternoon, around 4 P.M., and lower in the morning hours, around 4 A.M. (Figure 9-2). However, asthmatics can have day-to-night PEF variation as high as 50%.

Diagnosis of Asthma

- Consistent clinical history
- Reversible airflow obstruction by pulmonary function testing
- Exclusion of other diseases

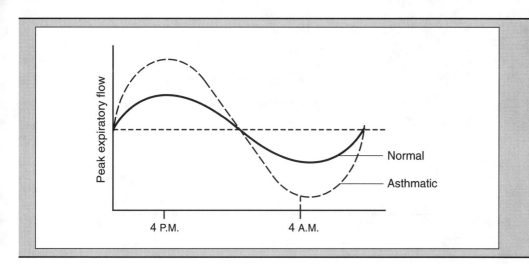

FIGURE 9-2
Circadian variation of airflow in normal and asthmatic patients.

Patients frequently suffer acute exacerbations of their symptoms on exposure to nonspecific stimuli such as exercise, respiratory irritants (e.g., strong smells, perfumes, laundry detergents, infections, air pollution, etc.), and cold air. Specific irritants, such as allergens, may also cause acute exacerbations of symptoms (Table 9-3).

Laboratory studies help form the physician's clinical impression of asthma. Pulmonary function tests (including spirometry) and lung volumes may show evidence of airflow obstruction (see Chapter 4). This airflow obstruction is revealed by decreases in the forced expiratory volumes, the forced vital capacity (FVC), the forced expiratory volume in 1 second (FEV_1), and the FEV_1/FVC ratio (Figure 9-3).

Table 9-3
Asthma Triggers

BRONCHOSPASTIC	INFLAMMATORY
Pharmacologic Agents	**Allergens**
Histamine	House dust mites
Methacholine	Animal dander
	Pollen
Physical Factors	Cockroaches
Exercise	
Hyperventilation	**Occupational Exposures**
Plicatic acid (cedar)	Toluene diisocyanate
Cold dry air	
Nonisotonic aerosol inhalation	**Infections**
	Viruses
Irritants	Bacteria
Environmental tobacco smoke	
Noxious gases	
Strong smells	
Emotional Stress	
Other Factors	
Rhinitis/sinusitis	
Gastroesophageal reflux	
Sensitivity to aspirin, NSAIDs*, sulfites	
Nonselective topical/systemic beta-blockers	

* Nonsteroidal anti-inflammatory drugs.

Modified from National Asthma Education Program Expert Panel: Guidelines for the diagnosis and management of asthma (Expert Panel Report 2). Bethesda, MD: National Institutes of Health, 1997.

FIGURE 9-3
Changes in forced expiratory volume in 1 second (FEV_1) and forced vital capacity in normal and acute asthmatics. Note the smaller volume exhaled in 1 second between the normal and the asthmatic.

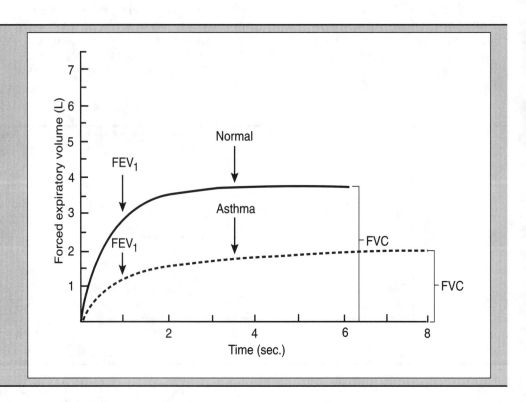

More specifically, the airflow response to inhalation of a bronchodilator, such as a beta-receptor agonist, may show a significant improvement in the expiratory flow rates. Airway obstruction is considered to be reversible if the FEV_1 or FVC is increased by at least 200 mL and is 12% greater than its baseline value after an inhaled β_2-adrenergic receptor agonist is given.

The lung diffusion capacity for carbon monoxide (D_LCO) (single breath) (see Chapter 4) is normal in asthma and may be helpful in differentiating asthma from emphysema.

The D_LCO is typically decreased in patients with emphysema, whereas it is usually normal in patients with bronchitis and asthma.

If spirometry, lung volumes, and D_LCO are normal, bronchoprovocation tests can be helpful in diagnosing airway hyperresponsiveness. Airway hyperresponsiveness may be elicited by several different bronchoprovocation tests, including inhalation of histamine or methacholine as well as isocapnic hyperventilation of cold air. Challenge tests with these agents are usually performed by having the patient inhale progressively higher concentrations of the agent.

The most common drug used is nebulized methacholine. The concentration that decreases the FEV_1 by 20% is called the PD_{20} or provocative dose. In asthmatics, the PD_{20} generally is less than 8 mg/mL. A positive methacholine challenge test establishes the presence of airway hyperresponsiveness and, with consistent history and symptoms, establishes the diagnosis of asthma.

Other tests that help establish the diagnosis include chest x-ray and evaluation of sputum. In asthma, the chest x-ray commonly is normal, but it may show hyperinflation of the lungs. Chest x-rays are useful in helping rule out disorders that may mimic asthma. The sputum and peripheral blood frequently show increases in eosinophils, whether the asthma has been shown to have an allergic or nonallergic component; these tests are helpful and supportive but are nonspecific.

Wheezing is a nonspecific sign that reflects airway narrowing, and may be present in a number of other disease states. The differential diagnosis of asthma includes COPD (emphysema, chronic bronchitis), upper airway obstruction, pulmonary embolism, congestive heart failure, hypersensitivity reaction, foreign body aspiration, vocal cord dysfunction, and idiopathic hyperventilation (Table 9-4).

COPD: emphysema, chronic bronchitis
Upper airway obstruction
Pulmonary embolism
Congestive heart failure
Hypersensitivity reaction
Idiopathic hyperventilation
Foreign body aspiration
Vocal cord dysfunction

Table 9-4
Asthma Differential Diagnosis

Differentiating between asthma and COPD may be difficult because of the presence of bronchospasm in some patients with COPD, as well as the failure of marked reversibility in some patients with asthma. Chronic bronchitis is usually characterized by a cough and mucus production for a minimum of 3 months per year for two consecutive years. Emphysema is a diagnosis that truly can be made only at autopsy because the definition is pathologically based. Pathologically, emphysema is characterized by enlarged respiratory air spaces and destruction of the alveolar capillary wall. When evaluating a patient for asthma, one must consider these different diagnoses in order to avoid a misdiagnosis and associated long-term morbidity and mortality.

■ PULMONARY FUNCTION CHANGES IN ASTHMA

The inflammation in asthma, which causes the pathologic abnormalities in the airway, results in airway narrowing, increased airflow resistance, and airflow obstruction. Airway smooth muscle contraction, which is a reversible abnormality, further contributes to the airway narrowing and resulting airflow obstruction.

Asthma is characterized by reversible airflow obstruction, and during asymptomatic periods there may be no demonstrable airflow obstruction. On the other hand, during symptomatic periods there are usually significant alterations in spirometry, lung volumes, and gas exchange.

In chronic severe asthma, airflow resistance is increased and maximal expiratory flow rates are reduced whereas lung volumes—especially functional residual capacity and residual volume—may be elevated. In less severe chronic asthma, lung volumes are usually normal.

In an acute exacerbation of asthma, there is typically an obstructive pattern on pulmonary function testing. Airway obstruction results in reductions in FEV_1 and the FEV_1/FVC ratio. The forced vital capacity may be normal or low, usually depending on the severity of asthma and air trapping. Patients who have a prolonged expiratory phase on the exhaled volume-time curve have an increased expiratory-to-inspiratory time ratio. The expiratory limb of the flow-volume loop is curvilinear and is probably caused by progressive closure of many airways during expiration.

Acute airflow obstruction in asthma tends to cause hyperinflation. The pattern of abnormal lung volumes is usually large elevations in residual volume and functional residual capacity with a more modest rise in total lung capacity.

The precise mechanisms leading to hyperinflation are poorly understood. The increase in functional residual capacity might have several causes. The first cause may be related to progressive airway closure of peripheral airways resulting in a reduction of their contribution to elastic recoil. The equilibrium between the elastic recoil of the chest and that of the lung occurs at a higher lung volume. This manifests as a shift in the static volume-pressure curve upward and leftward, resulting in an increased functional residual capacity. The second cause of hyperinflation is an increase in tonic activity of the inspiratory muscles, which are thought to be active throughout expiration, producing a greater radial retractile force on the airway walls and increasing the size of the airway lumen. A third cause is dynamic hyperinflation, which is the inability of the patient with obstructive disease to exhale completely the present breath before the next inhalation occurs. This leads to "breath stacking" and progressive hyperinflation until an equilibrium is attained between the amounts of air inhaled and exhaled.

The airway obstruction in asthma produces hyperinflation to increase the airway size and overcome the increased airflow resistance. This hyperinflation reduces airway resistance but at the expense of an increase in elastic work required. The lung hyperinflation shifts the pressure-volume curve upward, where the lung is less compliant. Therefore, it requires more work by the patient to breathe at a higher lung volume. If this condition is prolonged and severe, respiratory failure may result, and the patient may require mechanical ventilation.

▌EFFECTS OF AIRFLOW OBSTRUCTION ON CARDIAC FUNCTION

Airflow obstruction, which leads to increases in intrathoracic pressures, also has effects on cardiac preload and afterload. The higher negative inspiratory pressures in the chest are transmitted to the heart, causing proportional reductions in intracardiac pressures, and an increase in ventricular afterload. On the following beat, the ventricles may not develop enough force to maintain arterial pressure. This results in pulsus paradoxus, which is a transient drop in blood pressure with each inspiration but a return to its previous level at expiration. The severity of the pulsus paradoxus, measured as the difference in the systolic blood pressures during expiration and inspiration, is roughly proportional to the severity of airflow obstruction. The severity of the pulsus paradoxus is also affected by the force-generating ability of the respiratory muscles, which may result in a relatively low pulsus paradoxus in a fatigued patient.

▌GAS-EXCHANGE ABNORMALITIES

The gas-exchange abnormalities observed in acute asthma may show a reduction (hypoxemia) in partial pressure of oxygen (PO_2) with a reduction (hypocapnia) or an increase (hypercapnia) in the partial pressure of carbon dioxide (PCO_2). The most common syndrome of abnormalities is hypoxemia and hypocapnia with a respiratory alkalosis. The hypoxemia is roughly proportional to the severity of the airflow obstruction as reflected by the FEV_1. The predominant mechanism producing hypoxemia is ventilation-perfusion mismatch along with small and varying degrees of shunt, which can be corrected with low supplemental oxygen concentrations. In asthma, the airways are not homogeneously obstructed, which leads to poor ventilation in some alveoli, and the blood perfusion is altered by hyperinflation and hypoxic vasoconstriction, resulting in blood that has a low oxygen saturation. Collapsed airways associated with mucus plugging may cause significant shunt and require higher oxygen concentrations. An increase in PCO_2 may result from respiratory muscle fatigue and severe V/Q mismatch. The PCO_2 does not correlate with the severity of airflow obstruction, especially when the FEV_1 is less than 20% of predicted.

SPECIAL CATEGORIES OF ASTHMA

Special forms of asthma include aspirin-induced asthma, exercise-induced asthma, and occupational asthma.

ASPIRIN-INDUCED ASTHMA

The response induced by the ingestion of aspirin in sensitive individuals may consist of nasal congestion, eye irritation, or an asthma exacerbation, and usually occurs quite rapidly within approximately 30 minutes. Approximately 4% to 20% of asthmatics are sensitive to aspirin and related compounds, especially nonsteroidal anti-inflammatory drugs. Nasal polyposis and chronic rhinosinusitis occur in approximately 90% of those patients with aspirin sensitivity, and together with asthma are known as Samter's syndrome. There is no known familial predilection for aspirin sensitivity. Furthermore, it is not known to be associated with atopy as with an IgE-mediated mechanism. The mechanism appears to be an inhibition of the enzyme cyclooxygenase and the shunting of the arachidonic acid metabolites through the leukotriene pathway, resulting in increased production of the leukotrienes C_4, D_4, and E_4, the slow-reacting substances of anaphylaxis. Thus, drugs that inhibit the enzyme cyclooxygenase may cause an asthma exacerbation.

EXERCISE-INDUCED ASTHMA

Exercise-induced asthma (EIA) can be defined as a reversible decrease in airflow obstruction that occurs after exercise. EIA can be seen in up to 90% of asthmatics and in select populations such as some normal relatives of asthmatics and some patients with allergies. As with asthma, the common symptoms are wheezing, shortness of breath, cough, and chest tightness. However, the symptoms typically start several minutes after the cessation of exercise and usually improve within 1 hour. The typical fall in airflow is seen maximally from 5 to 15 minutes after exercise and resolves within 1 hour. The mechanism of EIA is thought to be associated with the exchange of heat and water that occurs in the airways during and after exercise. During exercise, the airways cool down while minute ventilation increases, thus cooling and drying the lower airways. Resting results in a rapid rewarming of the airways, which leads to bronchoconstriction, the exact mechanism of which is unclear. Theories include changes in airway osmolality, resulting in mast cell degranulation and smooth muscle constriction, and hyperemia of the airway wall vessels during rewarming, resulting in airway edema and obstruction.

EIA can be prevented or reduced in severity by attenuating the degree of heat exchange and inhibiting airway smooth muscle contraction. This can be done by using a warm-up period, which produces a refractory period, and beta-receptor agonists or the cromones (cromolyn sodium and nedocromil sodium) prior to exercise.

OCCUPATIONAL ASTHMA

Many substances in the workplace have been implicated in the development of asthma, including a variety of animal proteins, grain and wood dusts, cotton dusts, chemical compounds such as isocyanates and hydrides, metal salts, and various pharmaceuticals. The mechanisms for this form of asthma are not clearly established. It is important to determine if a relationship exists between a person's asthma and the workplace to avoid the offending material and decrease morbidity. Some people have persistent asthma despite removal of the inciting substance.

Clinically, inhalation of a suspected allergen or occupational irritant has been used to evaluate a patient with suspected but difficult-to-prove sensitivity to these antigens. It is rarely performed, because the allergen or occupational irritant usually can be identified and the test may result in severe reactions or death.

Case Study:
Resolution

A presumptive diagnosis of diffuse airflow obstruction is made on the basis of the patient's consistent history, physical exam, and laboratory information. The patient is treated with aerosolized albuterol delivered with a hand-held nebulizer for a total of four treatments, after which he shows considerable improvement in his symptoms and wheezing. He is also given intravenous methylprednisolone. His peak flow improves to 450 L/min. His significant response to beta-receptor agonist treatment supports the diagnosis of asthma.

The patient is discharged to home on tapering oral corticosteroids and given instructions to have a follow-up visit with a physician for further asthma education, treatment, and evaluation of possible allergy.

■ ASSESSMENT OF SEVERITY

Symptoms and signs are not accurate indicators of the severity of the acute asthma attack. Measurement of expiratory flow rates, including peak expiratory flow rate, is the most reliable predictor of severity. However, it may be difficult to use in patients with very severe airflow obstruction. The extremes of arterial blood gases (i.e., hypercapnia and acidosis) indicate a poor prognosis but are not as predictive as the measurement of flow rates. The predictors of impending death in asthma include alteration in consciousness, physical exhaustion, a "silent" chest, carbon dioxide retention, and evidence of barotrauma including pneumothorax and pneumomediastinum.

■ THERAPY FOR ACUTE AND CHRONIC ASTHMA

The treatment of asthma includes two broad categories of drugs: bronchodilators, which relax airway smooth muscle, and anti-inflammatory agents, which decrease the influx of inflammatory cells and the release and/or effects of chemical mediators from cells. Bronchodilators include short- and long-acting β-adrenergic receptor agonists, methylxanthines, and anticholinergics. The anti-inflammatory agents include corticosteroids, the cromones (cromolyn sodium and nedocromil sodium), and the leukotriene modifiers (Table 9-5). Environmental control measures such as allergen avoidance are always included in asthma treatment. Immunotherapy for chronic asthma can be considered in select cases. Supportive therapy for acute asthma includes oxygen, and therapy for severe cases with respiratory failure includes mechanical ventilation.

Table 9-5
Medications for Treatment of Asthma

BRONCHODILATORS	ANTI-INFLAMMATORY AGENTS
β_2-receptor agonists	Environmental control
Theophylline	Corticosteroids
Ipratropium bromide	Cromolyn sodium
	Nedocromil sodium
	Leukotriene modifiers
	Allergen immunotherapy

The therapeutic goals for asthma are to 1) reduce asthma mortality and morbidity; 2) reverse airway hyperreactivity; 3) control asthma symptoms; and 4) allow resumption of normal activity. The types of medications used in the treatment of acute and chronic asthma are discussed below.

MEDICATION DELIVERY

In asthma, therapy may be given orally or by inhalation. The preferred route of therapy is by inhalation. Inhalation therapy delivers smaller doses of medication directly to the lungs, often with greater efficacy and lower risk of side effects. Inhalation therapy can be performed through a small-volume nebulizer or a metered dose inhaler. Nebulizers deliver approximately 10% of the dose to be aerosolized to the lungs; metered dose inhalers also deliver small doses to the lungs. A tube spacer device attached to metered-dose inhalers is used to enhance aerosol drug delivery to the lungs.

BETA-ADRENERGIC RECEPTOR AGONISTS

In the treatment of asthma, the first-line therapy should be an inhaled β_2-receptor agonist. These drugs produce rapid bronchodilation within minutes and with minimal side effects. Stimulation of the β_2 receptors in various tissues of the lung, such as smooth muscle cells and other inflammatory cells, produces a complex series of biochemical events. The β_2-receptor agonists are representative of the group of sympathomimetic agents, which act on the beta receptors of the lung tissue to stimulate adenyl cyclase, an enzyme located on airway smooth muscle cells, and to increase intracellular cyclic adenosine monophosphate (AMP). The increase in cyclic AMP in the airway smooth muscle cells results in bronchodilation.

Beta-adrenergic receptor agonists that are more selective for the β_2 receptor are generally preferred. Drugs such as albuterol are β_2-receptor selective, resulting in decreased extrapulmonary side effects, especially cardiac side effects. Some newer beta-receptor agonists such as salmeterol have a longer duration of action (12 hours) than albuterol (4 to 6 hours), making them useful for controlling nocturnal asthma.

These sympathomimetic drugs can be given by three different routes: oral, parenteral, and inhalation. Inhaled beta-receptor agents tend to be preferred because of the direct delivery to the site of action in the airways, which results in fewer local and systemic side effects.

ANTICHOLINERGICS

Anticholinergic drugs are another group of bronchodilator agents used in certain cases of asthma. They include ipratropium bromide and glycopyrrolate. The most commonly used ipratropium bromide causes bronchodilation through a decrease in cholinergic or vagal tone of the airways by blocking postganglionic vagal pathways. It blocks the bronchoconstricting effects of acetylcholine by competing for muscarinic receptor sites. This blockade decreases the level of cyclic guanosine monophosphate (GMP), resulting in smooth muscle relaxation.

Anticholinergic drugs are less potent bronchodilators than the β_2-receptor agonists and have a slower onset of action, making the beta-receptor agonists more appropriate for first-line therapy. These are safe drugs because they have poor systemic absorption, resulting in few side effects. Therefore, they can be useful in patients with significant cardiac disease, older patients with fixed airway disease, and patients who have a poor response to β_2-receptor agonists.

THEOPHYLLINE

Theophylline is a methylxanthine that, for unclear reasons, acts both as a mild bronchodilator by relaxing airway smooth muscle and possibly as an anti-inflammatory agent. However, owing to the conflicting data on its efficacy, a narrow therapeutic window, and medication interactions, theophylline is used mostly as a third-line agent in the treatment of more severe patients after conventional anti-inflammatory agents and bronchodilators have been optimized.

Inhibition of phosphodiesterase has long been considered the mechanism of action of methylxanthine therapy. Recently, however, this mechanism has been refuted, and the true mechanism remains to be elucidated. The effectiveness of theophylline is related to its blood concentration, which is optimal between 5 and 15 µg/mL. Above such concentrations, the incidence of gastrointestinal, cardiac, and neurologic toxicity becomes unacceptable. Theophylline has a log-linear dosage response curve whose slope varies from one patient to another. Careful individualization of dosage is required to minimize toxicity. Certain conditions and medications may significantly alter the drug levels of theophylline (Table 9-6).

ANTI-INFLAMMATORY AGENTS

Anti-inflammatory agents used in asthma management include cromolyn sodium, nedocromil sodium, leukotriene modifiers, and the corticosteroids. Cromolyn sodium is an anti-inflammatory agent used most commonly in children. It is a drug that is given by inhalation as a powder or an MDI on a prophylactic basis. Although its mode of action is not fully understood, proposed mechanisms have included stabilization of mast cell

	INCREASED CLEARANCE	DECREASED CLEARANCE

Table 9-6
Factors Affecting Theophylline Clearance
	Enzyme induction P450
	  Rifampin
	  Phenobarbital
	  Ethanol
	  Smoking
	    Tobacco
	    Marijuana
	  Childhood
		Enzyme inhibition P450
		  Cimetidine
		  Erythromycin
		  Clarithromycin
		  Ciprofloxacin
		  Allopurinol
		CHF, liver disease
		Pneumonia
		Viral infection
		Old age

membranes and prevention of mediator release. It may also have effects on other inflammatory cells. It can prevent the early and late asthmatic responses to inhaled allergens as well as help prevent the increase in airway hyperresponsiveness following allergen inhalation. It has also been shown to protect against exercise-induced asthma and airway constriction resulting from inhalation of cold, dry air. It is not a bronchodilator, and thus its primary use is in prevention of attacks and not in the treatment of acute asthma attacks. It has no significant toxicity, but it may require several weeks of use before evidence of effectiveness appears, and it cannot be predicted who will respond.

Nedocromil sodium is another nonsteroidal anti-inflammatory medication used for treating asthma. Nedocromil sodium is more potent than cromolyn sodium in preventing bronchospasm resulting from inhaled allergens. Long-term usage has been shown to decrease nonspecific bronchial hyperreactivity, decrease symptoms, and improve airflow obstruction. The mechanism of action is not well understood, but it is thought to block chloride channels involved in cell activation in a number of inflammatory and airway cells. It has very few side effects and is effective in both allergic and nonallergic asthma, especially in adults.

Another group of anti-inflammatory agents that have recently been released for the treatment of asthma are the leukotriene modifiers. Leukotrienes are products of the arachidonic acid pathway that are potent bronchoconstrictors in humans. Arachidonic acid is converted by 5-lipoxygenase, the enzyme that catalyzes the oxidation of membrane arachidonic acid, to form the cysteinyl leukotrienes: LTA_4, which is converted to LTC_4, which in turn is converted to the most active metabolite, LTD_4 (Figure 9-4).

The leukotrienes, LTC_4, LTD_4 and LTE_4, of which LTD_4 is the most important, appear to produce their biological effects through the cysteinyl leukotriene-1 receptor ($CysLT_1$ receptor). The nonsteroidal anti-inflammatory drugs that decrease the leukotriene pathway mediators include the $CysLT_1$ receptor antagonists and the 5-lipoxygenase enzyme inhibitors. The 5-lipoxygenase inhibitors decrease the production of the leukotrienes by interfering with the binding of arachidonic acid to 5-lipoxygenase while the $CysLT_1$ receptor antagonists are specific competitive receptor blockers of the cysteinyl leukotriene activity. These drugs have been shown to reduce both day and night symptoms and to improve airflow obstruction. Moreover, they have been shown to reduce bronchoconstriction resulting from exercise, aspirin, and allergen inhalation. Although their role is not yet clearly defined in the treatment of asthma, they have shown promise in the treatment of mild to moderate chronic asthma.

Corticosteroids are the cornerstone of anti-inflammatory therapy. They reduce the airway inflammation and the airway hyperresponsiveness. These medications may have many possible effects on the inflammatory process, but it is not clear how they decrease the inflammation of asthma. Corticosteroids can inhibit the late asthmatic response, reduce recruitment and activation of inflammatory cells, increase β_2-receptor number, and decrease microvascular permeability and mucus production. Their anti-inflammatory effects probably require the production of new proteins, and therefore these effects may not become apparent for 6 to 12 hours. These drugs may be given by inhalation, orally, or parenterally. Chronic use of oral corticosteroids may have significant side effects. The inhaled route, using a spacer device, produces the fewest side effects.

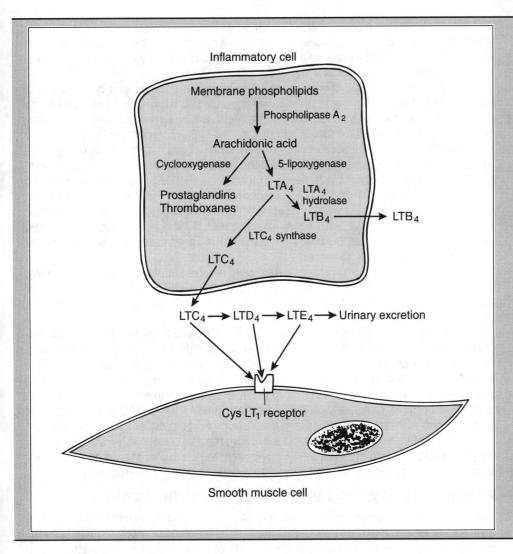

FIGURE 9-4
Leukotriene production and sites of action. The cysteinyl leukotrienes, LTC_4, LTD_4, and LTE_4, are predominantly produced by mast cells and eosinophils while LTB_4 is predominantly released by neutrophils and macrophages. The majority of the enzyme machinery is clustered on the nuclear membrane, which is the key site for the initiation of leukotriene synthesis. A cell stimulus activates phospholipase A_2 (PLA_2), which cleaves arachidonic acid from nuclear membrane phospholipid pools. The released arachidonic acid is bound by 5-lipoxygenase activating protein (FLAP) and then presented to 5-lipoxygenase (5-LO). The 5-LO enzyme converts arachidonic acid to an unstable intermediate, LTA_4. LTA_4 is converted to LTB_4 by a hydrolase or to LTC_4 by a synthase and then secreted out of the cell. The LTC_4 can then be further converted to LTD_4 and LTE_4, all of which may bind with specific receptors on target cells (e.g., smooth muscle cells, nerve cells, endothelial cells and epithelial cells).

PHARMACOLOGIC MANAGEMENT OF ACUTE ASTHMA EXACERBATION

There are several medications used in the treatment of acute asthma (Table 9-7). The treatment of acute severe asthma depends heavily on the initial intervention with aerosolized β_2-receptor agonist therapy. Repeated administration of a β_2-receptor agonist by a hand-held nebulizer every 20 minutes for up to three doses achieves at least as much bronchodilation as subcutaneous epinephrine or terbutaline with the same rapidity of onset and with less potential for toxicity. This is true even for individuals who have severe airflow obstruction and those who have been receiving chronic inhaled β_2-receptor agonist therapy prior to their acute exacerbation. Administration of β_2-receptor agonist by means of a metered-dose inhaler with a tube spacer delivery system may be as effective as administration with a hand-held nebulizer. Subcutaneous epinephrine and terbutaline are rarely used. They are generally reserved for patients who are unable or unwilling to use inhalation therapy.

Mainstay of Therapy for Acute Asthma Exacerbation

- Aerosolized β_2-receptor agonists
- Corticosteroids
- Oxygen

Inhaled β_2-receptor agonists
Systemic corticosteroids
Anticholinergics
Theophylline
Oxygen
Mechanical ventilation

Table 9-7
Treatment of Acute Severe Asthma

Theophylline administered intravenously, as a single agent, is a weak bronchodilator with a small potential benefit whereas the risk of toxicity is substantial. Therefore, it should be reserved for the most severe asthmatics who are already being treated aggressively with inhaled bronchodilator therapy.

Inhaled anticholinergic therapy such as ipratropium bromide can be used in the management of acute asthma. In some patients, ipratropium bromide administered with a hand-held, small-volume nebulizer or an MDI with a tube spacer delivery system may have a bronchodilatory effect that is additive to that of β_2-receptor agonist therapy.

Corticosteroid therapy accelerates recovery and reduces the incidence of mortality from acute asthma. Moreover, corticosteroid therapy has been shown to decrease the rate of asthma relapse in patients with recurrent asthma. It should be used for patients who are corticosteroid dependent, for those presenting with severe asthma, and for those who respond poorly to emergency room treatment. In the hospital, corticosteroids can be given orally or parenterally, with equal effectiveness. As the acute asthma stabilizes, generally by 48 to 72 hours, the oral corticosteroid (i.e., prednisone) can be tapered over 1 to 2 weeks to prevent recurrence.

During acute asthma attacks, patients should receive supplemental oxygen therapy, especially because β_2-receptor agonists also cause transient dilation of the pulmonary vasculature, thereby worsening ventilation-perfusion relationships and precipitating hypoxemia.

Asthmatics who require mechanical ventilation have a high mortality. During mechanical ventilation, the combination of airflow obstruction, which produces lung hyperinflation, and large increases in dead space, which produce a need for high ventilation to maintain an adequate arterial PCO_2, creates the problems of very high lung-distending pressures and the potential for barotrauma. It has been recommended that mechanical ventilation be used principally to provide an adequate arterial PO_2, which is usually accomplished with a modest increase in the inspired oxygen concentration. The amount of minute ventilation should be adjusted to achieve the most reasonable PCO_2 levels with the lowest lung-distending pressures. Lung-distending pressures should be monitored, and the patient should be frequently evaluated for evidence of barotrauma.

PHARMACOLOGIC MANAGEMENT OF CHRONIC ASTHMA

The most recent guidelines for the treatment of chronic asthma, issued by the National Institutes of Health (NIH) in 1997, are based on a stepwise approach to management. Patients are categorized according to the severity of their clinical symptomatology and airflow obstruction and their response to treatment. The categories of severity include intermittent, mild persistent, moderate persistent, and severe persistent asthma (Table 9-8). Increasing severity of clinical symptoms, especially frequency, or airflow obstruction, based on spirometric or peak flow measurements, requires increasing medication.

The NIH guidelines provide algorithms for the treatment of patients with asthma (Table 9-9), including recommended dosages and sequencing of medications as well as asthma education and monitoring of airflow obstruction. The guidelines, although a good

---

Table 9-8
Classification of Severity of Chronic Asthma

Intermittent
Symptoms no more than twice weekly
Nighttime symptoms no more than twice monthly
PEF and FEV_1, 80% or more*

Mild Persistent
Symptoms more than twice weekly but less than once daily
Nighttime symptoms more than twice monthly
PEF and FEV_1, more than 80%; variability, 20–30%*

Moderate Persistent
Symptoms daily
Nighttime symptoms more than once weekly
Daily use of short-acting β_2-receptor agonist
PEF and FEV_1, 60–80%; day-night variability, more than 30%*

Severe Persistent
Continual symptoms
Frequent nighttime symptoms
Physical activities limited
Frequent exacerbations
PEF and FEV_1, less than 60%; variability, more than 30%*

* Defined as the best function (measured as a percentage of predicted) that can be achieved without medication. Variability refers to average day-night variation.

Adapted from National Asthma Education Program Expert Panel: Guidelines for the diagnosis and management of asthma (Expert Panel Report 2). Bethesda, MD: National Institutes of Health, 1997.

SEVERITY OF DISEASE	LONG-TERM PREVENTIVE TREATMENT	QUICK RELIEF TREATMENT
Intermittent	None needed	ß₂-receptor agonist
Mild persistent	**Inhaled steroid (low dosage), nedocromil,** or **cromoglycate** Alternatives to consider: leukotriene modifier[a] and theophylline	ß₂-receptor agonist
Moderate persistent	**Inhaled steroid (medium dosage)** or inhaled steroid (low to medium dosage) and long-acting bronchodilator[b] If needed, increase inhaled steroids (medium to high dosage) and add long-acting bronchodilator	ß₂-receptor agonist
Severe persistent	**Inhaled corticosteroid (high dosage)** Long-acting bronchodilator Oral corticosteroids	ß₂-receptor agonist

Table 9-9
General Guidelines for Treatment of Chronic Asthma

Note: Preferred treatments are in boldface type; environmental control measures should be implemented at all disease severities.

[a] Position in therapy not fully established.
[b] Long-acting bronchodilators include **long-acting inhaled ß₂-receptor agonist,** sustained-release theophylline, and long-acting β₂-receptor agonist tablets.

Adapted from National Asthma Education Program Expert Panel: Guidelines for the diagnosis and management of asthma (Expert Panel Report 2). Bethesda, MD: National Institutes of Health, 1997.

starting point for the treatment of asthma, are limited because of the absence of information comparing the efficacies of various classes of drugs in patients with different severities of disease.

Environmental control measures or avoidance of known asthma triggers (allergens and irritants) may help to reduce the amount of required therapy. Certain forms of exercise, performed in cold weather, may have to be modified. A warm-up period prior to exercise is essential, and exercises such as swimming in a warm, moist environment may be preferable. Aspirin and other nonsteroidal anti-inflammatory drugs may precipitate exacerbations in some asthmatics and should be avoided. Esophageal reflux can potentially induce bronchospasm. Xanthines such as caffeine and theophylline can reduce lower esophageal tone and worsen esophageal reflux. Measures such as elevating the head of the bed, reducing caffeine intake, and using antacid therapy before sleep often help reduce acid reflux and may reduce asthma symptoms.

Patients with intermittent symptoms are treated with an inhaled β₂-receptor agonist medication, such as albuterol, by metered-dose inhaler on an as-needed basis. When the use of the inhaler β₂-receptor agonist becomes frequent and on a daily basis, an inhaled anti-inflammatory therapy should be added and β₂-receptor agonist therapy continued on an as-needed basis. The role of anticholinergic therapy in chronic asthma remains undefined.

Anti-inflammatory medications include the corticosteroids, cromolyn sodium, nedocromil sodium, and the leukotriene modifiers. Cromolyn sodium is helpful in some patients who show persistent mild asthma or have an atopic component to their disease. Because of the prophylactic action of cromolyn, a 4- to 6-week trial of routine use may be necessary to demonstrate efficacy. Cromolyn has been commonly used in pediatric patients whereas the more potent nedocromil has been used more commonly in adults.

The leukotriene modifiers, zafirlukast and zileutin, may be helpful for mild to moderate disease, although their specific place in asthma treatment is unclear at this time.

Inhaled corticosteroids, delivered by a metered-dose inhaler, are instituted when symptoms remain uncontrolled by a β₂-receptor agonist. They are the most potent of the anti-inflammatory drugs and are generally the initial medications prescribed for adults. A tube spacer delivery system should always be used with inhaled steroids because it enhances efficacy and reduces medication-related adverse effects.

In general, persistent asthma should be treated with short-acting β₂-receptor agonists and inhaled anti-inflammatory therapy, reserving the addition of long-acting bronchodilators such as theophylline and salmeterol for those patients who are not satisfactorily stabilized. Salmeterol and theophylline may be especially helpful in controlling nocturnal symptoms.

Mainstay of Chronic Asthma Therapy

- Environmental control
- β₂-receptor agonists
- Anti-inflammatory agents
  Corticosteroids (inhaled and oral)
  Nonsteroidal agents

Systemic corticosteroid therapy should be reserved for severe persistent or uncontrolled asthma after the previously mentioned therapies have already been attempted and optimally managed without success. However, after improvement and stabilization of the asthma, attempts should be made to continue to taper the oral corticosteroids to the lowest effective dosage.

■ COMPLICATIONS OF ASTHMA

ACUTE COMPLICATIONS

The complications of acute asthma attacks include pneumothorax, pneumomediastinum, arrhythmias, atelectasis, and respiratory muscle failure, as well as death. Death from asthma is a rare complication but has been increasing worldwide in recent years. It continues to occur in young people, usually because the severity of the disease is not appreciated. Other complications during acute attacks include those resulting from medications such as theophylline. Acute respiratory infection may also be a complication of a prolonged attack.

CHRONIC COMPLICATIONS

An important complication of chronic asthma is irreversible airflow limitation leading to decreased ability to exercise. The development of irreversible changes is related to the severity and duration of the disease. Severe airflow limitation may occur at any point in the airways and may be attributable in part to a loss of elastic recoil.

Bronchiectasis develops in a few patients, especially those with allergic bronchopulmonary aspergillosis or mucoid impaction.

Allergic bronchopulmonary aspergillosis (ABPA) is a complication of chronic asthma characterized by a history of cough productive of golden-brown sputum plugs. The asthma is characterized by episodes of severe recurrent exacerbations. There may be chest pain and occasional fever. Abnormalities in chest x-rays include transient infiltrates, especially in the upper lung fields, associated with central bronchiectasis and sometimes atelectasis or collapse. Usually there is associated eosinophilia, increased serum IgE, and a positive skin prick test and serum-precipitating antibodies to the fungus *Aspergillus fumigatus*. Microscopic examination of the sputum may show fungal mycelia and large numbers of eosinophils. Repeated or untreated attacks can lead to bronchiectasis with fibrosis and death from extensive disease. The associated asthma usually requires treatment with oral corticosteroids.

Complications of Acute Asthma Exacerbation

- Barotrauma
    Pneumomediastinum
    Pneumothorax
- Segmental or lobar lung collapse
- Respiratory failure
- Cardiac arrhythmia
- Death

Complications of Chronic Asthma

- Irreversible airflow obstruction
- Bronchiectasis
- Allergic bronchopulmonary aspergillosis

■ REVIEW QUESTIONS

1. Which one of the following statements about exercise-induced asthma is false?

   (A) Common symptoms include chest pain, wheezing, and shortness of breath.
   (B) The hallmark of exercise-induced asthma is a decrease in measured expiratory airflow (by peak flow meter or spirometry) that follows exercise and usually resolves spontaneously.
   (C) Only about 50% of asthmatics have exercise-induced asthma.
   (D) The β_2-receptor agonists inhaled approximately 15 to 20 minutes prior to exercise are the most effective drugs for prevention of EIA.
   (E) EIA is more common during skiing than during swimming.

2. Which one of the following is not a pathologic finding in chronic asthma?

   (A) Airway smooth muscle hypertrophy
   (B) Increased airway eosinophils
   (C) Basement membrane thickening
   (D) Microinfarcts and fibrosis of the airway interstitium
   (E) Desquamation of the airway epithelium

3. A 25-year-old man complains of a cough that is worse at night and started approximately several months ago. He denies heartburn symptoms, recent "cold," or nasal congestion. His mother has mild asthma. He has a cat at home. His physician suspects asthma. His chest x-ray and spirometry are normal. The next step in the evaluation of this patient should be to

   (A) administer ipratropium bromide by means of a metered-dose inhaler.
   (B) perform a methacholine challenge test.
   (C) obtain sputum for an eosinophil count.
   (D) start immunotherapy for presumed cat allergy.
   (E) start oral theophylline therapy.

4. A 21-year-old woman with asthma presents with complaints of cough and chest tightness, which have been occurring four times a week, requiring her to inhale a β_2-receptor agonist using a metered-dose inhaler. She notes waking up from sleep approximately three times per month with similar symptoms. She has been noncompliant with her medications in the past. She has no pets and does not smoke. Evaluation for environmental triggers is unrevealing. The most appropriate next step in her treatment is to add

   (A) oral theophylline.
   (B) oral low-dosage prednisone.
   (C) the long-acting β_2-receptor agonist salmeterol.
   (D) an inhaled corticosteroid.
   (E) inhaled ipratropium bromide.

5. A 65-year-old man with asthma is admitted to the hospital with a severe acute exacerbation over several days. The most appropriate medications for treating his acute attack are

   (A) inhaled β_2-receptor agonist, inhaled ipratropium bromide, and theophylline.
   (B) inhaled β_2-receptor agonist, cromolyn sodium, and oral corticosteroids.
   (C) inhaled β_2-receptor agonist, inhaled ipratropium bromide, and oral corticosteroids.
   (D) inhaled β_2-receptor agonist, acetylsalicylic acid, and inhaled steroids.
   (E) inhaled β_2-receptor agonist, oral corticosteroids, and zafirlukast.

◼ ANSWERS AND EXPLANATIONS

1. The answer is C. A majority of asthmatics (approximately 70% to 90%) have exercise-induced asthma that can cause significant limitation of their activities. The maximal decrease in airflow occurs 5 to 15 minutes after exercise is completed. Because inhalation of cold, dry air is a stronger inducer of bronchospasm than inhalation of warm, moist air, exercise-induced asthma is more common in cold weather sports such as skiing than in warm weather sports such as swimming. Inhaled β_2-receptor agonists, cromolyn, or nedocromil can be used to prevent exercise-induced asthma. Cromolyn and nedocromil are thought to be slightly less effective. Theophylline and anticholinergics are effective in some patients. Corticosteroids have no effect on EIA when used immediately before exercise. However, long-term therapy can modify the severity of EIA.

2. The answer is D. Microinfarcts are not present in asthma inflammation but may be present in a vasculitic process. Fibrosis does not occur in the interstitium of the lung in asthma but is found in the interstitial lung diseases (e.g., idiopathic pulmonary fibrosis, hypersensitivity pneumonitis) and occupational lung diseases (e.g., asbestosis, berylliosis). The other choices are present in the airway inflammation of asthma.

3. The answer is B. The patient appears to have cough-variant asthma. He does not appear to have common causes of chronic cough such as nasal congestion causing postnasal drip, a chronic pneumonia or airway lesion by chest x-ray, a recent upper respiratory tract infection, or acute bronchitis. Confirmation of the asthma is required. Because pulmonary function tests are normal, a bronchoprovocation test using the drug methacholine is indicated. If the test is negative and the patient has active respiratory symptoms, asthma is essentially excluded and other causes should be considered. Sputum eosinophil count is only supportive evidence for asthma. The patient may have a hypersensitivity to cat antigen, but this would require confirmation by allergy skin tests. If he is positive to cat allergen, environmental control measures, such as removal of the cat, should be instituted. Neither theophylline nor ipratropium bromide is the first drug of choice for treatment of asthma.

4. The answer is D. The patient has frequent symptoms not completely controlled by the β_2-receptor agonist. Because asthma is an inflammatory disease and because its severity in this case would be graded as at least mild persistent, an anti-inflammatory medication such as an inhaled steroid should be added. Oral corticosteroids would not be appropriate, because the disease is mild at this time and the side effects are significant. Ipratropium bromide and theophylline are bronchodilators and would not target the inflammation causing the underlying problem. Theophylline may be considered later if the patient has persistent symptoms.

5. The answer is C. Inhaled β_2-receptor agonist, which is the most rapidly acting bronchodilator, inhaled ipratropium bromide, and oral corticosteroids are the first-line medications for the hospitalized asthmatic. The addition of an anticholinergic drug may cause more bronchodilation, especially in severely obstructed patients, and may produce fewer cardiac side effects in the older patient (as in this case). Option A contains no systemic corticosteroid. Option B includes cromolyn sodium, which is not helpful in the acute attack. In option D, aspirin may be dangerous if the patient is aspirin-sensitive, and inhaled steroids have not been shown to be effective in the acute attack. In option E, zafirlukast has not been shown to be effective in the acute attack although it can be continued during the attack.

◼ SUGGESTED READING

Barnes PJ: A new approach to the treatment of asthma. *N Engl J Med* 321:1517–1527, 1989.

Barnes PJ: Inhaled glucocorticoids for asthma. *N Engl J Med* 332:868–875, 1995.

D'Alonzo GE, Ciccolella DE: Nocturnal asthma: physiologic determinants and current therapeutic approaches. *Curr Opin Pulm Med* 2:48–59, 1996.

McFadden ER Jr: Exercise-induced asthma. *N Engl J Med* 330:1362–1366, 1994.

McFadden ER Jr, Gilbert IA: Asthma. *N Engl J Med* 327(27):1928–1937, 1992.

National Asthma Education Program Expert Panel: Guidelines for the diagnosis and management of asthma (Expert Panel Report 2). Bethesda, MD: National Institutes of Health, 1997, pp 1–86.

Weinberger M, Hendeles L: Drug Therapy Theophylline in asthma. *N Engl J Med* 334:1380–1388, 1996.

Chapter 10

CHRONIC OBSTRUCTIVE PULMONARY DISEASE

Friedrich Kueppers, M.D.

■ CHAPTER OUTLINE

Learning Objectives
Introduction
Case Study
Causes of COPD
Mechanisms of Airway Obstruction
Clinical Aspects of COPD
Epidemiology of COPD
Treatment
Review Questions

■ LEARNING OBJECTIVES

At the completion of this chapter, the reader should:
• Understand the double nature of COPD.
• Be able to correlate structural abnormalities and function disturbance in COPD patients.
• Understand the pathophysiologic origins of the clinical symptoms of COPD.

■ INTRODUCTION

Two components of COPD:

1. Chronic Bronchitis
2. Airways Obstruction

Enlargement of submucosal glands resulting in an increased Reid index.

Typical Case History

Chronic obstructive pulmonary disease (COPD) is commonly defined as the presence of chronic bronchitis and emphysema in the same patient. Chronicity in the narrower sense, as used here, means the presence of cough and increased respiratory secretions for at least 3 months in each of two successive years.

The two disorders that comprise COPD—chronic bronchitis and emphysema—differ greatly in pathology and anatomic site and are easily distinguished from each other by the pathologist. Bronchitis is characterized by inflammation of the bronchi, as evidenced by edema and by the presence of polymorphonuclear granulocytes and monocytic white cells (lymphocytes and macrophages) within the bronchial walls and in the bronchial lumen. Another hallmark of chronic bronchitis is the increased branching and hypertrophy of submucosal mucus glands. This finding is quantifiable as the so-called Reid index, which measures the proportion of the total bronchial wall thickness that is occupied by submucosal glands. Normally, this ratio is less than 0.4. In chronic bronchitis, it is greatly increased and can serve as a useful indicator of the chronicity of the condition (Figure 10-1).

The second component of COPD is emphysema, which is defined as an abnormal permanent enlargement of the airspaces distal to the terminal bronchioli and destruction of the alveolar walls (Figure 10-2).

If the two components of COPD are so easy to distinguish, why are they combined under the term COPD? The reason is that they form a characteristic disease entity, as exemplified by the following case study.

Case Study

Localization of emphysema by computer assisted tomography (CT)

J.R., a 55-year-old office worker, sees his family physician because he is concerned about increasing shortness of breath. He complains about cough and increased sputum production for the last 5 years. J.R. started to smoke at age 15 and, until he stopped smoking 2 years ago, smoked an average of one pack of cigarettes per day; thus his cumulative cigarette load is 38 pack-years (one pack per day for 38 years).

His physician orders a chest x-ray and pulmonary function tests. The chest x-ray shows hyperinflation, flattened diaphragms, and increased retrosternal airspace. There are also suggestions of bullous changes and possibly scar formation at the apices of both lungs. The pertinent findings of the pulmonary function tests are shown in Table 10-1. An arterial blood-gas determination is also performed while the patient is breathing room air. The results are shown in Table 10-2.

In order to better localize and characterize the bullous changes in the upper lobes of the lungs, a computed tomography (CT) scan is obtained. It confirms the impression from the plain chest film that indeed most of the emphysematous and bullous changes are located in the upper lobes—particularly at the apices (Figure 10-4). The remaining portions of the lungs show emphysematous changes, but there is no predominance of any particular area. The essential features necessary to establish a diagnosis of COPD are summarized in Table 10-3.

Table 10-1
Results of Pulmonary Function Tests for Case Study

Parameter	Predicted	PRETREATMENT Best	PRETREATMENT % Predicted	POSTTREATMENT Best	POSTTREATMENT % Predicted	% Change
Spirometry (BTPS)						
FVC (liters)	4.05	4.15	103	4.34	107	5
FEV_1 (liters)	2.72	1.77	65	2.03	75	15
FEV_1/FVC (%)	69	43		47		
Lung Volumes						
VC (liters)	4.05	4.15	103	4.34	107	5
TLC (liters)	6.02	8.41	140	8.04	134	−4
RV (liters)	2.42	4.26	176	3.70	153	−13
RV/TLC (%)	41	51	124	46	112	−10

Interpretation of Spirometry:
The forced vital capacity (FVC) is normal. The forced expiratory volume (FEV_1), however, is moderately decreased. The FEV_1/FVC ratio is considerably decreased; normally it should be at least 70%.

Lung Volumes:
The total lung capacity (TLC) is greatly increased and so is the residual volume (RV), indicating hyperinflation and air trapping.

Following the application of albuterol (a bronchodilator) by inhalation, it should be noted that FEV_1 increases and RV decreases significantly.

These results show that J.R. has moderately severe airway obstruction that is largely fixed but to a small degree (approximately 15%) is reversible by bronchodilator medications. The increased RV is consistent with emphysema.

Table 10-2
Arterial Blood-Gas Determination for Case Study

PARAMETER	RESULTS	UNIT	NORMAL VALUES
pH	7.369	—	7.37–7.43
PCO_2	48.8	mmHg	35–45
PO_2	67.0	mmHg	76–96 (room air)
Bicarbonate	28.4	mEq/L	23–27
Base excess (BE)	+2.5	mEq/L	0 ± 2.5
Hemoglobin	17.0	GM%	12–16
Oxygen saturation (% O_2 Hb)	93.4	%	<94

The results show moderate hypoxemia and a mild respiratory acidosis (elevated PCO_2) that is largely compensated by the increased bicarbonate concentration. It should also be noted that the hemoglobin content is increased as a compensatory mechanism in hypoxemia.

History

☐ Smoking: age at initiation, quantity smoked per day, whether or not still smoker (if not, date of cessation)

☐ Environmental (chronological): may disclose important risk factors

☐ Cough (chronic productive): frequency and duration, whether or not productive (especially on awakening), presence or absence of blood

☐ Acute chest illnesses: frequency, productive cough, wheezing, dyspnea, fever

☐ Dyspnea

Physical Examination

☐ Chest

Airflow Obstruction Evidenced By:
Prolongation of forced expiratory time
End-expiratory wheezes during auscultation on slow or forced breathing

Severe Emphysema Indicated By:
Overdistention of lungs in stable state, low diaphragmatic position
Decreased intensity of breath and heart sounds

Severe Disease Suggested by (Characteristic, not Diagnostic):
Pursed-lip breathing
Use of accessory respiratory muscles
Indrawing of lower interspaces

Laboratory

☐ Chest x-ray: diagnostic only of severe emphysema but essential to exclude other lung diseases

☐ Spirometry (pre- and postbronchodilator): essential to confirm presence and reversibility of airflow obstruction and to quantify maximum level of ventilatory function

☐ Lung volumes

☐ Carbon monoxide diffusing capacity: not necessary except in special instances (e.g., dyspnea out of proportion to severity of airflow limitation)

☐ Arterial blood gases: not needed in stage I airflow obstruction ($FEV_1 \geq 50\%$ predicted); essential in stages II and III airflow obstruction ($FEV_1 < 50\%$ predicted); in very severe airflow obstruction, major monitoring tool

☐ Alpha$_1$-antitrypsin determination when there is evidence of predominant basilar emphysema

Modified from: Official statement of the American Thoracic Society. Standards for the Diagnosis and Care of Patients with COPD. *Amer J Respir Crit Case Med* 1995; 152, S82.

Table 10-3
Diagnosis of COPD

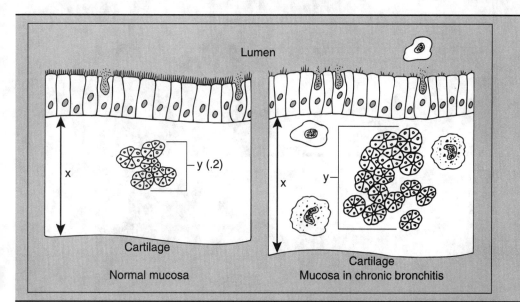

Lumen

x

y (.2)

Cartilage

Normal mucosa

x

y

Cartilage

Mucosa in chronic bronchitis

FIGURE 10-1
SCHEMATIC REPRESENTATION OF THE BRONCHIAL WALL WITH CHRONIC BRONCHITIS. (A) Normal bronchial wall. (B) Chronic bronchitis. Note: thickening of the wall as due to edema, presence of inflammatory white blood cells within the wall in the bronchial lumen, loss of ciliated cells, loss of cilia, hyperplasia of the submucosal glands that can be expressed as the Reid index (area occupied by the submucosal glands expressed as proportion of the submucosal wall area y/x); in chronic bronchitis it is often greater than 0.4, normal; 0.2.

FIGURE 10-2

PULMONARY HISTOLOGY OF EMPHYSEMA. (A) Panacinar: destruction of alveolar walls distributed throughout the parenchyma. (B) Centrilobular: destruction of alveolar walls centered around the bronchioli. In the right upper corner they are somewhat compressed but otherwise intact alveoli.

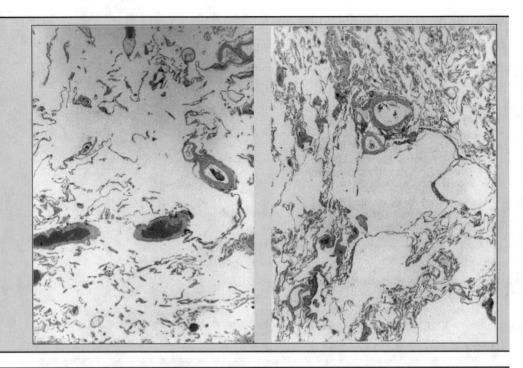

FIGURE 10-3

HIGH RESOLUTION COMPUTER-ASSISTED TOMOGRAPHY OF THE CHEST OF PATIENTS WITH EMPHYSEMA. (A) Scan at the level of the upper lobes of a smoker with characteristic bullous changes. (B) Scan through the lower lobes of a patient with emphysema associated with alpha$_1$ antitrypsin deficiency with characteristic bullous changes.

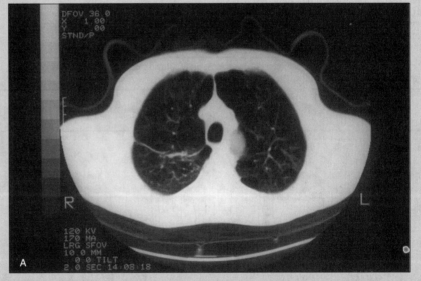

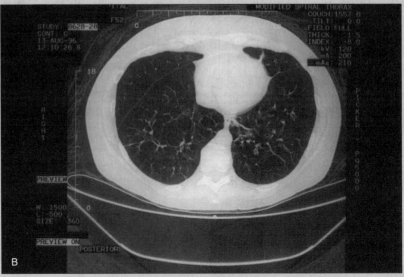

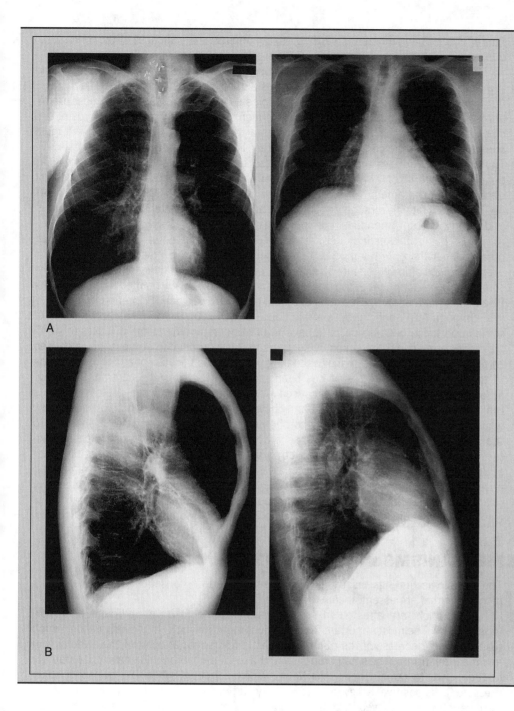

FIGURE 10-4
CHEST X-RAY OF A PATIENT WITH EMPHYSEMA. (A) Left: Anterior-posterior view. Note the loss of tissue and perfusion at the bases of the lung. Also note the flattening and low position of the diaphragms indicating hyperinflation. Right: Chest X-ray of a healthy individual is seen for comparison. (B) Left: Lateral view of the chest of the same patient. Note the anterior-posterior increase of the chest diameter and the increased retrosternal air space with loss of tissue. Loss of tissue is also seen at the bases. Note the flattened and low positioned diaphragms. Right: Lateral view of a normal chest for comparison.

■ CAUSES OF COPD

COPD is a good example of a multifactorial disease, which means that many factors, both environmental and constitutional (i.e., genetic) work together to produce the disease.

The most prominent environmental factor is tobacco smoke—especially cigarette smoke. Smoking, according to some estimates, accounts for 80% to 90% of the risk of developing COPD in a smoker's lifetime. The mechanism by which cigarette smoke produces lung damage is probably chronic inflammation of the airways—particularly the terminal bronchioli. Granulocytes and macrophages that accumulate in and around these bronchioli may be responsible for centrilobular emphysema. The term "centrilobular" implies that most of the destruction occurs around the terminal bronchioli in the center of a lobule (see Figure 10-2). Smoking-associated emphysema tends to affect predominantly the apical portions of the lung.

Secondhand smoke or passive smoking is also a risk factor for COPD, although to a lesser degree than the more concentrated smoke to which the active smoker is exposed.

Tobacco smoking: A major cause of COPD

Alpha₁ Antitrypsin deficiency, a genetic cause

This effect has been much more difficult to document clearly because of the difficulty of quantitating the passive exposure.

Other risk factors for COPD include air pollution, excessive exposure to dust, and some occupational exposure to noxious gases and airborne particles.

Among the genetic factors, alpha₁-antitrypsin (A1AT) deficiency is the most prominent. A1AT is an inhibitor of several proteolytic enzymes including elastase, trypsin, and chymotrypsin. The deficiency is inherited as a recessive trait. Patients with the most common type of deficiency have approximately 10% of the normal blood level of A1AT. The onset of shortness of breath, often associated with chronic bronchitis in A1AT deficiency, occurs somewhat earlier, between the ages of 35 and 45 years (somewhat depending on the amount of smoking), than do other types of COPD. However, A1AT deficiency is relatively rare: only about 1% of all white COPD patients are A1AT deficient, and among African-Americans it is approximately 100 times less common.

A1AT has other distinct features as well. The type of emphysema is *panacinar*, meaning that the entire acinus is involved in the destructive process. There is also a preponderance of lower lobe involvement, in contrast to the smoking-associated emphysema that is predominant in the upper lobe and is pathologically defined as centrilobular (see Figure 10-3 showing CT scans of apical (A) and lower lobe (B) predominance).

Elastase/protease hypothesis of emphysema

Although A1AT deficiency is a rare cause of COPD (about 1%; see above), it is of some importance because of its impact on our understanding of the disease. In A1AT deficiency, circumstantial evidence suggests that the associated emphysema is caused by proteolytic/elastolytic damage to the lung parenchyma because of a lack of inhibition of those enzymes. Therefore, it has been proposed that even the common smoking-associated emphysema could be caused by an imbalance between protease and its inhibitor(s). Cigarette smokers frequently have chronic bronchitis, which attracts many white blood cells—particularly polymorphonuclear granulocytes and macrophages—to the lung. Granulocytes, on becoming necrotic, release large amounts of protease (elastase, cathepsin G, proteinase III), which in turn can digest elastin and possibly other structural proteins of the lung. This process can take place whenever there is an imbalance between protease and inhibitors—i.e., whenever there is an excess of protease in relation to the available inhibitors. This hypothesis therefore has wider application for explaining the pathogenesis of emphysema in situations other than A1AT deficiency.

■ MECHANISMS OF AIRWAY OBSTRUCTION

The pathologic findings discussed above lead to certain consequences in respiratory mechanics that are essential components of COPD.

Mechanical consequences of loss of lung elasticity: Decrease of bronchial diameter and slowing of expiratory airflow.

The bronchi are affected in several ways, leading to an impediment of airflow (obstruction). The most important factor is a loss in the elasticity of the lung tissue, which results from a decrease of the number of elastic fibers that are part of the alveolar wall and the interstitium. The small bronchi and the respiratory bronchioli have little stability of their own; to remain open—particularly on expiration, when the transpulmonary pressure turns positive—they depend entirely on the traction provided by the surrounding parenchyma (i.e., alveoli). Loss of elasticity therefore leads to early airway collapse on expiration and air trapping beyond the small airways—i.e., within the alveoli (Figure 10-4).

As discussed in Chapter 4, the force that drives the air during expiration is the alveolar pressure, which in turn is determined by the elasticity of the alveolar walls. Loss of elasticity therefore slows the expiratory air movement. Thus, it becomes clear how the loss of elasticity of the lung parenchyma results in expiratory slowing of airflow, early collapse of small airways, and air trapping. Additional factors that lead to airflow limitation are increased mucus production and mucosal edema of the inflamed airway, both of which decrease the effective lumen of the bronchi.

CLINICAL ASPECTS OF COPD

The clinical history of the common form of COPD is characterized by cough and sputum production for many years (two or more) associated with and preceded by cigarette smoking. Shortness of breath usually develops in the fifth or sixth decade of life. There are exacerbations of bronchitis that are characterized by cough and increased production of purulent sputum, fever, leukocytosis, and increased shortness of breath. The intervals between these exacerbations become shorter as the disease progresses with time. Late complications are bronchiectasis (widening of the bronchi as a result of chronic inflammation), major impairment of gas exchange with hypercapnia (elevated blood carbon dioxide) or hypoxia (decreased oxygen content in blood), pulmonary hypertension (increased blood pressure in the pulmonary artery), and failure of the right ventricle, which is not able to produce the high pressures needed to sustain the pulmonary circulation.

> Chronic Bronchitis: Cough and sputum production for at least 3 months of each of two successive years.

PHYSICAL EXAM

Depending on the stage of COPD, characteristic physical findings can be recognized by the examining physician. Slowing of the expiratory flow can be noticed by auscultation of the airflow over the trachea. The respiratory sounds are reduced in intensity and seem distant. Hyperinflation of the lungs may be recognized by the lower position and the decreased movement of the diaphragm. The anterior-posterior diameter of the chest is increased, giving rise to the term "barrel chest" (Figure 10-5).

> Slowing of expiratory airflow: Hyperinflation

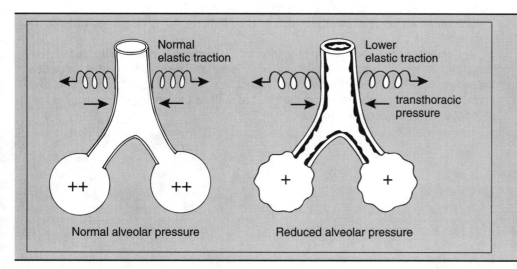

FIGURE 10-5
SCHEMATIC REPRESENTATION OF THE FACTORS THAT LEAD TO AIRWAY OBSTRUCTION IN COPD. (A) Normal airway. (B) Bronchus in COPD. The coiled springs represent the traction by the elastic parenchyma that keeps the airway open on expiration. Other factors are secretions within the airways (inflammation), increased thickness of the bronchial walls, and reduced alveolar pressure due to loss of elasticity of the alveolar walls.

The clinical history, with the physical exam and the appropriate pulmonary function tests, defines COPD (see Table 10-1) as a clinical and pathophysiologic entity. Although we have a good understanding of the pathophysiology of the disease, there are still substantial gaps in our knowledge of the factors that cause or contribute to COPD.

▍EPIDEMIOLOGY OF COPD

The prevalence of COPD in the population is difficult to measure, and the numbers are frequently revised. In the last decade, there has been a tendency to revise the numbers upward; since 1982, there has been an increase of more than 40% in the estimated number of cases of COPD. One reason is that the diagnosis is currently made more accurately and a distinction is made between asthma and COPD. Most current estimates of the prevalence of COPD in the adult white male population range from 4% to 6%. Estimates for women are lower, ranging from 1% to 3%, but the prevalence for women will almost certainly increase when those who increased cigarette smoking reach the fifth or sixth decade of life. Cigarette smoking among women has increased substantially, beginning in the 1960s. The trend toward a greater prevalence of COPD in women is already apparent.

> Prevalence of COPD:
>
> 4–6% in men
> 1–3% in women
> Prevalence increases with age

Estimates of mortality rate for COPD have also increased during the last decade. In 1991, the mortality rate was 18.6 per 100,000 persons, which represented an increase of 33% since 1979. In 1985, COPD was considered the underlying cause of 3.6% of all deaths and was thought to be a contributing factor in 4.3% of all deaths. The mortality rates for men and women are similar before age 55. At age 70, however, the rate for men increases to more than twice the rate for women, and it increases even more later in life. COPD ranks fourth among all causes of death.

■ TREATMENT

The emphysematous changes, the loss of elasticity, and the fixed airway obstruction cannot be altered, and thus therapy must be concentrated on those components of COPD that can be influenced.

Treatment of reversible components.

If there is a reversible component of airway obstruction (i.e., active constriction), bronchodilators should be used. The major bronchodilators are β_2 agonists (i.e., albuterol) and their derivatives that are available as inhaled formulations and as slow-release tablets. Anticholinergic agents (i.e., ipratropium) are also effective bronchodilators and have the additional advantage of reducing the quantity of respiratory secretions without increasing their viscosity. Ipratropium is available as an inhaled medication.

Theophylline (a potent phosphodiesterase inhibitor) is another medication with bronchodilator activity but with a mechanism of action that differs from that of β_2 agonists and anticholinergic agents. In addition to its relaxing effect on the smooth bronchial muscles, theophylline improves the pulmonary circulation and diaphragmatic action. It probably has an anti-inflammatory effect as well.

Airway inflammation can be treated with corticosteroids either as inhaled preparations or as systemic medications (i.e., prednisone).

Chronic bronchitis and especially acute exacerbations should be treated with appropriate antibiotics.

Antipneumococcal vaccination is an important prophylactic measure because *Streptococcus pneumoniae* is the most common organism that is responsible for the bronchitis component of COPD. Yearly vaccination against viral influenza (the "flu shot") is also indicated. It is useful in preventing the "flu" as well as preventing the bronchitis that often follows the initial viral infection.

■ REVIEW QUESTIONS

1. The increased incidence of COPD during the last decade can be attributed to

   (A) an increase in asthma
   (B) increased cigarette smoking in women
   (C) more accurate diagnosis
   (D) improved ascertainment of the disease in minority patients

2. Airway obstruction in COPD is caused mainly by

   (A) early collapse of the alveoli
   (B) reduced elasticity of the lung parenchyma
   (C) loss of lung capillaries
   (D) loss of bronchial wall stability

3. Emphysema in A1AT deficiency is, among other features, characterized as

   (A) a destructive process of the respiratory bronchioli
   (B) multiple capillary thrombi
   (C) a destructive process of the alveolar walls
   (D) the early presence of pulmonary hypertension

4. The elastase/protease hypothesis of emphysema states that

   (A) environmental agents stimulate elastase production in the lung.
   (B) elastase in tobacco smoke destroys lung parenchyma.
   (C) tobacco smoke lowers the elastic recoil of the lung.
   (D) elastic fibers are destroyed by elastase.

■ ANSWERS AND EXPLANATIONS

1. The answer is C. In earlier epidemiologic studies, COPD often was not distinguished from asthma and simple bronchitis, and therefore the reported prevalence was too low.

2. The answer is B. The alveoli do not collapse early and the bronchial walls are not weak in COPD. The mechanism of collapse or narrowing of the airways is the loss of elastic traction from the surrounding elastic tissue including the alveoli.

3. The answer is C. It is thought that leukocytic elastase attacks alveolar walls and the surrounding elastic fibers directly.

4. The answer is D. It is thought that leukocytic elastase lowers lung elasticity by destroying the elastic fibers.

■ SUGGESTED READING

Burrows B, et al.: The course and prognosis of different forms of chronic airways obstruction in a sample of the general population. *N Engl J Med* 317:1309–1314, 1987.

Crapo RO: Pulmonary function testing. *N Engl J Med* 331:25–30, 1994.

Ferguson GT, Cherniack RM: Management of COPD. *N Engl J Med* 328:1017–1022, 1993.

Chapter 11

SARCOIDOSIS

Daniel Shade, Jr., M.D.

Gerald O'Brien, M.D.

■ CHAPTER OUTLINE

Learning Objectives
Case Study: Introduction
Introduction
Incidence of Sarcoidosis
Etiology/Pathophysiology of Sarcoidosis
Clinical Manifestations of Sarcoidosis
Diagnosis and Assessment of Disease Activity
Case Study: Continued
Prognosis
Treatment
Case Study: Resolution
Summary
Review Questions

■ LEARNING OBJECTIVES

At the completion of this chapter, the reader should:
- Know the incidence and demographic characteristics of sarcoidosis.
- Understand the roles of the various effector cells in the initiation and maintenance of sarcoidosis.
- Understand the mechanisms underlying the formation of granulomas in sarcoidosis.
- Be familiar with the manifestations and clinical course of sarcoidosis.
- Understand how to use immunologic modifying agents in the treatment of sarcoidosis.

Case Study:
Introduction

G.C. is a 31-year-old African-American man who is referred to your clinic for further work-up of a markedly abnormal chest x-ray discovered during a routine pre-op evaluation prior to arthroscopic knee surgery. The patient states that he was well until 1 month ago, when he twisted his left knee during a basketball game. He denies cough, chest pain, weight loss, or dyspnea. His sister has asthma, but the rest of his immediate family is healthy. G. C. admits to smoking tobacco "occasionally," as well as to social alcohol use. He denies illicit drug use. He has no pets, and works as a short-order cook at a local diner.

On physical examination, the patient appears to be well nourished and in no distress. His ophthalmic and neurologic exams are grossly normal. His cardiac exam reveals no murmurs, rubs, or gallops. Examination of the thorax is significant for scant rales at both lung bases. There is a painful, erythematous, nodular rash on the anterior aspect of the lower extremities bilaterally. The remainder of the examination is entirely normal, except for a markedly swollen and tender left knee. Laboratory tests sent from his primary physician reveal normal hematologic and chemistry studies, including electrolytes and liver profile. An angiotensin-converting enzyme (ACE) level sent by the primary physician is still pending. The chest x-ray shows minimal, hazy, bilateral interstitial infiltrates and bilateral hilar lymphadenopathy (Figure 11-1). A purified protein derivative (PPD) and anergy panel are applied, and both are nonreactive.

FIGURE 11-1
The patient's film exhibits bilateral hilar lymphadenopathy.

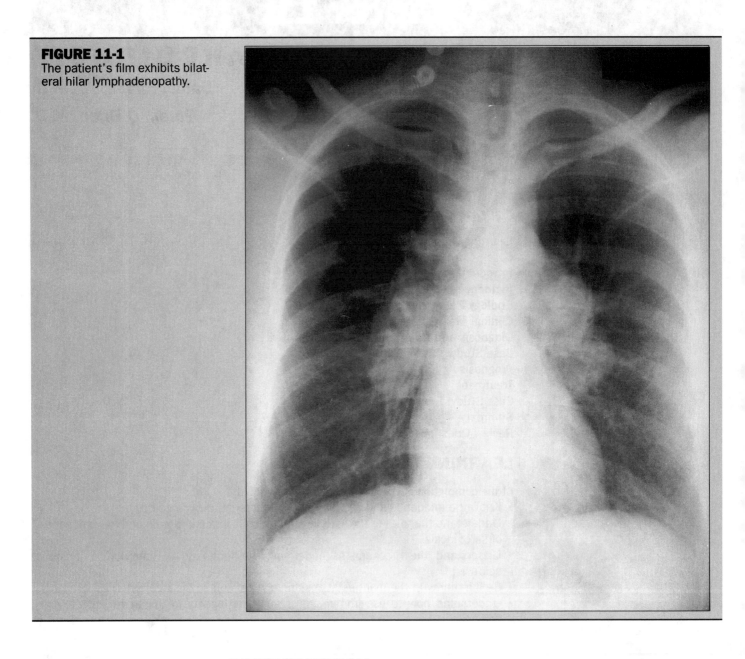

■ INTRODUCTION

Sarcoidosis (also called sarcoid) is a multisystem disorder with protean manifestations. It is characterized by a fluctuating course with exacerbations and/or spontaneous remissions that may resolve or progress to fibrosis. It is thought that sarcoidosis represents an imbalance of the immune system with localized hyperreactive aggregations of effector cells responding to an unknown antigen. Although sarcoidosis has been described in the literature for many years, a definitive understanding of its etiology, clinical course, and prognosis remains elusive.

■ INCIDENCE OF SARCOIDOSIS

Many patients with sarcoidosis are asymptomatic.

The exact incidence of sarcoidosis is difficult to assess because many patients are asymptomatic and are detected only during routine screening. Estimates range from 1.4 to 64 cases per 100,000 depending on the population studied. Larger proportions of cases are found in more temperate climates than in tropical regions, with Scandinavian series reporting the highest prevalence rates.

Sarcoidosis is more common in females and in African-Americans (but not in African or South American blacks). A striking example of this occurs in the United States, where blacks are affected more than whites, and black women are 17 times more likely to have sarcoidosis than white women. The incidence of sarcoidosis in Asian populations is quite low. The average age is 20 to 40 years, although a few cases at the extremes of age have been reported. Some of the abovementioned characteristics may be affected by selection biases within the reporting groups.

The typical sarcoidosis patient is 20 to 40 years old, female, and black.

ETIOLOGY/PATHOPHYSIOLOGY OF SARCOIDOSIS

Sarcoidosis is characterized by an intense inflammatory response to an unknown antigen. In light of the fact that the lungs are almost always affected, even if not clinically evident, it is thought that the offending agent may be inhalational. Various infectious agents have been proposed (Table 11-1), but culture data and documentation of person-to-person transmission are lacking. There is literature that implicates tumor antigens—germ cell tumor antigens, for example—in the initiation of the inflammatory response. The possibility of a genetic link has also been considered, because there have been a few cases of sarcoidosis in twins as well as in nontwin family members. However, this appears to occur quite sporadically, and its significance is not yet understood.

The inciting antigen for sarcoidosis is still unknown.

Mycobacterium tuberculosis
Nontuberculous mycobacterium
Yersinia enterocolitica
Cell-wall deficient organisms (mycoplasma-like organisms)
Borrelia burgdorferi
Nocardia
Fungi

Table 11-1
Infectious Agents Associated with Sarcoidosis

Regardless of the inciting antigen, it is clear that the tissue destruction and clinical manifestations seen in sarcoidosis are caused by a heightened local immune reaction, which may progress from an intense alveolitis to classic granuloma formation to end-stage fibrosis. In affected areas, massive recruitment and proliferation of immune effector cells take place. The increase in the number of cells is thought to result from both redistribution from the peripheral blood and in situ proliferation mediated by cytokines emitted from activated macrophages and T cells. This will be discussed in detail below.

In the lung, the influx and production of immune cells in active sarcoidosis are first seen as an alveolitis with a cellular composition that is much different from that observed in normal lung lavages. The composition of normal bronchoalveolar lavage (BAL) fluid is 90% macrophages, 9% lymphocytes, and less than 1% polymorphonuclear cells (PMNs). In contrast, in active sarcoidosis the BAL fluid contains 60% macrophages and 40% lymphocytes, of which 90% are T cells (Table 11-2). The T cells themselves exhibit a reversal of the pattern observed in the periphery, with 50% T_H (helper, or CD_4) cells, 25% T_S (suppressor, or T_S) cells, and only 10% B lymphocytes. The elevated T_H/T_S ratio observed in sarcoidosis is much larger than that seen in other processes where the normal ratio is also reversed, such as in drug reactions, amyloidosis, and pneumoconiosis. This is a distinctive immunologic feature of sarcoidosis.

The increase in immune cells in the lung is thought to be secondary to

- redistribution from peripheral blood
- in situ proliferation

	NORMAL (%)	SARCOIDOSIS (%)
Macrophages	90	60
Lymphocytes	9	40
Polymorphonuclear cells	< 1	—

Table 11-2
BAL Fluid Composition

The increased number of T_H cells are activated, or up-regulated, and secrete cytokines that recruit more effector cells into the area. The absolute number of T_S cells found in areas of inflammation is normal, although the relative proportion is decreased. The T_S cells function normally, but they do not proliferate as T_H cells do in response to cytokines such as interleukin-2 (IL-2), although in normal states they are able to respond to this stimulus. It has been postulated that this may represent a difference in cellular antigen recognition and processing by the lymphocytes.

Macrophages constitute a component of the mononuclear phagocytic system and are derived from monocytes and migrate to their respective tissues, where they act as powerful immune regulators by secreting chemoattractant cytokines and by acting as antigen-presenting cells. Macrophages also play a direct role in cytotoxic reactions against foreign antigens.

In the normal lung, macrophages represent the major type of cell recovered with BAL. During the active phase of sarcoidosis, the proportion of macrophages recovered decreases as a result of the massive influx and proliferation of T_H cells, but the absolute number of macrophages is increased as a result of redistribution and in situ proliferation.

In sarcoidosis, the macrophages express three times as many class II MHC receptors (which are required to present antigen to T_H cells) as nonactivated control cells express. In addition, macrophages secrete increased amounts of complement and of cytotoxic agents such as free radicals and cytokines. Type IV collagenase, an enzyme that disrupts the basement membrane, is also produced in great amounts by activated macrophages in sarcoidosis and may facilitate the entry of migrating effector cells into the inflammatory matrix.

Polymorphonuclear cells (PMNs) play a crucial role, especially in the later stages of the disease, as the inflammatory process proceeds from an alveolitis to granuloma formation and, if progressive, possibly to tissue destruction with fibrosis. PMNs are attracted to the site by signals sent by macrophages and lymphocytes. Interleukin-1 (IL-1), interleukin-8 (IL-8), tumor necrosis factor (TNF), and leukotriene B_4 have all been implicated as possible signals. Once recruited into the area, PMNs secrete powerful lysosomal enzymes and oxygen intermediates that have toxic effects on the surrounding tissue. The PMNs also play a role in altering connective tissue metabolism, which may also contribute to the development of pulmonary fibrosis. Recovery of significant numbers of PMNs on BAL is considered by some to portend a poor prognosis.

> Polymorphonuclear cells and macrophages, once recruited to the lung, release toxic substances that damage surrounding tissue.

Humoral activity is also up-regulated, with activation of B lymphocytes and resultant hypergammaglobulinemia. This up-regulation is thought to be a result of mediators secreted by activated T cells.

Cytokines are low-molecular-weight molecules released by many cells that exert powerful influences on the growth and functioning of other inflammatory cells. As discussed above, macrophages and lymphocytes secrete a myriad of cytokines that serve to "fuel the fire" in the inflammatory milieu by up-regulating the migration and proliferation of various cells. Table 11-3 lists some pertinent cytokines.

Table 11-3
Major Cytokines in Sarcoidosis

CYTOKINE*	SOURCE	MAIN ACTIONS
IFN	Activated macrophages, T cells	Regulates B cells, antiviral activity, activates cytotoxic cells
IGF-1	Activated macrophages	Mesenchymal cell growth
TNF	Macrophages	Antitumor, antiviral, metabolic functions, cell recruitment
IL-1	Macrophages, endothelial cells, fibroblasts	Stimulates T cells, PMN recruitment
IL-2	Activated T cells, NK cells	Promotes cytokine production, cell proliferation and activation, immunoglobulin synthesis (B cells)
IL-6	Macrophages, T cells, fibroblasts	Immunoglobulin synthesis
IL-8	Macrophages	Cell recruitment

* IFN = interferon; IGF-1 = insulin-like growth factor; TNF = tumor necrosis factor; IL = interleukin.

> Immunologic events occurring in the lung are the opposites of those occurring in the peripheral blood.

Interestingly, in sarcoidosis the cellular events that occur in the peripheral blood are the exact opposites of those observed at sites of active disease. In the blood, there is a decrease in the absolute number of T_H cells, with a decrease in the T_H/T_S ratio. Some investigators consider these findings to be supportive of the redistribution theory of effector cells seen at disease sites. The in vitro response of T cells to mitogen is decreased as well. Both factors may contribute to the hyporesponsiveness to skin antigen testing (delayed-type hypersensitivity reactions—i.e., PPD skin test) that is characteristic of sarcoidosis.

The accumulation of inflammatory cells in the lung may progress to form the hallmark of sarcoidosis—the non-necrotizing granuloma (Figure 11-2). The granuloma is a sharply circumscribed collection of fibroblasts and epithelioid cells, with mononuclear cells at the periphery, that forms as a response to a sustained antigenic challenge, as discussed above. T_H cells predominate in the center, whereas T_S cells occupy the periphery and probably act to slow the inflammatory process. Figure 11-3 depicts events thought to occur in the formation of granulomas. The presence of non-necrotizing granulomas is suggestive but is not pathognomonic for sarcoidosis, because they may be seen in other disorders (Table 11-4).

> Cutaneous anergy is common in sarcoidosis.

Mycobacterial disease
Fungal infection
Extrinsic allergic alveolitis
Celiac disease
Crohn's disease
Whipple's disease
Pneumoconiosis
Drug reaction
Foreign body reaction
Syphilis
Berylliosis

Table 11-4
Other Conditions Associated with Non-Necrotizing Granulomas

In sarcoidosis, granulomas usually are located in the upper two-thirds of the lung fields with a predilection for perilymphatic (bronchovascular) structures, but can occur anywhere in the lung parenchyma, blood vessels, airways, and pleural surfaces. Granulomas may regress spontaneously or progress to overt pulmonary fibrosis.

Not all patients progress to end-stage pulmonary fibrosis. It is thought that fibrosis results from both exuberant reparative processes and continued antigenic stimulation with sustained inflammatory actions and tissue damage. As stated previously, the influx of effector cells—particularly PMNs—is facilitated by cytokines emitted by T lymphocytes and macrophages, and by basement membrane disruption caused by type IV collagenase secreted by macrophages. The PMNs are then capable of causing membrane damage and eventual fibrosis by releasing their powerful lysosomal enzymes and reactive oxygen species. Fibroblasts then lay down a dense collagen framework that solidifies the fibrotic pattern (Figure 11-4).

FIGURE 11-2
The non-necrotizing granuloma
characteristic of sarcoidosis.

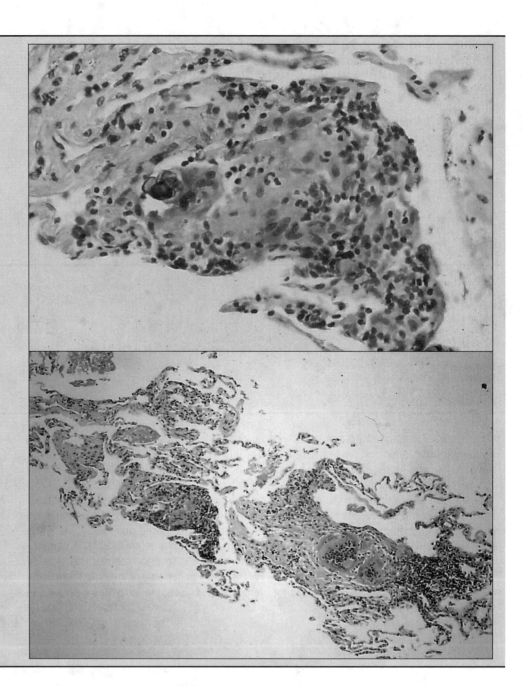

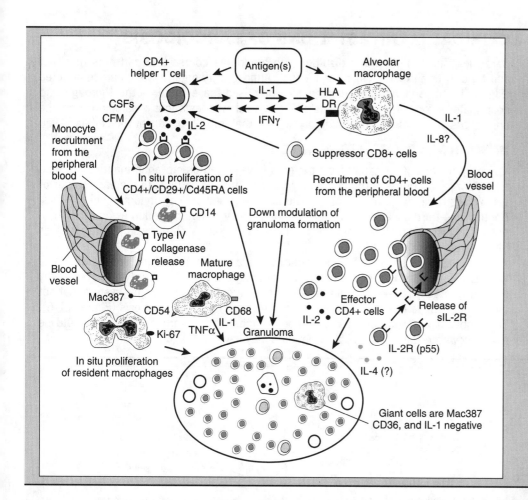

FIGURE 11-3
Mechanisms thought to be important in the formation of granulomas.

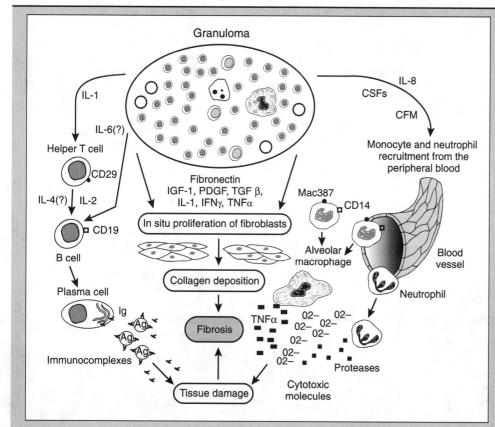

FIGURE 11-4
Mechanisms in the establishment of pulmonary fibrosis.

■ CLINICAL MANIFESTATIONS OF SARCOIDOSIS

Sarcoidosis is a multisystem disorder with a variable course that can present either acutely or with an insidious, chronic onset. Almost every organ system can be affected (Figure 11-5), and optimal management of this disease requires the thorough and coordinated efforts of many specialists. The clinical manifestations of sarcoidosis are the end results of the intense inflammatory activity that initially occurs at the cellular level.

INTRATHORACIC MANIFESTATIONS

Approximately 90% of sarcoidosis patients have intrathoracic abnormalities at some time during the course of the disease. Up to one-third of patients in the early stages of sarcoidosis have few or no symptoms and are diagnosed only by abnormal chest x-rays. Another one-third experience nonspecific pulmonary symptoms, such as cough or dyspnea. The last group of patients (the final one-third) have systemic complaints, such as fever, myalgias, or weight loss.

The classic chest x-ray findings are bilateral and symmetric hilar and paratracheal lymphadenopathies. Parenchymal involvement may either accompany lymphadenopathy or occur by itself. These abnormalities have been grouped into a staging system that not only is descriptive but also may impart information regarding prognosis (Figure 11-6). The probability of spontaneous remission is higher in the earlier stages. It should be noted, however, that 5% to 10% of patients may have normal chest x-rays.

One-third of all patients are asymptomatic, one-third have nonspecific complaints, and one-third have systemic complaints.

Up to 10% of patients may have normal chest x-rays.

FIGURE 11-5
Organ systems affected in sarcoidosis.

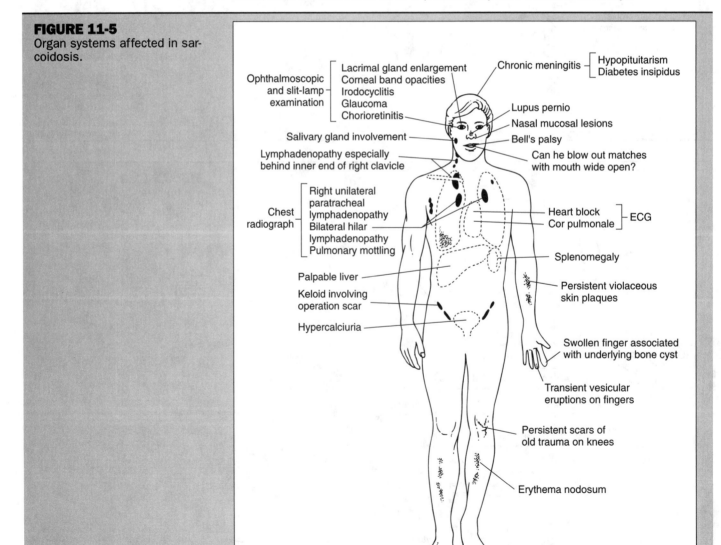

Other intrathoracic abnormalities occur less frequently and include bronchial compression by lymph nodes or granulomas, endobronchial granulomas, cavities with mycetoma formation (a possible cause of massive hemoptysis), bronchiectasis and bullae formation, fibrosis, and, rarely, pleural effusions. Myocardial sarcoidosis is rare but may cause conduction system abnormalities, arrhythmias, or cardiomyopathies.

EXTRATHORACIC MANIFESTATIONS

Skin involvement may occur in approximately 10% to 40% of patients and usually manifests itself as erythema nodosum or lupus pernio. Erythema nodosum is an immune-complex–related condition that presents as a painful panniculitis with red, tender lesions over the shins and calves. Lupus pernio is a chronic bluish purple elevation that affects the nose, cheeks, and ears. The upper respiratory tract may also be involved.

Ocular sarcoidosis is common, occurring in up to 25% of all cases, and can lead to blindness if undetected. The major manifestations are uveitis, conjunctival granulomas, and dry eyes as a result of lacrimal gland infiltration.

Almost any area of the nervous system can be affected by sarcoidosis. The most common presentation is cranial nerve palsy. Facial palsies indicating facial nerve (seventh cranial nerve) involvement are the predominant findings.

Renal failure may occur and is usually secondary to hypercalcemia and hypercalciuria induced by granuloma production of vitamin D metabolites, that enhance calcium reabsorption by the intestine. Overt granulomatous infiltration of the kidneys by granulomas that leads to renal failure is rare.

Other major clinical manifestations of sarcoidosis are listed in Table 11-5.

Table 11-5
Some Extrathoracic Manifestations of Sarcoidosis

Dermatologic
Erythema nodosum
Lupus pernio
Subcutaneous nodules (granulomas)

Ophthalmic
Granulomatous conjunctivitis
Granulomatous uveitis
Iritis
Chorioretinitis with and without nodules
Optic neuritis
Sicca/lacrimal gland involvement

Nervous System
Cranial nerve involvement (especially cranial nerve 7)
Basilar meningitis
Pituitary masses

Renal
Hypercalcemia (10–20% of patients)
Hypercalciuria (25–60% of patients), possible nephrocalcinosis
Granulomatous involvement

Hepatic
Hepatomegaly (20% of patients)

Cardiac
Conduction abnormalities
Pericarditis
Cardiomyopathy

Spleen
Splenomegaly (20% of patients)

Rheumatologic
Arthralgias (usually ankles or wrists)
Loffgren's syndrome (erythema nodosum, bilateral hilar adenopathy, and arthralgias)

Bone
Cysts (especially short bones of hands and feet)

FIGURE 11-6
Stages of sarcoidosis. (A) Stage 1: bilateral hilar lymphadenopathy. (B) Stage 2: pulmonary hilar lymphadenopathy and pulmonary infiltrates. (C) Stage 3: pulmonary infiltrates only. (D) Stage 4: pulmonary fibrosis.

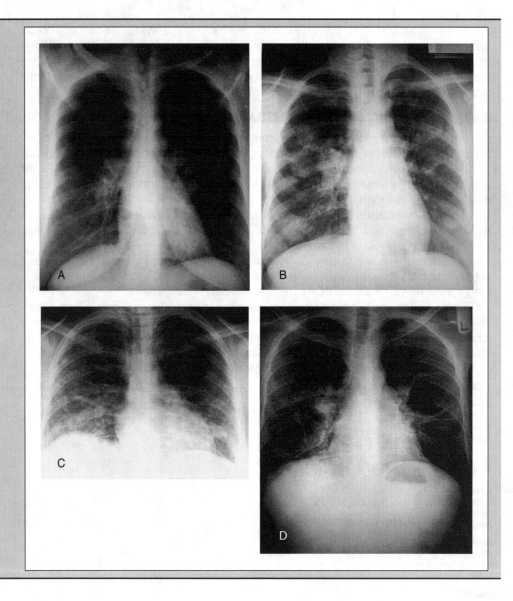

■ DIAGNOSIS AND ASSESSMENT OF DISEASE ACTIVITY

Diagnosis of sarcoidosis is easily made on clinical suspicion alone in an asymptomatic 20- to 40-year-old patient with bilateral hilar lymphadenopathy, especially if erythema nodosum and uveitis are present. In more difficult clinical scenarios, tissue diagnosis is required to establish the diagnosis and rule out more ominous entities such as lymphoma and tuberculosis. Although many tissues can be biopsied and yield satisfactory results, transbronchial biopsies obtained by bronchoscope have a high yield (up to 90%) and are highly specific. The yield increases with stage-to-stage progression of the disease and with the number of biopsies obtained.

The time-honored history and physical exam should be meticulously employed to help rule out other causes of noncaseating granulomas such as hypersensitivity pneumonitis and berylliosis.

Laboratory tests are nonspecific (Table 11-6) but may help support the diagnosis. Angiotensin converting enzyme (ACE) is produced by sarcoid granuloma and is elevated in 40% to 80% of patients with sarcoidosis. ACE levels tend to decrease with regression and treatment of the disease. This enzyme is nonspecific, however, and can be elevated in miliary tuberculosis, histoplasmosis, and leprosy as well as other disease processes (Table 11-7). For this reason, ACE levels may be used to track the course of disease over

Transbronchial biopsies have a high yield that increases with

- stage of disease
- number of biopsies taken

time in a patient, but should not be used as a screening tool. Bronchoalveolar lavage (BAL) is likewise nonspecific, although, as mentioned previously, the percentage of lymphocytes is usually elevated. BAL also may be used to rule out other disease entities, such as tuberculosis.

| Anemia |
| Leukopenia |
| Thrombocytopenia |
| Eosinophilia |
| Hypergammaglobulinemia |
| Hypercalcemia |
| Hypercalciuria |
| Increased ACE level |

Table 11-6
Potential Laboratory Abnormalities in Sarcoidosis

| Sarcoidosis |
| Miliary tuberculosis |
| Histoplasmosis |
| Leprosy |
| Pneumoconiosis |
| Berylliosis |
| Hypersensitivity pneumonitis |
| Gaucher's disease |
| Idiopathic pulmonary fibrosis |
| Lymphangioleiomyomatosis |

Table 11-7
Causes of Elevated ACE Level

Pulmonary function tests (PFTs) include measurements of airflow and lung volume as well as diffusion capacity. In sarcoidosis, PFT abnormalities are common, with the earliest changes being caused by the exuberant inflammatory reaction in the lung. As pulmonary scarring begins, the earliest PFT findings include reductions in lung volumes, or a restrictive pattern. A reduced diffusion capacity (D_LCO) may also be present early in the course of the disease. Obstructive patterns such as those observed in emphysema or asthma may be encountered if granuloma or inflamed lymph nodes impinge on the airways. In addition, some patients with sarcoidosis exhibit hyperresponsive airway narrowing (an obstructive pattern such as that in asthma) in response to provocative testing. PFTs, however, correlate poorly with x-ray findings and clinical findings because the pulmonary functional reserve is so large. Figure 11-7 shows typical PFT findings in sarcoidosis.

Pulmonary Function Tests

- Lung volumes
- D_LCO
- Airflow obstruction (mild)

Gallium-67 scanning is a radionuclide study that detects areas of inflammation in the lung with a sensitivity of 80% to 90% but a specificity of only about 50%. Other sources of inflammation, such as toxin-induced reactions, infectious agents, and neoplasms, can result in positive scans.

A difficult problem that has confounded clinicians for years is the lack of specific tests for assessment of disease activity in sarcoidosis. Ideally, such tests would provide information regarding the patient's prognosis as well as the response to therapy. The best markers available remain careful serial clinical examinations and chest radiography. ACE levels, although helpful in monitoring response to therapy, do not correlate well with prognosis. Inflammatory markers, such as gallium scans and BAL fluid analysis, do not predict the course of the disease. Measurement of gas exchange during cardiopulmonary exercise testing, although a sensitive test for detecting subtle abnormalities that may not be evident on baseline PFTs, does not seem to correlate with the course and prognosis of sarcoidosis. High-resolution computed tomography (HRCT), by distinguishing between fibrotic and irreversible changes in the thorax from areas of active inflammatory disease, may prove to be a useful adjunct to the physical exam and history in determining indications and responses to treatment.

Not Helpful in Predicting the Course of the Disease

- ACE levels
- Gallium scans
- BAL fluid analysis
- Initial cardiopulmonary exercise testing

FIGURE 11-7
Typical pulmonary function tests in a sarcoidosis patient, demonstrating reduced lung volumes (TLC = total lung capacity; RV = residual volume), reduced diffusion capacity (D_LCO), and intact airflow [normal forced expiratory volume in 1 second (FEV_1)/forced vital capacity (FVC)].

			Pre-RX		Post-RX		
Race:	Female/Black	Temp/Pres: 29 C / 761 mmHg					
ht:	67 in. 170 cm	Physician: DR. KAFAFKA					
weight:	192 lb 87 kg	Tested by: C. GROOMS					
		Pred	Best	%Pred	Best	%Pred	%Chg
Spirometry	**(BTPS)**						
FVC	Liters	4.32	3.22 *	74	3.09 *	71	-4
FEV1	Liters	3.48	2.47 *	71	2.47 *	71	0
FEV1/FVC	%	80	77		80		
FEF25-75%	L/sec	3.91	2.08 *	53	2.40 *	61	15
FEF50%	L/sec	4.50	2.59 *	58	3.01	67	16
FEF75%	L/sec	2.22	0.71 *	32	0.85 *	38	20
FEF200-1200	L/sec	6.39	4.74	74	4.72	74	-0
PEF	L/sec	7.05	5.35	76	5.47	78	2
FIVC	Liters	4.32	3.14 *		2.99 *		
MVV	L/min	121	107	88	111	92	4

			Pre-RX		Post-RX		
		Pred	Avg	%Pred	Avg	%Pred	%Chg
Lung volumes	**(BTPS)**						
VC	Liters	4.32	3.22 *	74	3.09 *	71	-4
TLC	Liters	5.80	4.81 *	83	4.23 *	73	-12
RV	Liters	1.75	1.59	91	1.14	65	-28
RV/TLC	%	28	33	120	27	98	-18
FRC N2	Liters	2.83	2.35	83	1.89	67	-20

Diffusion	**(HB = 13 g/dL CO Hb = 3%)**			
DLCO	mL/min/mmHg	28.7	18.8 *	65
DL Corr	mL/min/mmHg	28.7	21.4 *	75
DLCO/VA	L/min/mmHg	4.83	4.84	100
VA	Liters		3.89	

* = OUTSIDE 95% CONFIDENCE INTERVAL
Calibration: PRED: 3.19 ACTUAL: EXP 3.20   INSP 3.20
IPS-OL1O-06   IPS-OH10-05   N-1804-4

Comments:
BRONCHODILATOR: PROVENTIL WITH INSPEREASE DELIVERY SYSTEM.
patient effort and cooperation

Case Study:
Continued

Your initial concern regarding this asymptomatic young man is that he could have stage 2 sarcoidosis, but more ominous diseases, such as tuberculosis and lymphoma, are also possible. Accordingly, a chest CT is ordered and reveals nonspecific interstitial changes bilaterally, as well as bilateral hilar lymphadenopathy and right paratracheal lymphadenopathy. There is no evidence of pulmonary fibrosis. PFTs, consisting of measurements of airflow capacity, and lung volumes as well as diffusion capacity, are significant only for a very mild decrease in diffusion capacity (Figure 11-8). A cardiopulmonary exercise test is ordered and reveals a mild decrease in peak exercise capacity and a marked decrease in oxygen saturation at peak exercise. A fiberoptic bronchoscopy is ordered to make a definitive diagnosis. Biopsy results are positive for noncaseating granuloma. All cultures on biopsied material are negative, and there is no evidence of malignancy. The ACE level returns and is mildly elevated. An extensive ocular exam is performed and is within normal limits.

	Predicted	Actual
Spirometry		
FEV$_1$ (Liters)	3.50	3.33
FEV$_1$/FVC (%)	82	80
Lung volumes		
VC (Liters)	4.52	4.20
TLC (Liters)	6.0	5.59
Diffusion		
D$_L$CO (ml/min/mmHg)	31.0	20.0*

* = outside 95% confidence interval

FIGURE 11-8
Initial pulmonary function tests in our patient show only reduced diffusion capacity.

PROGNOSIS

Sarcoidosis may remit spontaneously or progress to end-stage and irreversible disease. It is known that the radiographic staging has some prognostic potential. Stage 1 disease resolves in 60% to 80% of patients, stage 2 remits in 50% to 60%, and stage 3 resolves in only 30% of cases. Table 11-8 lists some factors known to be associated with a poor prognosis in sarcoidosis.

Elderly (age of onset more than 40 years)
Black race
Symptoms lasting more than 6 months
Splenomegaly
Absence of erythema nodosum
Involvement of more than three organ systems
Stage 3 disease

Table 11-8
Factors Associated with a Poor Prognosis in Sarcoidosis

TREATMENT

The decision to treat sarcoidosis is often difficult because the clinical course is variable and unpredictable, and because most of the agents used to treat the disease are associated with significant side effects. There are guidelines that can assist the decision-making process. Indications for the initiation of treatment are shown in Table 11-9.

Severe ocular involvement
Severe cardiac involvement
Severe neurologic involvement
Malignant hypercalcemia
Symptomatic stage 2 disease
Stage 3 disease

Table 11-9
Indications for the Initiation of Treatment in Sarcoidosis

Historically, corticosteroids, which have powerful anti-inflammatory capabilities and therefore may interrupt the aforementioned heightened immune response characteristic of sarcoidosis, have been considered the first-line agents. In addition, corticosteroids, particularly inhaled corticosteroids, may improve the airway hyperresponsivity observed in a minority of sarcoidosis patients. The duration of treatment necessary to produce clinical improvement and prevent relapse is still unknown, despite the use of these drugs for many years. Systemic corticosteroids have many adverse side effects, including osteoporosis, impaired glucose metabolism, glaucoma, delayed wound healing, and, because they down-regulate cell-mediated immunity, increased susceptibility to opportunistic infections. Other anti-inflammatory agents reported on occasion to be useful in treating sarcoidosis include methotrexate, cyclophosphamide, azathioprine, cyclosporine, and hydroxychloroquine.

Agents Used to Treat Sarcoidosis

- Corticosteroids
- Methotrexate
- Azathioprine
- Cyclosporine
- Hydroxychloroquine

Lung transplantation has also been used with success to treat end-stage sarcoidosis. Interestingly, there have been a few reported cases of sarcoidosis occurring in the transplanted lung.

Case Study:
Resolution

G.C. has asymptomatic stage 2 sarcoidosis. He is released without medication to close follow-up and does well for 8 months until he complains of blurred vision and occasional wheezing. During physical examination, an intense uveitis is noted on slit-lamp exam. The bibasilar rales noted on the initial examination are still present, but now the patient exhibits expiratory wheezing on forced exhalation. The erythema nodosum observed on the initial exam is still present. His chest x-ray is unchanged. The serum ACE level is now moderately elevated, and his repeat PFTs show a further decrement in diffusion capacity, mild airflow obstruction, and moderate decreases in lung volumes (Figure 11-9). In the light of the patient's new subjective pulmonary and ocular complaints, and significant objective progression of the disease, he is started on a course of systemic corticosteroids and is released to close follow-up.

FIGURE 11-9
Subsequent pulmonary function tests reveal decreases in airflow, lung volumes, and diffusion capacity.

	Predicted	Actual
Spirometry		
FEV_1 (Liters)	3.50	2.98*
FEV_1/FVC (%)	82	72
Lung volumes		
VC (Liters)	4.52	3.80*
TLC (Liters)	6.0	5.43*
Diffusion		
D_LCO (ml/min/mmHg)	31.0	16.0*

* = outside 95% confidence interval

■ SUMMARY

Many features of sarcoidosis remain enigmatic despite years of active and intense research. Still, with advances in cellular and molecular biology, the important roles of immunologic effector cells in establishing and propagating the disease in response to an unknown signal have been elucidated. On a macroscopic level, the consequences of this exuberant activity are widespread and can affect almost every organ system. The knowledge that sarcoidosis is primarily immunologic in origin has led to the use of powerful immunologic modifying agents in its treatment to good effect, but, much more needs to be understood about the etiology and natural course of the disease.

▮ REVIEW QUESTIONS

1. A 32-year-old black man is referred to your office with an abnormal chest x-ray. On review, the x-ray shows evidence of bilateral hilar and right paratracheal lymphadenopathy. The remainder of the lung fields are normal. The patient feels well and denies cough, weight loss, night sweats, and fever. Physical exam is entirely normal. The best course of action is to

   (A) order a repeat chest x-ray.
   (B) send a serum ACE level.
   (C) schedule the patient for a transbronchial lung biopsy.
   (D) order a gallium scan.

2. Bronchoalveolar lavage fluid (BAL) from patients with active sarcoidosis can be expected to show

   (A) a marked influx of macrophages.
   (B) a reversal of the peripheral pattern with a high T_S/T_H ratio.
   (C) a reversal of the peripheral pattern with a high T_H/T_S ratio.
   (D) many acid-fast bacilli.

3. S.L. is a 40-year-old black woman recently diagnosed with sarcoidosis confirmed by transbronchial lung biopsy. Her chief complaint is increasing dyspnea on exertion, especially when climbing stairs. On PFT, the most common abnormality would be

   (A) an obstructive pattern with reduced airflows.
   (B) reduced lung volumes and absolute diffusion capacity (D_LCO).
   (C) hypercapnia.
   (D) variable intrathoracic obstruction.

4. A 67-year-old Japanese man comes to your office complaining of shortness of breath of 1 year's duration. Occasionally, after coughing, he notes blood-streaked sputum on his handkerchief. He has lost 35 pounds over the last 6 to 7 months. He admits to smoking two packs of cigarettes for 40 years. His primary physician noted hilar lymphadenopathy and bilateral nodular lesions on routine chest x-ray. PFTs were ordered and revealed severe airflow obstruction with hyperinflation and air trapping. The diffusion capacity was moderately reduced. The physician presumptively diagnosed sarcoidosis, started the patient on systemic corticosteroids, and referred him to your clinic for further treatment. Your best course of action is to

   (A) discontinue the corticosteroids and order a bronchoscopy.
   (B) discontinue the corticosteroids and order repeat PFTs.
   (C) increase the dosage of corticosteroids.
   (D) order an exercise test with measurement of oxygen saturation.

5. A 29-year-old black woman is referred to your clinic for dyspnea and vague substernal chest pain of 3 months' duration. Her physical exam is unremarkable, but a chest x-ray reveals bilateral hilar and paratracheal lymphadenopathy with hazy interstitial infiltrates at both lung bases. A fiberoptic bronchoscopy is ordered, and 2 days later the pathologist calls to say that the preliminary report of the biopsied material reveals noncaseating granulomas. Cultures are still pending. Based on these findings, which one of the following statements is true?

   (A) Glucocorticoid therapy should be initiated immediately for symptomatic sarcoidosis.
   (B) Skin testing to assess possible exposure to tuberculosis may be unreliable.
   (C) A trial of glucocorticoid therapy should be started after culture results and final pathology results are back.
   (D) The patient should be released and close follow-up should be arranged.

■ ANSWERS AND EXPLANATIONS

1. The answer is C. This case illustrates many of the presenting features of classic stage 1 sarcoidosis. Fully 30% of patients are asymptomatic on initial diagnosis. The majority of cases are found in blacks in the 20- to 40-year age group, and women are the most commonly afflicted. Although other entities such as tuberculosis and lymphoma must be considered in this age group, the striking lack of symptoms and normal physical exam strongly suggest the diagnosis of sarcoidosis. Close follow-up, would also be an acceptable course of action and would serve to exclude other diagnoses as well as permit early treatment if sarcoidosis were to become symptomatic. Most clinicians, however, would opt for definitive diagnosis by transbronchial lung biopsy, especially if treatment is warranted later in the patient's course. An ACE level and a gallium scan are not specific for sarcoidosis, although they are abnormal in the majority of cases and can be used as markers of disease activity.

2. The answer is C. It is thought that sarcoidosis represents a marked recruitment of immune cells from the periphery to the lungs in response to antigenic stimulation. The cells, predominantly T_H cells, elaborate cytokines that serve further to attract other immune cells to the lung. The pattern of cells recovered from BAL is the reversal of that seen in the peripheral blood, where cutaneous anergy is often observed. The pathology seen in sarcoidosis is a result of the exuberant influx of cells and release and degranulation of destructive enzymes into the lung. If persistent, the process may progress to form granuloma or overt pulmonary fibrosis.

3. The answer is B. Although PFTs do not track disease activity in sarcoidosis reliably, the earliest and most common findings are reduced lung volumes (restrictive pattern) and reduced absolute diffusion capacity. The reduced diffusion capacity is usually from parenchymal destruction and obliteration of the capillary-alveolar interface, but may on occasion be secondary to direct involvement of pulmonary vasculature by disease. An obstructive pattern is sometimes observed and is usually a result of airway compression by granulomas. A subset of sarcoidosis patients have hyperreactive airways that may also lead to an obstructive pattern. Variable intrathoracic obstruction may be detected on a flow-volume loop as truncation of the expiratory limb, but is rare unless bulky disease is present. Hypercapnia, seen on an arterial blood gas, is rare except in extensive, end-stage fibrotic disease.

4. The answer is A. This elderly Asian patient does not fit the usual demographic profile of the typical sarcoidosis patient. In addition, his symptoms as well as the tests ordered by the primary physician do not support a diagnosis of sarcoidosis. The marked systemic complaints and long smoking history suggest an underlying malignancy. Hemoptysis is rare in sarcoidosis, but can be seen if the patient is colonized or infected with fungus, such as aspergilloma. Very rarely, granuloma may cause hemoptysis by directly invading blood vessels. The chest x-ray, while demonstrating hilar lymphadenopathy, also suggests malignancy. The pulmonary function tests exhibit obstruction, with a decrease in diffusion capacity that is consistent with COPD, as suggested by the patient's long smoking history. Corticosteroids should be discontinued, and attempts to establish a diagnosis of lung cancer should be undertaken immediately.

5. The answer is C. Although noncaseating granulomas are classically associated with sarcoidosis, their presence is not pathognomonic for this disease. Indeed, many diseases, including tuberculosis and malignancy, may be associated with noncaseating granulomas. Sarcoidosis is, therefore, a diagnosis of exclusion, and therapy should be initiated only when certain other entities have been ruled-out. A PPD test may be negative even if the patient has been exposed to tuberculosis, because many sarcoidosis patients have cutaneous anergy.

Chapter 12

INTERSTITIAL LUNG DISEASES

Yaroslav Lando, M.D.

Gerald O'Brien, M.D.

■ CHAPTER OUTLINE

Learning Objectives
Case Study: Introduction
Introduction
Clinical Features and General Approach to the Patient with
  Interstitial Lung Disease
Case Study: Continued
Case Study: Continued
Case Study: Resolution
Examples of Interstitial Lung Disease
Summary
Review Questions

■ LEARNING OBJECTIVES

At the completion of this chapter, the reader should:

- Know and understand the clinical manifestations common to all forms of interstitial lung diseases.
- Know and understand the impact of interstitial lung disease on pulmonary function, respiration, exercise, and gas exchange.
- Understand how inflammation of the lung develops and may lead to fibrosis.
- Be familiar with the immunopathogeneses of specific examples of interstitial lung diseases.
- Understand the clinical approach to and treatment of a patient with suspected interstitial lung disease.

Case Study:
Introduction

A 62-year-old truck driver presents to your office complaining of shortness of breath. He has been in good health all his life, but has noticed a gradual worsening in his abilities to perform activities of daily living. His symptoms began about 6 months ago and initially consisted of dyspnea with heavy exertion only. Now, however, he can barely walk across the room without feeling short of breath. He denies fever or chills, and he has an occasional cough, but no sputum production. His past medical history reveals hypertension and peptic ulcer disease; there is no history of arthritis or of lung, heart, or kidney disease. He once smoked one pack of cigarettes per day for about 10 years, but he quit 25 years ago. He drives a truck, and his routes are mostly in the Pennsylvania-Ohio-Michigan area. His current medications include an H_2 antagonist and a calcium channel blocker.

On examination, the patient is comfortable at rest but gets dyspneic walking from the chair to the examination table. His oral mucous membranes are moist and without lesions, and his neck reveals no lymphadenopathy or jugular venous distention. A lung exam demonstrates fine, dry, end-inspiratory crackles at both lung bases, without wheezing or rhonchi. Breath sounds are bronchovesicular in quality. His heart is regular in rate and rhythm, with a normal first and a loud second heart sound, especially over the pulmonic valve area. There are no murmurs or rubs. An abdominal exam is benign, and the extremities are without cyanosis or edema, but he has nail bed clubbing. His skin is normal, and there are no joint abnormalities.

Case Study:
Continued

Routine chemistry and hematology studies are normal, as is his urinalysis. Resting pulse oximetry is 91% on room air, and falls to 80% with walking. Electrocardiogram shows normal sinus rhythm with evidence of right ventricular strain. A routine chest x-ray is shown in Figure 12-1.

FIGURE 12-1
Plain chest x-ray (posteroanterior view) of patient presented in case study.

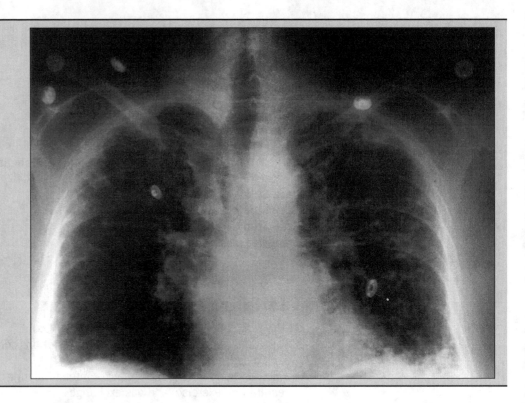

■ INTRODUCTION

The term "interstitial lung disease" is a misnomer because these disorders actually involve the alveoli as well as the interstitium.

Most interstitial lung disorders begin with some type of injury, leading to inflammatory and reparative processes.

The interstitial lung diseases constitute a heterogeneous group of more than 100 inflammatory and fibrotic disorders (Table 12-1). The term "interstitial lung disease" is somewhat of a misnomer, because it implies involvement of only the interstitial spaces of the lung parenchyma. Although the diseases in this category have the potential of infiltrating the interstitial compartment of the lung, most of them begin within the alveoli. Generally, the alveolar-capillary basement membrane sustains some type of injury, which increases its permeability and enables serum contents to enter into the alveolar space. An inflammatory reaction follows as part of the reparative and regenerative process of the endothelial and epithelial surfaces. In this reaction, inflammatory cells release proinflammatory and profibrotic mediators, resulting in fibroblastic proliferation and excessive collagen deposition. This process progresses from the alveolar spaces to the small airways, including the alveolar ducts and the respiratory and terminal bronchioles.

Because more than 100 disorders fit the description of interstitial lung disease, it is not the objective of this chapter to discuss all of them. We hope the reader will learn and understand the clinical manifestations common to all forms of interstitial lung disease. We will emphasize the effects of interstitial lung disease on pulmonary function, respiration, lung gas exchange, and exercise. The reader should understand how inflammation of the lung develops and potentially leads to fibrosis and the immunopathogenesis of specific types of interstitial lung disease. Finally, we will go over the clinical approach to and treatment of the patient suspected of having interstitial lung disease.

Fibrotic Disorders of Unknown Etiology

Acute interstitial pneumonia	Idiopathic pulmonary fibrosis	Lymphocytic interstitial pneumonia
Bronchiolitis obliterans/ organizing pneumonia	Autoimmune hemolytic anemia	Idiopathic thrombocytopenic purpura
Cryoglobulinemia	Inflammatory bowel disease	Celiac disease
Whipple's disease	Primary biliary cirrhosis	Chronic active hepatitis
Cryptogenic cirrhosis		

Disorders Related to Primary or Systemic Disease

Sarcoidosis	Eosinophilic granuloma	Amyloidosis
Lymphangioleiomyomatosis	Tuberous sclerosis	Neurofibromatosis
Lymphangitic carcinoma	Gaucher's disease	Niemann-Pick disease
Adult respiratory distress syndrome	Bone marrow transplantation	AIDS
Postinfection	Wegener's granulomatosis	Giant cell arteritis
Respiratory bronchiolitis	Cardiogenic edema	Pulmonary veno-occlusive disease
Alveolar proteinosis	Diffuse alveolar hemorrhage	Lipoid pneumonia
Bronchioalveolar carcinoma	Pulmonary lymphoma	Chronic aspiration
Eosinophilic pneumonia	Alveolar microlithiasis	

Disorders Related to Collagen Vascular Disease

Scleroderma	Polymyositis-dermatomyositis	Systemic lupus erythematosus
Rheumatoid arthritis	Ankylosing spondylitis	Mixed connective tissue disease
Primary Sjögren's syndrome	Behçet's syndrome	

Drug Induced (Antibiotics)

Nitrofurantoin	Sulfasalazine	Cephalosporins

Drug Induced (Antiarrhythmics)

Amiodarone	Tocainide	Propranolol

Drug Induced (Anti-inflammatory Agents)

Gold	Penicillamine

Drug Induced (Chemotherapeutic Agents)

Mitomycin C	Bleomycin	Busulfan
Cyclophosphamide	Chlorambucil	Melphalan
Methotrexate	Azathioprine	Cytosine arabinoside
BCNU/CCNU	Procarbazine	Nilutemide

Drug Induced (Other)

Dilantin	L-Tryptophan	Bromocriptine
Radiation	Oxygen	Paraquat

Occupational and Environment-Related (Inorganic)

Silicosis	Asbestosis	Talc pneumoconiosis
Kaolin pneumoconiosis	Aluminum oxide fibrosis	Berylliosis
Hard metal fibrosis	Coal worker's pneumoconiosis	Baritosis (barium)
Polyvinyl chloride pneumoconiosis	Stannosis (tin)	Antimony pneumoconiosis
Silicosiderosis (iron oxide)	Shale pneumoconiosis	

Occupational and Environment-Related (Hypersensitivity Pneumonitis)
(See Table 12-8.)

Table 12-1
Classification of Interstitial Lung Diseases

CLINICAL FEATURES AND GENERAL APPROACH TO THE PATIENT WITH INTERSTITIAL LUNG DISEASE

Because exact criteria vary from disease to disease, diagnosis requires a history and a physical exam. The history should include the duration of symptoms, the rate of disease progression, and the presence or absence of fever, hemoptysis, and extrathoracic symptoms. There must be a careful search for exposures associated with pneumoconioses, hypersensitivity pneumonitis, or drug-induced syndromes. A survey for extrathoracic abnormalities on physical examination is important as well.

HISTORY

The most disturbing symptom in patients with interstitial lung disease is usually progressive dyspnea, although nonproductive cough is generally present as well (Table 12-2). Substernal or pleuritic chest pain occurs in some types of interstitial lung disease (e.g., sarcoidosis). Wheezing, although unusual, has been reported (e.g., in chronic eosinophilic pneumonia), and hemoptysis is rare. The majority of patients with interstitial lung disease have symptoms with chronicity of months to years, and progress at various

The most common symptoms are dyspnea and a nonproductive cough.

rates. However, in some interstitial lung diseases the onset of symptoms is relatively acute (days to weeks), and these disorders are frequently mistaken for atypical pneumonias. Occasionally, patients present with spontaneous pneumothorax in diseases such as sarcoidosis and eosinophilic granuloma. Some patients initially present with nonrespiratory symptoms or have manifestations of extrathoracic disease, such as rash (sarcoidosis, drug reactions), telangiectasia (scleroderma), uveitis (ankylosing spondylitis, sarcoidosis), arthritis (connective tissue diseases), and glomerulonephritis (Goodpasture's syndrome).

Table 12-2 **Presentation of Interstitial Lung Disease**	**Respiratory Manifestations** Progressive dyspnea Cough (usually nonproductive) Chest pain (substernal or pleuritic) Wheezing Hemoptysis Pneumothorax **Nonrespiratory Manifestations** Rash Telangiectasia Uveitis Arthritis Glomerulonephritis

PHYSICAL EXAMINATION

Bibasilar crackles are commonly heard on lung auscultation.

The classic physical finding in a patient with interstitial lung disease is dry crackles heard best at both lung bases (Table 12-3). Clubbing of fingers and toes, if found, generally indicates very advanced fibrotic disease. Signs of pulmonary hypertension and cor pulmonale, such as jugular venous distention, a loud second pulmonic heart sound, and peripheral edema, can appear with advanced scarring and worsening hypoxia. Signs of multisystem involvement (kidneys, heart, skin) may be present as well.

Table 12-3 **Physical Exam Findings in Patients with Interstitial Lung Disease**	Bibasilar crackles Clubbing (fingers and toes) Jugular venous distention Loud second pulmonic heart sound Peripheral edema Signs of multisystem involvement (kidneys, heart, skin)

CHARACTERISTIC RADIOGRAPHIC FEATURES

Chest X-Ray. The most practical and logical way of identifying and defining the disease is with a standard chest x-ray. Many different terms (reticular, reticulonodular, ground glass) have been used to describe the parenchymal patterns associated with interstitial lung disease in an attempt to improve diagnostic specificity. Unfortunately, these patterns (Table 12-4) have been poorly predictive of histology. Occasionally, however, the chest x-ray alone or in combination with other findings can strongly suggest or be diagnostic of a given disorder.

There is a wide variety of radiographic presentations. Infiltrates range from focal to diffuse, from lower- to upper-lobe predominant, and from purely interstitial to alveolar patterns.

The most typical feature that appears on chest x-ray is bilateral symmetric infiltrates. These infiltrates can be separated into those that result in an alveolar pattern and those that produce primarily interstitial change. An alveolar pattern consists of a diffuse or patchy homogeneous infiltrate, with poorly defined nodules and air bronchograms, that obliterates normal structures (heart border, diaphragm). An interstitial radiographic pattern usually occurs when the lung interstitium becomes infiltrated and widened by inflammatory cells, smooth muscle proliferation, and collagen deposition. Interstitial infiltrates can vary in appearance. A "ground glass" pattern describes a hazy appearance obscuring the lung parenchyma that makes detection of discrete lesions difficult. A nodular pattern (with miliary nodules as small as 2 to 3 mm) is frequently mixed with networks of linear shadows and is described as reticulonodular. Kerley's B lines (short horizontal lines at the lung periphery) represent thickened interlobular septa and appear

		Table 12-4 **Chest Radiographic Findings** **in Interstitial Lung Disease**

Pleural Involvement
Lymphangitic carcinoma
Drug-induced (nitrofurantoin)
Radiation pneumonitis
Asbestosis (effusion, pleural thickening, calcified
    plaques, mesothelioma)
	Lymphangioleiomyomatosis (chylous pleural
	    effusion)
	Sarcoidosis
	Collagen vascular disease	

Hilar/Mediastinal Lymphadenopathy Sarcoidosis	Lymphoma	
Hilar Nodal Eggshell Calcification Silicosis	Sarcoidosis	
Kerley's B Lines Lymphoma Lymphangioleiomyomatosis Chronic left ventricular failure	Lymphangitic carcinoma Pulmonary veno-occlusive disease	
Pneumothorax Eosinophilic granuloma Tuberous sclerosis	Lymphangioleiomyomatosis Neurofibromatosis	
Increased Lung Volumes Lymphangioleiomyomatosis Sarcoidosis Neurofibromatosis Interstitial lung disease superimposed on COPD	Tuberous sclerosis Eosinophilic granuloma Chronic hypersensitivity pneumonitis	
Subcutaneous Calcinosis Scleroderma	Polymyositis-dermatomyositis	

to be caused by obstruction of the pulmonary lymphatics. Finally, a honeycomb pattern, with air containing cystic spaces 5 to 10 mm in diameter surrounded by thickened walls, indicates an underlying advanced fibrotic change.

The location of the reticulonodular infiltrates and honeycomb changes in many interstitial lung diseases is typically in the lower lung zones. Loss of volume can be observed. On the other hand, some interstitial lung diseases, especially ones with granulomatous inflammation, are known to exhibit radiographic abnormalities in the upper lung zones. It is important to point out that classification of the radiographic infiltrates of interstitial lung disease into purely alveolar and interstitial categories is done for descriptive purposes only. Many of these diseases present with a mixed radiographic appearance.

When the infiltrates are not diffuse, their location can be of diagnostic utility. Collagen vascular disorders, hypersensitivity pneumonitis, asbestosis, and idiopathic pulmonary fibrosis (IPF) tend to be lower-lobe-predominant diseases. Sarcoidosis, uremia, congestive heart failure, and Goodpasture's syndrome are examples of midlung-predominant diseases. Upper-lung-predominant diseases are easier to recognize by remembering the mnemonic "ASSET," (which stands for **A**nkylosing spondylitis, **S**ilicosis, **S**arcoidosis (note the overlap with midlung processes), **E**osinophilic granuloma or eosinophilic pneumonia, and **T**uberculosis.

Computed Tomography (CT) Scan.
Pulmonary parenchymal imaging is greatly enhanced by the thoracic CT scan. It provides a more accurate assessment of the type, duration, and severity of interstitial lung disease, compared with the plain chest x-ray. The imaging is even further improved when a high-resolution CT (HRCT) scan, which examines small volumes of lung tissue at a time, is obtained. This can help characterize the presence or absence of cysts, honeycombing, septal line prominence, hilar or mediastinal adenopathy, and the distribution of lesions (upper versus lower, peripheral versus central).

High-resolution CT scan is very helpful in characterizing the extent of parenchymal involvement.

PHYSIOLOGIC ALTERATIONS

Although there are some differences among the many disorders in the interstitial lung disease category, overall the pathophysiologic features of all of them are quite similar

Case Study:
Continued

Let's get back to our dyspneic truck driver. At this point, you have finished your initial examination and are pondering his case. You have a middle-aged male with cough and dyspnea on minimal exertion, who is hypoxemic at rest and with ambulation, and has a remarkably abnormal chest x-ray (see Figure 12-1). You see decreased lung volumes on both posteroanterior and lateral x-rays, with an increase in interstitial markings bilaterally, concentrated more in the lower lobes, forming a reticulonodular pattern. The pulmonary arteries appear prominent. You now want to proceed with further evaluation of his lung disease.

To quantify the severity of his disease process, you obtain an arterial blood gas (ABG), pulmonary function tests (PFTs), and an HRCT scan of his thorax. The ABG shows a pH of 7.46, a PCO_2 of 32 mmHg, and a PO_2 of 61 mmHg (alveolar-arterial gradient of 49), suggesting a mild respiratory alkalosis and pronounced hypoxemia. PFT data, shown in Figure 12-2, are significant for a decreased forced vital capacity (FVC) and forced expiratory volume in one second (FEV_1), a normal FEV_1/FVC ratio, a decreased total lung capacity (TLC), and a decreased carbon monoxide diffusion capacity (D_LCO). These data suggest a moderate-to-severe restrictive disease with an impairment in gas exchange. Figure 12-3 demonstrates this patient's chest CT scan. Extensive bilateral lower lobe patchy ground glass densities are seen. There is no evidence of enlarged lymph nodes or of significant pleural disease. The pulmonary arteries appear prominent.

FIGURE 12-2
Pulmonary function test results of patient presented in case study.

				Pre-Rx		Post-Rx		
Spirometry (BTPS)		Best %Pred	Pred	Best	%Pred	%Chg		
FVC	Liters		3.98	1.60	40	1.71*	43	7
FEV1	Liters		2.93	1.19*	41	1.31	45	10
FEV1/FVC	%		73	74		77		
FEF25-75%	L/sec		3.70	0.77*	25	1.13*	37	47
FEF50%	L/sec		3.05	1.04	28	1.43	39	38
FEF75%	L/sec		1.35	0.27	20	0.34	25	26
FEF200-1200	L/sec		6.46	0.87*	13	1.47*	23	69
PEF	L/sec		7.56	3.13*	41	3.86	51	23
MVV	L/min		128	41*	32	60*	47	46
				Pre-Rx		Post-Rx		
			Pred	Avg	%Pred	Avg	%Pred	%Chg
Lung Volumes (BTPS)								
VC	Liters		3.98	1.60*	40	1.71	43	7
TLC	Liters		5.52	3.10*	56	2.88	52	-7
RV	Liters		1.96	1.50	76	1.17	60	-22
RV/TLC	%		36	48*	134	41	114	-15
FRC N2	Liters		2.74	1.68	61	1.48	54	-12
ERV	Liters			0.18		0.31		72
IC	Liters			1.22		1.32		8
Diffusion	(Hb = 11.4 g/dl	CO	Hb = 2%)					
DLCO	Ml/min/mmHg		24.2	6.7*	28			
DL Corr	Ml/min/mmHg		24.2	8.7*	36			
DLCO/VA	L/min/mmHg		4.01	2.82	70			
VA	Liters			2.37				

* = Outside 95% Confidence interval
Calibration :   Pred : 3.29   Actual : Exp 3.23   Insp 3.27
IPS-0H10-05   N-1804-4

(Table 12-5). Because their pathology commonly involves inflammation and fibrosis of the alveoli and the alveolar walls, the following abnormalities are generally observed: 1) decreased lung compliance; 2) decreased lung volumes; 3) impairment of carbon monoxide diffusion capacity; 4) small airway abnormalities without generalized airflow obstruction; 5) gas-exchange abnormalities; and, in some cases, 6) pulmonary hypertension.

Lung Compliance and Ventilation Inflammation and fibrosis of the alveolar walls, which are frequently observed in interstitial lung disease, alter the dispensability of the lungs. Lung compliance is decreased (increased stiffness), requiring greater

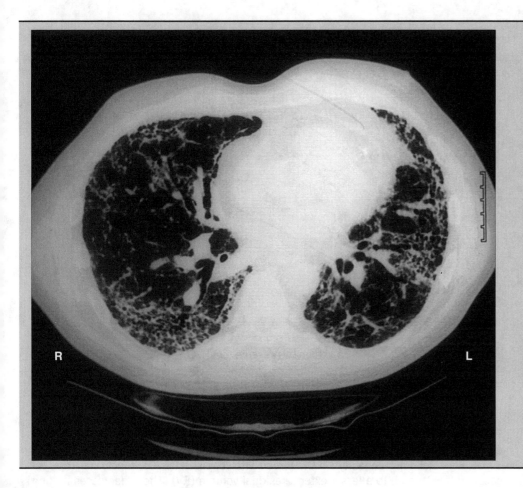

FIGURE 12-3
Thoracic CT scan of patient presented in case study.

Lung Compliance and Ventilation
Decreased lung compliance
Increased lung elastic recoil pressure
Increased work of breathing
Rapid, shallow breathing pattern

Pulmonary Function Studies
Normal (in early disease)
Reduced lung volumes
Normal, supernormal, or reduced FEV_1/FVC ratio
Reduced diffusion capacity

Gas Exchange
Hypoxemia (resting and with exercise)
Normocapnia
Increased alveolar-arterial gradient

Pulmonary Hypertension
Elevated right atrial and ventricular pressures
Cor pulmonale

Table 12-5
Physiologic Alterations in Patients with Interstitial Lung Disease

transpulmonary pressures to achieve any given lung volume. The pressure-volume curve is shifted down and to the right (Figure 12-4), and lung elastic recoil pressure is much higher than normal at all volumes. The patient's work of breathing is increased, because wider swings of transpulmonary pressures are needed to distend the stiffer lungs so as to achieve a normal tidal volume during inspiration. As a result, these patients develop a rapid, shallow breathing pattern (smaller tidal volume and higher respiratory frequency) in order to minimize the work of breathing while still maintaining adequate alveolar ventilation.

Lung compliance is decreased, the pressure-volume curve is shifted down and to the right, and lung elastic recoil pressure is elevated.

FIGURE 12-4
Pressure-volume curves characteristic of various pulmonary diseases. With progression of interstitial lung disease, its curve is shifted down and to the right.

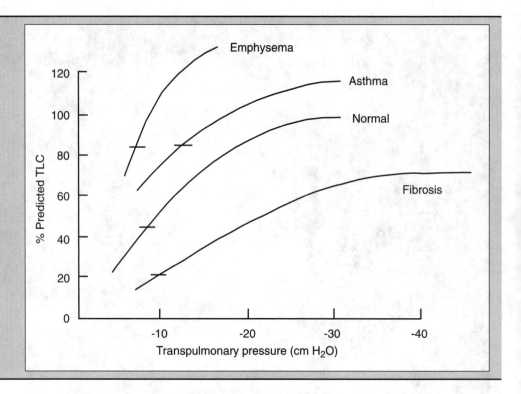

Pulmonary Function Tests. In the early stages of most interstitial lung diseases, PFTs tend to be normal. With disease progression, lung volumes are reduced—especially total lung capacity (TLC), forced vital capacity (FVC), functional residual capacity (FRC), and, to a lesser extent, residual volume (RV). These decreases in lung volumes are direct consequences of worsening lung compliance. At TLC, the inspiratory muscle force is balanced by the lung's inward elastic recoil, and because the recoil pressure is increased in interstitial lung disease, this balance occurs at a lower lung volume, causing TLC to be reduced. Similarly, at FRC, the chest wall's outward elastic recoil is counterbalanced by the lung's inward elastic recoil. Again, owing to greater elastic recoil pressure of the lung, this balance occurs at a lower lung volume, thereby causing a lower FRC.

Restriction (proportional reductions in all lung volumes) is the predominant pulmonary function abnormality found in interstitial lung disease. The FEV_1/FVC ratio (which, if reduced, generally diagnoses obstruction) is usually normal, or even supernormal as a result of increased lung recoil. However, because the pathologic process occurring in the alveolar walls also frequently affects the small airways, a mixed pattern of restriction and significant airflow obstruction can be seen in some disorders (e.g., sarcoidosis and eosinophilic granuloma). Diffusion capacity of carbon monoxide (D_LCO) is also affected in interstitial lung disease. D_LCO is decreased as a result of destruction of the alveolar-capillary interface by inflammation and fibrosis, resulting in a decrease in the surface area available for gas exchange.

PFT abnormalities can vary from only a mild reduction in D_LCO to severe reductions in lung volumes and airflow obstruction.

Gas Exchange. The most common gas-exchange abnormality observed in interstitial lung disease is hypoxemia without hypercapnia. In fact, arterial PCO_2 is generally low (except at end-stage), because patients are able to compensate by increasing their minute ventilation. This combination of hypoxemia and hypocapnia affects the alveolar-arterial (A-a) gradient (Figure 12-5), which is commonly increased in interstitial lung disease. Two factors contribute to the development of hypoxemia: 1) increased areas of low ventilation-perfusion matching and intrapulmonary shunting, and, to a lesser extent, 2) diffusion limitation.

Hypoxemia with an elevated A-a gradient is the most common gas-exchange abnormality.

Hypoxemia is worse during exercise. Although the mechanism of this worsening is not completely clear, limitation of oxygen diffusion may play a significant role. The combination of impaired gas diffusion and decreased transit time of each red cell at the

$$A\text{-}a = 713 \times F_iO_2 \times \frac{Pa\,CO_2}{0.8} - P_aO_2$$

where F_iO_2 is a fraction of inspired oxygen concentration,
P_aCO_2 is arterial partial pressure of carbon dioxide, and
P_aO_2 is arterial partial pressure of oxygen.

FIGURE 12-5
Formula for the alveolar-arterial (A-a) gradient.

alveolar-capillary interface may prevent complete equilibration of alveolar and arterial PO_2 (Figure 12-6). The worsening of gas exchange with exercise tends to correlate best with the severity of the underlying disease.

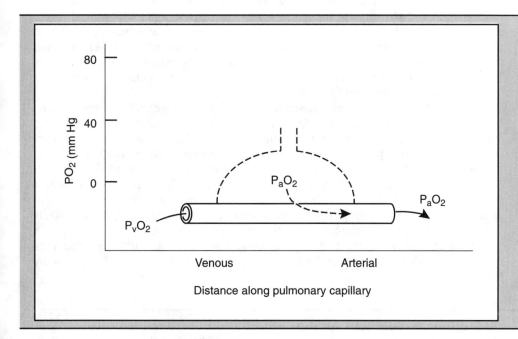

FIGURE 12-6
Schematic of the alveolar-capillary interface. Impaired gas diffusion and decreased transit time of each red cell across this interface may prevent complete equilibration of alveolar and arterial oxygen concentrations. P_aO_2 = arterial partial pressure of oxygen, P_AO_2 = alveolar partial pressure of oxygen, P_vO_2 = venous partial pressure of oxygen.

Pulmonary Hypertension. As each interstitial lung disease progresses, many patients develop pulmonary hypertension and cor pulmonale. The mechanisms of these physiologic abnormalities are hypoxic vasoconstriction and obliteration of the small pulmonary vessels by the fibrotic process within the alveolar walls. Pulmonary hypertension becomes even more marked with exercise as a result of worsening hypoxemia and a limited ability of the capillary bed to distend and recruit additional vessels to accommodate exercise-induced increases in cardiac output.

It is now time to proceed further in an attempt to make a specific diagnosis of your patient's lung disease. So far, you know that he has moderately severe restrictive lung disease with significant hypoxemia and possible pulmonary hypertension, most likely related to the nonhomogeneous parenchymal infiltrates found on the radiographic studies. What is your differential diagnosis of his interstitial lung disease? It seems that there are a hundred possibilities. Does he have some type of chronic infection? Is this sarcoidosis, scleroderma, or lupus? Or does he have a hypersensitivity pneumonitis from an unusual fungus growing inside his truck?

On careful review of all the available information, you begin to eliminate various disease entities from your differential diagnosis. His truck routes are through the Pennsylvania-Ohio-Michigan area, which has a high concentration of histoplasmosis, but

Case Study:
Continued

his normal white blood cell count and lack of fever and sputum production make an infectious etiology less likely. There are no extrapulmonary signs and symptoms to suggest a multisystem disorder such as a connective tissue disease or a pulmonary-renal syndrome. He is not taking any medication that is known to cause drug-induced lung disease. You order bloodwork to analyze serum markers for collagen vascular disorders and sarcoidosis. Because the available data have not identified a specific disease process, and the serum markers are neither sensitive nor specific, you recommend that the patient undergo fiberoptic bronchoscopy with bronchoalveolar lavage and transbronchial lung biopsies.

DIAGNOSIS AND ASSESSMENT OF DISEASE ACTIVITY

In an appropriate clinical scenario, fiberoptic bronchoscopy with BAL and transbronchial lung biopsies can be very helpful in making the diagnosis.

Fiberoptic bronchoscopy is safe and easy to perform, and can be a helpful diagnostic procedure in the evaluation of interstitial lung disease. Visual findings are rare, but can sometimes be helpful (e.g., many small white nodules in endobronchial sarcoidosis, or inflammation and strictures of the major airways in Wegener's granulomatosis). Bronchoalveolar lavage (BAL) by itself is not diagnostic, but can be extremely helpful in conditions such as eosinophilic granuloma (Langerhans' histiocytes in lavage fluid cells), asbestosis (asbestos bodies in lavage fluid), hypersensitivity pneumonitis (proliferation/transformation of lymphocytes in lavage fluid), and chronic eosinophilic pneumonia (greater than 30% eosinophil count in lavage fluid).

In patients undergoing bronchoscopy for evaluation of interstitial lung disease, transbronchial biopsies should be obtained. Evaluation of the biopsies can be diagnostic in disorders such as sarcoidosis (noncaseating granulomas), lymphangitic tumor (malignant cells), and eosinophilic pneumonia (eosinophilic parenchymal infiltration), and can be combined with the clinical picture to yield confident diagnoses in others (Table 12-6). For example, a diagnosis of idiopathic pulmonary fibrosis (IPF) can be concluded with a transbronchial biopsy that demonstrates the absence of tumor, granuloma, or infection in an appropriate clinical setting. The biopsy is not interpretable, however, if the tissue is "read" as normal or as consistent with an interstitial pneumonitis.

Thoracoscopic or minithoracotomy open-lung biopsy is the gold standard for making the diagnosis.

The gold standard technique for diagnosing many patients with interstitial lung disease is the open thoracotomy. This can be done by a relatively small incision or by thoracoscopy.

Table 12-6
Interstitial Lung Disease Diagnosis by Transbronchial Lung Biopsy

Frequent (open-lung biopsy usually not required)	
Sarcoidosis	Lymphangitic carcinoma
Eosinophilic pneumonia	Alveolar proteinosis
Bronchoalveolar carcinoma	Berylliosis

Infrequent (open-lung biopsy often required)	
Eosinophilic granuloma	Amyloidosis
Wegener's granulomatosis	Pulmonary lymphoma
Hypersensitivity pneumonitis	Lymphocytic interstitial pneumonia
BOOP	

Quantifying the amount of alveolitis and fibrosis can be very helpful in predicting disease reversibility and response to therapy.

It is very useful to identify the extent of inflammatory activity in any given interstitial lung disease. The greater the amount of active inflammation (alveolitis), the greater its potential to respond favorably to treatment. Inflammation of the lower respiratory tract usually precedes and causes subsequent fibrosis. The symptoms and physiologic derangement of interstitial lung disease can result from either inflammation or fibrosis; those resulting from inflammation are generally reversible, whereas those resulting from fibrosis are not. Quantification of inflammatory activity may provide an index of reversibility for a patient's disease and an indication of the likelihood of the patient subsequently developing pulmonary fibrosis. Proposed indices of inflammation vary from disease to disease. In sarcoidosis, for example, elevated lymphocyte counts in BAL fluid, increased gallium scan activity, elevated serum angiotensin-converting enzyme (ACE), and protein electrophoresis levels can provide helpful information regarding the extent of inflammation.

EFFECTIVENESS OF THERAPY

Treatment (Table 12-7) obviously varies depending on the disease, but for many disorders, unfortunately, there is little evidence of therapeutic efficacy. Examples of some accepted and controversial therapies include 1) steroids for IPF, sarcoidosis, and hypersensitivity pneumonitis (controversial, depending on the extent of active inflammation); 2) cyclophosphamide and steroids for Wegener's granulomatosis; and 3) cyclophosphamide and plasmapheresis for Goodpasture's syndrome. Treatment is rarely indicated for asbestosis. Supplemental oxygen, however, is one form of treatment that unquestionably is indicated for any patient with severe interstitial lung disease. Supplemental oxygen has been shown to reduce mortality in patients with chronic obstructive pulmonary disease (COPD) and arterial PO_2 less than 55 mmHg (at rest, exercise, or sleep), significant polycythemia (hematocrit greater than 55 to 60), or evidence of cor pulmonale. This finding has been extrapolated to patients with interstitial lung disease. Also, prophylaxis with pneumococcal and influenza A vaccines is indicated for all patients with significant interstitial lung disease. The final option for patients with moderate to severe lung disease not responding to medical therapy and without significant extrathoracic involvement is lung transplantation.

> Treatment depends on the specific disorder. Supplemental oxygen should be provided for every patient with hypoxemia or cor pulmonale.

Supportive (adequate nutrition and hydration)
Vaccination
Treatment of complications (e.g., infections)
Corticosteroids
Cytotoxic drugs
Plasmapheresis
Oxygen
Transplantation

Table 12-7
Therapeutic Options for Patients with Interstitial Lung Disease

Case Study: *Resolution*

Our dyspneic truck driver is now back in your office after having a bronchoscopy. His airways appeared normal, and the BAL fluid did not reveal significant eosinophilia, lymphocytosis, or elevated red blood cell count. BAL fluid bacterial, viral, and fungal cultures were negative, and there were no malignant cells. Transbronchial lung biopsies did not reveal evidence of granulomas or eosinophilic infiltrates, but demonstrated scant areas of fibrotic tissue. Serum markers, previously sent, were all negative. After reviewing all the subjective and objective information on this case, you make a clinical diagnosis of IPF (with areas of alveolitis based on the CT scan appearance). You recommend systemic steroid therapy, but the patient is reluctant, having heard of its multiple potential side effects. He undergoes an elective thoracoscopic lung biopsy. The biopsy demonstrates dense lymphocytic infiltration of the interstitium and accumulation of alveolar macrophages and type II pneumocytes within alveolar spaces, which helps support your diagnosis. You initiate a course of prednisone and prescribed supplemental oxygen. The patient returns several weeks later, reporting some improvement in his dyspnea and cough. He still requires supplemental oxygen, but feels stronger and able to return to work.

▪ EXAMPLES OF INTERSTITIAL LUNG DISEASE

Although numerous, diverse, and somewhat nebulous, these disorders tend to share many clinical features. More often than not, they are grouped together on the basis of these features. Most of these disorders are described in detail here; others are reviewed in other chapters of this book.

HYPERSENSITIVITY PNEUMONITIS

Hypersensitivity pneumonitis is an immunologically mediated disorder. It is caused by repeated inhalation of an aerosol containing a specific organic dust or chemical. Many of the known antigens (Table 12-8) are ubiquitous and can be separated into five categories: 1) antigens related to agriculture (e.g., thermophilic *Actinomyces* from moldy hay or

Hypersensitivity pneumonitis is caused by repeated inhalation of a specific aerosolized chemical or organic dust.

grain, causing farmer's lung); 2) antigens related to animals (e.g., bird proteins from droppings or feathers, causing bird breeder's lung); 3) antigens related to contaminated water (e.g., *Aureobasidium pullulans* or other microorganisms from contaminated water, causing humidifier or air conditioning lung); 4) antigens related to wood products (e.g., oak, cedar, and mahogany dust, causing woodworker's disease); and 5) antigens related to chemicals (e.g., isocyanates from polyurethane foam, varnish, or lacquer, causing chemical worker's lung). The resultant clinical syndrome may be acute and self-limited or chronic and progressive.

Table 12-8
Antigens Associated with Hypersensitivity Pneumonitis

DISEASE	ANTIGEN	SOURCE
Antigens Related to Agriculture		
Farmer's lung	Thermophilic *Actinomyces*	Moldy hay, grain
Bagassosis	Thermophilic *Actinomyces*	Moldy sugar cane (bagasse)
Malt worker's lung	*Aspergillus fumigatus, Aspergillus clavatus*	Moldy barley
Mushroom worker's lung	Thermophilic *Actinomyces*	Mushroom compost
Cheese washer's lung	*Penicillium casei*	Moldy cheese
Coffee worker's lung	Coffee bean dust	Coffee beans
Miller's lung	*Sitophilus granarius*	Infested wheat flour
Fish meal worker's lung	Fish meal dust	Fish meal
Compost lung	*Aspergillus*	Compost
Potato riddler's lung	Thermophilic *Actinomyces, Micropolyspora faeni, Thermoactinomyces vulgaris, Aspergillus* species	Moldy hay around potatoes
Tobacco worker's disease	*Aspergillus* species	Mold on tobacco
Wine grower's lung	*Botrytis cinerea*	Mold on grapes
Lycoperdonosis	Puffball spores	Lycoperdon puffballs
Antigens Related to Animals		
Bird fancier's, breeder's, or handler's lung	Bird proteins	Avian droppings or feathers
Pituitary snuff taker's lung	Animal proteins	Pituitary snuff
Furrier's lung	Animal fur dust	Animal pelts
Japanese summer house pneumonitis	*Trichosporon cutaneum*	House dust, bird droppings
Antigens Related to Contaminated Water		
Air conditioning or humidified air lung	*Aureobasidium pullulans*	Contaminated water in system
Sauna taker's lung	*Aureobasidium* species	Sauna water
Hot tub lung	*Cladosporium* species	Ceiling mold
Tap water lung	Unknown	Contaminated tap water
Cephalosporium pneumonitis	*Cephalosporium*	Contaminated basement sewage
Antigens Related to Wood Products		
Sequoiosis	*Aureobasidium, Graphium* species	Redwood sawdust
Woodworker's lung	Wood dust, *Alternaria*	Oak, cedar, mahogany dust
Maple bark disease	*Cryptostroma corticale*	Maple bark
Suberosis	Cork dust mold	Cork dust
Woodman's disease	*Penicillium* species	Oak, maple trees
Wood trimmer's disease	*Rhizopus, Mucor* species	Contaminated wood trimmings
Thatched roof disease	*Saccoromonospora viridis*	Dried grass and leaves
Familial pneumonitis	*Bacillus subtilis*	Contaminated wood dust
Antigens Related to Chemicals		
Chemical worker's lung	Isocyanates	Polyurethane foam, varnish, lacquer
Lab worker's pneumonitis	Male rat urine	Laboratory rats
Pauli's pneumonitis	Pauli's reagent	Laboratory reagent
Detergent worker's disease	*Bacillus subtilis* enzymes	Detergent

The histologic picture of this disease process is distinctive but not pathognomonic. It begins with an acute inflammatory alveolitis in which neutrophils predominate. After about 3 days, neutrophil counts fall and the alveolar walls become infiltrated with lymphocytes, leading to granuloma formation. If progression to a chronic, fibrotic stage occurs, it is indistinguishable from IPF. Generally there are no distinct features that allow the pathologist to suspect a particular causative agent.

There are several theories regarding the pathogenesis of hypersensitivity pneumonitis. Type III immune-complex-mediated injury has been implicated on the basis of the following observations: 1) all individuals with hypersensitivity pneumonitis have serum IgG precipitating antibody, which fixes complement when exposed to a specific antigen; 2) serum antibody titers are higher in persons with more severe disease; and 3) skin testing produces an Arthus-type reaction in 4 to 8 hours. However, for the following reasons, this disease does not fit well as a classic type III immune reaction: 1) complement levels are consistently normal during the acute disease or following antigen challenge; 2) there is no immune complex or complement demonstrated within the parenchyma of the affected lung; and 3) asymptomatic exposed individuals also have significant IgG antibody titers to the antigen, suggesting that they may simply be markers of antigen exposure rather than mechanisms of disease. Moreover, experimental animal data suggest that the development of hypersensitivity pneumonitis is a cell-mediated phenomenon (type IV immune or delayed hypersensitivity reaction, mediated by T lymphocytes) and not a humoral phenomenon. Evidence suggests that T lymphocytes in the lower respiratory tract become sensitized to a particular organic antigen. They may then release mediators that attract macrophages and possibly induce them to form granulomas.

Clinical presentation of hypersensitivity pneumonitis is variable, depending on host factors and on the intensity, frequency, and duration of the exposure. The acute syndrome is marked by fever, cough, and dyspnea, which begin 4 to 6 hours after exposure and peak over the next 24 hours. The subacute syndrome presents over days to weeks and is marked by severe and progressive cough and dyspnea. The most common radiographic presentation is finely nodular diffuse infiltrates. Pleural disease, hilar adenopathy, cavitation, and calcification are absent. In the latter phases of the disease, honeycombing of the lung, indicative of end-stage fibrosis, may become evident.

The diagnosis depends on obtaining a history of exposure to a recognized antigen, the presence of a specific serum antibody to this antigen, and BAL fluid lymphocytosis with a CD4/CD8 ratio of less than 1:1. Therapy is based on avoiding contact with the antigen. Usually the symptoms resolve spontaneously, but the syndrome also responds nicely to systemic steroids. Chronic disease can theoretically develop in persons with multiple acute illnesses.

DRUG-INDUCED INTERSTITIAL LUNG DISEASE

Interstitial lung disease frequently represents a complication or toxicity of many prescription drugs (Table 12-9). Because the list of offending medications expands yearly, we will discuss the general principles of drug-induced interstitial lung disease and mention the major agents that have been responsible.

Agents That Cause Direct Tissue Toxicity.
Chemotherapeutic agents form the largest category of drugs associated with disease of the alveolar wall. The agents that have been most commonly implicated in the development of lung disease are bleomycin, busulfan, methotrexate, cyclophosphamide, and nitrosoureas. In general, the risk of developing lung disease is directly correlated with a drug's cumulative dosage. On average, development of interstitial lung disease occurs months to years after drug use. Busulfan is specifically known to cause lung disease years after the onset of therapy.

The pathogenesis of interstitial lung disease induced by chemotherapeutic drugs is not known, but most likely involves the direct toxic effect of the drug on the parenchymal cells (an exception is methotrexate, which may have a hypersensitivity mechanism). Histologic samples of lung tissue from patients with chemotherapy-induced interstitial lung disease frequently show atypical type II alveolar epithelial cells with large nuclei. The remaining pathologic findings are similar to those found in other interstitial lung diseases. Fever and dyspnea are the most common symptoms of this disease. Peripheral eosinophilia can be seen in patients on methotrexate.

The diagnosis is primarily based on clinical suspicion. Occasionally, if a lung biopsy is done to rule out infectious etiologies, the presence of atypical epithelial cells without infectious agents suggests a drug-induced process. Therapy is based on discontinuing the use of the drug. Systemic steroids give variable results.

The pathogenesis of hypersensitivity pneumonitis is not clear. Two distinct mechanisms hypothesized are type III immune-mediated injury and type IV cell-mediated injury.

History of a known antigen exposure is very important to making the diagnosis.

Favorable prognosis: symptoms either resolve spontaneously or respond well to steroids.

Chemotherapeutic agents are the most common group of drugs causing direct tissue injury.

Diagnosis is based on clinical suspicion.

Table 12-9
Classification of Drugs That Induce Interstitial Lung Disease

Antibiotics
Nitrofurantoin (acute and chronic use)   Sulfasalazine

Anti-inflammatory Agents
Aspirin   Gold
Penicillamine   Methotrexate

Cardiovascular Agents
Amiodarone   Tocainide

Chemotherapeutic Agents
Bleomycin   Mitomycin-C
Busulfan   Cyclophosphamide
Melphalan   Chlorambucil
Azathioprine   Cytosine arabinoside
Methotrexate   BCNU/CCNU
Procarbazine   Zinostatin
Etoposide (VP-16)   Vinblastine

Agents That Induce Systemic Lupus Erythematosus
Procainamide   Isoniazid
Hydralazine   Hydantoins
Penicillamine

Illicit Drugs
Heroin   Methadone
Talc   Dextropropoxyphene

Miscellaneous Agents
Oxygen   Radiation
Hydrochlorothiazide   L-tryptophan
Drugs inducing pulmonary infiltrates
   and eosinophilia

Agents That Cause Hypersensitivity-Type Injury. Nitrofurantoin has been associated with both acute and chronic lung reactions. The two processes are unrelated. An acute process is a hypersensitivity reaction producing fever, pulmonary infiltrates, pleural effusions, and peripheral eosinophilia. The chronic process presents insidiously as a nonspecific interstitial pneumonitis and fibrosis similar to those of other end-stage interstitial lung diseases. Methotrexate is another example of an agent that causes a hypersensitivity reaction, which is an exception to chemotherapeutic medication.

Unknown Mechanism. Amiodarone is an antiarrhythmic agent that has been available in Europe since 1962, but no adverse pulmonary effects were reported until 1980. Although it has many systemic side effects, the most serious is interstitial pneumonitis, which has been reported in up to 6% of patients taking the drug. The mechanism of amiodarone toxicity is unclear, but it produces an unusual pathology, with foamy alveolar macrophages and type II pneumocytes containing lamellar inclusions that consist of any one of a number of phospholipids.

The incidence of pulmonary toxicity from amiodarone varies, but averages about 4%. The majority of patients who develop amiodarone pneumonitis have been taking the drug for at least several months. Most are receiving at least 400 mg per day. Symptoms include dyspnea, nonproductive cough, and occasionally low-grade fever. The chest x-ray initially shows subtle, asymmetrically increased lung markings that may be limited to the upper lobes. If the drug is continued and the disease progresses, a diffuse interstitial and/or alveolar pattern develops.

The diagnosis can be made by showing foamy alveolar macrophages and type II pneumocytes with lamellar inclusions in BAL fluid, but improvement after the drug is withdrawn and systemic steroids are added often supports a clinical diagnosis.

Amiodarone-induced toxicity usually occurs with higher dosages and prolonged use.

CONNECTIVE TISSUE/COLLAGEN VASCULAR DISORDERS ASSOCIATED WITH INTERSTITIAL LUNG DISEASES

Most collagen vascular diseases are associated with inflammatory reactions of the pulmonary parenchyma that may lead to diffuse pulmonary infiltrates (Table 12-10). In many of these disorders, the lung injury is physiologically, histologically, and radiographically

Rheumatoid arthritis
Systemic lupus erythematosus
Progressive systemic sclerosis (scleroderma)
Polymyositis/dermatomyositis
Sjögren's syndrome
Mixed connective tissue disease
Ankylosing spondylitis
Psoriatic arthritis
Behçet's disease
Relapsing polychondritis

Table 12-10
Connective Tissue/Collagen Vascular Disorders Associated with Interstitial Lung Disease

indistinguishable from idiopathic pulmonary fibrosis, especially at end-stage. It is important to try to make this distinction to avoid unnecessary lung biopsies. We will describe the four most common connective tissue diseases associated with interstitial lung disease.

Rheumatoid Arthritis (RA). There are six pulmonary syndromes associated with rheumatoid arthritis: 1) diffuse parenchymal fibrosis, 2) inflammation of the pleural surface, 3) parenchymal nodules, 4) pulmonary vasculitis, 5) Caplan's syndrome (rheumatoid pneumoconiosis), and 6) bronchiolitis obliterans. Persons who have some type of pulmonary involvement are more likely to have a systemic disease with subcutaneous nodules, peripheral eosinophilia, systemic vasculitis, high titers of rheumatoid factor, and reduced levels of complement than are patients without lung disease.

> Patients with pulmonary involvement are more likely to have systemic disease.

Overall, less than 5% of patients with RA have interstitial infiltrates on chest x-ray. However, as many as 30% of persons with RA have significant decreases in diffusion capacity (D_LCO), even in light of a normal chest x-ray. Lung biopsy in this group demonstrates the presence of mild interstitial fibrosis. Initially, patients are asymptomatic, even in the presence of an abnormal chest x-ray. As the disease progresses, dyspnea, nonproductive cough, and digital clubbing develop. The course of rheumatoid interstitial lung disease is not well defined. Typically, the disease progresses insidiously over a period of years. The patient usually presents in the fifth or sixth decade of life. Very few die of respiratory failure.

> Radiographically, visible disease is not as common as a reduction in D_LCO.

The diagnosis is generally clinical, based on the presence of RA and insidious onset of interstitial infiltrates. Conversely, fever and the rapid onset of pulmonary complaints make lung biopsy mandatory. Therapy is essentially supportive (i.e., oxygen), because less than 10% of patients demonstrate a response to systemic steroids.

> Most patients present in the fifth or sixth decade.

Progressive Systemic Sclerosis (PSS). PSS is characterized by its involvement of multiple organs. Skin is universally involved, followed in order of decreasing frequency by involvement of the peripheral vasculature, GI tract (esophagus), lung, heart, and kidney. Lung disease can manifest itself in three ways: 1) interstitial fibrosis, 2) pulmonary hypertension with or without interstitial fibrosis, and 3) chronic recurrent aspiration pneumonitis as a result of esophageal dysmotility. Postmortem examinations reveal nearly all patients with PSS to have interstitial lung disease, but this is recognized in only about half the individuals ante mortem.

> Pulmonary manifestations of PSS include interstitial fibrosis, pulmonary hypertension, and recurrent aspiration pneumonitis.

Histologically, nonspecific interstitial fibrosis is found in PSS. The alveolar septa are replaced by fibrous tissue with little cellular infiltration. In the later stages of the disease, pleural, interlobar, and peribronchial disease may be present. Arteriolar thickening with medial hypertrophy or concentric intimal proliferation has also been found.

The radiographic findings are nonspecific, with diffuse bilateral pulmonary infiltrates predominating at the lung bases. As the disease progresses, a reduction in lung volumes can be appreciated on serial chest x-rays. Cystic lesions and honeycombing often occur. Pleural effusions are rare.

Symptomatic interstitial lung disease is rarely the presenting manifestation of PSS. But as the disease progresses, respiratory symptoms develop in most patients and consist of dyspnea, nonproductive cough, and chest pain. Elevated rheumatoid factor, erythrocyte sedimentation rate, antinuclear antibody titers, and hypergammaglobulinemia are present in 25% to 80% of patients.

Diagnosis, in most instances, is clinical, based on the presence of diffuse pulmonary infiltrates in a patient with typical cutaneous features of PSS. Biopsy is not necessary. Treatment is supportive only.

Interstitial lung disease is not as common as pleural involvement in SLE.

Systemic Lupus Erythematosus (SLE). SLE is a chronic inflammatory disease that can affect skin joints, kidneys, nervous system, serous membranes, and the lungs. The intrathoracic manifestations of SLE occur frequently, but in contrast to other connective tissue diseases, interstitial lung disease is distinctly uncommon. Pleural involvement, including effusion, is present in more than 40% of patients, whereas acute lupus pneumonitis occurs in less than 30%. Patients usually present with fever, tachypnea, and hypoxia, and have poorly defined alveolar infiltrates on chest x-ray. Infection is the most common etiology of pneumonitis in a lupus patient. Diagnosis of SLE-related interstitial lung disease is based on appropriate clinical syndrome. Therapy is mostly supportive, though a trial of high dosage systemic steroids can be attempted.

Mixed Connective Tissue Disease (MCTD). MCTD is a syndrome with overlapping clinical features of PSS, SLE, RA, and polymyositis/dermatomyositis. Pulmonary dysfunction occurs in 80% of these patients, with the majority of patients experiencing no symptoms. About 30% develop diffuse interstitial infiltrates, predominantly in the middle and lower lung fields. Pathologic changes are a combination of chronic inflammation and fibrosis of alveolar septa. Diagnosis of MCTD-related interstitial lung disease is based on appropriate clinical syndrome. Biopsy is not necessary. Symptomatic therapy has been tried with systemic steroids and cyclophosphamide.

ALVEOLAR HEMORRHAGE SYNDROMES

Alveolar hemorrhage syndromes constitute a very large group of disorders with some overlap with the systemic vasculitides. The etiologies of these syndromes can be separated into two groups: those with a histologic entity known as capillaritis and those without this inflammatory lesion (Table 12-11).

Table 12-11
Etiologies of Diffuse Alveolar Hemorrhage

Disorders Associated with Pulmonary Capillaritis
Wegener's granulomatosis
Systemic necrotizing vasculitis
Connective tissue diseases
Mixed cryoglobulinemia
Behçet's syndrome
Henoch-Schönlein purpura
Goodpasture's syndrome
Pauci-immune glomerulonephritis
Immune complex-associated glomerulonephritis

Disorders Not Associated with Pulmonary Capillaritis
Idiopathic pulmonary hemosiderosis
Systemic lupus erythematosus
Goodpasture's syndrome
Diffuse alveolar damage
Penicillamine
Mitral stenosis
Coagulation disorders
Pulmonary veno-occlusive disease
Pulmonary capillary hemangiomatosis
Lymphangioleiomyomatosis
Tuberous sclerosis
Trimellitic anhydride

Capillaritis is an inflammatory lesion of the alveolar interstitium associated with alveolar hemorrhage.

Capillaritis is an inflammatory lesion of the alveolar interstitium associated with several systemic vasculitides. The interstitium is invaded by neutrophils resulting in fibrinoid necrosis. Integrity of the alveolar capillary membrane is lost, and leakage of red blood cells and neutrophils into alveolar spaces occurs. Hemosiderin-laden macrophages and collections of free hemosiderin within the alveoli become prominent after an acute bleed.

To diagnose alveolar hemorrhage, bronchoscopy is done with sequential lavage of 20-mL aliquots.

The most prominent symptoms of alveolar hemorrhage are cough, dyspnea, and hemoptysis. It is not uncommon, however, for hemoptysis to be absent on presentation, even in cases of extensive intra-alveolar bleeding. The duration of symptoms is usually short, lasting from days to weeks, before patients seek medical attention. Depending on the etiology, these symptoms can become recurrent. Systemic manifestations that may accompany pulmonary symptoms (again, depending on the etiology) are fever, sinusitis, inflammatory ocular disease, arthritis, glomerulonephritis, and signs referring to a cutaneous vasculitis. The findings on chest x-ray are those of diffuse or focal patchy alveolar infiltration, which can also be confirmed by thoracic CT scan. Interstitial infiltrates appear with recurrent and chronic hemorrhage. All patients have an iron deficiency anemia and elevation of white blood cell count, platelet count, and the erythrocyte sedimentation rate (the last particularly in disorders associated with capillaritis). To make the diagnosis of alveolar hemorrhage in the appropriate clinical setting, bronchoscopy is done with sequential lavage of 20-mL aliquots. If the number of red blood cells increases with each aliquot, alveolar hemorrhage is indicated.

Some alveolar hemorrhage disorders associated with capillaritis include, in decreasing order of frequency, Wegener's granulomatosis, systemic necrotizing vasculitis, several connective tissue diseases (e.g., SLE), mixed cryoglobulinemia, Behçet's syndrome, and Henoch-Schönlein purpura. We will discuss one of these disorders—systemic necrotizing vasculitis—in detail.

SYSTEMIC NECROTIZING VASCULITIS

Systemic necrotizing vasculitis is a variant of polyarteritis nodosa and is second in frequency to Wegener's granulomatosis as a cause of pulmonary capillaritis and diffuse alveolar hemorrhage. However, unlike polyarteritis nodosa (which does not cause diffuse alveolar hemorrhage), only the small blood vessels are involved, asthma and hypertension are absent, and there is relative sparing of the abdominal viscera. The lungs are involved in 20% to 30% of the cases, and the potential hemorrhage tends to be severe and often life threatening. As in other systemic vasculitides, there are coexisting glomerulonephritis, elevation of the erythrocyte sedimentation rate, nonspecific increases in the titers of autoantibodies such as antinuclear and rheumatoid factors, and the presence of circulating immune complexes.

Some alveolar hemorrhage disorders not associated with capillaritis include, in decreasing order of frequency, idiopathic pulmonary hemosiderosis, Goodpasture's syndrome, diffuse alveolar damage, disorders caused by several drugs and toxins, mitral stenosis, pulmonary veno-occlusive disease, and lymphangioleiomyomatosis. We will discuss two of the more common disorders.

GOODPASTURE'S SYNDROME

Known as "anti-basement membrane antibody disease," this diagnosis is reserved for patients with alveolar hemorrhage and glomerulonephritis, in whom this antibody appears in the serum and is bound to kidney and lung basement membranes. In up to 80% of the cases, renal and pulmonary diseases coexist, and in the remainder, renal disease exists in isolation. Most commonly it affects males in their twenties to thirties, and tends to cause significant, recurrent alveolar hemorrhage, especially in smokers.

> In Goodpasture's syndrome, pulmonary involvement coexists with renal disease in 80% of the cases.

Histologically, Goodpasture's syndrome appears similar to idiopathic pulmonary hemosiderosis, but has been reported to have capillaritis associated with it. Electron microscopy demonstrates that the basement membranes of the lung and kidney are diffusely fragmented and contain electron-dense deposits, indicating the presence of immune reaction product. It has been clearly shown that the pathogenesis of Goodpasture's syndrome is from antibodies attacking the basement membranes, but the stimulus for this reaction remains unknown. The clinical onset of this disease has been related to various respiratory infections (especially influenza A-2), hydrocarbon exposure, and tobacco use.

> Pathogenesis of Goodpasture's syndrome is related to specific antibodies attacking basement membranes.

Presenting symptoms are usually respiratory in nature and consist of hemoptysis, cough, and dyspnea. Fatigue from iron deficiency, microscopic hematuria, and proteinuria are common as well. Patients often exhibit pallor and have crackles and rhonchi on lung exam. Chest x-ray reveals patchy or diffuse dense alveolar infiltrates. As in idiopathic pulmonary hemosiderosis, these infiltrates resolve after an acute bleed, but leave residual reticulonodular changes. There are patients with Goodpasture's syndrome whose chest x-rays are abnormal, but whose urinalyses and renal functions are normal.

The diagnosis is generally made by detecting anti–glomerular basement membrane antibodies in the serum, kidney, or lung in an appropriate clinical setting. Tissue is best obtained from the kidney, even with normal renal function. Lung biopsy is rarely neces-

> Diagnosis of Goodpasture's syndrome is made by detecting serum anti–glomerular basement membrane antibodies and by kidney biopsy. Lung biopsy is not necessary.

sary. Treatment consists of systemic steroids and cyclophosphamide, with plasmapheresis reserved for patients with rapid deterioration of renal function.

DIFFUSE ALVEOLAR DAMAGE

This clinical disorder follows a variety of infectious, drug-induced, and other types of injury to the epithelial lining and alveolar-capillary basement membranes. It is in the category of alveolar hemorrhage syndromes because serum and red blood cells enter the alveolar space following an injury and result in significant hemoptysis. The interstitium becomes edematous and type I alveolar epithelial cells are sloughed. Chronic inflammation and fibroblastic proliferation occur even early in this process. However, the influx of neutrophils in this disorder is not as intense as it is in pulmonary capillaritis. With time, collagen deposits form, and the disease begins to resemble both a usual interstitial pneumonitis and an organizing pneumonia.

IDIOPATHIC CAUSES OF INTERSTITIAL LUNG DISEASE

> More than half of all patients with interstitial lung disease have no identifiable etiology.

Unfortunately, more than half of all patients with interstitial lung disease suffer from a process with which no etiology has been identified, even though their disease may carry a specific name. Idiopathic disorders can be separated into two groups: those with multisystem involvement and those with pulmonary involvement only. Multisystem diseases include sarcoidosis and vasculitides (e.g., Wegener's granulomatosis and Churg-Strauss vasculitis), and diseases primarily of the lung include idiopathic pulmonary fibrosis (IPF), eosinophilic granuloma (EG), idiopathic pulmonary hemosiderosis, chronic alveolar proteinosis, and bronchiolitis obliterans with organizing pneumonia (BOOP). We will discuss some of these disorders in detail.

Vasculitides

> Wegener's granulomatosis can involve any part of the respiratory tract, including the pleura.

Wegener's Granulomatosis. Wegener's granulomatosis is a syndrome of granulomatous inflammation involving the upper and lower respiratory tracts, and is associated with a glomerulonephritis. The entire respiratory tract can be involved. Grossly visible nodules that tend to cavitate can be found anywhere from nasal septum to pleura. Typical pathologic features are granulomatous inflammation and necrosis within the small airways, in small to medium-sized arteries and veins, and in the extravascular space. The earliest lesion is one of collagen micronecrosis (less than 1 mm in diameter) followed by accumulation of histiocytes to form a granuloma. Eventually, this inflammatory response progresses to areas of macronecrosis (greater than 1 mm in diameter) and then to fibrosis. Although Wegener's granulomatosis is considered to be a primary vasculitis, this pathologic process is not restricted to blood vessels. It can also involve the bronchial tree, pleura, or pulmonary parenchyma.

> The majority of Wegener's granulomatosis patients present with upper airway symptoms.

Clinical features of Wegener's granulomatosis are frequently multisystemic. The majority of patients present with upper airway symptoms, such as sinusitis, otitis media, rhinitis, epistaxis, oral ulcers, and hearing impairment. Most have abnormal chest x-rays, but few notice respiratory symptoms (dyspnea, cough, hemoptysis, chest pain). Rarely patients can present with alveolar hemorrhage. Pulmonary disease usually precedes renal involvement, but occasionally both organ systems are affected simultaneously. The kidney is involved in about 85% of the patients, and renal failure is the most important complication of Wegener's granulomatosis. Other signs and symptoms at initial presentation are fever, weight loss, arthritis, skin rash, and ocular inflammation. Joint discomfort is generally polyarticular and symmetric, never deforming, often involving the knees, ankles, and small joints of the feet. Ocular involvement includes uveitis, conjunctivitis, and episcleritis. Cardiac involvement can occur and includes congestive cardiomyopathy, acute myocarditis, and pericarditis.

> The kidney is involved in about 85% of patients with Wegener's granulomatosis.

> The most common chest x-ray finding in Wegener's granulomatosis is cavitary pulmonary nodules.

As mentioned, many of these patients have chest x-ray abnormalities, but the diffuse reticulonodular abnormality of interstitial lung disease is rarely seen. The most common finding on chest x-ray is pulmonary nodules that tend to cavitate. Pleural effusions have been demonstrated, but hilar adenopathy is extremely rare. The diagnosis of Wegener's granulomatosis, in the appropriate clinical setting, is established by tissue biopsy. Open-lung biopsy by thoracoscopy is the procedure of choice. The presence of antineutrophilic cytoplasm antibodies (ANCAs) is a highly specific and moderately sensitive marker of this disease. Therapy consists of systemic steroids and cyclophosphamide.

> The diagnosis of Wegener's granulomatosis is made by lung biopsy and by the presence of ANCAs in the serum.

Churg-Strauss Vasculitis. This syndrome is defined by the presence of peripheral eosinophilia and systemic vasculitis in a patient with bronchial asthma. Asthma, allergic rhinitis, blood eosinophilia, and an elevated serum IgE all suggest the occurrence of an allergic reaction. No specific antigen has been identified. A typical histologic presentation consists of tissue infiltration by eosinophils, necrotizing vasculitis of small arteries and veins, and extravascular granulomas.

Asthma is fundamental to the diagnosis of Churg-Strauss syndrome. It usually presents in adult years with an average onset of symptoms in the fifth decade of life. Typically, asthma precedes the onset of vasculitis by 8 to 30 years. The most common presenting symptoms are allergic rhinitis, fever, weight loss, arthralgias, and myalgias. Skin lesions including purpura, nodules, erythema, and urticaria are common, as well as involvement of the peripheral nervous system (mononeuritis multiplex). An elevated blood eosinophil count is a diagnostic feature of Churg-Strauss syndrome. In fact, up to 80% of circulating white blood cells may be eosinophils. The degree of eosinophilia and erythrocyte sedimentation rate (ESR) elevation correlate well with disease activity.

Chest x-ray is abnormal in nearly one-third of all patients. Various presentations are seen, including patchy migratory infiltrates, multiple bilateral nodules without cavitation, and interstitial lung disease. Pleural effusions are rare. Prognosis of the Churg-Strauss syndrome is very good. The treatment of choice is systemic steroids.

Lymphomatoid Granulomatosis. Lymphomatoid granulomatosis is a necrotizing angiocentric mononuclear cell inflammatory process. It is not a true vasculitis, but rather a lymphoproliferative process described as an extranodal T-cell lymphoma. Pulmonary disease is universal, although multiple organs (skin, nervous system) may be involved. Mortality is very high.

The histologic picture of this disease requires the presence of the following: 1) polymorphic lymphoid infiltrates consisting of atypical mononuclear cells, small lymphocytes, and plasma cells; 2) angiitis in the form of transmural infiltration of arterial and venous walls without focal necrosis; and 3) "granulomatosis," defined as focal necrosis within lymphoid nodules but without granulomatous inflammation.

This disease typically occurs in men in the fourth decade of life. Chest pain, dyspnea, and cough are the most common presenting symptoms. Skin involvement consists of a painful papular erythematous rash. Peripheral neuropathy and symptoms of a central nervous system mass lesion are the more common neurologic presentations. Most typical radiographic findings are either bilateral migratory infiltrates or multiple rounded densities suggestive of metastatic tumor. Diagnosis is made by open-lung biopsy. Prognosis is poor. Therapy consists of systemic steroids and cyclophosphamide.

Interstitial Lung Diseases with Pulmonary Involvement Only

Idiopathic Pulmonary Fibrosis (IPF). IPF is the second most common cause (following sarcoidosis) of chronic diffuse pulmonary infiltrates of unknown etiology. Five pathologic subtypes have been described: 1) usual interstitial pneumonitis; 2) usual interstitial pneumonitis with bronchiolitis obliterans; 3) desquamative interstitial pneumonitis; 4) lymphocytic interstitial pneumonitis; and 5) giant cell interstitial pneumonitis. All these histologic patterns can be found in a single patient.

Wide variability exists in the histologic pattern of IPF. Usually, the greater the histologic variability, the better the response to therapy. The pattern varies from dense alveolar septal fibrosis with little or no inflammation to a predominance of lymphocytes or plasma cells and minimal fibrosis. A "desquamative" reaction may also occur when alveolar macrophages and type II pneumocytes completely fill the alveoli, in association with only minimal fibrosis. The degree of fibrosis is the principal determinant of the response to therapy, with severe fibrosis being resilient to treatment while mild fibrosis tends to be more responsive.

The etiology of IPF remains relatively unknown, although several hypotheses have been discussed. One theory predicts an unidentified agent initiating an exaggerated inflammatory reaction that ultimately leads to fibrotic destruction of the alveolus. Alveolar macrophages are likely to be responsible for orchestrating these events. When stimulated by T lymphocytes, these macrophages attract neutrophils to the lung through production of neutrophil chemotactic factor and induce secretion of collagenase and

---

The triad of asthma, vasculitis, and peripheral eosinophilia identifies Churg-Strauss syndrome.

Lymphomatoid granulomatosis is a lymphoproliferative process described as an extranodal T-cell lymphoma.

The name "lymphomatoid granulomatosis" is somewhat of a misnomer, because this disease forms polymorphic lymphoid nodules, but without actual granulomas.

The greater the histologic variability in IPF, the better the response to therapy.

The degree of fibrosis is the principal determinant of the response of IPF to therapy.

myeloperoxidase. Macrophages also secrete fibronectin and a specific growth factor, which attract, immobilize, and stimulate replication of fibroblasts.

This proposed mechanism of IPF pathogenesis may work by way of immune complexes. This theory is supported by the following facts: 1) immune complexes are present in the serum and BAL fluid of patients with IPF, 2) IPF can be produced in animals by intratracheal instillation of immune complexes, 3) autoimmune collagen vascular diseases (as described earlier) are associated with lung fibrosis histologically identical to IPF, and 4) there are alterations in the quantities and qualities of various immune effector cells in lung specimens from these patients.

When Hamman and Rich first described this syndrome in 1935, they reported four patients who died from diffuse parenchymal fibrosis within 3 months of presentation. It is now known that there is wide variability in the natural history of IPF, and it is rare for the course to be either fulminant, as described by Hamman and Rich, or prolonged with survival exceeding 10 years. More commonly, there is an insidious progression with a 50% mortality (mostly respiratory) 4 to 6 years following presentation. About 10% of patients develop bronchogenic carcinoma during the course of the disease.

Age of onset varies, but averages about 60. Presenting symptoms are typically dyspnea and nonproductive cough of 2 years' duration. Patients who have had symptoms for less than 1 year at presentation seem to have a better prognosis, possibly because of a greater probability of having active inflammatory histopathology instead of end-stage fibrosis. About half the patients have constitutional symptoms of malaise and weight loss. Physical exam findings consist of tachypnea, crackles at the lung bases, clubbing, and exercise-induced cyanosis. Evidence of pulmonary hypertension becomes apparent late in the course.

The chest x-ray typically shows a diffuse reticular or reticulonodular pattern, more predominant at the bases. Pleural involvement is rare. In general, radiographic patterns correlate poorly with histology and do not distinguish inflammation from fibrosis. The exception is a honeycomb pattern that correlates well with end-stage fibrosis. Diagnosis of IPF can generally be made clinically once other etiologies (collagen vascular, infectious) have been ruled out. Occasionally, tissue is needed, in which case an open or thoracoscopic biopsy is the procedure of choice. Therapy for patients with active alveolitis is systemic steroids, with possible additions of azathioprine or cyclophosphamide. Patients with end-stage fibrosis are treated supportively.

Eosinophilic Granuloma. Eosinophilic granuloma of the lung is not a common disorder. It is also a relatively uncommon cause of diffuse pulmonary infiltrates, accounting for approximately 3% of patients with interstitial lung disease. As an entity, eosinophilic granuloma is usually included within the larger category of diseases termed histiocytosis X. The other two disorders within this category are Hand-Schüller-Christian disease and Letterer-Siwe disease. They are all histologically similar, with aggregations of abnormal histiocytes (Langerhans' cells) within the formation of a granuloma. These unique cells have cytoplasmic inclusions variously referred to as Langerhans' granules, Birbeck's granules, and histiocytosis X bodies. In eosinophilic granuloma of the lung, infiltration by these cells is generally limited to the lung, although discrete lesions occasionally may be found in bones. Histologically, there may also be infiltration of eosinophils, lymphocytes, macrophages, and plasma cells.

Persons with this disease tend to be young to middle-aged adults. They present with some combination of cough, dyspnea, chest pain, and/or hemoptysis. Many describe a flulike illness, and some have significant weight loss. Spontaneous pneumothorax can be a presenting feature and occurs in up to 50% of patients during the course of the disease. Chest x-rays are abnormal in essentially all patients. In fact, 20% to 30% of patients are asymptomatic with an abnormal chest x-ray. The radiographic features tend to be more prominent in the upper lung zones and have variable appearance (nodular, reticulonodular, interstitial, and alveolar). Some cases progress to extensive cystic disease and honeycombing. The natural history of the disease is variable, and in some patients can be self-limiting with stabilization of radiographic features over time. In others, however, it progresses to a significant functional impairment.

Diagnosis of eosinophilic granuloma can be made by bronchoscopy with BAL and

---

There is wide variability in the natural history of IPF; it is rare for the course to be either fulminant or prolonged.

About 10% of IPF patients develop bronchogenic carcinoma.

Unless there is a honeycomb pattern that correlates well with end-stage fibrosis, radiographic findings in IPF correlate poorly with histology.

Spontaneous pneumothorax can occur in up to 50% of patients with eosinophilic granuloma.

Radiographic features of eosinophilic granuloma tend to be upper lung zone predominant.

transbronchial biopsy in the patient with an appropriate clinical presentation. There is no effective treatment.

Bronchiolitis Obliterans with Organizing Pneumonia (BOOP). BOOP is an important etiology of diffuse pulmonary infiltrates. It is defined by the presence of intraluminal fibrosis of the small airways of the lung. Although it was once thought to be a rare disease, it is now being diagnosed and reported with increasing frequency. The etiology of BOOP is not entirely clear, although it has been associated with toxic fume exposure, postinfectious inflammatory residue, and connective tissue disease.

BOOP has a unique histologic appearance. There is patchy distribution of intraluminal fibrosis with plugs of connective tissue in respiratory bronchioles, alveolar ducts, and alveoli. This tissue is mostly a fibroblast stroma with minimal collagen deposition. Septal fibrosis is unusual, and honeycombing is absent. Interstitial infiltration with foamy macrophages and type II pneumocytes may be present. Cultures and special stains for microorganisms are negative. Because BOOP is quite distinct from IPF histologically, and is strikingly steroid responsive, it is important to make an early tissue diagnosis to differentiate these two entities.

BOOP affects all patients equally. Typically, the patient is middle-aged and presents with a subacute illness of 2 to 10 weeks' duration. Symptoms include nonproductive cough, fever, dyspnea, malaise, headache, and myalgias. Physical exam is unremarkable, with the exception of bibasilar crackles. Clubbing is rare. Chest x-ray is always abnormal. Typically, bilateral, patchy, alveolar infiltrates are present, which can be localized and lobar, simulating bacterial pneumonia. Occasionally, a classic interstitial reticular pattern is seen. Infiltrates can be fleeting, but never resolve completely. It is very unusual to see cavitary lesions or pleural effusions. There is an excellent correlation between radiographic appearance and histologic extent of the disease.

Diagnosis can be made clinically in the appropriate setting, but bronchoscopy should be done to rule out infectious etiologies. Rarely, tissue is needed. Treatment consists of systemic steroids.

Chronic Eosinophilic Pneumonia. Chronic eosinophilic pneumonia is a disease of middle-aged women, some with a history of asthma. It is typically described as a subacute pulmonary syndrome with diffuse pulmonary infiltrates and peripheral eosinophilia. Histologic appearance consists of accumulation of eosinophils and histiocytes within the alveoli, occasionally surrounded by amorphous material. This intraalveolar exudate frequently is associated with interstitial infiltration by the same two types of cells. Etiology is unknown, although a hypersensitivity reaction has been proposed.

A typical clinical presentation of chronic eosinophilic pneumonia consists of a subacute respiratory illness of more than 6 months' duration with symptoms (in decreasing order of frequency) of nonproductive cough, dyspnea, fever, and weight loss. Many patients are cigarette smokers. The classic radiographic pattern is described as "the photographic negative of pulmonary edema," because of the peripheral location (outer two-thirds of the lung fields) of its infiltrates. In a majority of patients, the disease is bilateral and primarily involves the upper lung zones. Significant peripheral eosinophilia, as high as 25%, is observed in almost 90% of the patients.

The diagnosis of chronic eosinophilic pneumonia can be confirmed by bronchoscopy with BAL and transbronchial lung biopsies, and patients respond well to systemic steroids.

▮ SUMMARY

The interstitial lung diseases are a very large group of pulmonary disorders. Many of them also have other organ system involvement. The keys to recognition and differentiation of these disorders are a thorough history and physical exam. Many diagnoses can be made purely on a clinical basis, although invasive techniques such as bronchoscopy and open/thoracoscopic lung biopsy are readily available if needed. Fortunately, several of these diseases are self-limiting, but many of the others have neither a good prognosis nor efficacious therapy. Supplemental oxygen should be offered to every hypoxemic patient with interstitial lung disease.

BOOP is a mixture of alveolar and small airway disease, demonstrating combined restrictive and obstructive physiology.

An excellent correlation exists between radiographic findings and the histologic extent of BOOP.

BOOP is strikingly responsive to steroid treatment.

The classic radiographic appearance of chronic eosinophilic pneumonia is described as "the photographic negative of pulmonary edema."

Significant peripheral eosinophilia is seen in almost 90% of chronic eosinophilic pneumonia patients.

▮ REVIEW QUESTIONS

1. G.D. is a 47-year-old man with a long history of bronchial asthma, who presents with several weeks of low-grade fevers, watery rhinorrhea, and myalgias. Physical exam findings are significant for diffuse urticaria and palpable purpura. Laboratory evaluation reveals a mildly elevated white blood cell count, 70% of which are eosinophils. Chest x-ray demonstrates diffuse, bilateral interstitial infiltrates. The most likely diagnosis is

   (A) idiopathic pulmonary fibrosis
   (B) Churg-Strauss vasculitis
   (C) chronic eosinophilic pneumonia
   (D) eosinophilic granuloma

Questions 2 and 3 refer to the following:
J.T. is a 33-year-old man with no significant past medical history who has had 3 to 4 weeks of fever, nonproductive cough, and progressive dyspnea. He has received several courses of outpatient antibiotic therapy without response. He now presents with worsening dyspnea requiring intubation and mechanical ventilation. Your evaluation reveals bibasilar crackles on lung auscultation, elevated white blood cell count, and bilateral patchy alveolar infiltrates on chest x-ray. Reviewing this patient's prior x-rays, obtained over the past month, you find fleeting infiltrates that never fully resolve.

2. Based on the given history, the next step in this patient's management should be

   (A) a trial of empiric intravenous antibiotic therapy
   (B) aggressive diuretic therapy
   (C) open-lung biopsy
   (D) fiberoptic bronchoscopy with BAL

3. Fiberoptic bronchoscopy with BAL is performed, and pending results, broad spectrum intravenous antibiotic coverage is initiated. Results of BAL reveal elevated white blood cell count with negative routine cultures and stains for microorganisms. After 1 week, there is no improvement in the patient's respiratory status. The next step in his management should be

   (A) thoracoscopic lung biopsy
   (B) repeat bronchoscopy with BAL to ensure that the initial negative findings were not a laboratory error
   (C) repeat bronchoscopy with transbronchial lung biopsy
   (D) continuation of current intravenous antibiotics

4. K.B. is a 35-year-old woman with a history of scleroderma involving skin on her face and hands, and Raynaud's disease. She now presents with a 6-month history of progressive dyspnea, nonproductive cough, and chest pain. Her chest x-ray demonstrates fine interstitial lower lobe infiltrates, suggesting new lung involvement of her systemic disease. You should

   (A) check serum levels of rheumatoid factor (RF), antinuclear antibody (ANA), and erythrocyte sedimentation rate (ESR) to confirm the diagnosis.
   (B) perform fiberoptic bronchoscopy with transbronchial biopsy to confirm the diagnosis.
   (C) evaluate the patient's need for supplemental oxygen.
   (D) refer the patient for thoracoscopic lung biopsy to confirm the diagnosis.

5. S.K. is a 79-year-old nursing home patient with a chronic indwelling bladder catheter and a history of frequent urinary tract infections and rheumatoid arthritis. He is brought for evaluation of dyspnea, which he experiences during transfer from his bed to the commode. He also complains of occasional nonproductive cough, but denies fevers or sputum production. His medication list includes aspirin, multivitamin, methotrexate, nitrofurantoin, and supplemental oxygen. His exam is remarkable for tachypnea of 28 breaths per minute and bilateral inspiratory crackles on lung auscultation. Chest x-ray reveals diffuse lung disease with a honeycomb pattern. You suggest

(A) fiberoptic bronchoscopy with transbronchial biopsy
(B) thoracoscopic lung biopsy
(C) a CT scan of the thorax
(D) discontinuation of methotrexate and substitution of a different antibiotic for the patient's recurrent urinary tract infections

6. G.C., a 43-year-old man with an obsessive-compulsive disorder and a long history of smoking, presents with hemoptysis, dyspnea, weakness, and fatigue. These symptoms were preceded by a flulike respiratory infection. His chest x-ray demonstrates diffuse bilateral infiltrates with an alveolar filling pattern. Renal dysfunction and antiglomerular basement membrane antibodies are found on laboratory analysis. To confirm the diagnosis of Goodpasture's syndrome, you recommend

(A) fiberoptic bronchoscopy with transbronchial biopsy
(B) renal biopsy
(C) thoracoscopic lung biopsy
(D) checking for presence of serum antinuclear antibodies (ANAs)

■ ANSWERS AND EXPLANATIONS

1. The answer is B. The described history of asthma and the coexisting systemic findings are not usually seen in idiopathic pulmonary fibrosis or eosinophilic granuloma. Although patients with chronic eosinophilic pneumonia usually have peripheral eosinophilia and can have histories of asthma, they do not present with palpable purpura and their x-rays usually have a "photographic negative of pulmonary edema" pattern.

2. The answer is D. The differential diagnosis in this case is very broad, but infectious etiology must be ruled out before a less common disorder is pursued. Fiberoptic bronchoscopy with BAL can be done quickly and safely at the bedside to obtain secretions from the affected lung segments. Given that this patient recently completed several courses of empiric antibiotic therapy, initiating a trial of empiric intravenous antibiotics may be too risky, because the more common respiratory pathogens have probably been eradicated and further empiric therapy may waste precious time. There is no reason to suspect congestive heart failure based on the given case, and so empiric diuretic therapy is not advised.

3. The answer is A. This is a complicated case of a very ill patient. Differential diagnosis is still broad and includes adult respiratory distress syndrome (ARDS), subacute onset of a hypersensitivity pneumonitis in response to an unknown antigen, acute onset of IPF, and BOOP. Continuation of antibiotics is not incorrect, but further diagnostic modalities should be employed. A repeat BAL may show a potential nosocomial respiratory superinfection, but it will not help in identifying the original cause of the patient's respiratory failure. Transbronchial biopsies would be helpful if sarcoidosis, lymphangitic carcinoma, and bronchioloalveolar carcinoma were suspected, but these disorders are not likely based on this patient's history and presentation. To identify potentially treatable disorders such as BOOP and hypersensitivity pneumonitis, an open-lung biopsy is needed, which now can be done by a thoracoscopic technique.

4. The answer is C. This patient has systemic scleroderma now involving the lungs. In this clinical scenario, this is the most likely diagnosis, and does not require tissue evaluation. Serum markers in option A are frequently elevated in this disease but are neither sensitive nor specific as diagnostic tools. As lung involvement worsens, however, patients often require supplemental oxygen (at rest or with exertion), and should be evaluated.

5. The answer is D. Both nitrofurantoin and methotrexate are known to cause interstitial lung disease in rare cases, and discontinuing them may be of benefit. Nitrofurantoin, especially, can cause a hypersensitivity-like pneumonitis that should resolve when the medication is discontinued. However, the main teaching point of this question is the fact that once radiographic honeycombing is seen, indicative of advanced, irreversible fibrosis, the etiology of the patient's lung disease becomes essentially unimportant to his prognosis. In this case, the patient's end-stage disease may have been idiopathic (IPF), as a result of nitrofurantoin and/or methotrexate, or related to another unidentified process.

6. The answer is B. Renal biopsy is the best modality for confirming the diagnosis of Goodpasture's syndrome.

■ SUGGESTED READING

DePaso WJ, Winterbauer RH: Interstitial lung disease. *Disease-a-Month* 37(2):61–133, 1991.

Raghu G: Interstitial lung disease: a diagnostic approach. *AJRCCM* (151):909–914, 1995.

Schwarz MI, Cherniack RM, King TE Jr: Diffuse alveolar hemorrhage and other rare infiltrative disorders. *In* Murray JF, Nadel JA, eds.: *Textbook of Respiratory Medicine*, vol. 2. Philadelphia: WB Saunders, 1994, pp. 1889–1903.

Schwarz MI, Cherniack RM, King TE Jr: Infiltrative and interstitial lung diseases. *In* Murray JF, Nadel JA, eds.: *Textbook of Respiratory Medicine*, vol. 2. Philadelphia: WB Saunders, 1994, pp. 1803–1826.

Weinberger SE: Interstitial diseases associated with known etiologic agents. *In* Weinberger SE, ed.: *Principles of Pulmonary Medicine*. Philadelphia: WB Saunders, 1986, pp. 132–143.

Weinberger SE: Interstitial lung diseases of unknown etiology. *In* Weinberger SE, ed.: *Principles of Pulmonary Medicine*. Philadelphia: WB Saunders, 1986, pp. 144–153.

Weinberger SE: Overview of the interstitial lung diseases. *In* Weinberger SE, ed.: *Principles of Pulmonary Medicine*. Philadelphia: WB Saunders, 1986, pp. 122–131.

Chapter 13

PATHOPHYSIOLOGY OF PULMONARY EMBOLISM

Michaela Stanciu, M.D.

Gilbert E. D'Alonzo, D.O.

▌ CHAPTER OUTLINE

Learning Objectives
Introduction
Case Study: Introduction
Pathophysiology and Risk Factors
Clinical Features
Case Study: Continued
Gas-Exchange Abnormalities
Hemodynamics
Pulmonary Infarction
Case Study: Continued
Diagnostic Tests
Case Study: Resolution
Management
Review Questions

▌ LEARNING OBJECTIVES

At the completion of this chapter, the reader should:

- Be able to describe the major risk factors for pulmonary embolism and describe how these factors are related to the known pathology of hypercoagulability.
- Understand the thromboembolic diagnostic process and appreciate how the process relates to the underlying pathophysiology of the condition.
- Understand how pulmonary embolism is treated.

▌ INTRODUCTION

About 100,000 patients die annually from PE.

Pulmonary embolism (PE), as a result of deep vein thrombosis (DVT), is commonly encountered in clinical practice. Recent estimates suggest that in the United States, on an annual basis, DVT occurs in 5,000,000 patients and there are 600,000 episodes of pulmonary embolism. Approximately 100,000 patients die annually from PE, and most of these deaths occur in situations where the correct diagnosis has not been considered and therapy has not been initiated. In fact, when the diagnosis is missed, the mortality is six times higher.

A better understanding of the pathophysiology of PE will hopefully lead to earlier diagnosis and treatment and reduce mortality. Furthermore, PE provides an excellent clinical example of a pathophysiology associated with an acute pulmonary vascular disease disturbance.

Case Study:
Introduction

A 67-year-old man with a diagnosis of lung adenocarcinoma presents to the emergency department (ED), extremely anxious and complaining of shortness of breath and chest discomfort. He nearly lost consciousness after getting out of bed to go to the bathroom, and his lightheadedness persisted as he became diaphoretic and dyspneic. Approximately 3 days prior to his ED visit, he injured his right leg. His lung carcinoma was diagnosed 12 months ago and he recently was told that he had recurrent disease with mediastinal lymph nodes recognized on a chest x-ray.

The patient is administered 100% oxygen by face mask and his arterial oxygen saturation is measured at 91% by pulse oximetry. He is found to be tachypneic (respiratory rate 38 breaths per minute), tachycardiac (150 per minute), and hypotensive with a blood pressure of 96/60 mmHg. While in the ED, he experiences hemoptysis, with a sputum productive of a very small amount of bright red blood. He complains of right lateral chest pain with deep inspiration. His dyspnea persists and his blood pressure improves with intravenous fluid resuscitation. Neck vein distention and an increased pulmonic component to the second heart sound with a very soft but variable gallop are found on auscultation of the heart. The variability of this gallop is associated with inspiration and expiration. The lungs are clear to auscultation, but breath sounds are decreased on the right side. There is a right thoracotomy scar. The abdominal exam is normal, and an examination of the lower extremities reveals a tender, swollen right calf.

■ PATHOPHYSIOLOGY AND RISK FACTORS

Classic thrombogenic triad:

1. Venostasis
2. Hypercoagulability
3. Vascular endothelial damage

More than 90% of clots that cause PE arise in the deep veins of the legs.

Only 50% of patients who are clinically suspected of having DVT have positive venograms, and less than 50% of patients with DVT present with the classic findings of leg edema, erythema, and pain in the lower extremities.

The symptoms of PE are often nonspecific, thus contributing to delay in diagnosis.

Venous thromboembolism can occasionally complicate the course of a seriously ill patient. However, this condition also may affect a previously healthy patient. A thrombus is formed in the vascular space from fibrin, blood cells, and platelets with potential to grow and break off, resulting in thromboembolism to the lung and other organs. In 1946, Rudolph Vircow first described the classic thrombogenic triad of 1) venostasis, 2) hypercoagulability, and 3) vascular endothelial damage. These three findings are often associated with the formation of a deep vein thrombosis (DVT), which can result in a subsequent embolic event. More than 90% of clots that cause PE arise in the deep veins of the legs at the knee level or higher, with a smaller percentage of clots coming from the deep veins of the pelvis, the inferior vena cava, and the right heart.

Only 50% of patients who are clinically suspected of having DVT have positive venograms, and less than 50% of patients with DVT present with the classic findings of leg edema, erythema, and pain in the lower extremities. This is why the diagnosis is often missed: at the time of the clinical examination, DVT is not generally entertained in those patients who have normal legs. This delay in diagnosis allows for the clot to extend and eventually break off, resulting in PE. Furthermore, the symptoms of PE are often nonspecific, thus contributing to delay in diagnosis.

Certain risk factors have been shown to be present in patients who develop DVT, with or without PE. The more factors that are present, the higher the likelihood of DVT development. The risk factors are often tightly associated with the components of Vircow's triad. There are a variety of common and uncommon risk factors and conditions that are associated with DVT and PE (Table 13-1).

Table 13-1
Common Risks Factors Associated with the Development of DVT and PE

Immobilization
Trauma/postoperative state
Congestive heart failure
Chronic obstructive pulmonary disease (COPD)
Malignancy
Obesity
Pregnancy
Hypercoagulable states:
    Protein C and S deficiencies
    Antithrombin III deficiency
    Lupus anticoagulant syndrome

■ CLINICAL FEATURES

The clinical presentation of PE is nonspecific and highly variable, depending on the degree of vascular obstruction, the size and location of the DVT, the age of the patient, and any preexisting cardiopulmonary factors. Early suspicion for PE is essential for the diagnosis of this condition.

The clinical signs and symptoms of PE are often dependent on the presence of cardiovascular and pulmonary disease. Cardiovascular and pulmonary compromise depends on the extent of embolic occlusion and the degree of preexisting cardiopulmonary disease. Thromboembolic occlusion of the pulmonary vascular bed affects lung tissue, gas exchange, the pulmonary circulation, and right and eventually left heart function.

Early suspicion for PE is essential for the diagnosis of this condition.

SYMPTOMS

Dyspnea and chest discomfort are the most common symptoms of acute PE. Anxiety, apprehensiveness, and a sensation of near-syncope are associated with more extensive embolization. Syncope is associated with massive life-threatening embolism. The degree of dyspnea and chest pain depends on the extent of embolization and the amount of existing cardiovascular and pulmonary reserve.

Dyspnea and chest discomfort are the most common symptoms of acute PE.

Dyspnea can be associated with hypoxia, enhanced central ventilatory drive, acidemia, or hypotension. Chest pain can be pleuritic or anginal in character. Pleuritic chest pain is classically associated with PE and generally follows a submassive embolic event and lung injury. The dull, heavy chest pain associated with pulmonary embolism can occur with either a submassive or massive embolic event in which right and left heart ischemia can occur. A small number of embolic patients experience loss of consciousness, a scenario generally associated with a massive event. The syncope is often associated with the acute development of pulmonary hypertension, right heart failure, and a hypotensive state. The incidence of symptoms associated with PE can be found in Table 13-2.

Table 13-2
Symptoms in Patients With Angiographically Diagnosed Acute PE

SYMPTOM	TOTAL PERCENT (N = 328)	PERCENT WITH MASSIVE EMBOLISM (N = 197)	PERCENT WITH SUBMASSIVE EMBOLISM (N = 130)
Chest pain	88	85	89
Pleuritic	74	64	85
Nonpleuritic	14	6	8
Dyspnea	85	85	82
Apprehension	59	65	50
Cough	53	53	52
Hemoptysis	30	23	40
Syncope	13	20	6

Adapted from Bell WR, Simon TL, De Mets DL: *Am J Med* 62:355–360, 1977.

SIGNS

Tachypnea is present in more than 90% of patients with acute PE. Tachycardia is found in only half of the patients, but both severe tachypnea and tachycardia are generally found in patients with massive pulmonary embolic events. When pulmonary hypertension develops acutely, right heart decompensation occurs and both an increased pulmonic component to the second heart sound and a right heart gallop rhythm can be heard on cardiac auscultation. The presence of hypotension and shock indicates acute cor pulmonale from a massive pulmonary embolism. This desperate scenario can be associated with acute right heart failure, which leads to passive liver congestion and abnormal liver function tests. At times, ascites can develop quickly. The common clinical signs associated with PE are listed in Table 13-3.

Tachypnea is present in more than 90% of patients with acute PE.

Table 13-3
Physical Findings in Patients with Angiographically Diagnosed Acute PE

SIGN	TOTAL PERCENT (N = 327)	PERCENT WITH MASSIVE EMBOLISM (N = 197)	PERCENT WITH SUBMASSIVE EMBOLISM (N = 130)
Tachypnea	92	95	87
Crackles	58	57	60
Increased S_2P*	53	58	45
Tachycardia	44	48	38
Fever	43	43	42
Diaphoresis	36	42	27
Gallop	34	39	25
Phlebitis	32	36	26
Edema	24	28	28
Cyanosis	19	25	9

* S_2P = pulmonic component of second heart sound.

Adapted from Bell WR, Simon TL, De Mets DL: *Am J Med* 62:355–360, 1977.

Case Study:
Continued

Laboratory data are as follows. Chest x-ray reveals a faint right lung infiltrate peripherally, electrocardiogram shows right axis deviation (Figure 13-1), and an arterial blood gas drawn while the patient is breathing 100% oxygen by face mask indicates a pH of 7.50, a PCO_2 of 20 mmHg, a PO_2 of 60 mmHg, and an oxygen saturation of 90%. Other laboratory results include normal serum electrolytes; blood urea nitrogen (BUN), 35 mg/dL; creatinine, 1.6 mg/dL; lactate dehydrogenase (LDH), 299 units per liter; creatine phosphokinase (CPK), 300; total bilirubin, 2.2 mg/dL; alkaline phosphatase, 312 units per liter; hemoglobin, 10 gm/dL; hematocrit, 31%; white blood count, 12.8/mm³; platelet count, 246,000/mm³; and normal prothrombin time and activated partial thromboplastin time.

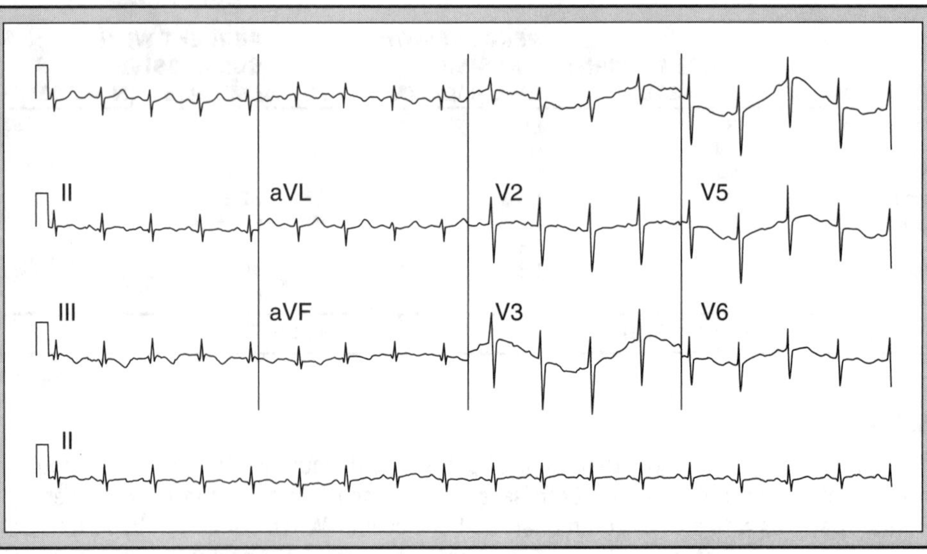

FIGURE 13-1
Electrocardiogram showing tachycardia and right axis deviation.

CHEST RADIOGRAPHY

Chest x-ray changes seen that accompany PE are subtle and generally nonspecific.

Often the chest x-ray changes that accompany PE are subtle. In fact, 12% of chest x-rays are normal. The chest x-ray can help exclude other diagnoses, such as pneumonia, heart failure, and pneumothorax. However, there is no clear feature that is helpful in diagnosing or excluding the diagnosis of PE. There are two radiographic signs that are representative of the vascular changes associated with PE. The first sign is oligemia of a section of lung parenchyma, which is known as Westermark's sign. This area of pulmonary hypolucency is the result of a marked reduction in blood flow through the pulmonary vasculature blocked by thrombus. The second sign is a unilateral enlargement of the right or left pulmonary artery. Each of these x-ray findings is found in only a minority of patients. Another sign that is often discussed as being associated with PE is a rounded density with blurred margins above the diaphragm known as the Hampton's hump. This finding is associated with pulmonary hemorrhage or infarction and can be seen in up to 25% of patients with acute PE. Chest x-ray findings associated with acute PE are found in Table 13-4.

Table 13-4
Chest Radiographic Findings in Patients with Acute PE (N = 128)

FINDING	PERCENT OF PATIENTS
Lung parenchyma	
Consolidation	41
Atelectasis	20
Pleural effusion	28
Diaphragm elevation	41
Pulmonary vessels	
Distention of proximal pulmonary arteries	23
Focal oligemia	15
Heart	
Left ventricular enlargement	16
Right ventricular enlargement	5

Adapted from *Circulation*: 47(suppl II):1–108, 1973.

ELECTROCARDIOGRAM

The most common electrocardiographic findings associated with acute PE are a normal study and sinus tachycardia, both of which are nonspecific. A variety of other changes that can occur are found in Table 13-5. The classic pattern—S1, Q3, T3 with right axis deviation—usually indicates the presence of right heart compromise, but is found in only 11% of patients with acute PE.

Normal A-a DO_2 makes the diagnosis of PE much less likely.

Table 13-5
Electrocardiographic Findings in Patients with Acute PE (N = 132)

FINDING	PERCENT OF PATIENTS
Sinus tachycardia	43
T-wave inversion	40
Sinus tachycardia segment depression	33
Low voltage in frontal plane	16
Left axis deviation	12
S_1-Q_3-T_3 pattern	11
Sinus tachycardia segment elevation	11
Right bundle branch block	11
Premature ventricular contractions	9
P-pulmonale	4
Right axis deviation	5
Atrial fibrillation	3

Adapted from *Circulation*: 47(suppl II):1–108, 1973.

ARTERIAL BLOOD GASES

A low arterial oxygen tension (P_aO_2) is a common finding in acute PE. However, a normal P_aO_2 does not exclude a diagnosis of PE, because 5% to 10% of cases have this finding. Hypocarbia, or a low P_aCO_2, is frequently present in PE. Patients with PE have a marked abnormality in gas exchange that leads to hypoxemia. The hypoxemia, as well as the resulting changes in flow and pressure that are occurring within the chest, can stimulate the respiratory system to hyperventilate. This hyperventilation leads to hypocarbia.

The degree of hypoxemia correlates with the severity of PE.

A more useful indicator of abnormal gas exchange is the alveolar-arterial oxygen gradient (A-a DO_2). Even patients who have normal or near-normal arterial P_aO_2 have evidence of increased A-a DO_2. In fact, a normal A-a DO_2 makes the diagnosis of PE much less likely. Patients with massive PE, who suffer shock with loss of consciousness, can retain carbon dioxide. It has been shown that the degree of hypoxemia correlates with the severity of PE. In general, an arterial blood gas can help increase the suspicion of PE, but other tests are necessary to solidify the diagnosis.

GAS-EXCHANGE ABNORMALITIES

Experimental data suggest that the mechanisms responsible for abnormal gas exchange in acute PE are ventilation-perfusion inequality and physiologic shunt.

The mechanisms responsible for abnormal gas exchange in acute PE are ventilation-perfusion inequality and physiologic shunt.

Right-to-left shunting of blood flow has been shown to occur in the pulmonary vascular bed following acute PE. If the arterial blood-gas measurement is performed on room air and then again after the patient has been breathing 100% oxygen, the presence of shunt can be suggested when there is little improvement in P_aO_2 during the administration of the highest concentration of inspired oxygen. Why shunt develops has not been fully explained, but one possibility is that secondary to PE, pulmonary hypertension develops and preexisting pulmonary arterial-venous anastomoses open. Some clinical investigators have suggested that the development of atelectasis distal to the embolic event with subsequent reperfusion of blood to that area can lead to physiologic shunt. Atelectasis can result from the loss of alveolar surfactant. Atelectasis may be related to certain mediators released at the time of the embolic event. When an area of lung tissue is hypoperfused and alveolar hypocarbia results, reflex pneumoconstriction and bronchiolar constriction result from a loss of surfactant following the embolic event, which may be humorally mediated ("airshift" concept). Another possible mechanism for shunt development might be associated with the development of pulmonary hypertension, right heart dysfunction with subsequent right atrial pressure elevation, and opening of an intracardiac shunt. A potentially patent foramen ovale can be found in normal individuals. The right heart high-pressure state during thromboembolism can lead to the opening of the patent foramen ovale that was present but not functional because it was closed under the preexisting low-pressure state.

As mentioned previously, arterial blood gases can be performed while the PE patient is breathing room air and 100% oxygen. If there is a substantial improvement in oxygenation with the administration of 100% oxygen, a degree of ventilation-perfusion inequality should be suspected. It is believed that ventilation-perfusion inequality plays a more important role as a mechanism of hypoxemia following acute PE. An increase in the number of low-ventilation-perfusion-ratio lung units is responsible for the hypoxemia that occurs. The formation of these low units is similar to that of shunt, with the exception of the intracardiac shunt.

Dead space as related to lung gas exchange is defined as lung tissue that is ventilated but nonperfused or very poorly perfused. An increased dead space–tidal volume (V_D/V_T) ratio can result in a widening of the alveolar-arterial carbon dioxide gradient. The V_D/V_T ratio can increase following PE, and measuring this ratio can provide further evidence for the diagnosis of acute PE. Recognizing abnormal gas exchange in PE is important, and the mechanisms for these abnormalities are multifactorial, but none of these findings is "diagnostic" of PE.

■ HEMODYNAMICS

Hemodynamic compromise—specifically, hypotension and shock—can be associated with an acute PE and often signals a massive embolic event. However, patients with preceding underlying cardiopulmonary disease can have less-than-massive embolic events and still experience hypotension and shock. When 25% of the lung vascular bed is obstructed by clot, the mean pulmonary arterial pressure begins to increase above 20 mmHg. Following a massive obstructive vascular event, where the pulmonary vascular bed is greater than 50% obstructed, there is not only an increase in pulmonary arterial pressure but also a decrease in cardiac output. The acute change in mean pulmonary arterial pressure necessary for sustaining life should be no higher than 40 mmHg. Pressures higher than 40 mmHg are often associated with vascular collapse and death. Patients with serious underlying cardiovascular and/or pulmonary disease can generally tolerate much smaller vascular occlusions before developing severe hypoxemia or shock, or both. Left ventricular function depends on right ventricular function, so biventricular failure can occur.

■ PULMONARY INFARCTION

Sometimes, a pulmonary embolic event leads to pulmonary infarction, or the death of lung tissue. Pulmonary infarction occurs infrequently because of the lung's blood supply, receiving oxygen from both the bronchial and pulmonary arterial circulations, as well as from alveolar oxygen. When infarction occurs, it usually develops at the periphery of the lung, where the bronchial circulation tapers off. Therefore, lung infarction generally occurs following more peripheral embolic distribution and is not generally associated with a large, centrally occlusive clot. Large, centrally occlusive clots are associated with shock and death, whereas more peripheral emboli are known to be associated with pleuritic chest pain, hemoptysis, and more stable hemodynamics.

Case Study:
Continued

Our patient is suspected of having a serious pulmonary embolic event. Intravenous continuous heparin is instituted, and further diagnostic testing is pursued. A ventilation-perfusion lung scan is performed (Figure 13-2A and B).

Ventilation is assessed following the administration of a radioactive gas mixed with oxygen. After the patient breathes this mixture, the radioactive gas equilibrates throughout the lung and multiple views of each lung are obtained. These images reflect lung units that are being ventilated and often correspond with the chest x-ray. Then, a perfusion scan is performed by injecting a solution of radioactive albumin that equilibrates throughout the lung circulation, producing an image of the pulmonary arterial bed. The ventilation and perfusion portions are compared, and areas of lung that are ventilated but not perfused are suggestive of PE.

When the ventilation-perfusion lung scan indicates a high probability of PE, there are multiple areas, bilaterally, of perfusion defects with normal ventilation. The greater the number of mismatched defects, the higher the likelihood of PE. Our patient has a high-probability scan for pulmonary embolism.

A venous ultrasound of the lower extremities is performed (Figure 13-3). A right femoral and popliteal thrombus with free-floating clot is evident, as is a left calf thrombus.

Because of hypotension, an echocardiogram is performed. Left ventricular function is normal, with an estimated ejection fraction of 45%. There is moderate right ventricular hypertrophy with some dilatation and wall motion hypokinesis. Mild tricuspid regurgitation is present, and the estimated systolic pulmonary arterial pressure is 50 mmHg.

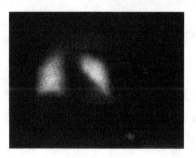

Ventilation (V̇)
A   (Xenon-133/Gas)

Perfusion (Q̇)
(Technetium–99m MAA, I.V.)

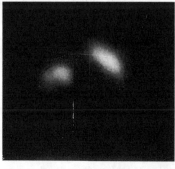

Ventilation (V̇)
B   (Xenon-133/Gas)

Perfusion (Q̇)
(Technetium–99m MAA, I.V.)

FIGURE 13-2
(A) Normal ventilation-perfusion (V̇/Q̇) lung scan. Homogeneous distribution of either Xenon gas or microaggrated technetium. (B) V̇/Q̇ lung scan indicating high probability for PE. Absence of Q̇ right upper lobe, left lower lobe and right lower lobe with normal V̇ bilaterally.

FIGURE 13-3
(A) Venous ultrasound results for a normal patient. The vein (V) and artery (A) are imaged in transverse without compression (left). With compression (right), the vein lumen is obliterated and the walls of the vein oppose, whereas the thicker-walled high-pressure artery remains visible. (B) Venous ultrasound results for a patient with acute DVT. The superficial femoral artery (A) and superficial femoral vein (V) are visualized without compression (left). There appear to be intraluminal echos in the vein. With compression (right), the vein walls do not oppose and the intraluminal material appears more echogenic. This is consistent with acute DVT.

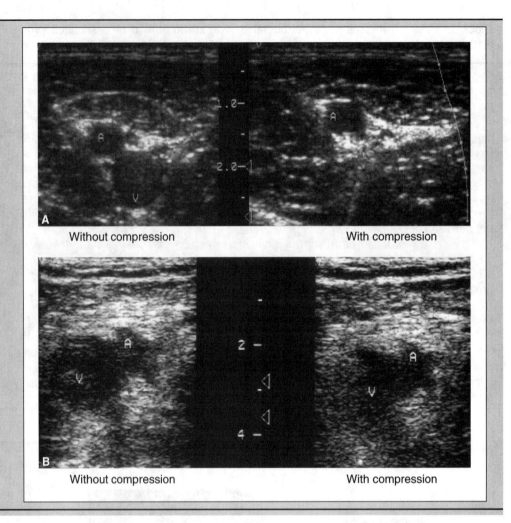

Without compression   With compression

Without compression   With compression

▍DIAGNOSTIC TESTS

Venography is considered the gold standard for the diagnosis of DVT of the lower extremities.

Venography is considered the gold standard for the diagnosis of DVT of the lower extremities. This test can visualize the entire venous system of the lower extremity after intravenous injection of contrast medium. The high degree of accuracy of this study is balanced by its invasiveness. It is also expensive and can induce phlebitis. Venography is reserved for select patients for whom less invasive studies have failed to confirm a diagnosis.

The noninvasive studies, impedance plethysmography and Doppler ultrasound imaging, are commonly employed in the evaluation process for DVT of the lower extremities. Impedance plethysmography measures changes in calf blood volume indirectly by measurement of alterations in electrical resistance through the legs in an effort to detect changes in blood flow into and out of the legs. Thigh cuff inflation leads to temporary venous obstruction, and the volume response in the calf is indirectly measured during inflation and deflation of the cuff. This test accurately diagnoses DVT in the proximal veins of the lower extremities—that is, veins above the popliteal space—but it is not as helpful in detecting calf vein disease. This test is inexpensive and has been well standardized. As a noninvasive test, it has become a commonly employed procedure for the diagnosis of proximal leg DVT.

Doppler ultrasound of the lower extremities evaluates variations in sounds and visual images, which represent changes in lower-extremity blood flow. As with impedance plethysmography, Doppler ultrasound requires both performance and interpretive skills. It is useful in diagnosing proximal leg clots by demonstrating an absence of normal vascular compressibility because the venous segment is thrombosed (see Figure 13-3), as found in our patient. Like impedance plethysmography, Doppler ultrasound is a highly reliable test for determining DVT.

Figures 13-4 and 13-5 show a step-by-step practical approach to the diagnosis of DVT and PE, respectively.

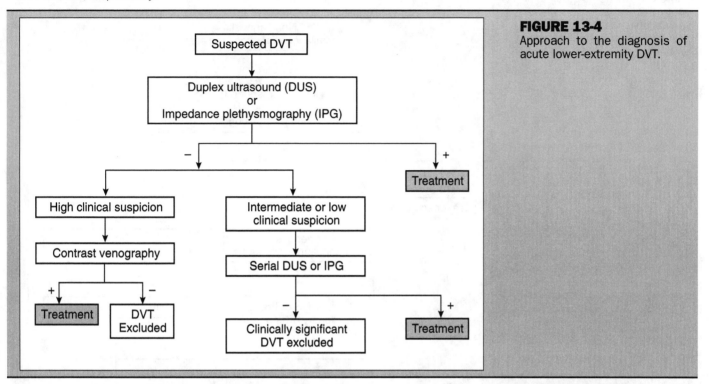

FIGURE 13-4
Approach to the diagnosis of acute lower-extremity DVT.

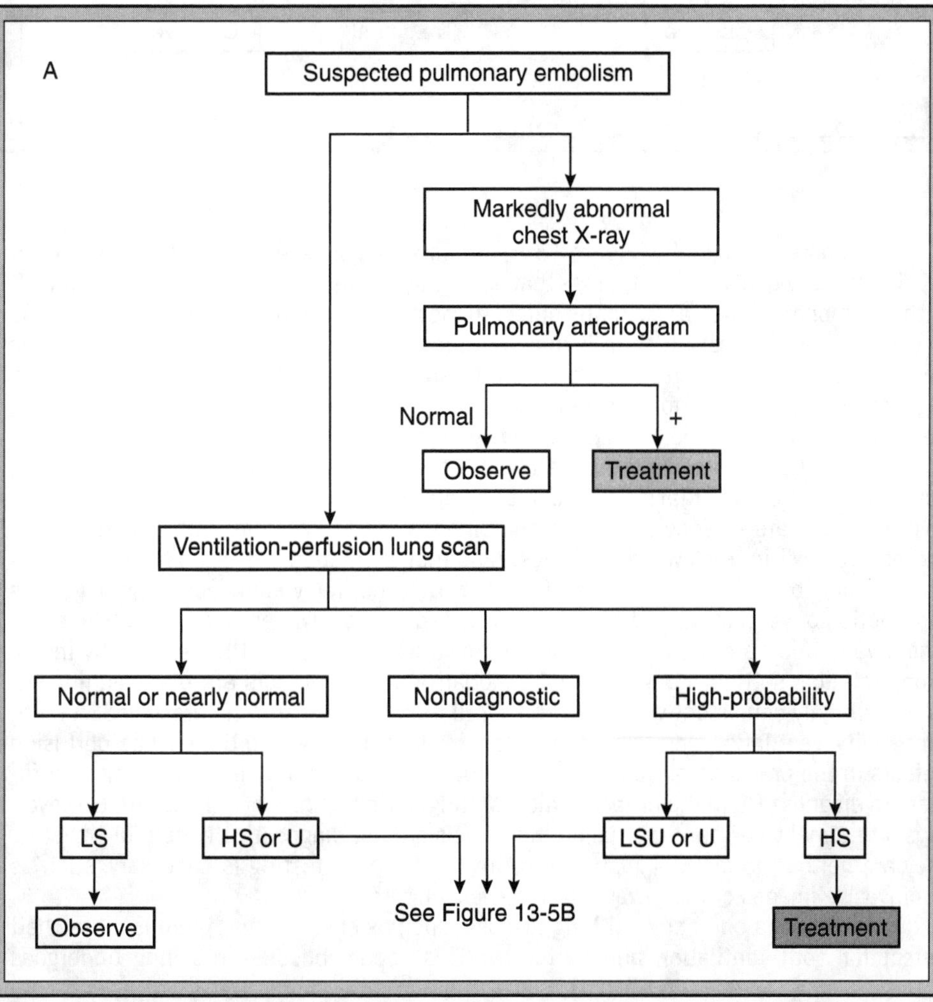

FIGURE 13-5A
Approach to the diagnosis of acute PE in patients with apparent clinical stability.

FIGURE 13-5B
Approach to the diagnosis of acute PE in patients whose ventilation-perfusion lung scans are other than normal or high-probability.

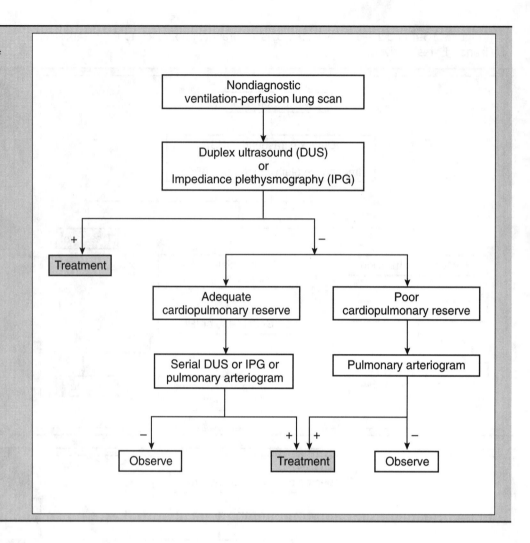

Pulmonary arteriogram remains the gold standard for the diagnosis of PE.

Perfusion defects to lung segments or lobes are more significant, and are highly consistent with PE when ventilation to those areas is preserved.

A high-probability interpretation is sufficient to diagnose PE in the proper clinical setting. Most abnormal ventilation-perfusion lung scans are not diagnostically helpful.

Pulmonary angiography (Figure 13-6) remains the gold standard for the diagnosis of PE. There are two diagnostic findings that are highly consistent with PE: an abrupt cut-off of the pulmonary vessel, and a filling defect in the presence of incomplete obstruction. As in venography, contrast medium is injected directly into the pulmonary artery, and this invasive procedure, which is associated with significant but low morbidity, requires a highly trained physician for performance and interpretation. Therefore, angiography is performed only when other, less invasive tests remain ambiguous.

For most patients, as for the patient in our case study, the ventilation-perfusion lung scan has become the initial study of choice when PE is suspected, because it is noninvasive and accurate—especially when combined with studies that help document the presence of DVT in the lower extremities. A normal ventilation-perfusion lung scan rules out the diagnosis of PE. This type of study should normally show nearly homogenous distribution of ventilation and perfusion. As noted previously, perfusion defects in areas where ventilation are normal, or nearly normal, signify possible PE—especially in the proper clinical setting. Lung segment or lobar perfusion defects are more significant, findings highly consistent with PE when ventilation to those areas is preserved. A high-probability ventilation-perfusion lung scan is described as multiple lobar perfusion defects in the presence of normal ventilation. A high-probability interpretation is sufficient to diagnose PE in the proper clinical setting, as in the case of our patient. However, most abnormal ventilation-perfusion lung scans are not diagnostically helpful—that is, they are neither normal nor high probability, and further testing is necessary, such as noninvasive images of the lower-extremity vasculature.

When there is parenchymal lung disease, such as emphysema, there is a matched defect for both ventilation and perfusion. This occurs because the lung undergoes

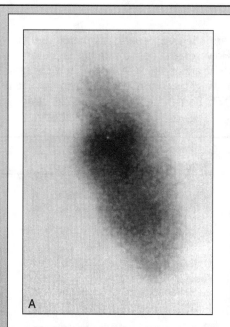
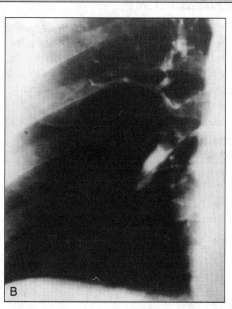

FIGURE 13-6
Perfusion lung scan in a patient with pulmonary embolism, proven by pulmonary angiography (B), showing absent perfusion to right lung.

hypoxic vasoconstriction, and areas of nonventilated or poorly ventilated lung are not being perfused.

As previously mentioned, intravenous heparin was initiated and thrombolytic therapy was considered. An inferior vena cava filter (Greenfield filter) was placed in order to prevent further PE from occurring (Figure 13-7). This option was chosen, in addition to using heparin for initial anticoagulation, because of the presence of a free-floating clot, a high-risk factor for recurrent embolization. In this patient who has hypotension and serious acute pulmonary hypertension, a second embolic event could be fatal.

Thrombolytic therapy is rejected at this point to avoid the risk of intracranial bleeding, because there is the possibility that metastatic brain cancer could develop from his pulmonary malignancy.

Case Study:
Resolution

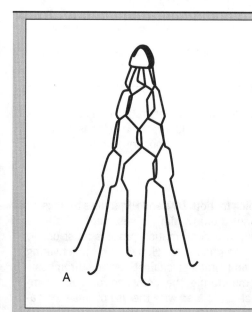
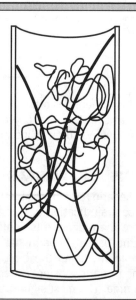

FIGURE 13-7
(A) Greenfield inferior vena cava (IVC) filter. (B) Bird's nest IVC filter.

■ MANAGEMENT

Both DVT and PE are treated with systemic heparin therapy. Heparin is generally administered by a continuous intravenous infusion. However, the best treatment is preventative, but this is not always possible. In patients who are at high risk for DVT, low dosages of standard heparin therapy or low-molecular-weight heparin (LMWH) can be used prophylactically to prevent the formation of DVT. So can certain mechanical devices (prophylactic measures) (Table 13-6).

> Both DVT and PE are treated with systemic heparin therapy.

Table 13-6
Incidence of Thromboembolic Events after Surgery or Trauma or with Certain Medical Conditions and Recommended DVT Prophylaxis

RISK GROUP AND THROMBOEMBOLIC INCIDENCE		RECOMMENDATION
Low Risk Under 40 years old Minor surgery (< 60 min duration) Bedridden, uncomplicated Medical patients, pregnancy		Early ambulation and graduated-compression stockings (GCS)
Incidence (%):		
Distal DVT	2-6	
Proximal DVT	0.4-1.0	
PE	0.2-1.0	
Fatal PE	0.002	
Moderate Risk[a] Over 40 years old Abdominal, pelvic, thoracic surgery Myocardial infarction, cardiomyopathy, previous thromboembolism		Early ambulation and low-dosage heparin (LDH) or low-molecular-weight heparin (LMWH) or intermittent pneumatic compression (IPC)[b]
Incidence (%):		
Distal DVT	8-40	
Proximal DVT	1-8	
PE	1-8	
Fatal PE	0.1-0.4	
High Risk[a] Elderly Extended surgery duration Hip and major knee surgery Fractured hip Extensive trauma including soft-tissue injury and multiple fractures[c] Stroke		PIC and LDH or LMWH and early ambulation
Incidence (%):		For elective hip and major knee surgery, use low-dosage warfarin or adjusted-dosage heparin or LMWH and IPC with early ambulation
Distal DVT	40-80	
Proximal DVT	10-20	
PE	5-10	
Fatal PE	1-5	

[a] Risk is increased further by the following factors: obesity, prolonged bedrest, estrogens, and venous varicosities.
[b] IPC is the prophylactic method of choice for neurosurgery, ophthalmologic surgery, certain urologic procedures, or when the bleeding risk is considered to be high.
[c] Consider early placement of vena cava filter.

Additional therapies other than anticoagulation include general medical supportive care, such as supplemental oxygen and medications to support the cardiovascular system. Occasionally, surgical intervention, in the form of pulmonary thrombectomy, is necessary.

HEPARINS AND WARFARIN

Standard heparin remains the treatment of choice for both DVT and PE, unless there is an absolute contraindication to using anticoagulant therapy. Many times, heparin is initiated before the diagnosis is confirmed. However, a confirmation process must occur, because the use of heparin has significant complications. Heparin, by inactivating antithrombin III, slows the clotting process and protects against further thrombosis formation. Heparin dosing is regulated by monitoring the activated partial thromboplastin time. The most significant side effect associated with the use of this medication is bleeding. Continuous infusion of heparin, carefully regulated, may reduce the incidence of bleeding as a complication.

> Standard heparin remains the treatment of choice for both DVT and PE.

Low-molecular-weight heparins (LMWHs) are now being used in the treatment of DVT and are under consideration as therapy for PE. These heparins, which consist of smaller molecules of standard heparin, have a high affinity for certain blood clotting factors but also work by inhibiting antithrombin III. A standard dose of LMWH is administered and coagulation parameters do not have to be monitored. The principal side effect of this medication is bleeding.

Warfarin is an oral anticoagulant that is used for long-term anticoagulation, after the initial use of heparin. Warfarin acts by inactivating the vitamin K–dependent coagulation factors (II, VII, IX, and X, and protein C, which acts with protein S). The effect of warfarin is initially delayed, until the vitamin K–dependent factors are depleted and the patient becomes therapeutically anticoagulated. Heparin is continued until warfarin is therapeutic. The prothrombin time is monitored on a regular basis in order to optimize therapy and reduce the risk of complications, specifically bleeding. The complications of heparin and warfarin are listed in Table 13-7.

> Warfarin is an oral anticoagulant that is used for long-term anticoagulation, after the initial use of heparin.

Complications of Heparin
Hemorrhage
Decreased platelets (autoimmune)
Osteoporosis
Hyperkalemia (distal RTA)
White clot syndrome (arterial clot)
Hypoaldosteronism
Alopecia
Allergy
Complications of Warfarin
Hemorrhage
Warfarin-induced skin necrosis
Embryopathy (at 6–12 weeks' gestation)

Table 13-7
Complications of Heparin and Warfarin

THROMBOLYTIC THERAPY

Streptokinase, urokinase, and tissue plasminogen activator are three thrombolytic medications that have been approved for treatment of DVT and PE. These medications lyse or dissolve clots, and their use has been focused on massive PE or severe extensive bilateral lower-extremity thrombosis. The principal side effect of these medications, as for other anticoagulants, is bleeding. The risk of intracranial bleeding seems to be higher with these medications than with heparin and warfarin.

VENA CAVA INTERRUPTION AND EMBOLECTOMY

Inferior vena cava (IVC) interruption is rarely indicated, because anticoagulation is highly effective. For patients who have a high risk of bleeding or who are actively bleeding, and for whom there is an absolute contraindication for anticoagulation, vena cava interruption by use of a filter is recommended. This filter is inserted into the IVC, below the renal veins, using a percutaneous approach under local anesthesia. Table 13-8 lists the indications for IVC interruption. When the filter is in place in the IVC, it acts as a mechanical barrier against further embolization of clots. Surgical pulmonary embolectomy or lower-extremity deep vein embolectomy is rarely performed, but would be considered in the case of life-threatening massive PE or a severe extensive lower-extremity venous clot that has not responded to medical intervention.

Acute pulmonary embolism in a patient who has an absolute contraindication to anticoagulation
Following serious trauma where there is a high embolic risk and little patient reserve
When DVT or PE reoccurs despite adequate anticoagulation
Large free-floating clot in the deep venous system
Patients with pulmonary hypertension secondary to chronic pulmonary embolic disease

Table 13-8
Indications for Inferior Vena Cava Interruption

▌REVIEW QUESTIONS

Questions 1–3

A 66-year-old man with a history of prostate cancer, 2 weeks after a transurethral prostatic resection (TURP) and 5 days after being discharged to home, presents to the ED with acute onset chest pain, diaphoresis, and near-syncope that began while he was sitting at the dining room table with his family. In the ED he is tachycardic and tachypneic, with a temperature of 100.6°F, a blood pressure of 98/56, and a pulse oximetry on 100% oxygen by face mask of 95%. Examination reveals jugular venous distention, regular sinus rhythm with increased pulmonic second sound (P_2), clear lungs, and a normal abdomen. The lower extremities show evidence of chronic venous stasis, edema, and calf pain.

1. Which one of the following is the finding most likely to aid in the diagnosis of DVT?

   (A) Edema
   (B) Calf pain
   (C) Chronic venous stasis
   (D) Lower-extremity Doppler evidence

2. The most frequent ECG finding in the presence of PE is

   (A) S1-Q3-T3 pattern and P-pulmonale
   (B) sinus tachycardia segment depression and elevation
   (C) atrial fibrillation
   (D) sinus tachycardia

3. The gold standard for the diagnosis of PE is

   (A) Doppler ultrasound of the legs
   (B) ventilation-perfusion scan
   (C) pulmonary arteriogram
   (D) venogram of the lower extremities

■ ANSWERS AND EXPLANATIONS

1. The answer is D. Only 50% of patients who have clinically suspected DVT have it confirmed by Doppler ultrasound or venography. The signs and symptoms of DVT are nonspecific.

2. The answer is D. Tachycardia and normal are the most frequent ECG findings in the presence of PE. The classic S1-Q3-T3 pattern is rare, being present in only 10% of the cases.

3. The answer is C. The lower-extremity venogram remains the gold standard for diagnosis of DVT, but has been widely replaced by Doppler ultrasound because of its noninvasive but accurate results. The V/Q scan remains the study of choice for diagnosis of PE, but in most cases it is indeterminate, leading to the use of the gold standard, the pulmonary arteriogram.

Chapter 14

LUNG CANCER

David S. Kukafka, M.D.
John M. Travaline, M.D.

■ CHAPTER OUTLINE

Learning Objectives
Case Study: Introduction
Epidemiology of Lung Cancer
Etiology of Lung Cancer
Clinical Presentation of Lung Cancer
Case Study: Continued
Diagnostic Work-up of Lung Cancer
Major Histologic Types of Lung Cancer
Staging of Lung Cancer
The Solitary Pulmonary Nodule
Therapy for Lung Cancer
Case Study: Continued
Complications of Lung Cancer
Case Study: Resolution
Prognosis in Lung Cancer
Review Questions

■ LEARNING OBJECTIVES

At the completion of this chapter, the reader should:
- Know the epidemiologic factors and risks for lung cancer.
- Know the diagnostic approach and work-up for patients with possible lung cancer.
- Understand the basic histology of lung cancer as related to clinical practice.
- Know the basic classification and staging of lung cancer.
- Understand the various treatment modalities for lung cancer.
- Be able to recognize the complications and systemic manifestations of lung cancer and paraneoplastic syndromes.

Case Study:
Introduction

L.B., a 58-year-old man with a 10-year history of hypertension, presents to his physician with a 3-month history of cough productive of intermittent blood-tinged sputum. He admits to smoking one pack of cigarettes per day since he was 17 years old. For the last 10 years, he has had a chronic morning cough with yellow sputum, but over the last 3 months has been coughing more frequently, occasionally producing blood flecks mixed with white-colored sputum. In addition, he notes a 10-lb weight loss, decreased appetite, and a voice that sounds "more gravelly." He denies exposure to tuberculosis and notes a negative skin test on a routine testing while he was in the service at age 20.

On physical examination he is comfortable at rest, with a respiratory rate of 20 breaths per minute. Examination of head, ears, eyes, nose, and throat is unremarkable. There was no adenopathy in the neck. A lung exam reveals normal, equal breath sounds. The rest of his exam is normal. There is no digital clubbing.

Chest x-ray reveals normal lung fields and a normal cardiac silhouette. Lab data reveal normal chemistries, with a mild increase in white blood cell count. Results of pulmonary function studies are shown in Table 14-1. The flow-volume loop is shown in Figure 14-1.

Table 14-1	PARAMETER	ACTUAL	% OF PREDICTED
Pulmonary Function Data for Patient in Case Study	FVC	3.86 L	92
	FEV$_1$	2.01 L	62
	FEV$_1$/FVC*	60%	—

* FEV$_1$/FVC is less than 75%, indicating an obstructive pattern.

FIGURE 14-1
Abnormal flow-volume loop for patient in case study, showing truncation of the expiratory limb, which is indicative of an intrathoracic obstruction.

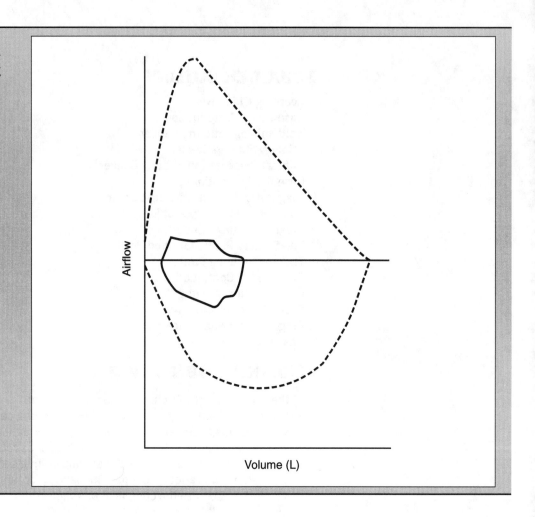

Airflow

Volume (L)

EPIDEMIOLOGY OF LUNG CANCER

Lung cancer is the leading cause of cancer death.

Lung cancer is the most frequent cause of cancer death in the United States, producing approximately 28% of all cancer deaths. It is estimated that nearly 180,000 persons in 1996 were newly diagnosed with lung cancer, and there were more than 150,000 lung cancer deaths in 1996. Lung cancer is also the leading cause of cancer death in women. Despite increased knowledge, therapies, and an enormous amount of research effort, there has been no significant change in the survival rate for patients with lung cancer over the past two decades.

ETIOLOGY OF LUNG CANCER

Cigarette smoking and asbestos exposure produce the greatest risks for the development of lung cancer.

Cigarette smoking accounts for approximately 85% of bronchogenic cancer. The risks of smoking are directly related to the number of cigarettes smoked per day, the number of years one smoked, the depth of inhalation, the age of initiation of smoking, and the amount of tar in the cigarettes smoked. Predisposing factors for lung cancer related to smoking, and the relative risks for developing lung cancer, are shown in Table 14-2. If we assign a value of 1 to the risk of lung cancer in someone who has had no exposure to

FACTOR	RELATIVE RISK	Table 14-2
Nonsmoker	1	Factors and Relative Risks for
Smoker, 1 to 2 packs per day	42	Lung Cancer
Ex-smoker	2 to 10	
Passive smoke exposure	1.5 to 2	
Asbestos exposure	5	
Asbestos and tobacco	90	

tobacco smoke and has never smoked, then the risk for a person who smokes one to two packs of cigarettes per day is approximately 42. Although cigar and pipe smokers have an increased risk for lung cancer, it is substantially less than that of cigarette smokers. Moreover, ex-smokers are estimated to have a risk value of 2 to 10.

There is also evidence that persons exposed to passive or "second-hand" smoke are at increased risk for lung cancer. For example, it is estimated that nonsmoking wives of smokers have approximately 1.5 to 2 times the normal risk for development of lung cancer. Asbestos exposure is another risk factor that increases one's chance of developing lung cancer. Moreover, the relative risk is significantly higher when smoking is added to asbestos exposure. A nonsmoker, for example, exposed to asbestos has about 5 times the normal risk of developing lung cancer. In contrast, a person who is exposed to asbestos and also smokes has a risk value of more than 90. Certain chemicals, which include chloromethyl ether, nickel, arsenic as found in glass, paints, and pesticides, and aromatic hydrocarbons found in the petroleum industry, as well as ionizing radiation, are listed among the occupational carcinogens for lung cancer.

There is also evidence for radon, which is a naturally occurring decay product of uranium, being associated with an increased risk for lung cancer. When radon is inhaled, it may contribute to the risk of bronchogenic cancer.

CLINICAL PRESENTATION OF LUNG CANCER

The clinical presentation of lung cancer may range from an unexpected finding on a chest x-ray to problems that a patient may suffer from local airway effects, mediastinal involvement, or metastases. Local airway involvement of lung cancer typically presents as cough, hemoptysis, dyspnea, or wheezing. Manifestations of mediastinal spread of lung cancer include 1) hoarseness as a result of direct recurrent laryngeal nerve invasion; 2) superior vena cava syndrome, which produces plethora, fullness, and dilated neck veins resulting from compression of the superior vena cava with reduction of venous return; and 3) diaphragm paralysis secondary to tumor compression of the phrenic nerve as it courses through the mediastinum. Metastatic disease may present with general symptoms such as weight loss, cachexia, fever, and fatigue, or with specific complaints related to distant tumor involvement such as bone pain, bone fractures, or seizures.

A thorough history of the patient often provides clues to the extent of lung cancer.

Hoarseness may be a sign of mediastinal involvement by lung cancer.

The expiratory limb of the flow-volume loop of the patient suggests large airway obstruction (see Figure 14-1). This abnormality, in conjunction with his history of hemoptysis, weight loss, and an unremarkable chest x-ray, leads to use of fiberoptic bronchoscopy. Bronchoscopy reveals a fungating mass measuring 1 by 2 cm on the anterolateral wall of the distal trachea (Figure 14-2). A biopsy is performed, confirming the diagnosis of squamous cell carcinoma. A chest computed tomography (CT) scan demonstrates local invasion of mediastinal vascular structures by tumor mass.

Case Study:
Continued

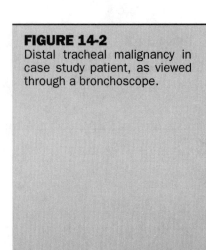

FIGURE 14-2
Distal tracheal malignancy in case study patient, as viewed through a bronchoscope.

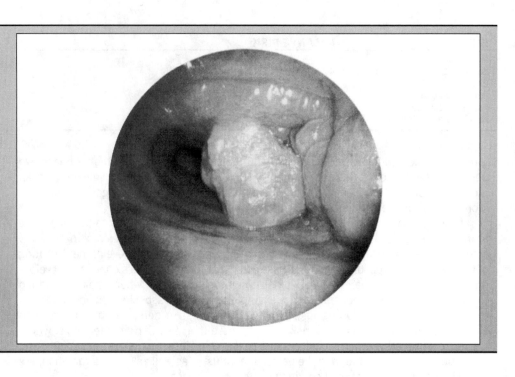

DIAGNOSTIC WORK-UP OF LUNG CANCER

Radiographic stability of a lung mass or nodule for at least 2 years greatly diminishes the likelihood that it is malignant.

The diagnostic work-up of lung cancer should begin with the physician asking the following two questions: 1) does this patient have a detectable lung cancer, and 2) if this patient has lung cancer, what is its type and stage? As in all areas of clinical medicine, the evaluation of the patient begins with a history and physical examination. In evaluating a patient for possible lung cancer, other diagnostic modalities that are used include sputum cytology, radiographic imaging techniques such as chest x-rays, CT scans of the chest and other areas, and magnetic resonance imaging. In addition, bronchoscopy, mediastinoscopy, thoracentesis, and radionuclide scanning are also frequently employed.

The history and physical examination should begin with an assessment of the patient's performance status. Questions as to how functional a patient is are important in helping to assess how well the patient may do with lung cancer, and perhaps help decide whether the patient is able to tolerate therapy that may be associated with major side effects and toxicity. Attention to whether a patient has gained or lost weight is also important, as are inquiries into the signs or symptoms previously mentioned that may be present to assess for the presence of metastatic disease.

Review of chest x-rays is extremely important in the evaluation of a patient being worked up for suspected lung cancer. An x-ray that shows a past abnormality is crucial in this process. If an abnormality on a chest x-ray has been present for 2 or more years without any change in its size, it most likely represents some process other than lung cancer. Moreover, certain patterns of calcification may suggest a benign process. Certain chest x-ray abnormalities suggest specific lung cancer cell types (Table 14-3). Centrally located lesions, especially when found with atelectasis or postobstructive pneumonia, hilar adenopathy, or cavitation, suggest squamous cell carcinoma. Adenocarcinoma typically presents as a peripheral nodule, with occasional pleural or chest wall involvement, and hilar adenopathy. Small cell lung carcinoma typically presents with a rapidly enlarging hilar or perihilar mass with extensive hilar or mediastinal adenopathy. Bronchoalveolar cell carcinoma, a subtype of adenocarcinoma, frequently shows a multicentric pattern of alveolar infiltrates.

Table 14-3
Typical Chest X-Ray Appearance of Cancer by Cell Type

CANCER HISTOLOGY	CHEST X-RAY FEATURES
Adenocarcinoma	Peripheral solitary nodule
Squamous cell	Central lesion
Small cell	Hilar or perihilar mass
Bronchoalveolar cell	Multicentric pneumonic pattern

Anorexia and weight loss are found in approximately one-third of patients at the time of presentation with lung carcinoma. Weakness is also common, and fever may be present and may be related to the underlying tumor itself or be a manifestation of a complication of the tumor, such as bronchial obstruction producing a postobstructive pneumonia. Heterotrophic osteoarthropathy or digital clubbing may be observed in about one-third of the patients presenting with lung carcinoma.

After the history, physical examination, and review of the x-rays have been completed, a complete blood cell count, urinalysis, liver function tests, and serum calcium should be obtained.

Bronchoscopy is also a valuable tool in the evaluation process, particularly if a "central" tumor or tumor in the proximal large bronchi exists. This procedure may produce a diagnostic yield higher than 90% for directly visualized central tumors of the airway. More peripheral tumors, or tumors in the lung parenchyma, not able to be visualized by bronchoscopy, however, are less likely to be diagnosed with this procedure, and may require additional invasive diagnostic procedures, such as a transthoracic needle aspiration or perhaps open thoracotomy with direct surgical biopsy.

> Bronchoscopy is frequently performed to obtain a biopsy and establish the diagnosis of lung cancer.

■ MAJOR HISTOLOGIC TYPES OF LUNG CANCER

The major histologic types of lung cancer can be divided into two broad categories: 1) small cell lung carcinoma and 2) non–small cell lung carcinoma, which includes squamous cell carcinoma, adenocarcinoma including the bronchoalveolar subtype, and large cell carcinoma. Table 14-4 lists the major types of lung cancer and the associated prevalence of each type.

> The two major categories of lung cancer are small cell and non–small cell lung carcinoma (SCLC and NSCLC).

TYPE	APPROXIMATE PREVALENCE
Small cell lung carcinoma	25%
Non–small cell lung carcinoma	
Squamous cell carcinoma	30%
Adenocarcinoma	20%
Bronchoalveolar cell carcinoma	15%
Large cell carcinoma	10%

Table 14-4
Classification and Approximate Prevalence of Lung Cancer

Histologically, small cell lung carcinoma (SCLC) typically appears as very small cells with very little cytoplasm (Figure 14-3). Clinically, these cells are usually manifested grossly by central masses and lymphadenopathy in the thorax. Endoscopically they may appear to have mucosal or submucosal invasion. SCLC accounts for approximately 25% of all lung cancers. It is staged and treated differently than NSCLC.

> The most common type of lung cancer is NSCLC.

Non–small cell lung carcinoma (NSCLC) includes squamous cell carcinoma, adenocarcinoma, and large cell carcinoma. Squamous cell carcinoma typically arises from the squamous epithelium in the proximal bronchi. Histologically there is keratinization or "pearls," which are flattened cells surrounded by a central core of keratin. These "pearls" are a distinctive feature of squamous cell carcinoma (Figure 14-4). Histologically, intercellular bridges may also be noted. Hypercalcemia, as discussed later, is a very common paraneoplastic syndrome associated with squamous cell carcinoma, and is secondary to the elaboration of a substance similar to parathyroid hormone (PTH). Squamous cell carcinoma is the least likely lung cancer to metastasize. Over 50% of patients who die from squamous cell carcinoma have disease confined solely to the thorax.

> NSCLC includes squamous cell carcinoma, adenocarcinoma, and large cell carcinoma.

Adenocarcinoma, on the other hand, is derived from bronchial gland cells. Clinically it is a tumor that is most commonly found in the periphery of the lung, and typically metastasizes to the liver, adrenal glands, bone, and central nervous system. At autopsy, in fact, the brain is involved in over one-half of the cases. Adenocarcinomas are associated with a variety of paraneoplastic syndromes produced by the tumor cells secreting growth hormone, corticotropin, calcitonin, or follicle-stimulating hormone (FSH). Hypertrophic osteoarthropathy (digital clubbing), which is sometimes painful, is frequently seen with adenocarcinoma as in other types of NSCLC.

> Hypercalcemia is most commonly associated with squamous cell carcinoma.

Large cell carcinoma is a type of NSCLC that cannot be histologically classified as either adenocarcinoma or squamous carcinoma by light microscopy. There are two subtypes of large cell carcinoma: giant cell carcinoma and clear cell carcinoma. Clear cell carcinoma has features that resemble those of renal cell carcinoma.

FIGURE 14-3
Photomicrograph demonstrating the typical histologic appearance of small cell lung carcinoma.

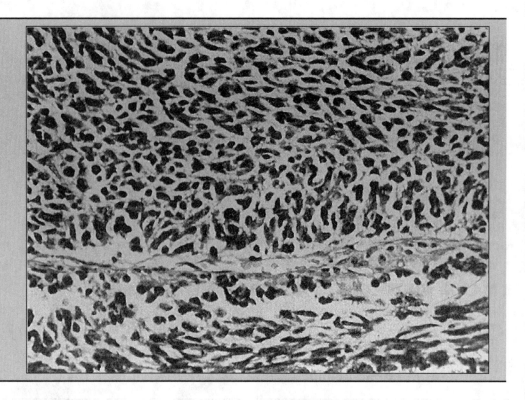

FIGURE 14-4
Photomicrograph demonstrating the typical histologic appearance of squamous cell carcinoma. Note the presence of a squamous "pearl."

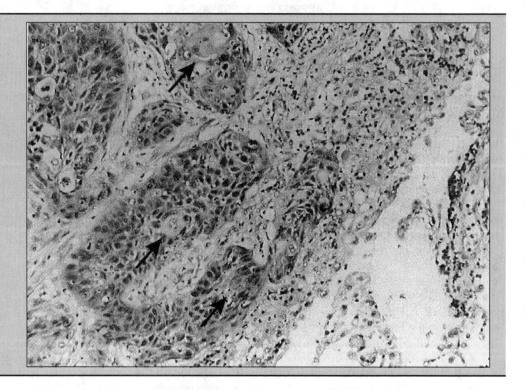

▌STAGING OF LUNG CANCER

The staging for lung carcinoma varies depending on whether the patient has the small cell or the non–small cell variety of cancer. SCLC is typically staged as either limited—that is, a tumor that is confined to one hemithorax or can be incorporated into one radiation port—or extensive—that is, a tumor that extends beyond one hemithorax. Staging for NSCLC, however, is based on a system that incorporates the size of the tumor, the presence and location of lymph node involvement by the cancer, and the presence or absence of metastasis. These three components define the TNM system, where T stands for tumor size and location, N for nodal involvement, and M for metastasis (Table 14-5). The TNM system helps the clinician estimate the prognosis for a patient with lung carcinoma and select treatment options, and provides a basis for standardizing data reporting from clinical trials in lung cancer.

Stage 0	Carcinoma in situ
Stage IA	T1 N0 M0
Stage IB	T2 N0 M0
Stage IIA	T1 N1 M0
Stage IIB	T2 N1 M0 or T3 N0 M0
Stage IIIA	T1-3 N2 M0 or T3 N1 M0
Stage IIIB	T4 Any N M0 or Any T N3 M0
Stage IV	Any T Any N M1

T1 = tumor ≤ 3 cm; T2 = tumor > 3 cm; T3 = tumor invading chest wall; T4 = tumor invading mediastinum; N0 = no lymph node metastasis; N1 = ipsilateral hilar node metastasis; N2 = ipsilateral mediastinal node metastasis; N3 = contralateral node metastasis; M0 = no distant metastasis; M1 = distant metastasis.

Table 14-5
Staging for Non–Small Cell Lung Carcinoma

■ THE SOLITARY PULMONARY NODULE

A particularly common clinical situation is the patient with a solitary pulmonary nodule, which is defined as a single, well-circumscribed lesion smaller than 3 cm within the lung parenchyma. The differential diagnosis for a solitary pulmonary nodule is broad, but the most important diagnosis to establish is that of malignancy. The likelihood of a solitary pulmonary nodule being malignant in any patient increases with age, so that, for example, a patient who is over 50 years old and smokes has a chance of malignancy of more than 50%. Previous chest x-rays are useful, particularly if the lesion can be demonstrated to have been present and without growth for at least 2 years, again suggesting that the lesion is not malignant. In evaluating a patient with a solitary pulmonary nodule, a chest CT may be helpful in assessing for mediastinal adenopathy, which if present may suggest an alternative stage of disease.

Perhaps the most important point with respect to the evaluation and management of a solitary pulmonary nodule is to avoid a delay in diagnosis. This is often achieved by having the patient undergo thoracotomy for the purpose of sampling the nodule for diagnosis, and at the same time removing the nodule, giving the patient the greatest chance for cure from possible lung carcinoma.

■ THERAPY FOR LUNG CANCER

The therapy for lung carcinoma can be categorized on the basis of the histology of the cancer (Table 14-6). Patients with SCLC may undergo chemotherapy, radiation therapy, and possibly surgery. Chemotherapeutic agents used include alkylating agents, such as cyclophosphamide, carmustine (BCNU), and lomustine (CCNU); *Vinca*; alkaloids; and doxorubicin. The major toxicities from such chemotherapies include myelosuppression, alopecia, hemorrhage, cystitis, neurotoxicity, mucositis, and cardiac injury. Combined modality therapy with concurrent chest irradiation is an option for limited cases of SCLC. Prophylactic brain radiation is also sometimes given if a complete response to chemotherapy is achieved, so as to decrease the occurrence of brain metastasis.

Chemotherapy is the primary treatment for SCLC.

THERAPY	SCLC	NSCLC
Surgery	Limited role	Yes, depending on stage
Chemotherapy	Yes	Investigational protocols
Radiation therapy	Yes	Yes

Table 14-6
Therapy for Lung Cancer

For NSCLC, surgery is the best option when it can be offered. Radiation therapy for patients with nodal involvement is important, either preoperatively or postoperatively. Palliative radiation therapy for symptoms of pain, hemoptysis, or superior vena cava syndrome is also important in NSCLC. The exact role of chemotherapy in NSCLC remains experimental and is currently undergoing intense investigation.

Case Study:
Continued

The patient has stage IIIB lung cancer (see Table 14-5) and therefore is not a candidate for surgery. He is referred for radiation therapy and is also considered for palliative laser bronchoscopy to debulk the tumor in his airway and improve his airway function. Two weeks after his diagnosis, he notices progressive swelling of both arms. In addition, his wife notes that he has become lethargic.

He is admitted to the hospital. His exam is remarkable for bilateral upper-extremity swelling and facial and periorbital edema. Admission laboratory data are as follows: glucose, 110 mg/dL (normal); sodium, 136 mEq/L (normal); potassium, 4.2 mM (normal); creatinine, 1.2 (normal); and calcium, 15.5 mM (elevated). A CT scan of the head is normal. A CT scan of the thorax reveals progressive enlargement of a mediastinal tumor, with encasement of the superior vena cava (Figure 14-5).

FIGURE 14-5
Chest CT scan of case study patient, showing compression of the superior vena cava by a large tumor mass.

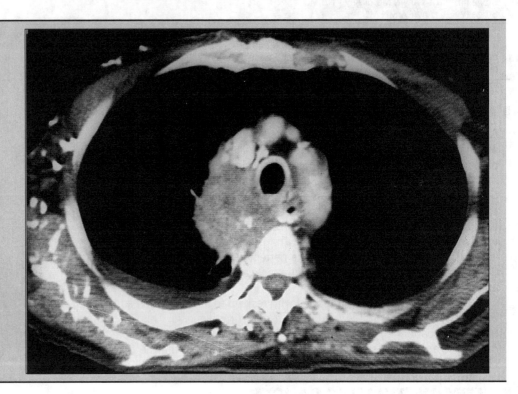

■ COMPLICATIONS OF LUNG CANCER

There are various complications of lung cancer that are either produced by mechanical effects of the cancer or associated with the primary cancer. Table 14-7 lists many of these complications.

Table 14-7
Complications of Lung Cancer

COMPLICATION	COMMON CELL TYPE	PREVALENCE	ASSOCIATED ABNORMALITIES
Pancoast's tumor	Squamous cell	2–5%	Horner's syndrome
SVC syndrome	Non–small cell		Facial swelling, dilated neck and chest wall veins
Central airway obstruction	Squamous cell		Flattened inspiratory or expiratory limbs of the flow-volume loop
Paraneoplastic syndromes:			
SAIDH	Small cell	5–10%	Hyponatremia
Hypercalcemia	Squamous cell		Lethargy, constipation
Eaton-Lambert syndrome	Small cell		Fatigability
Increased ACTH	Small cell	25%	Cushing's syndrome
Digital clubbing	Non–small cell		Pain, swelling

MECHANICAL/LOCAL COMPLICATIONS

Superior Vena Cava Syndrome. Superior vena cava (SVC) syndrome is a complication of lung carcinoma produced by the obstruction of the superior vena cava, typically by bronchogenic carcinoma. Early symptoms of this syndrome include facial fullness progressing to facial or arm edema, dilated veins over the anterior chest wall, jugular vein distention, and engorgement of the veins of the arms and hands. This complication usually responds very nicely to treatment of the underlying cancer with either radiation therapy or chemotherapy, depending on the type of carcinoma cell involved. In the case study, the typical findings of upper-extremity edema and facial fullness are present.

Pancoast's Tumor. Pancoast's tumor, by definition, is a tumor of the superior sulcus of the lung apex. It occurs in approximately 2% to 5% of patients with bronchogenic carcinoma. It is typically of a squamous cell variety, although it rarely can be associated with SCLC. It usually presents with symptoms of pain and sometimes upper-extremity weakness. It involves invasion of the brachial plexus with an incidence of approximately 40% at the time of presentation. Pancoast's tumor is frequently (about 60% of the time) associated with Horner's syndrome, which is the presence of ptosis, myosis, and anhidrosis. These findings are produced by invasion of the cervical sympathetic chain by the tumor.

Airway Lesions. Airway lesions may also complicate lung cancer. When lung cancer involves the airways, producing obstruction of the large airways, a characteristic pattern of the flow-volume curve may be observed, depending on the nature and location of the obstruction (Figure 14-6). For example, with a tumor in the extrathoracic airway, there is limitation of flow on the inspiratory portion of the flow-volume curve. This occurs because intratracheal pressure is lower than the surrounding atmospheric pressure on inspiration, thus flattening the inspiratory portion of the flow-volume curve. On expiration, however, intra-airway pressure exceeds the surrounding atmospheric pressure, thus producing a normal contour of the flow-volume curve on expiration. Conversely, with a tumor located within the intrathoracic airway, intra-airway pressure is greater than the surrounding pleural pressure on inspiration, and thus inspiratory flow is normal. On expiration, however, with an intrathoracic airway tumor, the surrounding pleural pressure is greater than the intra-airway pressure, producing a flattening of the expiratory portion of the flow-volume curve.

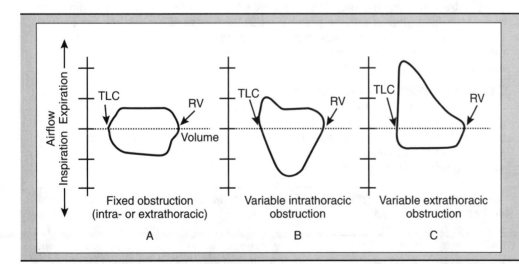

FIGURE 14-6
Representative examples of the various patterns of abnormal flow-volume loops found with intra- and extrathoracic airway obstruction.

PARANEOPLASTIC SYNDROMES

Paraneoplastic syndromes are extrapulmonary processes that occur in conjunction with lung cancer and cannot be explained by direct tumor extension. They appear to be caused by abnormal production of various substances or hormones in conjunction with the cancer cells. It is estimated that up to 20% of patients with lung cancer develop some type of paraneoplastic syndrome. These syndromes also tend to occur more commonly with SCLC. The reason for this is not certain, but may have to do with SCLC cells being embryologically similar to neuroendocrine cells, thus having a propensity to secrete hormonal substances.

Endocrinologic paraneoplastic syndromes include the syndrome of inappropriate antidiuretic hormone (SIADH) and excessive adrenocorticotropic hormone (ACTH) production. Hypercalcemia is an important paraneoplastic syndrome observed mostly in squamous cell cancer, and is attributable to the elaboration of a PTH-like factor. Hypertrophic osteoarthropathy is also associated with lung cancer, as is Eaton-Lambert syndrome, a neuromuscular syndrome characterized by progressive weakness and easy muscle fatigability.

> Paraneoplastic syndromes in lung cancer include SIADH, Cushing's syndrome, hypercalcemia, digital clubbing, and Eaton-Lambert syndrome.

SIADH. The syndrome of inappropriate antidiuretic hormone is the most common paraneoplastic syndrome associated with SCLC. Approximately 5% to 10% of SCLC patients may present with SIADH. Additionally, 40% to 50% can be shown to have subclinical abnormalities compatible with SIADH. The source of the antidiuretic hormone (ADH) may be the primary tumor or its metastasis.

Excess ACTH. The inappropriate release of ACTH is also a common paraneoplastic disorder observed in SCLC. Approximately 25% of patients with SCLC have elevated ACTH, although only 3% to 7% have Cushing's syndrome. The clinical features of this syndrome may be masked by underlying anorexia and weight loss from the tumor itself, so other signs of Cushing's syndrome, such as hypokalemia or hypertension (signs of mineralocorticoid excess), should be sought. Hyperpigmentation may be seen in 25% to 30% of these patients.

Hypercalcemia. Hypercalcemia is more likely to be caused by elaboration of a PTH-like substance in squamous cell carcinoma than by metastasis to bone. It is unusual in SCLC, and if it is present, one is more likely to be dealing with NSCLC or with hypercalcemia from a cause other than the cancer.

In the case study, the patient is found to have an elevated calcium level, and has become lethargic. Such a change in his mental status is probably caused by the hypercalcemia.

Hypertrophic Pulmonary Osteoarthropathy. Hypertrophic pulmonary osteoarthropathy, also commonly referred to as digital clubbing, is a common manifestation of intrathoracic malignancy. The reason for its development is unknown. Pain at the ends of the digits often accompanies this disorder, and suggests periosteal inflammation. Digital clubbing tends to be more common with adenocarcinoma and squamous cell carcinoma than with SCLC. Nonsteroidal anti-inflammatory agents appear to be effective in relief of the pain.

Eaton-Lambert Syndrome. The Eaton-Lambert syndrome is recognized as excessive muscle fatigability, especially of the lower extremities. It is similar to myasthenia gravis in that increased fatigability more so than weakness is the prominent feature. The diagnosis of this syndrome rests on electromyography, which demonstrates facilitation of action potentials with repeated muscle stimulation. Unlike other neuromyopathies, this syndrome typically responds to treatment of the underlying tumor.

Case Study:
Resolution

The patient is admitted to the hospital and receives radiation therapy to relieve compression of the SVC. He also receives intravenous saline and diuretic therapy for the hypercalcemia. He responds well to this treatment and is discharged from the hospital. He continues to decline in a general way, with a progressive loss of appetite, weight loss, and general debility. He died at home 2 months after his discharge from the hospital.

■ PROGNOSIS IN LUNG CANCER

The prognosis in lung cancer is determined largely by the extent of the disease at the time of diagnosis. For NSCLC, when surgery can be performed (usually for stage I and stage II carcinoma), the prognosis is better than for inoperable disease. For SCLC, although surgery is not the primary therapeutic intervention, disease that is limited has a greater likelihood of responding favorably to chemotherapy. Other factors that influence prognosis include the specific site of metastasis (liver metastasis portends a worse prognosis), performance status, weight loss, anemia, and the presence of other diseases.

Anemia is a poor prognostic indicator of lung cancer.

▌REVIEW QUESTIONS

1. The most common mechanism for hypercalcemia associated with lung carcinoma is

   (A) enhanced secretion of parathyroid hormone (PTH)
   (B) bone metastasis
   (C) elaboration of osteoclastic activation factor
   (D) elaboration of PTH-like substance

2. Match each of the following descriptions with the appropriate type of lung cancer from the list below. Typical presentations of lung cancer:

   (1) A tumor characterized histologically by very little cytoplasm visible by light microscopy and a clinical presentation manifested usually by a central mass and lymphoadenopathy, and accounting for approximately one-fourth of all lung cancers.
   (2) A 47-year-old man presents with a cough and a low-grade fever. He has no history of cigarette smoking. Chest x-ray shows a right lower lobe infiltrate. The patient is treated with antibiotics, and his fever goes away. Eight weeks later, his cough persists and the chest x-ray is unchanged.
   (3) The initial presentation chest x-ray of an 82-year-old man with a remote history of cigarette smoking shows a well-defined 2-cm nodule at the periphery of the left upper lobe. On physical examination, he is found to be a little confused and to have digital clubbing and focal tenderness of the L3 vertebra.

   (A) Small cell lung carcinoma
   (B) Squamous cell carcinoma
   (C) Adenocarcinoma
   (D) Large cell carcinoma
   (E) Bronchoalveolar cell carcinoma

3. Regarding solitary pulmonary nodules, which one of the following statements is false?

   (A) A chest CT scan may reveal mediastinal adenopathy not apparent on a chest x-ray.
   (B) Old chest x-rays are usually not helpful.
   (C) Thoracotomy may be appropriate for removing the nodule.
   (D) The probability of the nodule being malignant increases with age.

■ ANSWERS AND EXPLANATIONS

1. The answer is D. Hypercalcemia in lung cancer is most commonly seen with squamous cell carcinoma. The pathophysiology of hypercalcemia when associated with lung cancer is thought to be the elaboration of a PTH-like substance. PTH levels in patients with hypercalcemia of malignancy have been shown to be normal or undetectably abnormal. Bone metastasis may produce pain or fracture, or no symptoms at all. It is not a mechanism for hypercalcemia, however. Osteoclastic activation factor, or, more precisely, elaboration of various cytokines to produce hypercalcemia by osteolytic destruction, is a mechanism of hypercalcemia in metastatic disease such as breast cancer but not in lung cancer.

2. The answers are 1, A; 2, E; 3, C. Small cell lung carcinoma derives its appellation from its appearance under light microscopy. It accounts for approximately 25% of all primary lung cancers. It is typically a rapidly growing cancer and usually presents itself with mediastinal lymphadenopathy. It is treated primarily with chemotherapy. Surgery has little to no role in treatment.

Bronchoalveolar cell carcinoma of the lung is a subtype of adenocarcinoma. It is the lung cancer least associated with cigarette smoking. Its appearance clinically is that of a nonresolving lung infiltrate detected by chest x-ray.

This patient has a peripheral nodule and the suggestion of metastatic disease based on physical examination. Adenocarcinoma is more likely to be metastatic by the time a patient presents to a physician. Its appearance on chest x-ray is usually that of a peripheral nodule. Digital clubbing is more commonly observed in NSCLC than in SCLC.

3. The answer is B. In the evaluation of a solitary pulmonary nodule, the opportunity to review prior chest x-rays is extremely important. The differential diagnosis for solitary pulmonary nodule is very broad. Perhaps the most important diagnosis to exclude from the differential is that of malignancy. Malignant lung nodules grow over time. If it can be demonstrated that a solitary pulmonary nodule has not changed in size over a period of at least 2 years, it generally can be safely considered nonmalignant. Otherwise, evaluation should include a CT scan to assess for lymphadenopathy and/or the presence of other nodules perhaps not visible on chest x-ray. Thoracotomy to remove a nodule suspected of being malignant is the most definitive therapy for lung cancer and may be curative. The probability of a solitary pulmonary nodule being malignant is increased by age, a history of smoking, and its absence on previous chest x-rays older than 2 years.

■ SUGGESTED READING

ATS Statement. Pretreatment evaluation of non-small-cell lung cancer. *Am J Respir Crit Care Med* 156(1):320, 1997.

Carr DT, Holoye PY, Hong WK: Bronchogenic carcinoma. In Murray JF, Nadel JA, eds.: *Textbook of Respiratory Medicine*, Vol. 2. Philadelphia: WB Saunders, 1994, pp. 1528–1596.

Matthay RA (Guest Editor): Lung cancer. *Clin Chest Med* 14(1), 1993. Philadelphia: WB Saunders.

Mountain CF: Revisions in the international system for staging lung cancer. *Chest* 111(6):1710, 1997.

Pritchard RS, Anthony SP: Chemotherapy plus radiotherapy compared with radiotherapy alone in the treatment of locally advanced, unresectable, non–small-cell lung cancer. *Ann Int Med* 125(9):723, 1996.

Chapter 15

MYCOBACTERIAL DISEASES

Perwaiz H. Rahim, M.D.

Samuel L. Krachman, D.O.

■ CHAPTER OUTLINE

Learning Objectives
Case Study: Introduction
Introduction
Classification
Case Study: Continued
Tuberculosis
Case Study: Continued
Case Study: Continued
Case Study: Continued
Nontuberculous Mycobacteria
Case Study: Resolution
Summary
Review Questions

■ LEARNING OBJECTIVES

At the completion of this chapter, the reader should:

- Understand the classification of the mycobacteria, with an emphasis on the differences between *Mycobacterium tuberculosis* and the nontuberculous mycobacteria.
- Know the reasons for the increased prevalence of tuberculosis over the past decade, and be able to identify which groups of individuals are thus at an increased risk of developing active disease.
- Understand how tuberculosis is transmitted, and the immune-mediated mechanism that attempts to control the spread of the disease once an individual becomes infected.
- Understand the screening test used to identify individuals infected with tuberculosis, and how its interpretation is dependent on each individual's immune status.
- Be able to identify the signs, symptoms, and radiographic findings commonly associated with active tuberculosis.
- Understand the diagnostic techniques used to identify mycobacteria infections, including the use and interpretation of polymerase chain reaction (PCR) tests.
- Know the mechanism behind the development of drug resistance and the problems associated with the development of multidrug-resistant tuberculosis.
- Have a working understanding of the most common drug regimens used in the treatment of active tuberculosis and in preventative therapy, as well as the incorporated use of directly observed therapy.
- Better understand the association between HIV and immunodeficiency with the development of active tuberculosis.
- Better understand the nontuberculous mycobacteria that can cause diseases and the treatment of such diseases.

Case Study:
Introduction

R.J. is a 28-year-old black woman who was initially seen in the emergency room with chief complaints of increasing shortness of breath, cough productive of clear sputum, and occasional hemoptysis and associated fever for the past 7 days. R.J. denies any prior pulmonary problems such as asthma during childhood or recurrent pneumonia, and she denies any history of tuberculosis. She states that she had a PPD skin test done for work approximately 1 year ago, which was negative, but she reports that she has recently been around one of her sister's friends who is HIV positive and who was complaining of a cold and had a productive cough approximately 3 weeks ago.

▌INTRODUCTION

Over the past decade, TB has reemerged, with the number of new cases increasing by 14%.

The mycobacteria are a group of organisms that can cause severe parenchymal lung destruction and are a leading cause of death worldwide. *Mycobacterium tuberculosis* (TB) is the most prevalent, with the other forms of mycobacterium more commonly infecting patients with preexisting lung disease or those who are immunocompromised. Over the past decade, TB has reemerged as a serious national problem. Prior to 1984, the incidence of TB had been steadily declining over a period of several decades. From 1985 to 1993, the number of new cases *increased* by 14%. This increase seems to have been related to several factors, including 1) an association of TB with the human immunodeficiency virus (HIV) epidemic; 2) immigrants arriving from countries with a high prevalence of TB; 3) transmission among individuals who are in close contact with each other, such as in nursing homes and prisons; and 4) breakdown of the healthcare structure that had previously been effective in controlling the disease. In addition, recent reports of the emergence of multidrug-resistant organisms have led to a renewed interest in the health care system regarding more effective diagnosis and treatment of patients with active disease. New guidelines have been developed to help deal with these problems. This chapter reviews those aspects of the mycobacteria—particularly TB—that have led to a resurgence of TB, and also reviews the risk factors, diagnosis, treatment, and guidelines that have been developed to help deal with this often devastating group of diseases.

▌CLASSIFICATION

Mycobacteria are obligate aerobic organisms that grow and replicate intracellularly.

Mycobacteria are characterized by the fact that they are able to withstand being decolorized when an acid-alcohol mixture is applied to a slide previously stained with either Ziehl-Neelsen or auramine O (Figure 15-1). In addition, they are obligate aerobic organisms that grow and replicate intracellularly.

FIGURE 15-1
Acid-fast bacilli ("red snappers") seen on Ziehl-Neelsen staining of the sputum.

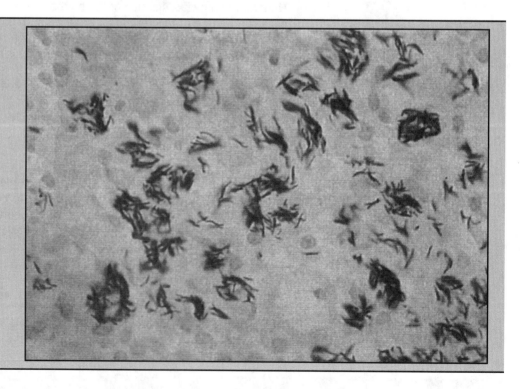

The mycobacteria are classified as either *Mycobacterium tuberculosis* complex or as nontuberculous mycobacteria. The *M. tuberculosis* complex includes *M. tuberculosis*, *M. bovis*, *M. africanum*, and *M. microti*. *M. bovis* and *M. africanum* rarely cause disease, and *M. microti* does not cause disease in humans.

The nontuberculous mycobacteria are generally classified on the basis of their growth rates as well as their ability to produce pigment [Runyon classification (Table 15-1)]. These classification systems are useful clinically because they can help identify pathogenic organisms and guide therapy.

GROUP	NAME	EXAMPLE
1	Photochromogens	*M. kansasii*
2	Scotochromogens	*M. scrofulaceum*
3	Nonchromogens	*M. avium* complex
4	Rapid growers	*M. fortuitum, M. chelonei*

Table 15-1
Runyon Classification of Non-tuberculous Mycobacteria

R.J. states that her fever has been as high as 102°F but denies any associated shaking chills. She does report night sweats requiring her to get up and change her clothes during the night. She states that the blood noted in her sputum is usually streaked and has been intermittent. She denies any occupational exposure history and is a nonsmoker.

Case Study:
Continued

■ TUBERCULOSIS

EPIDEMIOLOGY

With the introduction of antituberculosis medications in the 1940s, it was anticipated that the incidence of TB would decline steadily with the ultimate goal of totally eradicating the disease. This was partially realized in the United States with a 5.6% annual decline in the incidence of TB from 1953 to 1984. However, from 1985 to 1993, the number of new cases unexpectedly and dramatically increased by 14%, from 22,201 to 25,313 cases per year (Figure 15-2). This increase seemed to be related to at least four main factors: 1) the HIV epidemic; 2) immigrants arriving from countries where the incidence of TB is high; 3) transmission of TB in settings where people are closely congregated, such as prisons and homeless shelters; and 4) the breakdown of the healthcare system that in the past had closely monitored TB prevention and treatment.

In addition to the increase in active disease cases, the number of individuals infected with TB also significantly increased. It is estimated that 10 to 15 million people

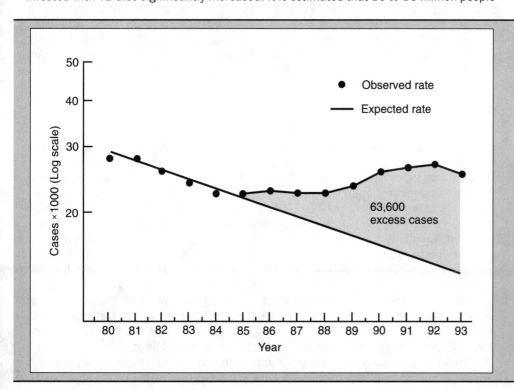

FIGURE 15-2
Expected and observed cases of tuberculosis in the United States between 1980 and 1993. Reproduced with permission from Centers for Disease Control: *Core Curriculum on Tuberculosis: What the Clinician Should Know*, 3rd ed. Atlanta: U.S. Department of Health and Human Services, 1994.

Approximately 10 to 15 million persons in the United States are infected with TB.

in the United States are infected with TB. Those most likely to become infected include 1) close contacts of persons with active disease; 2) foreign-born individuals from countries where TB is commonly found, including countries in Africa, Asia, and Latin America; 3) inhabitants of long-term facilities such as nursing homes; 4) the elderly; 5) intravenous drug abusers (IVDAs); 6) local groups with an increased prevalence, such as migrant farmworkers; and 7) healthcare workers subject to occupational exposure.

Certain groups that are infected also carry increased risks of developing active disease. These groups include: 1) HIV-infected persons (this is the strongest risk factor for developing active disease once infected, increasing the incidence 100-fold over that of individuals infected with TB only); 2) individuals recently infected (during the past 2 years); 3) persons with certain underlying medical illnesses (Table 15-2); 4) IVDAs; 5) patients with prior TB disease who were inadequately treated; and 6) racial and ethnic minorities (when compared with whites, Hispanics, Native Americans, and Alaskans are five times more likely, blacks eight times more likely, and Asians 10 times more likely to develop active disease).

Table 15-2
Conditions That Increase the Risk of Developing Active TB

Recent infection with TB
IVDA
HIV infection
Diabetes mellitus
Silicosis
End-stage renal disease
Prolonged steroid use
Hematologic/reticuloendothelial disease
Immunosuppressive therapy
Chest x-ray findings of previous untreated TB
Head and neck cancer
Intestinal bypass surgery/chronic malabsorption

TRANSMISSION

TB becomes aerosolized with coughing and sneezing, the rate of infection being 10% to 23% for close contacts.

TB becomes aerosolized when a person with active disease coughs or sneezes. These droplet nuclei are small (1 to 5 µm) and can become suspended in the air for up to several hours. People nearby can then inhale these particles and become susceptible to infection. Factors that can increase the risk of infection include the duration of exposure, a high burden of organisms in the infected patient, and an enclosed, poorly ventilated environment. Overall, the rate of infection for a close contact is 21% to 23%. Patients with multidrug-resistant TB or with HIV are no more infectious than other patients. The best method of decreasing the risk of infection is prompt isolation of patients with active disease and initiation of therapy.

PATHOGENESIS

TB is phagocytized by macrophages in the alveoli, with the immune system controlling the spread of infection by 2 to 10 weeks.

Once the air particles containing the TB organisms are inhaled, the smaller droplet nuclei are able to reach the alveoli. Larger particles become lodged in the larger airways. Once in the alveoli, the TB organisms are phagocytized by macrophages and are able to multiply. The bacilli are then able to spread to different organ systems by way of the lymphatics and the blood stream. The immune system is usually able to control the spread and contain replication of the bacilli within 2 to 10 weeks, which is about the same period of time required for a tuberculin skin test to become reactive. It does so by means of T-cell-mediated immunity (a delayed-type hypersensitivity) with the activation of T lymphocytes—specifically, CD4+ helper and CD8+ suppressor T cells. CD4+ helper T cells secrete interferon-γ, which activates the macrophages to destroy the bacilli within them by means of nitrogen intermediates such as nitric oxide. CD8+ suppressor T cells actually kill the macrophages that contain the bacilli, resulting in the formation of caseating granulomas—a finding characteristic of a delayed-type hypersensitivity reaction (Figure 15-3). The mycobacteria are unable to grow in this extracellular environment that is devoid of oxygen, and thus the infection is usually contained.

If the immune system is unable to keep the infection in check, active disease can develop. About 5% of infected individuals develop active disease within the first 2 years.

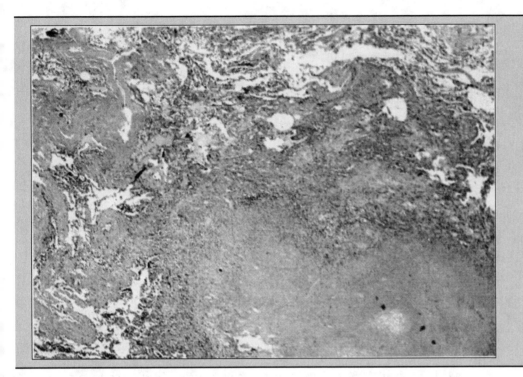

FIGURE 15-3
Granuloma formation with caseation noted in the center, surrounded by giant cells and epithelioid cells.

After that, another 5% develop active disease at some time during their lives. This is to be compared with HIV patients, whose risk of developing active disease is much higher once infected—10% each year compared with 10% over an entire lifetime for nonimmunosuppressed individuals infected with TB.

Although TB disease can involve many organ systems, the lungs are the most commonly involved, with 85% of patients having pulmonary involvement. Other organ systems that can be affected include the pleural space (pleural effusion), the bones and joints (septic arthritis), and the central nervous system (meningitis). TB can also present as a widely disseminated disease, referred to as *miliary TB*.

On physical exam, the patient's temperature is 101.8°F, her pulse is 88, and her respiratory rate is 14. Her blood pressure is 124/76. Her eyes are PEARLA (pupils equal and reactive to light and accommodation), EOMI (extraocular muscles intact). An ear exam shows her tympanic membranes to be intact bilaterally. Her mouth and throat are negative for erythema or exudate. Her neck is without palpable lymphadenopathy. Her heart is regular and her lungs are relatively clear to auscultation bilaterally. Her abdomen is soft, with positive bowel sounds, negative for organomegaly. Her extremities are negative for edema.

Case Study:
Continued

SCREENING

It is important to identify persons who are infected with TB in order to decrease the chance that these individuals will develop active disease in the future. This not only helps the person infected, but also prevents the spread of TB to others. Once identified, infected individuals can receive appropriate therapy. The Mantoux tuberculin skin test is the screening test used to identify infected individuals. It involves the intradermal injection of 0.1 mL of purified protein derivative (PPD) tuberculin (5 tuberculin units) into the anterior forearm surface. The diameter of the induration (not the erythema) that develops 48 to 72 hours later is measured in millimeters and recorded. The size of the tuberculin reaction that is considered positive depends on the patient group (Table 15-3). A reaction in one patient may be considered positive if only 5 mm in diameter, and in another patient negative if less than 15 mm. Thus, it is important to decide for each individual what should be considered a positive tuberculin reaction representing infection with TB.

The Mantoux tuberculin skin test is read at 48 to 72 hours and represents evidence of TB infection.

Table 15-3
Positive Tuberculin Skin Test

≥ 5 mm
Known or suspected HIV+
Close contact of person with active TB
IVDA (uncertain of HIV status)

≥ 10 mm
With certain medical conditions (HIV negative)
From country where TB is common
Underserved racial and ethnic groups/homeless
From long care facilities
Less than 4 years old

≥ 15 mm
No known risk factors for TB

One-third of HIV patients infected with TB are PPD negative.

It is also important to determine that the patient's immune system is functioning properly at the time the tuberculin skin test is performed so that a negative response can be interpreted in the proper context. This is why control antigens to *Candida* and/or mumps are placed on the opposite forearm—antigens to which most individuals have been exposed in the past and that should lead to a reaction. If there is no response to the controls, the person is considered *anergic*, and a negative tuberculin test may not be a true negative. For example, approximately one-third of HIV patients who are infected with TB are PPD negative. This could be related to their low CD4+ lymphocyte counts. However, this does not entirely explain the observation, because positive PPDs can occur in HIV patients with CD4+ counts that are very low (less than 200 per microliter).

From 10% to 25% of patients with active TB have negative PPD tests.

In addition, about 10% to 25% of patients with active TB disease have negative PPDs. This may be related to the fact that they have recently been exposed to and acquired the disease, and yet the 2-to-10-week period necessary to develop a positive skin response has not passed.

Another reason for the PPD to be nonreactive in someone infected with TB is that with time the lymphocytes lose their memory to recognize the antigen to which they were exposed many years earlier. Thus, in older individuals, a second PPD may need to be placed 1 to 3 weeks later to *boost* the immune system so that it recognizes the PPD antigen again. This is referred to as the *booster effect*.

DIAGNOSIS

Chest x-ray findings include infiltrates and/or cavities in the upper lobes or superior segments of the lower lobes.

A thorough initial history and physical examination are extremely important in correctly identifying patients with active disease in order to initiate appropriate therapy. Patients often present with symptoms of cough (which has often been present for a number of weeks) and hemoptysis. In addition, they complain of fever, chills, night sweats, loss of appetite, and associated weight loss. The history should include questions that look for risk factors such as exposure history, country of origin, race and minority status, and risk for HIV. On physical examination there may be evidence to suggest consolidation in the lungs and thus pneumonia, or the exam may be unrevealing. Radiographically, the chest x-ray may demonstrate an abnormality, most commonly at the apices, in the posterior segment of the upper lobe or the superior segment of the lower lobe. These abnormalities can range from a simple infiltrate to cavitary lesions of variable size and shape. Patients with HIV and TB can present with infiltrates in any lobe and with any distribution.

Obtain at least three daily sputum samples, with smears being positive in 40% to 70% of culture-positive cases.

To diagnose active pulmonary TB, one should obtain at least three separate sputum specimens, preferably early in the morning. If the patient is unable to cough up a specimen, sputum production can be induced with inhaled saline. Other methods of obtaining a specimen include the use of bronchoscopy and obtaining a gastric aspirate (although this is more commonly done in infants). If other organ systems are thought to be involved, examination of such specimens as cerebral spinal fluid, urine, and pleural fluid can be considered.

Once obtained, a specimen is initially stained on a slide and looked at microscopically. For sputum it is best first to digest, centrifuge, and thus concentrate the specimen. Traditional stains such as Ziehl-Neelsen and Kinyoun can be used to identify the acid-fast bacilli. Overall, sputum smears are positive in 40% to 70% of culture-positive cases of TB. In many hospitals the initial screening of a specimen is done using a fluorochrome stain, auramine O, with examination under a fluorescent microscope. This method is both faster and more sensitive than traditional staining methods.

Specimens are then inoculated on culture media, including Löwenstein-Jensen, which is egg based, or Middlebrook-Cohn, which is agar based. Cultures grown on these media are inspected every 2 to 3 days but may take up to 6 weeks to demonstrate growth. Radiometric culture systems place ^{14}C palmitic acid in the liquid growth media. As the mycobacteria grow, they liberate $^{14}CO_2$, which can be detected and measured. Growth can be detected earlier, usually within 10 to 14 days.

Newer techniques for identifying mycobacteria include the polymerase chain reaction (PCR) test, which uses small DNA primers that are complements for select regions of the mycobacteria DNA. Once bound, these segments are then amplified in the process. A probe specific for the DNA of a particular species [such as for TB or *Mycobacterium avium* complex (MAC)] is then used, and will bind to the amplified DNA if present. This entire process takes only a few hours. This technique has been used mostly to identify the species of mycobacterium from a culture once growth has been noted. More recently, its direct application to clinical samples (such as sputum) has been examined. Problems remain with the low sensitivity of the test, meaning that a number of samples are negative when tested with PCR, but eventually grow out mycobacteria on culture. However, if the acid fast bacilli (AFB) stain and PCR are both positive, the diagnosis of TB is established. In addition, if the AFB smear and PCR are both negative, it is unlikely that TB will grow from that specimen. It is when the two tests do not agree that the overall clinical picture needs to be considered in determining therapy. This situation of discordance points out why all specimens need to be cultured. In addition, all positive cultures for TB should have drug susceptibility testing performed to rule out resistance.

> PCR testing uses DNA primers to help identify mycobacteria infections.

R.J. is admitted to the hospital and placed in an isolation room. Anyone entering the room is required to wear a particulate respirator mask. A PPD is placed on her left forearm, and controls of Candida and mumps are placed on her right forearm, all of which are marked and documented in the chart. Each morning over the next 3 consecutive days, a sputum sample is collected and sent to the microbiology lab for evaluation. All three concentrated sputums are AFB smear positive when evaluated with a fluorochrome stain. In addition, a Ziehl-Neelsen stain is performed and shows the presence of AFB organisms. An HIV test is ordered, and the result is negative.

Case Study:
Continued

TREATMENT

Once diagnosed, patients with active disease should be started on appropriate therapy. The goal is to provide effective therapy in the shortest period of time. This is extremely important, because a lack of compliance and thus an incomplete course of therapy is one of the major mechanisms leading to the development of multidrug-resistant TB (MDRTB). It has been shown that approximately 25% of patients receiving therapy for active TB do not complete their therapy within a 12-month period.

All therapies involve the use of multiple drugs, because spontaneous chromosomal mutations occur when TB replicates. Many of these mutations involve the development of resistance to antimicrobials used in the treatment of TB. These mutations occur randomly and are not associated with continuous exposure to a certain antimicrobial. The spontaneous emergence of a mutation that is resistant to one antimicrobial is not usually associated with resistance to other, unrelated drugs. Mutations having resistance to either isoniazid (INH) or rifampin occur in approximately 1 in 10^8 to 1 in 10^9 replications. The probability of a spontaneous mutation having resistance to both drugs is the product of the two, or 1 in 10^{16}. Most patients with TB never have close to this number of organisms present, and thus the likelihood of having resistance to both drugs is negligible. Unfortunately, these probabilities do not hold when patients take their medications at suboptimal doses or on an irregular basis, or omit individual medications they are supposed to be taking. It is under these circumstances that multidrug-resistant strains can develop. In New York City, 33% of patients with active disease were resistant to one or more drugs, and 19% were resistant to both INH and rifampin.

> Lack of compliance with therapy is a major mechanism leading to development of multidrug-resistant TB.

> In New York City, 33% of patients have resistance to one or more drugs, and 19% are resistant to INH and rifampin.

In larger cities, 30% to 40% of new cases of active TB are secondary to recent infection.

The concern about MDRTB pertains not only to the individual with active disease but also to the possible spread to others that come in contact with that person. This disease process is much more difficult to treat effectively, even with the best available treatment, and has been associated with a high mortality rate. Unlike the classic scenario in which a patient develops active disease by reactivating a prior infection acquired years earlier, recent studies from New York and San Francisco have demonstrated that 30% to 40% of new cases of active TB represent recent transmission and thus primary disease. Thus, a person walking around the neighborhood with active TB that is multidrug resistant can easily transmit the disease to others and cause multiple cases of newly acquired MDRTB. This risk also applies to healthcare workers who come in contact with patients who have MDRTB.

When INH resistance is greater than 4%, most initial treatment regimens contain four drugs.

Because of the concern regarding drug-resistant organisms, most initial treatment regimens include four drugs—especially in areas of the country where the incidence of INH resistance is greater than 4%. The four drugs most commonly used for initial therapy are INH, rifampin, pyrazinamide (PZA), and ethambutol. The length of therapy for patients never previously treated is either 6 or 9 months. With the 6-month regimen, all four drugs are taken initially for the first 2 months. If the organism is susceptible, the final 4 months of therapy consist of INH and rifampin only. Although not as frequently used, the 9-month regimen consists of an initial 2 months on three medications (usually INH, rifampin, and either PZA or ethambutol) followed by INH and rifampin for the remaining 7 months. This regimen is sometimes used when the patient is unable to take one of the four drugs usually used (such as PZA with pregnancy). If susceptibility testing demonstrates multidrug resistance, the patient's regimen is individually adjusted, and therapy is often continued for a period of 12 to 24 months.

All TB drugs have associated adverse side effects that require monitoring (Table 15-4). This includes hepatotoxicity with the use of INH, rifampin, and PZA. All adults who are treated should have baseline liver function tests obtained prior to starting therapy. Second-line TB drugs are used when patients have MDRTB, or occasionally when they are unable to take one of the first-line drugs because of side effects. These second-line drugs generally have worse side-effect profiles and often require more intense monitoring.

Table 15-4
Adverse Reactions with TB Therapy

Hepatitis
With use of INH, rifampin, PZA
Baseline and monthly liver function tests

Optic Neuritis
With use of ethambutol
Monitor visual fields

Ototoxicity/Renal Toxicity
Streptomycin
Baseline and regular hearing and renal function checks

Directly observed therapy (DOT) has significantly improved patient compliance.

The use of directly observed therapy (DOT) has had a tremendous impact on patient compliance. Not only has it led directly to a decrease in the total number of new cases of TB, it has also resulted in a decrease in primary and acquired drug resistance as well as the number of relapses of patients being treated for MDRTB. Most commonly, DOT-treated individuals travel to designated centers where the treatments are administered and the patients are observed while taking them. They are given incentives to come to these centers, such as food vouchers and tokens for transportation. They are monitored closely in regard to their compliance, and intervention by the judicial court system can be implemented if necessary, including incarceration to allow continued DOT. DOT can be administered on a schedule of two or three times a week, after an initial period of daily therapy. All patients with questionable compliance should be encouraged to enroll in DOT.

Response to therapy should be monitored by repeating sputums monthly until they show no growth. Failure to become culture negative after 2 months should raise the issue of noncompliance versus drug resistance, and patients definitely should be enrolled in DOT and repeat sensitivities should be obtained.

PREVENTATIVE THERAPY

Certain individuals who are infected with TB, but show no evidence of active disease, may be candidates for preventative therapy (Table 15-5). Their PPDs are interpreted as reactive based on the criteria previously described. Preventative therapy substantially decreases the risk of developing active disease. Most commonly, INH is taken daily for a 6-month period, which decreases the risk of developing active disease by 69%. Children should receive 9 months of therapy, and patients with HIV, 12 months. Alternative therapies include rifampin for those who are unable to tolerate INH or who have INH-resistant organisms, although its effectiveness has not been studied. In patients exposed to persons with MDRTB, regimens should include at least two drugs, such as PZA and a quinolone, or be based on sensitivities. The risk of toxic side effects increases with age, particularly in those older than 35 years of age. Therefore, the risk-benefit ratio needs to be evaluated when deciding who should receive preventative therapy in this older age group.

> INH preventative therapy decreases the risk of developing active disease by 69%.

Positive PPD, Regardless of Age
Known or suspected HIV
Close contact with active TB
Chest x-ray shows previous untreated TB
IVDA
Certain medical conditions
Recent converter (within 2 years)

Positive PPD, Younger than 35 Years Old
From country where TB is common
High risk racial and ethnic groups, underserved
From long care facility
Children less than 4 years old
Homeless

Table 15-5
Preventative Therapy for TB

R.J. is then placed on a four-drug regimen consisting of INH, rifampin, PZA, and ethambutol. Baseline liver function tests are obtained prior to starting her medications. For the next 10 days, R.J. clinically improves, with a decrease in hemoptysis, and her temperature begins to decrease. After 14 days of daily therapy, R.J. is discharged after being enrolled in directly observed therapy (DOT) through the city health department.

Case Study:
Continued

BCG VACCINATION

Bacille Calmette-Guérin (BCG) is a vaccine that is administered, mostly outside of the United States, as a preventative therapy. BCG is derived from a strain of *M. bovis* that has been attenuated over years through serial passage in culture. Its effectiveness has varied widely, from 0% to as high as 76%, depending on the study. Because of the relatively low risk of infection in the United States, and this variable effectiveness, BCG is not routinely used in this country. It has been used in situations where infants and children are continuously exposed to a person with active disease and are unable to take INH preventative therapy. Problems arise in trying to interpret a PPD skin test in an individual who has received a prior BCG vaccination. The response is less likely to reflect the prior BCG vaccination 1) if it was given many years prior to the skin test; 2) if the response is a large induration; and 3) if the person comes from a country with a high incidence of TB. In these instances, prior BCG vaccination should be disregarded, active infection ruled out, and preventative therapy prescribed.

> BCG vaccine as preventative therapy has had variable effectiveness.

TUBERCULOSIS IN HIV-INFECTED PATIENTS

Approximately 10% to 30% of patients with TB are infected with HIV. In addition, the incidence of TB in HIV is about 100 to 300 times that of the general population. Immunosuppression associated with HIV infection is a major risk factor for the development of active tuberculosis. This risk includes reactivation TB as well as the development of primary disease after recent exposure to an infected individual. TB can often be the initial clinical manifestation of HIV disease. Extrapulmonary TB also occurs more

> From 10% to 30% of patients with TB have HIV infection.

frequently in those infected with HIV, being present in more than 70% of patients, compared with 24% to 45% in non-HIV TB cases. The most common forms of extra-pulmonary TB are lymphadenitis and miliary TB.

The length of therapy for active TB is the same as for non-HIV patients, but may be longer if the clinical and bacteriologic response to therapy is suboptimal. In one study it took a median of 10 weeks before sputum samples became negative. Overall, survival is poor, with a median survival of 16 months from the time of diagnosis of TB in HIV-infected patients. This probably reflects their underlying immune status at the time of diagnosis rather than infection with TB itself.

> The median survival of HIV patients diagnosed with active TB is 16 months.

Preventative therapy has been advocated for HIV patients who are anergic, as well as for those with positive PPDs, when the risk of infection is increased (i.e., area where the incidence of TB is high). Yet, a recent study of anergic HIV patients showed no significant difference in the incidence of active TB in those who took INH prophylaxis compared with a control group. Thus, the use of preventative therapy in anergic HIV patients remains controversial. *For more information on this topic, see Chapter 16, "HIV Infection and the Lung."*

■ NONTUBERCULOUS MYCOBACTERIA

In recent years, a number of mycobacteria other than TB have been found to be potential human pathogens. These organisms have been referred to as "atypical mycobacteria" or nontuberculous mycobacteria (NTM). An increase in the number of infections caused by NTM has occurred with the AIDS epidemic; especially noted is the increased number of HIV patients who have acquired *Mycobacterium avium* complex (MAC). As mentioned earlier, these organisms are classified on the basis of growth rate and the ability to produce pigment (see Table 15-1).

> Nontuberculous mycobacteria are also potential pathogens in humans.

Most of these organisms are acquired from environmental sources such as soil and water, with person-to-person transmission rarely occurring. Most NTM infections occur in patients who have underlying chronic lung diseases, such as chronic obstructive pulmonary disease (COPD), pneumoconiosis, bronchiectasis, and old TB. Thus, chest x-ray findings are often confused with those observed in TB patients, simulating cavitary lesions in the upper lobes where bullous disease is common, but usually with less parenchymal involvement. Many of these organisms may exist as saprophytes, and thus repeated positive sputum cultures, associated with symptoms and chest x-ray findings, are required to diagnose active disease.

> Many NTM infections occur in patients with underlying lung disease.

Mycobacterium kansasii most commonly occurs in middle aged white men with underlying lung disease as mentioned above. Symptoms are usually vague and include fever, malaise, and cough. CXRs demonstrate a predominance of upper lobe cavitary lesions. Treatment includes standard anti-TB medications based on sensitivities and is usually extended over an 18-24 month period.

MAC infections can occur in both HIV and non-HIV hosts. The symptoms and chest x-ray findings in non-HIV patients are similar to those found with *M. kansasii*. In patients with HIV, dissemination is most often found, with lung involvement playing a minor role. CD4+ counts are usually less than 100 per cubic centimeter. Most patients have symptoms related to the gastrointestinal (GI) system, such as nausea, vomiting, and diarrhea. Other commonly involved sites include bone marrow, blood, lymph nodes, and liver. Diagnosis is most commonly made by isolation of the organism from blood or the GI tract. Treatment for disseminated MAC in HIV patients includes at least two drugs, such as ethambutol and clarithromycin. Other drug combinations have been used. Recently, rifabutin prophylaxis has been shown to be effective at decreasing the incidence of MAC in HIV patients, but did not affect overall survival. Clarithromycin and azithromycin have also been used prophylactically.

Other NTM can cause disease in humans, including the rapid growers *M. chelonei* and *M. fortuitum*. Unlike the other NTM mentioned above, pulmonary disease usually occurs in patients with no underlying lung disease. Most patients are white, in their sixties, with cough and occasional fever and night sweats. Chest x-rays show patchy infiltrates, with cavitation noted in only 25% of cases. Treatment consists of antibiotics such as ciprofloxacin or sulfonamides, based on sensitivity testing.

Case Study:
Resolution

R.J. is placed on a twice-a-week DOT regimen, and monthly sputum samples are obtained to document her response to therapy and to rule out development of drug resistance. Drug susceptibility tests are performed on her AFB sputum cultures, which are shown to be sensitive to all drugs. After 2 months, her regimen is decreased to two drugs based on the sensitivities. R.J.'s family members and friends who have been exposed to her are PPD skin tested, and when these tests are positive, chest x-rays are obtained.

∎ SUMMARY

In conclusion, tuberculosis has reemerged as an important clinical pathogen causing significant morbidity and mortality worldwide. The increased number of new cases appears to be attributable to several factors, including the HIV epidemic and the increase in the number of immigrants arriving from countries with a high prevalence of TB. In addition, cases of MDRTB have increased in number and are often difficult to treat successfully. This has led to the development of new measures to improve compliance with therapy, such as DOT. Recent studies suggest that the institution of these programs may be making strides in controlling this disabling and often deadly disease.

▌REVIEW QUESTIONS

1. Which one of the following statements regarding the resurgence of TB as a major cause of disease in the United States is false?

   (A) The increased number of new cases of TB is in some part related to the immune deficiency associated with HIV disease.
   (B) Immigrants from other countries have the same risk of developing TB as that of U.S. citizens living in the inner cities.
   (C) The healthcare system was initially unable to monitor the increased number of new cases first evident in the mid 1980s.
   (D) Close contacts of patients with active disease have an increased risk of becoming infected.

2. Once aerosolized, the tuberculous organisms are inhaled by close contacts, reach the alveolus, and then

   (A) are destroyed by lymphocytes, which prevents the development of active infection.
   (B) cause no further problems as long as the host remains HIV negative.
   (C) are resistant to treatment because of the inability of antibiotics to reach the site of infection.
   (D) are phagocytized by macrophages, with the immune system usually able to control the spread and replication of the bacilli within a few weeks.

3. A 25-year-old third-year medical student has his yearly PPD test done at the student health center. He had one done approximately 1 year ago, and it was reportedly negative. Although he is now on clinical rotations in the hospital, he does not recall having any contact with patients having active TB. He has not felt ill and denies any cough or fever. His PPD is read at 48 hours and measures 12 mm. A chest x-ray is negative. Which one of the following would be the appropriate treatment for this student?

   (A) Treatment with an initial four-drug regimen pending cultures of induced sputums
   (B) No treatment necessary in this setting
   (C) Baseline liver function tests prior to starting a 6-month regimen of INH therapy
   (D) Pyrazinamide and a quinolone antibiotic for 6 months.

4. A 36-year-old white man, HIV positive since 1989 secondary to IV drug abuse, presents with a 5-day history of cough, SOB, and subjective fever. He states that his cough has been productive of white sputum but he denies hemoptysis. On physical examination his temperature is 101°F, his lungs are relatively clear to auscultation, and his chest x-ray shows an infiltrate in the right upper lobe. He denies any known exposure to TB, but has often slept in a homeless shelter. What is the appropriate initial management of this patient?

   (A) Admit the patient to an isolation room, obtain three daily sputum samples, place a PPD with controls, and start a four-drug regimen for TB as well as antibiotics for community-acquired pneumonia, pending test results.
   (B) Obtain a sputum sample and discharge the patient home on a four-drug regimen for TB.
   (C) Admit the patient, start him on a drug regimen of trimethoprim-sulfamethoxazole (Bactrim) and steroids, and schedule him for a bronchoscopy.
   (D) Start the patient on oral penicillin and see him in the office in approximately 1 week.

5. Which one of the following statements is incorrect regarding NTM infections?

   (A) They most commonly occur in patients with underlying pulmonary disease.
   (B) Most infections are acquired from the soil or water, rather than by person-to-person transmission.
   (C) Pulmonary-related complaints of cough and hemoptysis are the most common presenting symptoms of MAC infections in patients with HIV.
   (D) These organisms are classified on the basis of growth rate and the ability to produce pigment.

ANSWERS AND EXPLANATIONS

1. The answer is B. Immigrants, especially those from countries in Africa, Asia, and Latin America, where the incidence of TB is high, have an increased risk of developing active disease. The prevalence of active disease is greater in these countries than in the United States, and thus the risk of these infected individuals developing active disease, either as a primary process or by reactivation later in life, is increased.

2. The answer is D. After the aerosolized bacilli are inhaled and reach the alveoli, the first cells that attempt to control the infection are the macrophages. These cells phagocytize the bacilli, yet the tuberculous organisms are still able to replicate within these cells and can spread by way of the blood and lymphatics to other organs. Subsequent T-lymphocyte activation eventually prevents further replication and spread and keeps the organisms dormant and suppressed. It is only when the immune system is suppressed or overwhelmed that active disease can develop, leading to the destruction of the involved organ systems.

3. The answer is C. Based on the student's age, the increased risk of exposure in his work setting, and the size of his PPD response, preventative therapy is indicated. His lack of symptoms and a normal chest x-ray demonstrate that he has no evidence of active disease. Therefore, the appropriate treatment would be 6 months of INH therapy. Pyrazinamide and a quinolone would be appropriate if there had been a known exposure to a patient with multidrug-resistant TB, which is not the case here.

4. The answer is A. The patient belongs to a group considered to be at high risk for development of active TB. Although the chest x-ray could be consistent with a community-acquired pneumonia, TB needs to be ruled out. It would be helpful to know the patient's CD4+ cell count, but this is often not available when the patient is first evaluated. The most important measure to prevent the spread of TB is to place the patient in isolation immediately. After appropriate specimens have been obtained, and if the clinical suspicion remains high, treatment can be started and in this case consists of a four-drug regimen. It must be remembered that approximately 30% of HIV patients infected with TB will have negative PPD tests and that it may take up to 6 weeks for cultures to become positive. Thus, beginning therapy is not initially dependent on positive stain or culture results. Newer diagnostic techniques, such as PCR testing, may decrease the amount of time necessary for positive results to become available.

5. The answer is C. Most NTM infections occur in patients with underlying lung disease, such as COPD, pneumoconiosis, or old TB. HIV patients also have an increased incidence of developing MAC infections. Yet, most patients have disseminated disease, with the lung only incidentally involved. Most patients present with gastrointestinal symptoms, and cultures are most often positive from blood and stool specimens.

SUGGESTED READING

American Thoracic Society: Diagnosis and treatment of disease caused by nontuberculous mycobacteria. *Am Rev Respir Dis* 142:940–953, 1990.

American Thoracic Society: Rapid diagnostic tests for tuberculosis: what is appropriate use? *Am J Respir Crit Care Med* 155:1804–1814, 1997.

American Thoracic Society: Treatment of tuberculosis and tuberculosis infection in adults and children. *Am J Respir Crit Care Med* 149:1359–1374, 1994.

Barnes PF, Blouch AB, Davidson PT, et al: Tuberculosis in patients with human immunodeficiency virus infection. *N Engl J Med* 321:1644–1650, 1991.

Centers for Disease Control: *Core Curriculum on Tuberculosis: What the Clinician Should Know*, 3rd ed. Atlanta: U.S. Department of Health and Human Services, 1994.

Goble M, Iseman MD, Madsen LA, et al: Treatment of 171 patients with pulmonary tuberculosis resistant to isoniazid and rifampin. *N Engl J Med* 328:527–532, 1993.

Gordin FM, Matts JP, Miller C, et al: A controlled trial of isoniazid in persons with anergy and human immunodeficiency virus infection who are at high risk for tuberculosis. *N Engl J Med* 337:315–320, 1997.

Horsburgh CR: *Mycobacterium avium* complex infection in the acquired immunodeficiency syndrome. *N Engl J Med* 324:1332–1338, 1991.

Iseman MD: Treatment of multidrug-resistant tuberculosis. *N Engl J Med* 329:784–791, 1993.

Markowitz N, Hansen NI, Hopewell PC, et al: Incidence of tuberculosis in the United States among HIV-infected persons. *Ann Intern Med* 126:123–132, 1997.

Menzies D, Fanning A, Yuan L, et al: Tuberculosis among health care workers. *N Engl J Med* 332:92–97, 1995.

Weis SE, Slocum PC, Blais FX, et al: The effect of directly observed therapy on the rates of drug resistance and relapse in tuberculosis. *N Engl J Med* 330:1179–1184, 1994.

Chapter 16

HIV INFECTION AND THE LUNG

Ubaldo Martin, M.D.

Gerard J. Criner, M.D.

■ CHAPTER OUTLINE

Learning Objectives
Introduction
Case Study: Introduction
Pathogenesis of HIV Infection in the Lower Respiratory Tract
Case Study: Continued
Pulmonary Infections in HIV Disease
Case Study: Continued
Case Study: Continued
Noninfectious Pulmonary Diseases
Case Study: Resolution
Diagnostic Approach to Pulmonary Disease in the HIV Patient
Summary
Review Questions

■ LEARNING OBJECTIVES

At the completion of this chapter, the reader should:
- Understand the principal immunologic processes that affect the lungs in HIV infection.
- Appreciate the clinical presentations of infectious lung diseases in HIV patients.
- Recognize the noninfectious pulmonary complications of HIV infection.
- Be aware of the major diagnostic tests and therapeutic options used in the evaluation and treatment of HIV patients with infectious and noninfectious pulmonary complications.

■ INTRODUCTION

The acquired immune deficiency syndrome (AIDS) has emerged as a global pandemic in the last 15 years. Its etiologic agent, the human immunodeficiency virus (HIV), is a blood-borne retrovirus commonly transmitted through sexual intercourse, parenteral inoculation, or mother-to-infant transmission prenatally or during breast feeding. Two types of HIV have been recognized: HIV-1 and HIV-2. The two types vary in geographic distribution but are strikingly similar in transmission mode, pathogenicity, and clinical features.

> About 80% of AIDS patients have at least one pulmonary disorder, 90% of which are infectious.

The lungs are principal targets of the infectious and noninfectious complications of HIV infection. The spectrum of pulmonary diseases associated with HIV infection continues to broaden, with more than 80% of AIDS patients having pulmonary disorders of some nature, 90% of which are infectious. Prophylaxis for certain opportunistic infections and broader antiviral regimes has increased longevity in AIDS patients, thus resulting in a marked increase in the prevalence of pulmonary disorders. This chapter deals with the pathogenesis of HIV infection in the lower respiratory tract, specific pulmonary infectious and noninfectious diseases that occur in the HIV patient, and the overall diagnostic and therapeutic approach to the patient with HIV disease.

Case Study:
Introduction

J.D. is a 32-year-old white man who was diagnosed with HIV disease 3 years ago. He has no other significant comorbidities. He acquired HIV infection through unprotected heterosexual contact. He denies use of intravenous drugs or other risk factors. At the time of diagnosis, his CD4 cell count is 445 cells per cubic millimeter.

PATHOGENESIS OF HIV INFECTION IN THE LOWER RESPIRATORY TRACT

The respiratory environment is a unique milieu that becomes infected with airborne or blood-borne pathogens and local immune modulator cells, causing regional immunodeficiency.

The proclivity for lung disease in HIV patients is not completely understood. However, the respiratory system is a unique environment that may become infected with airborne or blood-borne pathogens, and may have regional immunodeficiency induced by the local secretion of pulmonary immune modulator cells (Figure 16-1). Regardless of the transmission route, the initial HIV infection appears to be caused by a single genotype. After several weeks of infection modulated by the host's initial immune response, 15 to 20 genetically distinct variants of HIV, also called quasispecies, can be found. The HIV retrovirus disseminates throughout the bloodstream, and viral particles called virions become trapped by secondary lymphoid tissues. Owing to the constant and close interaction of cells in the follicular areas, infection of the virus then proceeds from cell to cell. At some point, the cells become unable to trap or retain the viral particles, which become redistributed to tertiary lymphoid tissues such as the lung or liver.

FIGURE 16-1
Schematic showing how the human immunodeficiency virus propagates within the lung, inducing the development of opportunistic infections. Reproduced with permission from Zurlo J: Respiratory infections and the acquired immunodeficiency syndrome. Chapter 3 *in* Bone RG, ed.: *Pulmonary and Critical Care Medicine.* Boston: Mosby, 1997.

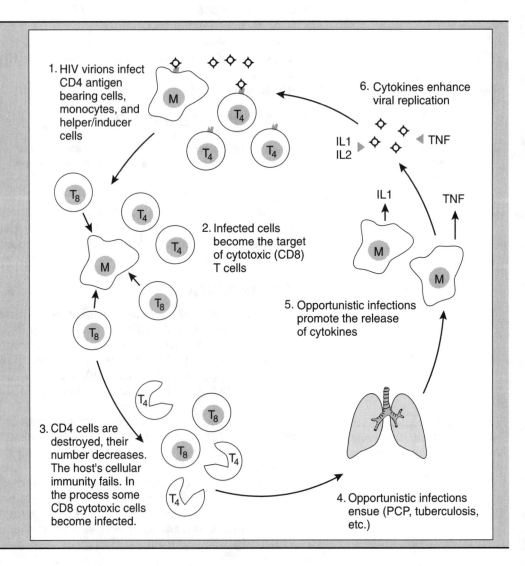

HIV virions probably reach the lung in various forms and by various routes. A migratory process allows T cells infected with HIV to reach the lung's lymphatic tissue. There is evidence of cell-free HIV particles reaching the lung by way of the microcirculation, crossing the alveolocapillary barrier, and infecting local cells. Infected T cells may also interact with other cells bearing specific receptors called CD4 cells. The CD4 receptor is thought to play a major role in the infection and propagation of HIV infection among cells. This receptor allows the integration of the viral genome from infected T cells into noninfected CD4+ cells other than T cells, such as alveolar macrophages and local lung lymphocytes. Finally, peripheral CD4+ monocytes (i.e., the precursors of macrophages) may migrate into the lung tissue, where they eventually differentiate into mature, chronically infected pulmonary macrophages.

CD4+ T cells help B cells develop into immunoglobulin-secreting plasma cells, thereby helping to activate other cells to become cytotoxic, and hence their name—helper, inducer, or cytotoxic T cells. Cytotoxic T cells are highly specific against HIV-infected cells and in theory should provide an effective means of controlling the spread of HIV among cells, but in fact they are one of the major targets of HIV. As HIV infection progresses, these cells become less efficient in their ability to control HIV spread, thereby enabling the virus to infect more cells. This lowers patient immunity and predisposes patients to the development of opportunistic infections.

> Cytotoxic T cells become less efficient in their ability to contain HIV infection, thus enabling the virus to infect more cells.

One of the most interesting aspects of HIV infection and its effect on the lung is the fact that the lung becomes a microenvironment composed of genetically different populations of viral particles. Once opportunistic infections occur, pulmonary macrophages are stimulated to produce cytokines such as interleukin-2 (IL-2), tumor necrosis factor (TNF), and interleukin-6 (IL-6), all of which act further to propagate viral replication throughout the lung. It is thought that local cytokine production in the lung plays an important role that further contributes to the susceptibility of the lung to infections.

In summary, in HIV disease, the lung becomes a microenvironment where virus replication readily occurs in response to a host of local factors. Cytotoxic cells initially attack and destroy HIV-infected cells, but eventually become infected and subsequently ineffective in controlling the virus, thereby fostering the development of opportunistic infections. Opportunistic infections then trigger a further release of local cytokines that potentiate viral replication, thereby creating a vicious cycle that leads to progressive destruction and depletion of the lung's immune system (see Figure 16-1).

> In HIV infection, the lung becomes a microenvironment where virus replication readily occurs in response to a multitude of local factors.

Case Study:
Continued

The patient was feeling fine until 3 days ago, when he noticed the onset of fever and chills associated with a cough productive of green sputum. Over the next 2 days he became progressively more short of breath and developed right-side chest pain that was worse on deep inspiration.

He is brought to the emergency department. He looks anxious and diaphoretic. His blood pressure is 100/65, his heart rate is 115, his respiratory rate is 28, and his temperature is 103.2°F. His oxygen saturation is 90% on room air. Lung auscultation reveals end-inspiratory crackles at the left base and bronchial breath sounds with egophony. The right base is dull to percussion.

Laboratory data reveal a white blood count of 17,000 with a marked left shift. Chest x-rays show right lower lobe consolidation.

Blood and sputum cultures are sent. Gram staining of sputum shows many gram-positive diplococci and abundant white blood cells. The patient is started on antibiotics. Two days later, blood cultures grow Streptococcus pneumoniae.

■ PULMONARY INFECTIONS IN HIV DISEASE

BACTERIAL INFECTIONS

In early HIV disease, when the CD4+ lymphocyte count is relatively well preserved, patients have an increased propensity to develop the same pulmonary infections that affect the general population (Table 16-1). More than one-third of all HIV patients develop a severe bacterial infection during the course of their disease; community-

> More than one-third of all HIV patients develop a severe bacterial infection during the course of their disease; community-acquired pneumonia may be the most frequent disorder.

acquired pneumonia may be the most frequent lung manifestation of HIV infection. In 1993, the Centers for Disease Control revised the case definition for AIDS and decided to include recurrent bacterial pneumonia as an inclusion criteria for the diagnosis of AIDS.

Table 16-1
Bacteria Found to Cause Pneumonia in HIV-Infected Patients

PATHOGEN	COMMUNITY-ACQUIRED	NOSOCOMIAL
Associated with B-Cell Abnormalities		
Streptococcus pneumoniae	X	X
Haemophilus influenzae		
Type B	X	
Nontypeable	X	
Associated with T-Cell Abnormalities		
Bordetella pertussis	X	
Rhodococcus equi	X	
Nocardia species	X	
Uncertain Relationship to Immunodeficiency		
Streptococcus agalactiae (group B)	X	
Staphylococcus aureus	X	X
Moraxella catarrhalis	X	X
Legionella species	X	
Mycoplasma pneumoniae	X	X
Klebsiella pneumoniae	X	
Haemophilus species	X	X
Enterobacter aerogenes	X	X
Pseudomonas aeruginosa	X	X

Modified from Zurlo J: Respiratory infections and the acquired immunodeficiency syndrome. Chapter 3 *in* Bone RG, ed.: *Pulmonary and Critical Care Medicine.* Boston: Mosby, 1997.

Although the effects of HIV infection on the impairment of cellular immunity are well known, it also appears to alter humeral immunity, resulting in a high incidence of high-grade lymphomas, hypergammaglobulinemia, and an inadequate response to antigenic stimulation, thereby resulting in insufficient production of antibodies after immunization. The resultant effect on B-cell dysfunction is responsible for the increased frequency of infections by encapsulated bacteria, such as *Streptococcus pneumoniae* and *Haemophilus influenzae*. Moreover, monocyte and macrophage function is affected, resulting in defective chemotaxis, phagocytosis, and intracellular killing. These factors increase the probability that infections with pathogens, such as *Staphylococcus aureus*, will occur. In addition, there is evidence supporting defective neutrophil function and inadequate complement activation as complementary factors enhancing the susceptibility to bacterial infections. In general, this constellation of findings predisposes the HIV-infected patient to an eightfold greater incidence of bacterial infections compared with the normal population. Bacterial organisms are now recognized as the most common type of organisms causing pneumonia when CD4 counts are greater than 250 cells per cubic millimeter.

The most common cause of community-acquired pneumonia is *Streptococcus pneumoniae*. The incidence of pneumococcal pneumonia among HIV-infected patients is 5 to 6 times greater than that of the general population. *Haemophilus influenzae* is the second most common pathogen and tends to occur more frequently in younger patients. Other pathogens reported to cause pneumonia include *Legionella pneumophila*, group B streptococci, *Nocardia asteroides*, and *Rhodococcus equi* (in patients who have been exposed to horses or other animals). In hospitalized patients who acquire pneumonia, nosocomial pneumonias secondary to gram-negative organisms or *Staphylococcus aureus* are most common.

The clinical presentation of bacterial pneumonia in the HIV-infected individual is similar to that observed in the general population and is hallmarked by the abrupt onset of fever, chills, cough productive of purulent sputum, dyspnea, and pleurisy. The chest radiograph shows that localized infiltration and consolidation are present on physical examination. In contrast to the general non-HIV-infected population, HIV-infected individuals have an increased frequency of multilobar involvement and a greater incidence of bacteremia (80% compared with a 20% risk of bacteremia with *Streptococcus pneu-*

Pneumococcal pneumonia occurs 5 to 6 times more commonly in HIV patients than in the general population.

Bacterial pneumonia presents much as in the general population and is characterized by the abrupt onset of fever, chills, dyspnea, and cough productive of purulent sputum.

moniae in the general population and a 25% incidence of *Haemophilus influenzae* bacteremia). Moreover, HIV-infected individuals have increased difficulty in eradicating infections and an increased incidence of relapses with the same types of pyogenic organisms.

Diagnostic evaluation for bacterial infections includes a chest x-ray, expectorated sputum with Gram stain, and, when appropriate, cultures of blood and pleural fluid. Initial antibiotic treatment usually consists of a third-generation cephalosporin with the addition of erythromycin, if *Legionella pneumophila* is suspected.

J.D. has had an uneventful recovery from pneumonia. He has been relatively healthy for 1 year and presents to the medicine clinic for a regular follow-up visit. His last CD4 count, performed 3 months prior to this visit, was 355 cells per milliliter. He relates that about 6 weeks ago he noticed the onset of cough. He attributed it initially to a common cold and was therefore not concerned. The cough persisted over several weeks and eventually became associated with general malaise, weakness, and loss of appetite. He has lost about 10 lb. Over the past 2 weeks, profuse sweating has occurred at night, and his cough, initially dry, is now productive of bloody sputum.

In the clinic, the patient has a temperature of 100.6°F, but the rest of his vital signs are within normal limits. He is in minimal respiratory distress and exhibits bitemporal muscle wasting. His lung examination reveals bilateral post-tussive rales. The right base is dull to percussion and decreased fremitus is detected.

Chest x-rays reveal bilateral reticular infiltrates and a large right pleural effusion. The patient is placed in respiratory isolation, and sputum samples are taken. A Ziehl-Neelsen stain of the sputum shows many acid-fast bacilli. The patient is started on four antituberculous drugs.

Case Study:
Continued

MYCOBACTERIAL INFECTIONS

Mycobacterium Tuberculosis. A major factor contributing to the recent rise in the incidence of tuberculosis (TB), which began in the United States in 1986, is the evolving number of cases of *Mycobacterium tuberculosis* in the HIV-infected population.

Tuberculosis develops by either progression of newly acquired infection or reactivation of latent disease. As previously mentioned, HIV has a profound effect on cell-mediated immunity, thereby limiting the HIV patient's ability to suppress direct progression from initial infection to frank disease. Therefore, HIV patients are more prone to present with recent tuberculous infections than immunocompetent individuals. In the latter, tuberculous infection is usually attributable to reactivation of latent disease. Moreover, HIV-infected individuals are more likely to present with disseminated extra-pulmonary manifestations of tuberculous disease, with symptoms resulting from involvement of liver, bone marrow, central nervous system, or lymphatic tissue by TB.

> HIV-infected patients are more prone to present with recent rather than latent infections of TB, with disseminated rather than focal pulmonary sites of involvement.

The suppression of cellular immune response in HIV patients also impairs their ability to react to tuberculin skin testing. As the CD4+ lymphocyte count falls, the ability to manifest a positive tuberculin skin reaction also decreases, thus resulting in a high prevalence of HIV patients with low CD4 counts having negative skin reactions to purified protein derivative (PPD) and other common antigens.

A wider variety of clinical presentations and radiographic findings make a diagnosis of TB somewhat problematic in the HIV-infected patient. Chest x-rays frequently do not reveal findings suggestive of TB infection, such as cavities, apical scarring, and pleural effusions, and may be normal in up to 10% of patients. The most common abnormalities include diffuse and focal infiltrates and mediastinal and hilar adenopathies—radiographic findings that are uncommon chest radiographic manifestations of TB in immunocompetent patients.

Presenting symptoms of tuberculous infection in the HIV patient include cough, fever, weight loss, and night sweats. Because of its virulence, TB usually presents in the earlier stages of HIV infection. Because TB is a common and preventable disease, chemoprophylaxis should be considered for all patients with documented HIV infection. All HIV patients with PPD skin reactions greater than 5 mm should receive prophylaxis against TB regardless of age once active disease has been excluded. Patients who are at

> All HIV-infected patients with PPD reactions greater than 5 mm should receive prophylactic therapy.

greater risk for TB include drug abusers, alcoholics, the homeless, past or present prison inmates, and patients from highly endemic areas. In addition, patients with histories of positive PPD tests who have never received treatment should receive chemoprophylaxis. Patients with chest x-ray abnormalities consistent with prior tuberculous infection, and close contacts of patients with active TB, should also receive therapy. Prophylaxis consists of either isoniazid (INH) or rifampin (in patients with suspected INH resistance) for a minimum of 6 to 12 months.

All HIV-infected patients who have evidence of tuberculous infection (i.e., acid fast bacillus positive (AFB) smear, positive DNA probe for *Mycobacterium tuberculosis*, or culture positive for *M. tuberculosis*), should receive a full treatment regime against *M. tuberculosis*. Therapy should consist of INH (300 mg/day), rifampin (600 mg/day), pyrazinamide (20 to 30 mg/kg/day), and ethambutol (15 to 25 mg/kg/day) during the first 2 months, followed by INH and rifampin for another 4 months to complete at least 6 months of therapy (Table 16-2). If the patient is noncompliant or the disease responds slowly to therapy, the duration of treatment should be prolonged. Therapy also should be prolonged if INH and rifampin cannot be used concurrently. HIV patients do not seem to differ significantly from the general population in outcome after effective treatment, and morbidity and mortality are surprisingly low with an effective regime. Culture results should help guide initial empiric antibiotic therapy once they become available after 6 to 8 weeks of growth.

Table 16-2
Centers for Disease Control Recommendations for the Treatment of Tuberculosis in HIV Patients with Known or Suspected Drug-Sensitive Organisms

DISEASE	REGIMEN	DURATION
Pulmonary	Isoniazid 300 mg/day Rifampin 600 mg/day[a] Pyrazinamide 20 to 30 mg/kg/day (during the first 2 months)	Continue for a minimum of 9 months and for at least 6 months after three cultures are negative[b]
Extrapulmonary or central nervous system	Same as above plus ethambutol 25 mg/kg/day	Same as above
Positive tuberculin skin test[c]	Isoniazid 300 mg/day	12 months

[a] The dosage should be 450 mg/day for patients weighing no more than 50 kg.
[b] For patients not receiving either isoniazid or rifampin, treatment should be continued for a minimum of 18 months and for at least 12 months after three cultures are negative.
[c] All patients with known purified protein derivative (PPD) positivity irrespective of age or those who are likely to be newly infected with an organism with a low likelihood of multiple drug resistance.

Modified from Zurlo J: Respiratory infections and the acquired immunodeficiency syndrome. Chapter 3 *in* Bone RG, ed.: *Pulmonary and Critical Care Medicine.* Boston: Mosby, 1997.

Outbreaks of multidrug-resistant (MDR) tuberculosis have emerged in New York, Miami, and Baltimore. These organisms carry a poor prognosis and a higher mortality, close to 75% in some reports. Prompt recognition and rapid institution of treatment may help to lower this high mortality. Epidemiologic data suggest that transmission occurs mainly in treatment centers where noncompliant individuals harbor resistant organisms that are easily spread in centers that house large numbers of immune-deficient patients. Supervised outpatient drug treatment programs should be advocated for patients considered to be at high risk for noncompliance.

***Mycobacterium Avium* Complex.** The closely related atypical mycobacterium species *M. avium* and *M. intracellulare* have been grouped together as the *Mycobacterium avium* complex (MAC). Approximately 25% to 35% of all HIV-infected individuals eventually develop MAC, with the risk of MAC infection increasing as the CD4+ T-lymphocyte cell count decreases. In patients with CD4 cell counts between 100 and 200 cells per cubic millimeter, the risk of MAC infection is about 3%. When patient CD4 counts fall to less than 100 cells per cubic millimeter, the risk increases to approximately 40%. More than 95% of patients with disseminated MAC infections have CD4+ lymphocytes that number 50 cells per microliter or less.

MAC infection occurs most often in patients with advanced HIV infection and seldom heralds the onset of the AIDS syndrome. MAC is typically cultured from blood and bone marrow, but lymph nodes, spleen, liver, stool, bone marrow, and sputum may also yield

MAC infection occurs more commonly in HIV patients with advanced disease and lower CD4 counts.

the diagnosis. MAC disseminates even in the early stages of infection, and the lungs, because they are frequently involved, are often the initial site from which the organism is identified. Most of the clinical manifestations of MAC infection are extrapulmonary, and pulmonary involvement by itself does not appear to alter the course of the disease.

MAC is a ubiquitous organism usually found in water and sewage and is known to cause disease in birds and mammals as well as in humans. It is not spread from person to person, but probably enters the body through the lungs or the gastrointestinal tract. Human infections are thought to arise as a result of environmental exposure.

A specific constellation of symptoms associated with MAC infection is difficult to determine, because MAC is usually diagnosed late in the course of HIV infection. It appears to be most commonly associated with a wasting syndrome consisting of fever, weight loss, chronic diarrhea, abdominal pain, progressive anemia requiring transfusions, malabsorption, and extrahepatic obstructive jaundice.

The diagnosis of MAC is made on the basis of blood cultures performed by peripheral leukocyte lysis and inoculation into a solid medium (Löwenstein-Jensen). More recently, diagnostic methods using DNA probes and polymerase chain reaction have shown promise in the earlier detection of *Mycobacterium avium* complex (i.e., several hours).

Treatment for MAC is complicated. Because patients usually present in the advanced stages of AIDS and frequently have multiple comorbidities, multiple drug combinations are usually necessary to control and/or eradicate the infection, and drug reactions are common. The newer macrolides, such as azithromycin, and clarithromycin, are the most active agents against MAC. They are used in combination with ethambutol, rifampin, rifabutin, clofazimine, ciprofloxacin, or the aminoglycosides. Lifetime treatment is usually required.

With the advent of antiretroviral therapy, AIDS patients are living longer with lower CD4 counts. Prophylaxis against MAC has been recommended for patients with CD4 counts less than 100 cells per cubic millimeter, and rifabutin, clarithromycin, and azithromycin have been proposed as effective agents.

Case Study:
Continued

The patient receives 6 months of antituberculous therapy. He is started on antiretroviral therapy. He is lost to follow-up for 2 years and then presents to the emergency department complaining of severe shortness of breath. He was fine until 3 weeks prior to this visit, when he first noticed some dry cough and minimal shortness of breath. He also has tactile fevers and fatigue. He denies chills or sputum production. His shortness of breath has progressively worsened and he is unable to perform even simple tasks without becoming extremely dyspneic.

The emergency physician evaluates him. The patient looks anxious. His respiratory rate is 30 breaths per minute, his heart rate is 125 beats per minute, and his oxygen saturation is 89% by pulse oximeter. His temperature is 99.8° F. He is using accessory respiratory muscles. Physical exam reveals oral thrush with minimal cervical adenopathy. His lungs are clear to auscultation. There is no abdominal tenderness and no hepatomegaly.

Chest x-rays show diffuse bilateral interstitial infiltrates. His white blood cell count is only 3.1×10^3 cells per cubic millimeter. An arterial blood gas is remarkable for a P_aO_2 of 59 mmHg with an alveolar-arterial gradient of 48 mmHg. The patient is started on high-dosage trimethoprim-sulfamethoxazole and steroids. He is placed on supplemental oxygen by face mask. The next day, a pulmonary consult is obtained, and the patient undergoes bronchoscopy and bronchoalveolar lavage.

The specimen obtained with lavage is stained with methenamine silver, showing multiple organisms consistent with Pneumocystis carinii.

PNEUMOCYSTIS CARINII PNEUMONIA

Pneumocystis carinii pneumonia (PCP) is the most common AIDS-related infection. It afflicts approximately 70% to 75% of all HIV-infected individuals and, despite early recognition and aggressive treatment, still carries a mortality of 10% to 20% per episode. Pneumocystis infection represents reactivation of latent infection because all humans are exposed to *P. carinii* during the first decade of life.

PCP is the most common AIDS-related infection.

Pneumocystis carinii is a eukaryotic organism previously thought to be a protozoan, but more recent studies have linked it to higher fungi. It is widely distributed throughout the environment, but mammals appear to be the only species capable of harboring it. Three forms of the organism exist—the trophozoite, cyst, and precyst forms. The trophozoite form appears to be the infecting particle. The trophozoite attaches to the type 1 pneumocyte and induces pathologic changes that cause the cells to degenerate, thereby inducing inflammation and decreasing the production of surfactant. As a result, the alveolar spaces become filled with cellular debris and microatelectasis develops, causing increased intrapulmonary shunting and hypoxemia.

Most cases of PCP develop when the absolute CD4+ lymphocyte count falls below 200 to 250 cells per cubic millimeter. Symptoms develop gradually and include fever, dyspnea, malaise, and nonproductive cough, but chills, chest pain, and productive sputum may also occasionally occur. Physical examination is notable for fever and tachypnea; lung auscultation is usually normal. The duration of symptoms is usually 1 month prior to presentation, and patients are often misdiagnosed with bronchitis.

The typical chest x-ray shows bilateral interstitial and alveolar infiltrates, although cavitary infiltrates, focal infiltrates, and nodular densities have occasionally been described. Apical infiltrates and the development of pneumothoraces have also been recognized with the advent of inhaled pentamidine for PCP prophylactic therapy. PCP should always be considered when an HIV-infected individual develops a pneumothorax, because 1% to 2% of patients with *P. carinii* infection develop this complication.

Arterial blood-gas analysis usually reveals an elevated alveolar-arterial oxygen gradient with hypoxemia, but may be normal in milder or earlier forms of the disease. Exercise-induced oxygen desaturation is common and often occurs with normal or near-normal gas exchange. If performed, pulmonary function studies usually demonstrate a reduced diffusion capacity, and lung gallium scanning may show diffuse lung uptake. Some investigators have reported elevations of lactate dehydrogenase, with the level correlating with disease severity.

The diagnosis depends on demonstration of the organism in respiratory secretions. Induced sputum can provide a diagnosis in 56% to 76% of patients if properly obtained and stained with toluidine blue or Giemsa stain. Moreover, the use of fluorescent antibody stains has been described recently. Bronchoalveolar lavage by means of flexible fiberoptic bronchoscopy is the diagnostic procedure of choice if sputum examination is nondiagnostic. Diagnostic yields of 85% to 100% have been reported, but yields may be as low as 62% in patients receiving prophylactic aerosolized pentamidine. Transbronchial lung biopsy is not affected by previous prophylactic pentamidine therapy and has a similar yield. Neutrophilia and increased interleukin-8 (IL-8) levels in bronchoalveolar fluid have prognostic value and indicate patients at high risk for a complicated course or fatal outcome.

> PCP is diagnosed by induced sputum analysis, followed by bronchoalveolar lavage by bronchoscopy or bronchoalveolar lavage and transbronchial lung biopsy.

The drug of choice for PCP is trimethoprim-sulfamethoxazole (TMP/SMX), in a 1 mg/5 mg ratio, 15 to 20 mg/kg/day given in three or four divided doses for 3 weeks. HIV-infected individuals treated with TMP/SMX have a high incidence of adverse reactions, which include fever, rash, leukopenia, thrombocytopenia, and renal dysfunction. If patients show no improvement after 5 to 7 days of drug therapy, or if drug toxicity develops, pentamidine is the alternative agent of choice. Pentamidine is usually given in a dosage of 3 to 4 mg/kg/day intravenously. Other options include dapsone, atovaquone, clindamycin-primaquine, and trimetrexate. If the patient has a P_aO_2 greater than 70 mmHg or an alveolar-arterial oxygen gradient greater than 35, the patient should be started on systemic steroids (Table 16-3). Patients should receive 40 mg of prednisone twice daily for 5 days, followed by 40 mg of prednisone daily for 5 days, then 20 mg of prednisone daily to complete 21 days of treatment. It is believed that corticosteroids decrease the inflammatory alveolitis that arises from *Pneumocystis carinii* infections.

Because of the high incidence of relapse, numerous prophylactic regimes for PCP have been advocated, such as TMP/SMX orally once a day, three times a week. Dapsone, fansidar, and aerosolized pentamidine have also been used for PCP prophylaxis. PCP prophylaxis should be offered to all AIDS patients who have had a prior episode of PCP or have an absolute CD4+ T-lymphocyte count of less than 200 cells per cubic millimeter.

Who benefits?	Adults or adolescents with PCP who have arterial $PO_2 < 70$ mmHg or A-a gradient > 35 mmHg
Initiation	Within 24 to 72 hours of beginning anti-PCP therapy
Dosage schedule	Prednisone, orally: days 1 to 5, 40 mg twice daily; days 6 to 10, 40 mg daily; days 11 to 21, 20 mg daily
Side effects	Increased frequency of oral herpes simplex lesions and oral thrush; no increase in the incidence of Kaposi's sarcoma or serious opportunistic infections

Table 16-3

Recommendations and Conclusions of the National Institutes of Health–University of California Expert Panel for Corticosteroids as Adjunctive Therapy for PCP in AIDS Patients

Modified from Zurlo J: Respiratory infections and the acquired immunodeficiency syndrome. Chapter 3 *in* Bone RG, ed.: *Pulmonary and Critical Care Medicine*. Boston: Mosby, 1997.

FUNGAL INFECTIONS

Before the advent of AIDS fungal infections were seen primarily in patients with hematologic malignancies, patients treated with chemotherapy, patients on immunosuppressive therapy, and patients being treated with high-dosage corticosteroids. Immune suppression in these circumstances was usually short-lived, quite unlike the case of HIV patients, who have profound and severe immune suppression on a prolonged basis.

Cryptococcosis. Cryptococcosis usually occurs in patients with CD4+ lymphocyte counts of less than 200 cells per microliter. Cryptococcosis is the most common and most important deep fungal infection complicating AIDS. It develops in 10% of all AIDS patients, and in 5% of patients it is the initial opportunistic infection that heralds the onset of AIDS.

Cryptococcus neoformans is an encapsulated fungus that exists in nature as a yeast. The capsule is composed of a polysaccharide that can be detected on direct smears by India ink preparation or in histopathologic preparations by mucicarmine staining. Although *C. neoformans* is the most common fungal pulmonary HIV infection, cases of isolated pulmonary involvement are rare. More than 75% of patients who present with cryptococcosis have meningitis with or without disseminated disease.

Common clinical presenting signs are fever, weight loss, and headache. Approximately 50% of patients also present with respiratory symptoms that include cough, dyspnea, and chest pain. Overall, sputum production is rare. Physical examination usually reveals dyspnea, rales, and lymphadenopathy, with the most frequent complaint being headaches without meningismus. Clinical presentations of clinical pulmonary cryptococcosis and PCP are strikingly similar, with both demonstrating respiratory symptoms that include the insidious onset of dyspnea, cough, and fever.

The chest radiograph usually demonstrates diffuse interstitial infiltrates, but cavitary lesions, lymphadenopathy, and pleural effusions may also be evident. The acute respiratory distress syndrome secondary to disseminated cryptococcosis has also been reported. Sputum examination has a low diagnostic yield, and bronchoscopy with bronchoalveolar lavage is the procedure of choice, with a diagnostic sensitivity of more than 80%. Serum cryptococcal antigens are present in more than 90% of cases, and bone marrow biopsy and blood cultures have a diagnostic sensitivity of approximately 90%. India ink preparation of cerebrospinal fluid (CSF) may also show the organism. A lack of inflammatory cells in CSF, a high CSF protein level, and a large burden of organisms in the CSF coupled with a change in mental status are all associated with a poorer prognosis.

Amphotericin B is the initial drug of choice. It is administered for several weeks with the cumulative dosage goal of 15 to 30 mg/kg. Fluconazole is an effective alternative agent for those intolerant to amphotericin B. Lifelong antifungal maintenance therapy is necessary for surviving patients. Mortality is 40% to 80% of patients with disseminated cryptococcosis, with median survival of 8 to 9 months.

Histoplasmosis. Approximately 5% of HIV patients who live in areas endemic for histoplasmosis, such as the Ohio and Mississippi river valleys, Puerto Rico, Haiti, South America, and Central America, develop disseminated histoplasmosis. *Histoplasma capsulatum* is a dimorphic organism that grows in nitrogen-rich soils. Infection occurs by inhalation of infectious micronidia, which develops into a yeast phase that causes pneumonitis. By means of the pulmonary route, the organisms then spread into the

Cryptococcosis is the most common deep fungal infection in HIV patients. It infects 10% of all AIDS patients and heralds the onset of AIDS in 5% of all patients.

Physical examination in cryptococcosis reveals headache without meningismus.

reticuloendothelial system and lymph nodes. A cell-mediated immune response then occurs, with the production of specific macrophages that engulf the fungi and form granulomas with central necrosis, fibrosis, and, ultimately, calcification. This protective response is partially or completely absent in patients with depressed T-cell function, thereby enabling the fungus to spread.

Most patients report weight loss as the initial symptom, with only 4% of patients having isolated pulmonary symptoms. As the illness progresses, patients develop cough and dyspnea. Sputum production is uncommon. Approximately 25% of patients present with hepatosplenomegaly. Gastrointestinal involvement is hallmarked by diarrhea and sometimes upper gastrointestinal bleeding secondary to ulceration. Disseminated intravascular coagulation can be seen in cases with rapid progression.

In 40% of patients, the chest x-ray is normal, but chest x-rays may show bilateral nodular infiltrates with or without lymphadenopathy. A chest x-ray pattern of diffuse small nodular infiltrates, similar to miliary tuberculosis, has also been reported.

Serologic testing for *Histoplasma capsulatum* may be useful in areas where background rates of zero positivity are very low. The sensitivity for precipitants to histoplasma is approximately 70% to 80%. Isolation of histoplasma is commonly reported from the blood (90%), bone marrow (90%), and respiratory tract (85%). A rapid diagnosis can usually be made by a histologic evaluation demonstrating characteristic organisms in lung or bone marrow tissue.

Testing for histoplasma polysaccharide antigen in serum or urine is both sensitive and specific in patients with progressive disseminated histoplasmosis. This can be seen by direct peripheral blood smear in up to 50% of patients.

Amphotericin B is the choice for initial treatment; however, mortality remains high at 20% to 50%, with relapses commonly found and life-long suppressive therapy required. In less severe cases, some data indicate that itraconazole may also be successful.

Coccidioidomycosis. Coccidioidomycosis is a relatively frequent diagnosis in AIDS patients living in endemic areas in the southwestern United States. It is a dimorphic fungus that grows as a mycelium. In tissue, it converts into the parasitic form of giant spherules that contain multiple endospores. When the endospores are released, they convert back into the spherule form.

Illness is relatively benign in HIV patients with relatively preserved T-cell function. In contrast, in severely compromised patients, the disease spreads rapidly with involvement of the respiratory tract. Patients develop cough productive of purulent sputum and fever. Approximately 25% to 35% of patients have meningitis at the time of presentation, with 5% demonstrating skin lesions.

Diffuse reticular infiltrates are the most common chest radiographic presentation; bulky hilar and mediastinal lymph node enlargement are also occasionally observed. The organism may be isolated from lymph nodes, blood, urine, and skin, as well as from pulmonary secretions. Contrary to histoplasmosis, specific antigen testing is not available.

Mortality is high, with 15% of patients dying despite aggressive medical therapy. Amphotericin B is the treatment of choice and should be promptly instituted. Fluconazole can be used for chronic suppression. Overall, the median survival is 1 to 5 months from the time of diagnosis.

Blastomycosis. *Blastomyces dermatitidis* is another dimorphic fungus. It is relatively uncommon in HIV patients but extremely aggressive when immune compromise is severe.

Patients usually present with a rapid progression of symptoms and deterioration of respiratory status. Respiratory symptoms include cough, purulent sputum, and dyspnea; meningeal signs are commonly found.

Chest radiographs demonstrate lobar infiltrates. Less commonly observed are nodules or diffuse interstitial infiltrates that may resemble PCP.

There is no specific fungal antigen test, and serologic tests lack adequate sensitivity and specificity. Demonstration of the characteristic yeast forms in respiratory secretions provides a quick and relatively specific diagnosis. Cultures of specimens require a long time to grow the fungi and should be considered confirmatory tests.

Amphotericin B should be used for primary therapy and continued until the patient shows clinical improvement. Once patients improve, itraconazole is given for lifetime therapy. Mortality is high, with 50% of patients dying within 2 months.

Aspergillosis. Aspergillosis has only recently been described as an infectious pulmonary complication of HIV disease and usually occurs in patients in the latter phases of their lives. Most patients are granulocytopenic and have been placed on broad-spectrum antibiotics or steroid therapy prior to aspergillosis infection. Dissemination of the fungus occurs in 30% of cases.

The lungs are the portals of entry for the spores. HIV patients may exhibit a wide variety of presentations, some of which are rarely seen in noncompromised hosts. Cavitary infiltrates are common with a predilection for the upper lobes. Cavities may increase in size up to 10 cm in diameter and rupture, resulting in pneumothorax or pyopneumothorax. Bronchial casts containing aspergillus organisms may be found when expectorated. As the disease progresses, pseudomembranes or ulcerations in the airway can develop, which may eventually cause airway obstruction.

Diagnosis is made by the presence of aspergillus in respiratory secretions in HIV-infected granulocytopenic patients. Amphotericin B is the primary drug treatment with itraconazole used for maintenance therapy. Mortality is extremely high (i.e., 60% to 70%) once tissue invasion occurs.

VIRAL INFECTIONS

Cytomegalovirus (CMV). Active CMV infections are found in 70% to 90% of HIV patients at autopsy. In some reports, CMV has been implicated as one of the major causes of death in at least 16% of patients who die from AIDS. However, because coexistent pathogens are frequently found in lungs at autopsy, it is not clear whether CMV by itself accounted for the lung disease or some other copathogen was responsible.

CMV is ubiquitous in the environment. Infection is very common among immunocompetent subjects, but it rarely progresses to clinical disease. After the initial infection, a latency period ensues wherein the virus remains in a quiescent state in peripheral leukocytes and organs such as the liver and spleen. Reactivation occurs at a later date as a consequence of immune suppression.

Clinical manifestations are typical but nonspecific for CMV infection. These include fever, nonproductive cough, dyspnea, and respiratory failure. HIV-infected individuals appear to have a more benign course than bone marrow recipients who contract the disease. The plain chest x-ray usually shows evidence of a diffuse interstitial infiltrate.

Secondary to the frequent presence of CMV in the lungs of patients with AIDS and its uncertain role in causing clinical disease, criteria for the diagnosis of CMV and pneumonitis must be adhered to strictly. These criteria include a compatible clinical and radiographic picture, exclusion of other pulmonary pathogens, recovery of CMV in the culture of lower respiratory tract secretions, and histologic evidence of CMV infection by means of intranuclear inclusions in lung tissue.

Ganciclovir is the treatment of choice for CMV pneumonitis. An induction dosage of 5 mg/kg twice daily for 14 days is followed by long-term maintenance with 5 mg/kg/day. Coadministration of CMV hyperimmunoglobulin does not appear to improve patient outcome. If the virus is resistant to ganciclovir, foscarnet is a second-line treatment. Valcyclovir, an oral agent, has also been investigated for CMV treatment.

Other Viruses. Several other viral infections of the lung have been reported in HIV patients. Herpes simplex virus has been reported to cause pneumonia, although it is an infrequent pathogen. Herpes simplex pneumonitis should be considered when histologic evidence of pulmonary infection exists and no other pathogen is identified. Other viruses, such as respiratory syncytial and parainfluenza viruses, have been reported but are not unique to this patient group. Yearly vaccination against influenza is recommended for HIV patients, but its effectiveness has not been objectively demonstrated.

CMV has been implicated in 16% of deaths in AIDS patients, but the presence of other infections or disorders clouds the significance of CMV as a pathogen.

NONINFECTIOUS PULMONARY DISEASES

KAPOSI'S SARCOMA

Kaposi's sarcoma is the most common malignancy in AIDS. Its frequency is 20,000 times higher in HIV patients than in the general population.

The emergence of Kaposi's sarcoma (KS) in homosexual patients in the 1980s was one of the events that led to the discovery of HIV/AIDS. It is the most common malignancy in patients with AIDS. Although this tumor is occasionally seen in the elderly and in renal transplant patients, its incidence is 20,000 times higher in the HIV population than in the general public. KS occurs in approximately 20% of infected homosexual men and in 2% of all other HIV-infected individuals. The pathogenesis of KS is unclear; HIV virus has not been found in the lesions. The tumor is believed to originate from the hyperproduction of angiogenesis factors or secondary to an occult infection. Recently, sequences of herpes virus 8 have been found in KS tissue.

KS usually presents as a multicentric disease with skin mucosa and GI tract involvement 50% of the time. KS-related lung disease usually is preceded by extrapulmonary disease manifestations.

KS usually presents as a multicentric disease involving skin, the mucosa, and internal organs—particularly the lymphatics and the gastrointestinal tract, which are involved 50% of the time. AIDS-associated KS usually presents with cutaneous disease, with skin lesions having a predilection for the face but sometimes observed on the genitalia, lower extremities, and torso. The lesions have a pink to bluish color and vary in size from several millimeters to centimeters. Patient symptoms are nondescript and include fever, weight loss, and malaise. Cough and dyspnea are also frequently reported. Patients may also present with hemoptysis and pleuritic chest pain. Physical examination is usually unremarkable. In some cases, wheezing as a result of endobronchial lesions or stridor caused by compression of the upper airway may be found.

Predominant chest radiographic findings include interstitial infiltrates with hilar lymphadenopathy, or ill-defined pulmonary nodular infiltrates. Pleural effusions may also be seen and may be unilateral or bilateral. The diagnosis of pulmonary KS usually requires an open-lung biopsy demonstrating spindle-shaped cells surrounded by vascular channels containing erythrocytes. Visualization of the typical macular plaques on visual inspection of the tracheobronchial tree is also considered adequate to establish the diagnosis in patients who present with the appropriate clinical findings.

The diagnosis of KS carries a poor prognosis, with median survival ranging from 2 to 10 months. The presence of pleural effusions, severe shortness of breath, low white blood count, and absence of cutaneous lesions are all considered poor prognostic factors. Patients with pulmonary KS show poor response to chemotherapy. Some studies have reported an improved survival in patients who have been treated with vinca alkaloids, bleomycin, and the anthracyclines. Transient responses have also been demonstrated with the use of whole-lung irradiation. More recent therapeutic research has focused on angiogenesis and growth factor inhibitors.

LYMPHOMA

Non-Hodgkin's lymphoma occurs in 5% of HIV patients and is comprised of multiple, highly malignant clones of B-cell origin.

The most common type of lymphoma affecting HIV patients is non-Hodgkin's lymphoma, which occurs in 5% of patients, a 60-fold increase when compared with the general population. Unlike non-Hodgkin's lymphoma in patients of normal immunity, this disease in HIV-infected individuals is comprised of multiple, highly malignant clones of B-cell origin. At the time of presentation, the disease is usually disseminated with extensive extrapulmonary involvement of the central nervous system, gastrointestinal tract, and bone marrow. Putative factors involved in the pathogenesis of this tumor include Epstein-Barr virus (EBV), chronic B-cell stimulation, and cytokine production.

Up to 30% of patients have intrathoracic disease, with the chest x-ray commonly showing interstitial nodular infiltrates, solitary pleural nodules, pulmonary thickening, pleural effusions, and mediastinal lymphadenopathy. Unusual presentations include solitary pulmonary nodules and endobronchial lesions.

The diagnosis can be obtained by flexible fiberoptic bronchoscopy and transbronchial lung biopsy, pleural biopsy, or thoracentesis, but often an open-lung biopsy is required. Prognosis is poor, with a mean survival of 4 to 6 months. Treatment with intensive chemotherapy has not been shown to be more effective than standard therapy. Newer investigational regimes include monoclonal antibodies against interleukin-6 and interferon therapy.

LYMPHOCYTIC AND NONSPECIFIC INTERSTITIAL PNEUMONITIS

Lymphocytic Interstitial Pneumonitis (LIP). LIP is a lymphoproliferative disorder characterized by diffuse infiltration of lymphocytes and plasma cells into the alveolar septae along lymphatic vessels. Besides afflicting HIV-infected patients, it has been found in patients with Sjögren's disease, systemic lupus erythematosus, thyroiditis, chronic active hepatitis, myasthenia gravis, and autoimmune hemolytic anemia.

The pathogenesis of this disease is not known, but it is believed that the lymphocytic and plasma cell infiltration of the alveolar interstitium suggests a response to chronic antigen load. Repeated Epstein-Barr virus (EBV) infections are thought to be the most likely etiology, because high titers of EBV antibodies have been demonstrated in HIV adult patients with LIP and HIV infection. Patients who have this disorder also appear to be more likely to have the human leukocyte antigen (HLA) DR5 phenotype, which further suggests an autoimmune basis for the disease.

The presentation is usually heralded by the insidious onset of cough, dyspnea, fever, malaise, and weight loss. The chest radiograph demonstrates bilateral lower lobe interstitial or reticular nodular infiltrates. Lymphadenopathy is uncommon in adults.

The diagnosis is difficult. Histologic examination of lung tissue is required. There is no definite treatment, but cases in children have been treated with corticosteroids with variable results. Some preliminary studies suggest that the antiretrovirals may favorably affect the course of the disease.

Nonspecific Interstitial Pneumonitis. Nonspecific interstitial pneumonitis has not been as well characterized as LIP. It is essentially a histologic diagnosis that is characterized by lymphocytic infiltrates surrounding the bronchi and vessels with alveolar interstitial involvement less pronounced than in patients with LIP. Some patients may also develop diffuse alveolar fibrosis. This disorder has been termed chronic interstitial pneumonitis because of the presence of mononuclear and lymphocytic infiltrates.

Patients usually have nonspecific respiratory symptoms or may be asymptomatic. More than 25% of patients characterized with this disorder have had concurrent Kaposi's sarcoma, have received previous experimental drug therapy for HIV infection, have had a prior history of PCP, or have been drug abusers.

Case Study:
Resolution

After his first episode of pneumocystis pneumonia, J.D. continues to be followed by an HIV specialist. His CD4 cell count has dropped to 135 cells per milliliter. He is started on TMP/SMX prophylaxis, but after several weeks he develops severe reactions that force his doctor to discontinue this therapy. He fails alternative drugs but tolerates aerosolized pentamidine. He remains stable for several months.

He has gone to the outpatient pharmacy to refill his medications when he suddenly feels short of breath and develops pain in his right hemithorax. The pain is sharp and worse during inspiration. He is rapidly transported to the emergency department.

The patient is afebrile, his respiratory rate is 35 breaths per minute, and he is tachycardic. His blood pressure is within normal limits. He was ambulating until today. He denies other symptoms, leg swelling, and leg pain. Physical examination reveals decreased breath sounds in the right lung, which is also noted to be hyperresonant to percussion. A chest x-ray shows a large pneumothorax.

PNEUMOTHORAX

Pneumothorax complicates approximately 2% of HIV-infected patients. The majority of patients who develop spontaneous pneumothorax have an underlying chronic pneumocystis infection, although some have interstitial lung disease resulting from nontuberculous or tuberculous mycobacterium, cytomegalovirus infection, and Kaposi's sarcoma involving the visceral pleura. Patients treated with aerosolized pentamidine for PCP prophylaxis are at higher risk, possibly because pentamidine tends not to deposit in the upper lobes, thereby creating apical areas of chronic subpleural pneumocystis infection that leads to lung destruction. Overall, large apical subpleural air cysts may rupture, causing a pneumothorax.

> Pneumothorax may occur in 2% of AIDS patients. PCP infection may have a role. Commonly, bilateral pneumothorax occurs and treatment is difficult.

Patients with AIDS have a tendency to have bilateral pneumothoraces with a high recurrence rate, especially those who have had prior pneumothoraces. Patients typically require prolonged hospitalization secondary to pneumothorax and have a high mortality owing mainly to failure of conventional therapy. In some series, mortality of patients admitted for spontaneous pneumothorax approaches 40%.

Spontaneous pneumothoraces are difficult to treat in HIV patients because of persistent bronchopleural fistula. Tube thoracostomy is unlikely to be successful. Open thoracotomy and surgical closure of persistent bronchopleural fistulas is indicated.

EMPHYSEMA

Cystic lesions of the lung tissue as well as emphysema have been described in HIV patients. The mechanisms by which these lesions develop is unknown, but some patients have been reported to have had prior PCP or chronic pneumonia, which may have induced lung destruction. In some patients, HIV-infected cells may have had a direct cytolytic effect on alveolar walls and pulmonary capillaries, causing emphysema. A recent study performing computed tomography (CT) examination of the chest in 55 AIDS patients showed that 42% had evidence of bullous disease. In comparison with patients who have cigarette-smoking-induced emphysema, patients with HIV disease and emphysema have signs of air trapping, hyperinflation, and markedly reduced diffusion capacity, but only mild signs of airway disease. Emphysema should be considered as an additional diagnosis in patients with HIV infection who present with dyspnea and no clear etiology.

PLEURAL EFFUSIONS

Pleural effusions may occur in 25% of patients hospitalized with AIDS. The mean age and risk factors of these patients do not differ from those of patients admitted without pleural effusions, but patients with pleural effusions overall tend to have lower CD4 counts. In most patients (66%), the pleural effusion is attributable to an infectious etiology, with bacterial pneumonia being most common (31%), followed by PCP (15%), *Mycobacterium tuberculosis* (8%), septic emboli (3%), and Nocardia, cryptococcosis, and MAC (3%). In the remaining patients who have noninfectious causes of pleural effusions, the most common etiologies are hypoalbuminemia, unsuspected cardiac failure, and Kaposi's sarcoma. Massive pleural effusions that develop in HIV patients usually are the result of Kaposi's sarcoma or tuberculosis.

PULMONARY HYPERTENSION

Pulmonary hypertension has been described as being more common in HIV-infected patients than in the non-HIV-infected population. A prospective evaluation of 74 HIV patients with cardiopulmonary disorders revealed pulmonary hypertension afflicting 8%. In comparison with females who developed primary pulmonary hypertension, those who developed pulmonary hypertension with HIV infection were more likely to be male, had a median age of 38 years, and exhibited pulmonary artery pressures ranging from 50 to 100 mmHg, systolic. Plexogenic pulmonary arteriopathy is the most common pathologic finding. It has been speculated that HIV or another retrovirus may damage the pulmonary epithelium or cause injury by releasing mediators that induce pulmonary hypertension. Currently, characterization of pulmonary hypertension in HIV-infected individuals is undergoing closer investigation.

▌DIAGNOSTIC APPROACH TO PULMONARY DISEASE IN THE HIV PATIENT

HISTORY AND PHYSICAL EXAMINATION

It is important to note that not all lung disease in HIV patients is related to HIV infection. HIV patients may present with exacerbations of asthma, chronic bronchitis, and upper respiratory tract infections that are similar in presentation and frequency to those in the normal immunocompetent population. In contrast, however, HIV-infected individuals are uniquely susceptible to bacterial pneumonias, particularly those caused by *Streptococcus pneumoniae* and *Haemophilus influenzae*. Bacterial infections present with a typical acute onset of fever, pleuritic chest pain, productive cough, and shortness of breath.

In addition to these usual pulmonary disorders, HIV-infected patients are predisposed to a unique spectrum of pulmonary diseases. Patients with opportunistic diseases caused by *Pneumocystis carinii*, and mycobacterial and fungal pneumonias, usually have a more gradual onset of systemic symptoms of fever, weight loss, and fatigue as well as respiratory symptoms of dyspnea and nonproductive cough. Patients with HIV infection who present with pulmonary Kaposi's sarcoma, or non-Hodgkin's lymphoma most likely already have the diagnosis established because of prior systemic manifestations of the disease.

If a patient is not already known to have evidence of or risks for HIV infection, a history detailing the patient's sexual lifestyle, medical history, use of intravenous drugs, or prior record of sexually transmitted diseases should be documented. Moreover, documentation of the patient's past travel history, place of origin, and occupational history may be helpful in diagnosing certain HIV-related infections.

> History taking in the HIV patient with pulmonary disease should document the patient's past medical, social, travel, and occupational history.

Certain physical findings may be helpful in establishing or suggesting a diagnosis of HIV infection. The presence of thrush or oral candidiasis may be presumptive evidence of HIV infection. Skin lesions, lymphadenopathy, and hepatosplenomegaly may indicate the presence of Kaposi's sarcoma, non-Hodgkin's lymphoma, or disseminated mycobacterial or fungal infections.

Examination of the thorax may be completely normal in patients with early or mild HIV-related lung disease. Localized consolidation of the lung may indicate the presence of acute bacterial pneumonia whereas more widespread diffuse rales indicates a disseminated infiltrative process. Evidence of a pleural effusion on examination may suggest the presence of Kaposi's sarcoma, tuberculosis, or hypoalbuminemia.

CHEST IMAGING

One of the most essential initial laboratory investigations of the HIV-infected patient is a chest radiograph. Certain abnormalities point to the various classes of disorders, as shown in Table 16-4. Three classes of common radiographic abnormalities are described: 1) diffuse reticulonodular infiltrates, 2) focal airspace consolidation, and 3) normal lungs. Intrathoracic lymphadenopathy and pleural effusion are less common than these three entities, but each of these abnormalities also suggests a separate differential diagnosis.

Table 16-4
Differential Diagnosis of Commonly Observed Chest Radiographic Patterns in HIV Patients

PATTERN	DISEASES
Diffuse reticulonodular infiltration	*Pneumocystis carinii* pneumonia Disseminated tuberculosis Disseminated histoplasmosis Disseminated coccidioidomycosis Lymphocytic interstitial pneumonitis
Focal airspace consolidation	Bacterial pneumonia Kaposi's sarcoma Cryptococcosis
Normal	*Pneumocystis carinii* pneumonia Disseminated *Mycobacterium avium* complex Disseminated histoplasmosis
Adenopathy	Tuberculosis Kaposi's sarcoma Disseminated *Mycobacterium avium* complex
Pleural effusion	Kaposi's sarcoma Tuberculosis Non-Hodgkin's lymphoma Pyogenic empyema

Modified from Zurlo J: Respiratory infections and the acquired immunodeficiency syndrome. Chapter 3 *in* Bone RG, ed.: *Pulmonary and Critical Care Medicine*. Boston: Mosby, 1997.

On occasion, chest CT may also be valuable, especially in evaluating mediastinal abnormalities, localized masses, or fluid collections. A chest CT may not only differentiate parenchymal from pleural or mediastinal abnormalities better than a conventional chest x-ray but may also provide a road map to biopsy or drainage procedures.

PULMONARY FUNCTION TESTING

Although pulmonary function tests (PFTs) are commonly abnormal in patients with pulmonary disease and HIV infection, the resulting disturbances are frequently similar and in most cases do not discriminate among the various etiologies. Therefore, pulmonary function testing is not routinely indicated in the evaluation of patients with obvious HIV-related pulmonary complications.

The major role of pulmonary function testing in HIV-infected patients is to aid in the selection of symptomatic patients with normal or near-normal chest x-rays who have abnormalities on pulmonary function testing that require further diagnostic evaluation.

Four types of functional disturbances have been detected on pulmonary function testing. These include 1) a restrictive ventilatory defect characterized by a low vital capacity; 2) impaired oxygenation with a low P_aO_2 or widened alveolar-arterial oxygen gradient, which is almost always present in patients with PCP during exercise; 3) a low carbon monoxide diffusion capacity, again commonly observed in patients with PCP; and 4) an obstructive ventilatory defect characterized by expiratory flow rate limitation, which has been associated with endobronchial Kaposi's sarcoma.

Moreover, pulmonary function testing may be helpful in selected HIV-infected patients in whom disorders of the airways, such as asthma and chronic bronchitis, produce symptoms that are not related to the HIV infection and require different treatment.

> Pulmonary function tests are usually abnormal and nonspecific in HIV patients. However, in symptomatic patients with normal chest x-rays, pulmonary function abnormalities may aid characterization of the patient's problem.

SPUTUM ANALYSIS

Sputum examination in HIV-infected patients may reveal both bacterial infections and certain types of opportunistic infections.

Most patients with HIV-related bacterial pneumonia have cough productive of purulent sputum. Examination of the sputum with Gram stain and culture is helpful in revealing the diagnosis and selecting the appropriate antimicrobial agent.

Sputum induction while patients inspire 3% to 5% saline solution generated by an ultrasonic nebulizer has also been shown to be effective in eliciting respiratory secretions and diagnosing PCP. Meticulous technique is required in collecting the specimen, as well as in processing and examining it, but several studies have shown sensitivities of 55% to 92% in detecting PCP by this method. The addition of indirect immunofluorescent staining using monoclonal antibodies directed against *Pneumocystis carinii* have been shown to improve further the sensitivity and specificity of this test.

BRONCHOSCOPY

If sputum induction is negative for identifying the etiology of the pulmonary disease in the HIV patient, flexible fiberoptic bronchoscopy remains the cornerstone diagnostic test. In the first few years of the HIV epidemic, both bronchoalveolar lavage and transbronchial lung biopsy were used to establish the diagnosis of a respiratory disorder. More recently, however, bronchoalveolar lavage by flexible fiberoptic bronchoscopy has been demonstrated to be easier to perform, with fewer complications, and has by itself a high yield in the diagnosis of PCP. Although bronchoalveolar lavage is not as effective as bronchoalveolar lavage plus transbronchial lung biopsy in diagnosing fungal and mycobacterial disorders, most authorities still recommend bronchoalveolar lavage as the initial test. If the initial bronchoscopic examination with bronchoalveolar lavage is nondiagnostic, most physicians elect to rebronchoscope the patient and perform transbronchial lung biopsy and a repeat lung lavage. Figures 16-2 to 16-4 show a diagnostic approach using bronchoscopy based on the radiographic abnormality in diagnosing the HIV patient.

OTHER TECHNIQUES

Percutaneous needle aspiration is of limited value for patients with diffuse lung disease because of its high propensity for complications (i.e., 50% incidence of pneumothorax). In patients who have focal mass lesions, transthoracic needle aspiration may be of benefit.

Similarly, open-lung biopsy, which is considered by some to be the gold standard diagnostic procedure for the evaluation of pulmonary diseases of unknown cause, has a limited role. Small studies that have looked at the role of open-lung biopsy in HIV patients who have undergone prior nondiagnostic bronchoscopy have shown that, although a new treatable infection or malignant diagnosis may be identified, the ultimate outcome of patients is not changed. Overall, open-lung biopsy is seldom performed in patients with HIV disease, because the yield in identifying treatable diseases has been low and the complication rate appears to be high. Further investigation is needed to clarify the role of this technique in the HIV patient group.

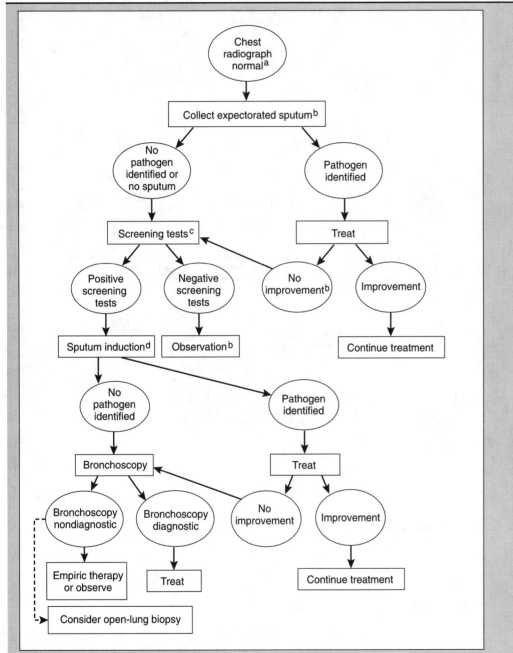

FIGURE 16-2

Algorithm for evaluation of the patient with pulmonary symptoms and a normal chest x-ray. [a] If PCP is suspected, treatment with antimicrobial therapy should be initiated while proceeding with diagnostic evaluation. [b] If the patient is severely symptomatic, bronchoscopy should be performed. [c] Tests to help detect the presence of pulmonary disease, especially PCP (i.e., blood gases, diffusing capacity). [d] If PCP or tuberculosis is suspected, sputum induction should be performed. Reproduced with permission from Zurlo J: Respiratory infections and the acquired immunodeficiency syndrome. Chapter 3 *in* Bone RG, ed.: *Pulmonary and Critical Care Medicine.* Boston: Mosby, 1997.

FIGURE 16-3
Diagnostic algorithm for evaluation of the patient who presents with focal infiltrates on chest x-ray. Reproduced with permission from Zurlo J: Respiratory infections and the acquired immunodeficiency syndrome. Chapter 3 *in* Bone RG, ed.: *Pulmonary and Critical Care Medicine*. Boston: Mosby, 1997.

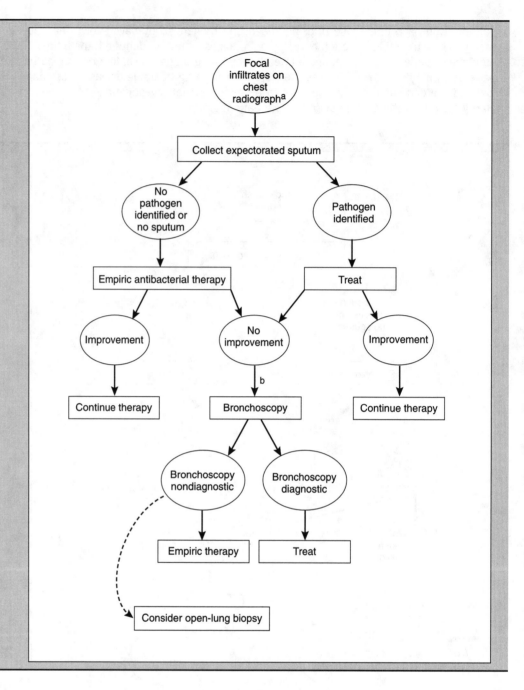

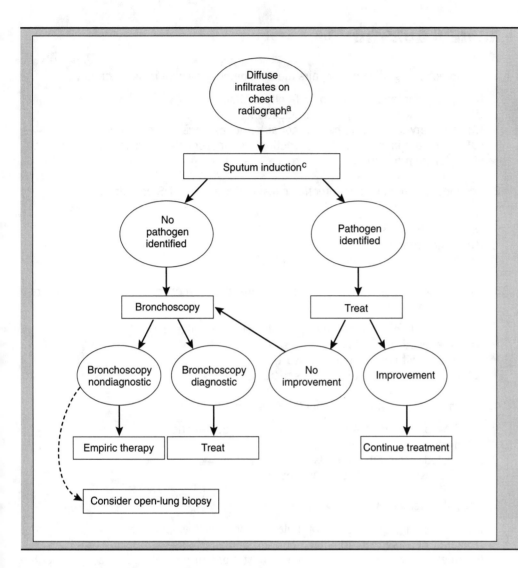

FIGURE 16-4
Algorithm for evaluation of the patient with diffuse infiltrates on chest x-ray. Reproduced with permission from Zurlo J: Respiratory infections and the acquired immunodeficiency syndrome. Chapter 3 *in* Bone RG, ed.: *Pulmonary and Critical Care Medicine*. Boston: Mosby, 1997.

■ SUMMARY

Patients with HIV infection who present with pulmonary disease exhibit a unique spectrum of common disorders that afflict the general population and selected disorders that are prone to afflict only those with HIV infection. The environment of the lung is a unique milieu that propagates HIV replication and induces local immune dysfunction that predisposes the lung to a variety of infectious and noninfectious complications.

A diagnostic approach to pulmonary disease in the HIV patient (see Figures 16-2 to 16-4) that includes a detailed history and physical examination along with chest imaging, sputum analysis, and flexible fiberoptic bronchoscopy should allow one to arrive at the correct pulmonary diagnosis so as to establish effective treatment.

∎ REVIEW QUESTIONS

1. HIV infection significantly impairs the lung defense mechanisms secondary to

   (A) an augmentation in cytotoxic T-cell function
   (B) a decrease in lung cytokine production
   (C) immunity to blood-borne, but not airborne, pathogens
   (D) a decrease in cytotoxic T-cell function over time coupled with an increase in local cytokine production

2. The most common type of infection causing disease in AIDS patients is

   (A) bacterial infections
   (B) viral infections
   (C) fungal infections
   (D) *Pneumocystic carinii* pneumonia (PCP)

3. HIV-infected patients who have disease caused by *Mycobacterium tuberculosis* are more likely to

   (A) have CD4 counts lower than 50 cells per cubic millimeter
   (B) have reactivation of latent disease
   (C) present with disseminated disease
   (D) not respond to antituberculous therapy

4. *Pneumocystic carinii* pneumonia (PCP) is

   (A) the most common AIDS-related opportunistic infection
   (B) diagnosed by culture results
   (C) treated with corticosteroids
   (D) diagnosed only by open-lung biopsy

5. Kaposi's sarcoma (KS) in HIV patients

   (A) arises from highly malignant multiple clones of B lymphocytes
   (B) rarely occurs in HIV-infected homosexual men
   (C) rarely exhibits extrapulmonary manifestations in patients diagnosed with pulmonary KS
   (D) has a poor prognosis, with median survival ranging from 2 to 10 months

■ ANSWERS AND EXPLANATIONS

1. The answer is D. Initially, cytotoxic T cells are highly active against HIV-infected cells, but eventually they become infected and their number decreases, with a concomitant decrement in function. As cell-mediated immunity deteriorates, the patient becomes more prone to opportunistic infections, which trigger the production of local cytokines. Enhanced viral replication thereby allows more cells to become infected.

2. The answer is A. HIV patients have an eightfold greater incidence of bacterial infections compared with the general population. *P. carinii* is the most common opportunistic infection in HIV patients, but bacterial infections are generally more frequent causes of disease.

3. The answer is C. HIV patients are more likely to have disseminated tuberculosis on presentation. Tuberculosis can present in patients with relatively preserved CD4 cell counts in comparison with patients who have *M. avium* complex (MAC), who usually develop diseases with CD4 counts less than 50. Non-HIV patients with tuberculosis usually have reactivation of latent disease, whereas HIV patients usually present with newly acquired disease. If placed on appropriate therapy, patients with HIV respond to antituberculous agents, and their outcomes do not differ significantly from those of non-HIV patients.

4. The answer is A. *P. carinii* is the most common opportunistic infection in HIV patients. Its diagnosis depends on demonstration of the organism in respiratory secretions. Induced sputum, bronchoalveolar lavage, and transbronchial biopsy have very high yields in HIV patients, where the number of organisms is high, and open-lung biopsy is therefore only rarely necessary. Corticosteroids are an important adjunctive therapy for PCP, probably because they decrease the magnitude of inflammatory alveolitis.

5. The answer is D. KS is believed to originate from hyperproduction of angiogenesis factors. It is more common in HIV-infected homosexual males than in other HIV patients. KS pulmonary involvement frequently signals disseminated disease. Prognosis at the time of diagnosis, especially in the presence of large pleural effusions, shortness of breath, low white blood cell count, and absence of cutaneous lesions, is extremely poor (2 to 10 months median survival).

■ SUGGESTED READING

Cohen PT, Sande MA, Volberding PA: *The AIDS Knowledge Base*. Waltham, MA: The Medical Publishing Group, a division of the Massachusetts Medical Society, 1990.

Libman H, Witzburg R: *HIV Infection. A Clinical Manual*, 2nd ed. Boston: Little, Brown, 1990.

Murray JF, Mills J: Noninfectious pulmonary complications in HIV disease. *Am Rev Resp Dis* 141:1582–1598, 1990.

Murray JF, Mills J: Pulmonary complications of human immunodeficiency virus, Part I. *Am Rev Resp Dis* 141:1356–1372, 1990.

Vander Els NJ, Stover DE: Approach to the patient with pulmonary diseases. *Clin Chest Med* 17:767–785, 1996.

White D, Stover D: Pulmonary complications of HIV disease. *Clin Chest Med* 17(4):621–822, 1996.

Zurlo J: Respiratory infections and the acquired immunodeficiency syndrome. Chapter 3 in Bone RG, ed.: *Pulmonary and Critical Care Medicine*. Boston: Mosby, 1997.

Chapter 17

SLEEP APNEA AND SLEEP-RELATED BREATHING DISORDERS

Samuel L. Krachman, D.O.

Thomas Berger, B.A., R.P.S.G.T.

■ CHAPTER OUTLINE

Learning Objectives
Case Study: Introduction
Introduction
Normal Control of Breathing
Case Study: Continued
Normal Sleep
Case Study: Continued
Control of Breathing During Sleep
Case Study: Continued
Sleep-Disordered Breathing
Case Study: Continued
Case Study: Continued
Case Study: Resolution
Summary
Review Questions

■ LEARNING OBJECTIVES

At the completion of this chapter, the reader should:

- Understand the normal control of breathing. This includes the central controller's role of processing afferent information from chemo- and mechanoreceptors, and its ability to exert an appropriate ventilatory response in order to maintain homeostasis.
- Understand normal sleep physiology, including the normal stages of sleep (non-REM stages 1 to 4 and REM sleep) and their distribution over the course of a night's sleep.
- Be familiar with the normal changes that occur in the control of breathing during sleep and how these changes impact gas exchange, breathing pattern, and airway resistance.
- Know how disease states—specifically, obstructive sleep apnea, congestive heart failure, and chronic obstructive pulmonary disease—can affect the normal control of breathing and manifest themselves by pathologic changes in breathing pattern during sleep.

Case Study:
Introduction

C.W. is a 48-year-old white man with a history of excessive daytime sleepiness for the past 5 years. His wife reports that he has snored loudly for the past 7 years, and that his snoring has become louder and more frequent over the past 2 years. His snoring has been so severe that he has often needed to leave the bedroom and sleep on the couch in order for his wife to get some rest. They have even thought of getting separate bedrooms because of the disruption his snoring has caused. C.W. usually goes to bed at approximately 11:00 P.M. and has no difficulty initiating sleep. During the night, besides the loud snoring, his wife has noticed episodes in which he has struggled to breathe. C.W. reports that he occasionally wakes up gasping during the night. In addition, he reports episodes of nocturia × 2 and occasional nocturnal sweating. He also thrashes about during the night, and finds the covers disheveled in the morning.

■ INTRODUCTION

To understand the different types of breathing disorders that occur during sleep, it is important first to learn about the normal control of breathing as well as normal sleep physiology. With this background, one can better understand how disease states can affect these normal mechanisms and lead to the observed signs and symptoms associated with these disorders.

■ NORMAL CONTROL OF BREATHING

The respiratory control center normally controls breathing and allows maintenance of homeostasis.

Normally, breathing is controlled by the respiratory control system, a complex system that enables homeostasis to be maintained. It can adjust to accommodate for marked changes in oxygen consumption and carbon dioxide production. Thus, the respiratory control system can maintain the arterial PO_2 (P_aO_2) and arterial PCO_2 (P_aCO_2) within narrow ranges, mostly by changes in minute ventilation.

CENTRAL CONTROLLER

The central respiratory controller is located in the medulla and is composed of the DRG and VRG.

The central respiratory controller is located in the medulla and is able to process information from adjacent chemoreceptors as well as from afferent neurons that terminate within it. It is composed of two aggregates of neurons: the dorsal respiratory group (DRG) and the ventral respiratory group (VRG) (Figure 17-1). Processed information from these two areas leads to a respiratory motor response, with projections to various respiratory muscle groups, including the diaphragm. The central controller appears to contribute to respiratory rhythmogenesis. There also seems to be input to the central controller from above, including the pons, which tends to smooth out respiration, as well as the cerebral cortex, which can have behavioral influences and affect functions such as those involved in speech.

SENSORS

Both chemo- and mechanoreceptors sense changes that require responses by the central controller in regards to altering respiration to maintain homeostasis. *Central chemoreceptors* are located in the ventrolateral area of the medulla and respond to changes in [H+] and PCO_2 in the extracellular fluid of the intracerebral interstitium. For example,

FIGURE 17-1
The central respiratory controller, located in the medulla, is composed of the dorsal respiratory group (DRG) and the ventral respiratory group (VRG).

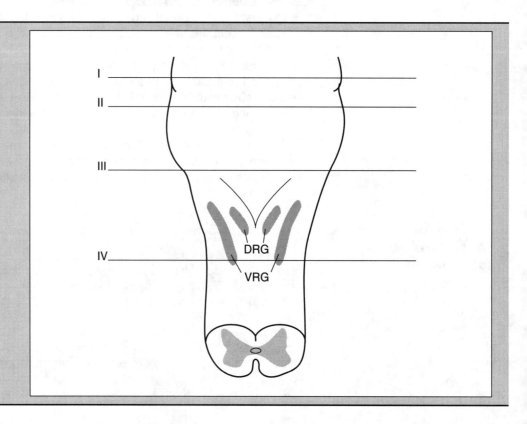

respiratory acidosis leads to an increase in P_aCO_2, with the carbon dioxide freely diffusing across the blood-brain barrier. This leads to increases in [H+] and PCO_2 around the central chemoreceptors and causes a linear increase in minute ventilation (Figure 17-2). Overall, the ventilatory response to changes in P_aCO_2 is the most important in regulating minute ventilation.

The ventilatory response to changes in P_aCO_2 is the most important response in regulating minute ventilation.

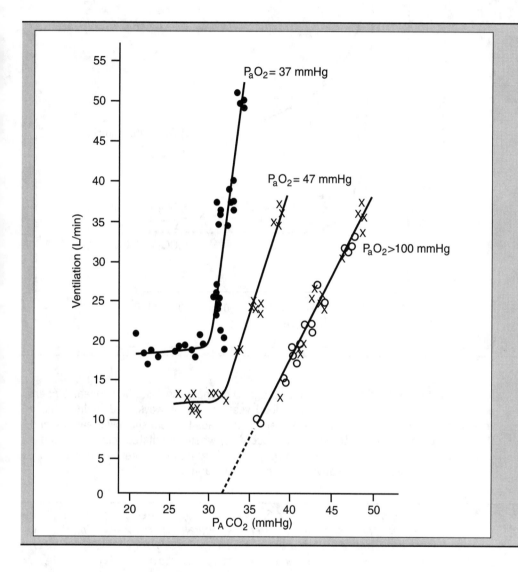

Peripheral chemoreceptors include the carotid bodies, a group of cells located at the bifurcation of the carotid arteries, which sense changes in P_aO_2. They contain glomus cells, which contain neurotransmitters such as dopamine and serotonin, and sustentacular cells, which may be similar to glial cells in the central nervous system. Glomus cells respond to hypoxemia and transmit afferent information by way of the carotid sinus nerve, which joins the glossopharyngeal nerve to reach the DRG. The carotid bodies are responsible for the ventilatory response to hypoxemia. They do not demonstrate increased activity until the P_aO_2 is less than 60 mmHg, thus demonstrating a hyperbolic ventilatory response (Figure 17-3). They do not play a major role in response to changes in P_aCO_2.

Mechanoreceptors, located within the lungs, upper airways, and respiratory muscles, send important sensory information that affects ventilation and maintains homeostasis. The *slowly adapting stretch receptors* are located within airway smooth muscle, and their stimulation helps terminate inspiration. The *rapidly adapting stretch receptors* (*irritant receptors*) are located in the airways between epithelial cells and respond to

Mechanoreceptors located in the lungs, upper airway, and chest wall supply important sensory information to the central controller to maintain homeostasis.

FIGURE 17-3
The ventilatory response to hypoxemia. Note that the response is hyperbolic, with an increase in ventilation not observed until the P_aO_2 is less than 60 mmHg in the setting of normocapnia. With hypercapnia, the ventilatory response is greater at any given level of P_aO_2. Reproduced with permission from Loeschcke HH, Gertz KH: Intracranieel chemorezeptoren mit wirkung out die atmung. *Pflugers Archiv* 267: 460–477, 1958.

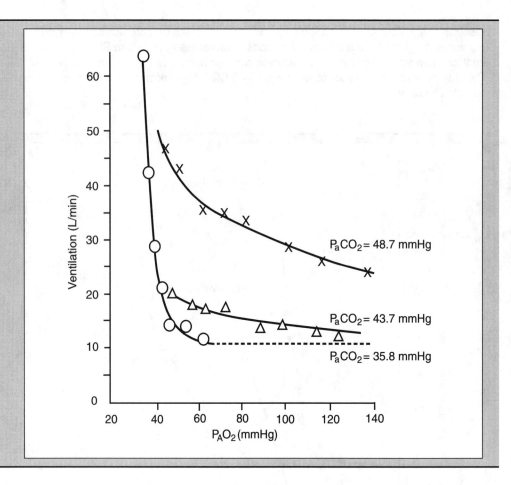

inhalation of noxious stimuli, leading to cough, bronchospasm, and tachypnea. *C fibers* are located in the lung parenchyma, blood vessels, and airways, and include the *J receptors*, whose stimulation by interstitial edema leads to rapid shallow breathing and the sensation of dyspnea. *Upper airway receptors*, when stimulated, can cause bronchospasm, coughing, and sneezing. *Muscle spindles*, although present in accessory muscles of respiration, are relatively lacking in the diaphragm.

Case Study:
Continued

C.W. usually awakens at approximately 6:00 A.M. and feels tired on awakening. He occasionally has morning headaches. C.W. reports generalized tiredness during the day. He says that he often falls asleep in front of his computer at work and has also fallen asleep during meetings recently. He denies any history of traffic accidents but has found himself falling asleep at traffic lights waiting for them to change.

■ NORMAL SLEEP

Normal sleep is composed of NREM (stages 1 to 4) and REM sleep.

Normal sleep is generally categorized as non–rapid eye movement (NREM) sleep and rapid eye movement (REM) sleep based on differences in several physiologic parameters. NREM sleep is further subdivided into stages 1 through 4, representing a continuum of sleep, with stages 3 and 4 [also referred to as delta or slow-wave sleep (SWS)] constituting a deeper and more restful sleep with a higher arousal threshold.

Although the brain is very active during REM sleep, this stage is characterized by inhibition of spinal motor neurons, leading to muscle atonia (referred to as tonic REM) with intermittent bursts of rapid eye movements and distal muscle twitches (referred to as phasic REM). REM sleep is also considered to be restful sleep, with a variable arousal threshold. Dreaming appears to be associated with REM sleep, which originates in the pons.

Most normal individuals take approximately 10 to 20 minutes to initiate sleep. Sleep onset usually occurs through stage 1, which is usually short-lived, accounting for only about 2% to 5% of total sleep time (TST). This stage then leads to stage 2, followed within 10 to 25 minutes by stages 3 and 4, with most of the SWS occurring during the first one-third of the night. SWS accounts for approximately 13% to 23% of TST and decreases normally with age. The first REM period is observed approximately 70 to 90 minutes into sleep, with the initial period lasting just a few minutes. REM periods then cycle every 90 minutes (predominantly alternating with stage 2 sleep, which accounts for 45% to 55% of TST), increasing in length and intensity as the night progresses. REM sleep accounts for 20% to 25% of TST (Figure 17-4).

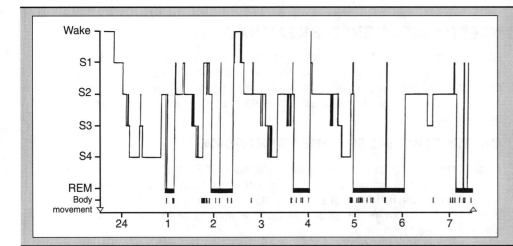

FIGURE 17-4
Histogram of sleep staging across the night in a normal young adult. Note the majority of stage 3 and stage 4 periods during the first third of the night. The first REM period occurs 90 minutes into sleep and cycles every 90 minutes, increasing in length as the night progresses.

Although most young adults sleep approximately 7½ to 8 hours per night, this is quite variable from individual to individual as well as from night to night. Most are able to maintain daytime performance and alertness if they receive not less than 5 hours of sleep. Besides quantity, continuity of sleep appears to be an important factor in maintaining alertness during wakefulness.

Most young adults can maintain daytime alertness and performance if they receive not less than 5 hours of sleep.

C.W. reports that since his job changed 2 years ago from a patrolman to a desk officer with the police force he has gained approximately 20 lb. Associated with this weight gain have been increasing symptoms of daytime sleepiness. He denies any history of thyroid disease and of head or nasal injuries. He reports that he does not drink any alcohol just prior to bedtime.

Case Study:
Continued

■ CONTROL OF BREATHING DURING SLEEP

Normal sleep onset can be associated with an alteration in breathing pattern. During the transition from wakefulness to sleep onset, there is a decrease in behavioral input to the respiratory control system, which was active but influenced by higher cortical inputs (such as those involved in speech, laughter, and coughing) during wakefulness. The hypoxic drive to breathe is decreased, and the ventilatory response to P_aCO_2 is damped as one enters NREM sleep. In addition, minute ventilation decreases, owing primarily to a decrease in tidal volume, and as a consequence P_aCO_2 increases 3 to 10 mmHg and P_aO_2 decreases 2 to 8 mmHg. Upper airway resistance is also noted to increase with sleep.

Many of these observed changes are sleep stage specific. The pattern of breathing can be periodic in nature in sleep stages 1 and 2. This occurs because, at sleep onset, one fluctuates between wakefulness and stages 1 and 2. During an arousal, the elevated P_aCO_2 associated with sleep precipitates hyperventilation in order to drive the P_aCO_2 down to the awake set point, commonly below the sleep apneic threshold. The breathing

At sleep onset, breathing can be periodic in nature as one vacillates between wakefulness and stages 1 and 2 of sleep.

pattern appears to be more regular during SWS. During REM, the breathing pattern is very irregular, with periods of hypoventilation noted during phasic REM.

Case Study:
Continued

On physical exam, the patient's blood pressure is 148/92, his pulse is 72, and his respiratory rate is 14. Nose exam shows no evidence of polyps. Mouth and throat exam shows a small oral pharynx but no anatomic abnormalities such as micrognathia or retrognathia. The patient's neck is short, and he has heavy jowls. His thyroid is not palpably enlarged. His heartbeat is regular. His lungs are clear to auscultation bilaterally. His abdomen is soft and symmetrically enlarged, with positive bowel sounds. His extremities are negative for edema.

■ SLEEP-DISORDERED BREATHING

Abnormal breathing patterns during sleep are observed in several disease processes, either as a primary or an associated finding. The effects of sleep disordered breathing on cardiovascular function, oxygenation, and sleep quality have been shown to increase morbidity, and in some cases mortality. Therefore, appropriate diagnosis and treatment are important.

OBSTRUCTIVE SLEEP APNEA SYNDROME

Obstructive sleep apnea syndrome (OSAS) has a reported incidence of 2% to 4% in the general population aged 30 to 60 years old.

Incidence. Obstructive sleep apnea syndrome (OSAS), manifested by recurrent episodes of airway obstruction during sleep, is a common form of sleep disordered breathing, with a reported incidence of 2% to 4% in middle-aged adults. The male-female ratio is about 8:1, with an increased prevalence in women following menopause, but with a continued male predominance.

Terminology. An *apnea* by definition is a complete lack of airflow for at least 10 seconds associated with a decrease in oxygen saturation (S_aO_2) of 4% or more (Figure 17-5). A *hypopnea* is defined as a decrease in airflow of at least 50% for 10 seconds or more, and is also associated with a decrease in S_aO_2 of 4% or more. Thus, a hypopnea represents only partial airway obstruction (Figure 17-6).

FIGURE 17-5
Obstructive apnea. Note the lack of airflow associated with continued effort to breathe, as demonstrated by the increasing esophageal pressure swings and abdomen and rib cage paradoxical movements. Reproduced with permission from Strollo PJ, Rogers RM: Obstructive sleep apnea. *N Engl J Med* 334:101, 1996.

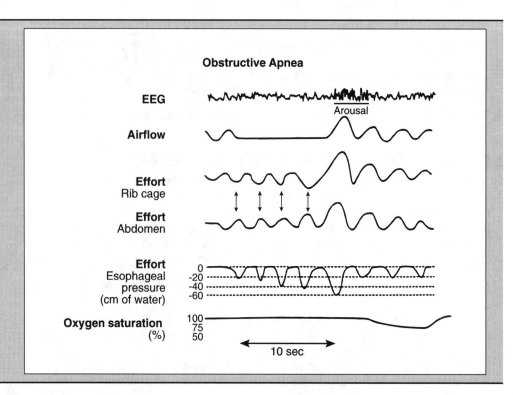

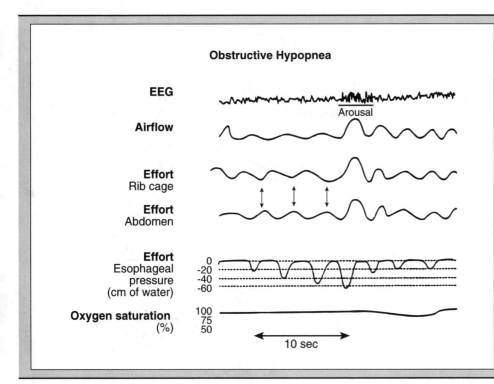

Obstructive Hypopnea

EEG

Arousal

Airflow

Effort
Rib cage

Effort
Abdomen

Effort
Esophageal
pressure
(cm of water)

0
-20
-40
-60

Oxygen saturation
(%)

100
75
50

10 sec

FIGURE 17-6
Obstructive hypopnea, as evidenced by a decrease in airflow of greater than 50%, associated with increasing respiratory effort. The decrease in oxygen saturation occurs following the event as a result of a delay in circulation time to the pulse oximeter on the patient's finger. Reproduced with permission from Strollo PJ, Rogers RM: Obstructive sleep apnea. *N Engl J Med* 334:101, 1996.

Pathogenesis. During normal sleep there is a decrease in central output to the upper airway dilator muscles that maintain upper airway patency during wakefulness. In patients with OSAS, whether owing to increased redundant tissue in the upper airway (as with obesity) or to another anatomic abnormality (such as a small or recessed chin), continued respiratory effort by the diaphragm leads to the development of subatmospheric pressure, and eventually obstruction, in the upper airway. The most common sites of obstruction in patients with OSAS are across from the soft palate (velopharynx) and farther down in the hypopharynx (Figure 17-7). Most patients have more than one site of obstruction.

The most common sites of obstruction in OSAS are the velopharynx and hypopharynx.

Toward the end of an apnea or hypopnea, increasing respiratory effort develops that eventually leads to arousal from sleep. The stimuli that lead to an increase in central controller output and increasing respiratory effort are probably multiple and include hypoxemia and hypercapnia as well as stimulation of mechanoreceptors in the chest wall. Whatever the stimuli, increasing respiratory effort is what ultimately leads to arousal from sleep. Repeated arousals during the night can fragment sleep, which may have an effect on the central controller. One study has demonstrated that a night of sleep deprivation decreases the central controller's output to upper airway dilator muscles during carbon dioxide rebreathing, which could predispose to upper airway obstruction and worsen the degree of apnea. Thus, in OSAS the central controller could be affected in a way that decreases its normal response to such stimuli as hypercapnia and hypoxia.

Symptoms and Signs. The most common complaint of patients with OSAS is excessive daytime sleepiness, which probably is attributable to the repeated arousals that occur throughout the night. The patient's daytime sleepiness can range from mild tiredness throughout the day to falling asleep inappropriately, such as while driving or talking on the phone. Other symptoms include nocturnal sweating, nocturia, personality changes noted by family members, decreased libido, morning headaches, esophageal reflux, and waking up gasping during the night. Family members and friends note loud snoring, often associated with witnessed apneas. On examination, two-thirds of patients are obese, and 50% to 60% have systemic hypertension. The upper airway may show enlarged tonsils or other anatomic abnormalities, but is more often normal. Lower-extremity edema can also develop in association with the development of pulmonary hypertension.

In OSAS, the most common symptom is excessive daytime sleepiness and the most common sign is loud snoring.

FIGURE 17-7
The most common sites of obstruction in OSAS are across from the soft palate in the oropharynx (referred to as the velopharynx) and farther down in the hypopharynx. Most patients have more than one site of obstruction.

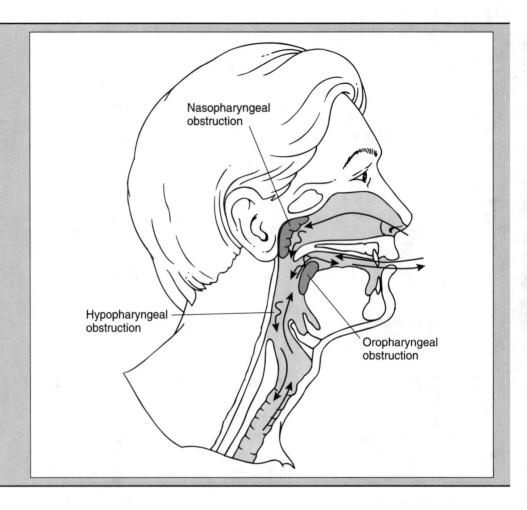

Nasopharyngeal obstruction

Hypopharyngeal obstruction

Oropharyngeal obstruction

Diagnosis. A full night sleep study, referred to as a *polysomnogram* (PSG), is performed to diagnose OSAS. This test consists of recordings that include electro-oculogram (EOG) to identify REM sleep, electroencephalogram (EEG) to stage sleep, airflow at the mouth and nose, thoracic and abdominal motion with breathing, electrocardiogram (ECG), and S_aO_2 (Figure 17-8). Apneas and hypopneas can be identified on these tracings as described above. The number of disordered breathing events during sleep is reported as the apnea-hypopnea index (AHI), which is the average number of apneas plus hypopneas per hour of sleep. An AHI greater than 5 is considered diagnostic for OSAS.

Cardiovascular consequences in OSAS include cyclic elevations in blood pressure and cardiac output as well as bradydysrhythmias.

Cardiovascular Consequences. During normal sleep, systemic blood pressure (BP) decreases approximately 10% to 15%, with the greatest reduction taking place during NREM stages 3 and 4. Similarly, heart rate decreases 5% to 10% during NREM sleep. Both heart rate and systemic BP fluctuate substantially during REM, with mean values approaching those observed during wakefulness. In patients with OSAS, cyclic increases in systemic BP are observed, with mean increases in systolic and diastolic pressures of 25%, with the specific magnitude being proportional to the severity of oxyhemoglobin desaturation associated with the apneic episodes. Pulmonary artery pressures demonstrate similar cyclic increases in patients with OSAS, which can lead to development of chronic pulmonary hypertension. Cardiac output (CO), which normally decreases approximately 10% during NREM sleep, is also affected. During an apnea, CO initially decreases, but after termination of the event it increases above baseline levels. Heart rate is also affected, with bradycardia noted with each apnea. This effect seems to be related to the severity of the oxyhemoglobin desaturation and to be secondary to an increase in vagal parasympathetic activity. Following each apnea, heart rate accelerates, leading to the characteristic sinus bradycardia-tachyarrhythmia that is often observed.

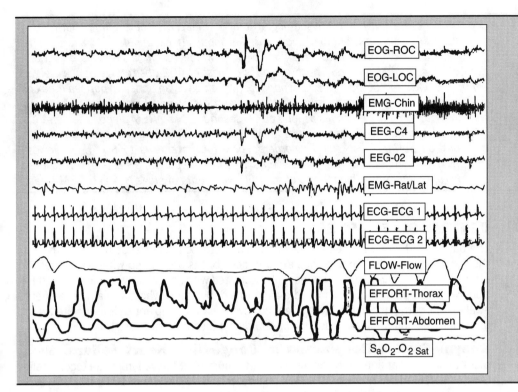

FIGURE 17-8
Typical sleep montage recorded during a PSG. The tracing demonstrates recordings of eye movements (EOG), chin electromyogram (EMG), EEG, anterior tibialis EMG, ECG, airflow at the nose and mouth, thoracic and abdominal movements, and oxygen saturation (S_aO_2).

Treatment. *Tracheostomy* is still probably the gold standard to which other forms of therapy are compared, although it is now rarely used as an initial treatment because of low patient acceptability and the associated morbidity. More recently, *nasal continuous positive airway pressure* (nasal CPAP) has become the most widely used treatment modality. It consists of a small nasal mask connected to a pressure device that acts as a pneumatic splint to keep the airway patent. After the initial diagnosis, the patient has a repeat PSG, during which the CPAP is gradually increased until there are no further apneic or hypopneic episodes. The patient then wears the device at home during the hours of sleep. Although effective, the overall compliance with CPAP has been only 40% to 60%. Another intervention is surgery such as *uvulopalatalpharyngoplasty* (UPPP), which basically enlarges the airway at the level of the soft palate. It is effective only about 50% of the time, because the obstruction in OSAS usually occurs at multiple levels. Other interventions include oral devices and medications, both of which have limited effectiveness.

The most common treatment for OSAS is nasal CPAP.

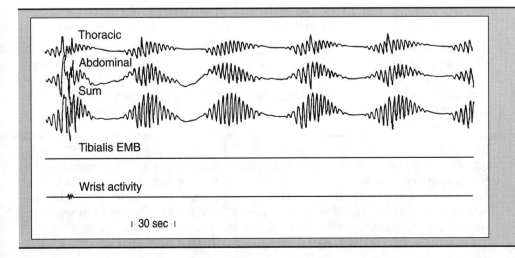

FIGURE 17-9
Cheyne-Stokes respiration in a patient with congestive heart failure. Note the crescendo-decrescendo alternation in tidal volume associated with central apneas. Reproduced with permission from Ancoli-Israel S, Engler RL, Friedman PJ, et al.: Comparison of patients with central sleep apnea: with and without Cheyne-Stokes respiration. *Chest* 106:780–786, 1994.

Case Study:
Continued

C.W. undergoes a full night polysomnogram at the Sleep Disorders Clinic. During the night he displays intermittent loud snoring that is not positional in nature. In addition, he has a total of 460 disordered breathing events, which result in arousals or oxygen desaturations of 4% or more. These episodes consist of 402 obstructive apneas, eight central apneas, and 50 obstructive hypopneas, which gives an apnea/hypopnea index of 62 per hour. The median duration of these sleep disordered breathing events is 25 seconds, but there are episodes as long as 60 seconds during REM sleep. The patient's initial oxygen saturation is 95% as measured by a pulse oximeter, and the average oxygen desaturation during these sleep disordered breathing events is to 80%. The lowest oxygen saturation noted during these events is 72%. The patient's sleep architecture is very disrupted, with significant decreases in the amounts of stage 3-4 and REM sleep.

CENTRAL SLEEP APNEA

The patient with central sleep apnea exhibits a decrease in central controller output to the muscles of respiration and thus experiences apneas associated with no respiratory effort. Idiopathic central sleep apnea, not associated with any underlying medical condition, most commonly occurs in middle-aged to elderly adults who complain of frequent awakenings during the night. More often, however, central sleep apnea is associated with an underlying condition such as CHF or neurologic disorders such as stroke.

Cheyne-Stokes respiration is a form of periodic breathing with a crescendo-decrescendo alternation in tidal volume separated by periods of apnea.

Cheyne-Stokes Respiration in Congestive Heart Failure. Sleep
disturbances in patients with congestive heart failure (CHF) have long been recognized. Sleep disordered breathing in CHF was first described by Cheyne in 1818 in a 60-year-old man with heart failure. In 1854, Stokes described a similar abnormal pattern of respiration leading to apnea. *Cheyne-Stokes respiration* (CSR) is described as a form of periodic breathing with a crescendo-decrescendo alternation in tidal volume separated by periods of apnea or hypopnea (Figure 17-9). The incidence of CSR is approximately 40% in CHF patients with left ventricular ejection fraction (LVEF) of less than 40%. It is rarely associated with less severe left ventricular dysfunction.

Pathophysiology of CSR. The exact mechanism responsible for the development of CSR in CHF still remains unknown, yet several theories have been proposed. An increased central sensitivity to P_aCO_2, referred to as an *increased controller gain*, appears to be one possible mechanism. This theory suggests that an increase in P_aCO_2 leads to an exaggerated ventilatory response that places the P_aCO_2 far below the apneic threshold, and an apnea occurs. The elevated P_aCO_2 that develops at the termination of the apnea again leads to an exaggerated ventilatory response, and the process repeats itself. Another candidate mechanism involves the lower volumes of stored carbon dioxide and oxygen caused by interstitial edema in the lungs, leading to a more unstable respiratory system (*underdamping*) with exaggerated changes in P_aCO_2 and P_aO_2 during transient changes in ventilation. In patients with CHF, a *circulatory time delay* can occur between the gas exchange occurring at the alveolar capillary membranes of the lungs and that occurring at the peripheral chemoreceptors (carotid bodies). Thus, the central respiratory control center is delayed in its response to the respiratory muscles, and CSR can develop.

Clinical Features and Diagnosis. Many patients with CSR present with symptoms of disturbed sleep, probably as a result of the multiple arousals that occur during the night. Thus, many patients complain of excessive daytime sleepiness. Others complain of frequent arousals during the night. Diagnosis is made with a full night PSG study, which demonstrates this characteristic breathing pattern, occurring predominantly during stages 1 and 2 of sleep.

Treatment. Patients with CSR secondary to CHF should first have their *medical therapy* optimized, because improvement in cardiac function can improve CSR. *Oxygen therapy* worn during sleep has also been shown to be effective. It appears to increase the body's oxygen stores and stabilize the respiratory control system. Nasal CPAP, similar to that used in OSAS, has been used in the treatment of CSR. Nasal CPAP has been shown to improve left ventricular function, possibly by the positive pressure it creates in the thorax. This pressure seems to be transmitted across the left ventricular muscle wall, and

in this way unloads the left ventricle. It also seems to decrease the tidal volume during breathing, which allows the P_aCO_2 to rise and stay above the apneic threshold.

C.W. returns for a nasal CPAP trial and a repeat PSG study while on nasal CPAP. During the night, the nasal CPAP is titrated up to a final level of 10 cm of water with resolution of all of his sleep disordered breathing events. His oxygen saturations are approximately 95% on this level of CPAP.

Case Study:
Continued

CHRONIC OBSTRUCTIVE PULMONARY DISEASE (COPD)

Patients with COPD have a higher incidence of death at night than in the daytime. One of the mechanisms thought to be responsible is the development of hypoxemia during sleep.

Incidence and Mechanism. It has been shown that approximately 27% of patients with COPD demonstrate significant oxygen desaturation during REM sleep, despite having awake P_aO_2 values higher than 60 mmHg (Figure 17-10). *Alveolar hypoventilation* appears to be the primary mechanism. During REM, hypotonia develops in the rib cage and abdominal muscles, and these patients then hypoventilate. Awake blood-gas values do not help identify which patients will desaturate during REM.

Approximately 27% of patients with COPD demonstrate significant oxygen desaturation during REM sleep.

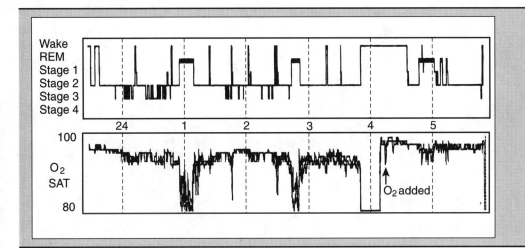

FIGURE 17-10
REM associated nocturnal oxygen desaturation (NOD) in a COPD patient with an awake P_aO_2 greater than 60 mmHg. Supplemental oxygen was added prior to the final REM period, preventing any further NOD.

Symptoms and Consequences. Patients with COPD and nocturnal oxygen desaturation (NOD) have very disrupted sleep, with difficulty initiating sleep as well as frequent arousals during the night. They also complain of excessive daytime sleepiness. COPD patients with REM-associated NOD appear to be the ones who develop chronic pulmonary hypertension. Whether NOD by itself is a predictor of survival remains uncertain.

Treatment. *Oxygen therapy* is the only form of therapy that has been shown to improve survival in patients with COPD. This applies to its use in patients who have daytime hypoxemia; thus far, supplemental oxygen has not been shown to affect survival in those patients with isolated nocturnal oxygen desaturation. It has been shown to improve sleep architecture, increasing stages 3 and 4 and REM and decreasing the time to sleep onset. Nocturnal *noninvasive positive pressure ventilation* (NPPV) involves the use of a positive pressure device that allows individual adjustment of the inspiratory and expiratory pressures. This allows the device to ventilate, instead of only maintaining airway patency as with CPAP. It is used most commonly for patients with elevated P_aCO_2. Although it was initially thought to rest chronically fatigued muscles and improve daytime function, it appears that its main effect involves resetting of the central respiratory control center's sensitivity to carbon dioxide, which has become blunted over time. Improved survival with NPPV has yet to be demonstrated.

| **Case Study:** *Resolution* | C.W. returns to the Sleep Disorders Clinic after being on nasal CPAP during the night for a 1-month period. He reports that he has been much more alert during the day and has no longer been falling asleep inappropriately at work. He states that with his increased energy he has been able to start a walking program and has actually lost 5 lb. His wife no longer complains of his loud snoring and has not asked him to leave the bedroom since he started nasal CPAP. C.W. will now follow-up on a regular basis in the Sleep Disorders Clinic. |

▌SUMMARY

In summary, sleep disordered breathing can occur as a primary disorder or be associated with an underlying disease state such as COPD or CHF. Its pathogenesis is often associated with abnormalities in the central respiratory controller. Disruption of normal sleep architecture often leads to the associated signs and symptoms observed in these patients. The effects of sleep disordered breathing on cardiovascular function and oxygenation are probably responsible for the increased morbidity, and in some cases mortality. Once the disorder has been diagnosed, effective treatments are available that may have an impact on overall survival.

■ REVIEW QUESTIONS

1. Which of the following statements about the control of breathing is *not* true?

   (A) The central controller is composed of the dorsal respiratory group (DRG) and the ventral respiratory group (VRG).
   (B) The most important regulator of minute ventilation is the ventilatory response to changes in P_aCO_2.
   (C) Central chemoreceptors respond primarily to changes in P_aO_2.
   (D) Mechanoreceptors are located within the lung parenchyma, upper airway, and respiratory muscles.

2. Which one of the following statements regarding REM sleep is false?

   (A) Muscle activity, especially in the limbs, is heightened in comparison with NREM sleep.
   (B) Dreams occur during REM sleep.
   (C) REM sleep is very restful sleep.
   (D) REM periods occur approximately every 90 minutes during the night and progressively increase in length.

3. The control of breathing changes with sleep onset in which one of the following ways?

   (A) The behavioral system increases its input in controlling ventilation.
   (B) The pattern of breathing becomes more regular during all stages of sleep.
   (C) Minute ventilation decreases, with an increase in P_aCO_2 and a decrease in P_aO_2.
   (D) Periodic breathing often occurs as patients fall asleep into stages 1 and 2.

4. The most common site(s) of obstruction in obstructive sleep apnea syndrome (OSAS) is (are)

   (A) the nasopharynx
   (B) the velopharynx and hypopharynx
   (C) the tonsillar pillars
   (D) the trachea

5. What percentage of patients with significant CHF (LVEF of less than 40%) have Cheyne-Stokes respiration (CSR) during sleep?

   (A) 30%
   (B) 40%
   (C) 80%
   (D) 100%

6. What is the main mechanism for the development of REM-associated nocturnal oxygen desaturation in patients with COPD?

   (A) The development of obstructive apneas
   (B) Nocturnal bronchospasm
   (C) The development of periodic breathing
   (D) Alveolar hypoventilation

■ ANSWERS AND EXPLANATIONS

1. The answer is C. The central chemoreceptors respond primarily to changes in PCO_2 and $[H^+]$ concentration in the extracellular fluid of the intracerebral interstitium. When these parameters increase, a linear increase in ventilation occurs.

2. The answer is A. Although the brain is very active during REM sleep, inhibition of spinal motor neurons leads to muscle atonia (except for the diaphragm). Episodes of rapid eye movements and muscle twitches occur periodically and are referred to as phasic REM. A condition known as REM sleep behavior disorder occurs when the spinal motor neurons are not inhibited and the patients physically act out their dreams.

3. The answer is C. As one enters sleep, the minute ventilation decreases as a result of a decrease in tidal volume. As a result, P_aCO_2 increases and P_aO_2 decreases. The apneic threshold for breathing in regard to P_aCO_2 is thus elevated. Periods of wakefulness that occur at sleep onset respond to the elevated P_aCO_2 by hyperventilation until P_aCO_2 decreases well below the sleep-related threshold. As sleep resumes, an apnea can occur until the P_aCO_2 again increases. This is reported to occur in 40% to 80% of normal individuals at sleep onset.

4. The answer is B. Most patients with OSAS have more than one site of obstruction, and this is probably one of the reasons that surgery (which usually addresses only one site of obstruction) is only 50% effective. The most common sites are the velopharynx (across from the soft palate) and farther down at the hypopharynx. The most common site in children is the tonsillar bed associated with tonsillar hypertrophy.

5. The answer is B. Approximately 40% of CHF patients with LVEF of less than 40% have CSR during sleep. It is uncertain why some patients develop CSR and others do not despite similar ejection fractions. Some believe it is a result of a difference in central controller gain, with those patients with CSR having higher controller gain than those without CSR.

6. The answer is D. The muscle atonia that occurs during REM leads to the development of alveolar hypoventilation and thus NOD. This occurs in approximately 27% of patients with COPD, despite having an awake P_aO_2 above 60 mmHg.

■ SUGGESTED READING

Fletcher EC, Miller J, Divine GW: Nocturnal oxyhemoglobin desaturation in COPD patients with arterial oxygen tensions above 60 mmHg. *Chest* 92:604–608, 1987.

Krieger J: Breathing during sleep in normal subjects. In Kryger MH, Roth T, Dement WC, eds.: *Principles and Practices of Sleep Medicine*. Philadelphia: WB Saunders, 1994, pp. 212–223.

Murray J: Control of breathing. In *The Normal Lung*. Philadelphia: WB Saunders, 1986, pp. 233–260.

Quaranta AJ, D'Alonzo GE, Krachman SL: Cheyne-Stokes respiration during sleep in congestive heart failure. *Chest* 111:467–473, 1997.

Shepard JW, Thawley SE: Localization of upper airway collapse during sleep in patients with obstructive sleep apnea. *Am Rev Resp Dis* 141:1350–1355, 1990.

Strollo PJ, Rogers RM: Obstructive sleep apnea. *N Engl J Med* 334:99–104, 1996.

Chapter 18

PLEURAL DISEASE

Kathleen J. Brennan, M.D.

■ CHAPTER OUTLINE

Learning Objectives
Introduction
Case Study: Introduction
Normal Anatomy and Physiology
Case Study: Continued
Pleural Effusions
Case Study: Continued
Management of Pleural Effusions
Pneumothorax
Case Study: Resolution
Review Questions

■ LEARNING OBJECTIVES

At the completion of this chapter, the reader should:

- Understand the normal anatomy and physiology of the pleura and the differences between parietal and visceral surfaces.
- Understand the basic principles behind pleural fluid formation and the factors that can alter either pleural fluid formation or resorption.
- Be able to differentiate between transudates and exudates, be able to cite common clinical examples of each, and understand the general approach to assessing a pleural effusion.
- Know the mechanisms involved in pneumothorax formation and be able to differentiate among the various types, know the conditions that predispose to secondary pneumothorax, and know the general approach to diagnosis and treatment of a pneumothorax.

■ INTRODUCTION

The pleura represents an important component of the respiratory system, not only as a site for primary disease but also as a structure frequently affected by underlying parenchymal processes. This chapter initially reviews normal pleural anatomy and physiology and then proceeds to discuss two common abnormalities of the pleural space: pleural effusions (fluid in the pleural space) and pneumothorax (air in the pleural space).

Case Study: Introduction

B.A., a 42-year-old woman with a history of dysfunctional uterine bleeding, presents with increased shortness of breath accompanied by left pleuritic chest pain. She was in her usual state of health until 2 weeks prior to her presentation in the emergency department, when she noted left-side chest pain and gradual onset of shortness of breath. The chest pain worsened with respiration and did not radiate. She also developed cough productive of purulent sputum with occasional blood streaks, accompanied by fevers, chills, fatigue, and malaise.

Her past medical history is significant for dysfunctional uterine bleeding noted over the past year. Her medication on admission is iron sulfate. She has a history of penicillin allergy. Her family history is significant for cardiac disease. Her social history reveals no prior tobacco or alcohol use. She works as a missionary for her church and had a negative tuberculin skin test within the past year.

■ NORMAL ANATOMY AND PHYSIOLOGY

PLEURAL ANATOMY

The pleura is divided into the visceral pleura, which covers the lung, and the parietal pleura, which lines the inner chest, the mediastinal structures, and the diaphragm.

The pleura is a smooth, semitransparent, serous membrane that lines the chest wall, lung, mediastinum, and diaphragm, and is divided into parietal and visceral surfaces (Figure 18-1). The parietal pleura covers the inner surface of the chest wall. In accordance with overlying intrathoracic structures, the parietal pleura is subdivided into costal, mediastinal, and diaphragmatic areas. The visceral pleura is the portion covering the surface of the lung. A thin layer of fluid is normally present between the visceral pleura and the parietal pleura and acts as a lubricant. The potential space between the visceral and parietal pleura layers is designated as the pleural space.

FIGURE 18-1
Diagram of the chest cavity, depicting the relationship between the visceral and parietal pleurae.

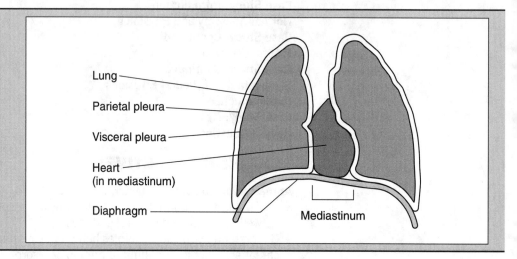

In humans, the visceral pleura has a single layer of mesothelial cells over a thick connective tissue layer through which run blood vessels and capillaries.

Under scanning electron microscopy, microvilli are present over the entire pleural surface. These microvilli are thought to increase the pleural surface area and participate in fluid exchange. In cross-sectional analysis, both the visceral pleura and the parietal pleura are lined with a single layer of mesothelial cells, overlying a layer of connective tissue (Figure 18-2). In contrast to many small mammals, humans have a relatively thick visceral pleura owing to the connective tissue layer under the mesothelial cells, which contains numerous blood vessels (capillaries) and lymphatics within the collagen matrix.

FIGURE 18-2
Schematic of a cross section through the pleura. The pleura consists of a single layer of mesothelial cells.

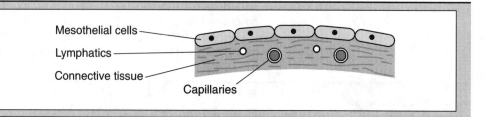

PLEURAL BLOOD SUPPLY

In humans, the visceral and parietal surfaces receive blood from systemic arterial sources. The parietal surface is supplied by capillaries from the local arterial supply. Intercostal arteries supply the costal pleura, the pericardiophrenic artery supplies the mediastinal pleura, and the superior phrenic and musculophrenic arteries supply the diaphragmatic pleura. Although there is some debate, the bronchial arteries are thought to supply the visceral pleura in humans.

PLEURAL LYMPHATICS

There is an extensive network of lymphatic vessels that run through the visceral pleura. These vessels run toward the hilum and penetrate the lung to join the bronchial lymphatic vessels by passing through the interlobar septa. The parietal pleura contains lymphatic vessels that communicate with the pleural space by means of stomas 2 to 6 mm in diameter. These round, slitlike openings are usually found in the mediastinal and intercostal pleurae. Some branches of parietal lymphatics contain dilated submesothelial branches called lacunas.

The costal pleural lymphatics drain toward nodes along the internal thoracic artery and dorsally toward the internal lymph nodes near the heads of the ribs. The mediastinal pleura is drained by lymph nodes that drain to the tracheobronchial and mediastinal nodes. Diaphragmatic pleural lymphatics drain into the parasternal, middle phrenic, and posterior mediastinal lymph nodes.

PLEURAL INNERVATION

Although the visceral pleura contains no pain fibers, sensory nerves are present in the parietal pleura. The parietal pleura covering the chest wall is supplied by the adjacent intercostal nerves. Therefore, stimulation of the coastal pleura or the outer portion of the diaphragmatic pleura refers pain to the adjacent chest wall. In contrast, the central portion of the diaphragm receives innervation from the phrenic nerve, and therefore stimulation of the pleura in this area refers pain to the ipsilateral shoulder.

> The visceral pleura contains no pain fibers. The parietal pleura is supplied by intercostal nerves with the exception of the central diaphragm, which is innervated by the phrenic nerve.

PHYSIOLOGY OF THE PLEURAL SPACE

The pleural space is approximately 7 to 24 mm in width and has a slightly negative pleural pressure between 0 and -5 cmH$_2$O when measured at functional residual capacity (FRC) or end-expiration. The negative pressure results from the opposing elastic forces of the chest wall (acting to spring outward) and lung (acting to collapse inward). Pleural pressure is not the same throughout the thorax. Pleural pressure is more negative in the superior thorax and decreases as one descends caudally to the inferior thorax. This gradient results from several factors: 1) the effect of gravity, 2) changes in the shapes of the chest wall and the lung in its superior-to-inferior direction, and 3) the weight of the intrathoracic structures themselves.

Pleural fluid is evenly distributed throughout the pleural space, and in normal conditions less than 5 mL is present. Pleural fluid can enter or exit the pleural space by way of capillaries or lymphatics of the parietal or visceral pleura, or through interstitial spaces.

Pleural fluid formation is best described by Starling's "law of transcapillary exchange," which dictates fluid movement across a membrane. Starling's law is expressed as

$$Q_f = L_p \times A[(P_{cap} - P_{pl}) - \sigma_d (\pi_{cap} - \pi_{pl})],$$

where Q_f is the flow of a liquid across a membrane; L_p is the filtration coefficient per unit area or the hydraulic water conductivity of that particular membrane; A is the surface area of the membrane; P and π are the hydrostatic and oncotic pressures, respectively, of the capillary (cap) and pleural space (pl); and σ_d is the solute reflection coefficient for protein, a measure of the membrane's ability to restrict the passage of large molecules.

Figure 18-3 depicts how the hydrostatic and oncotic pressures affect pleural fluid movement. If the hydrostatic pressure in parietal pleural blood vessels is $+30$ cmH$_2$O, and the hydrostatic pressure in the pleural space is -5 cmH$_2$O, there is an overall hydrostatic pressure gradient of $+35$ cmH$_2$O [$+30 - (-5) = 35$ cmH$_2$O] moving fluid out from the capillaries and into the pleural space. The oncotic pressure gradient between the parietal pleura and pleural space can be represented as $+34$ cmH$_2$O $- +5$ cmH$_2$O $= 29$ cmH$_2$O, acting to move fluid out of the pleural space and back into the capillaries. The overall difference between the hydrostatic and oncotic pressures ($35 - 29 = 6$ cmH$_2$O) is 6 cmH$_2$O in the direction of pleural fluid formation. The net gradient

> Fluid movement across the pleural membrane is dependent on Starling's law:
> $$Q_f = L_p \times A$$
> $$[(P_{cap} - P_{pl}) - \sigma_d (\pi_{cap} - \pi_{pl})]$$

across the visceral pleura is probably close to zero, but this has not been demonstrated. In summary, the movement of fluid across a membrane is a balance between 1) the hydrostatic and oncotic pressures in the pleural space and the visceral and parietal pleurae and 2) the filtration coefficient of the membrane.

Resorption of fluid from the pleural space occurs predominantly by means of lymphatics. The parietal pleural lymphatics can also remove proteins, cells, and particulate matter from the pleural space.

FIGURE 18-3
Diagram of the relationship between hydrostatic and oncotic pressure gradients across the pleura. See text for explanation. Modified from Light RW: *Pleural Disease*. Boston: Williams & Wilkins, 1995.

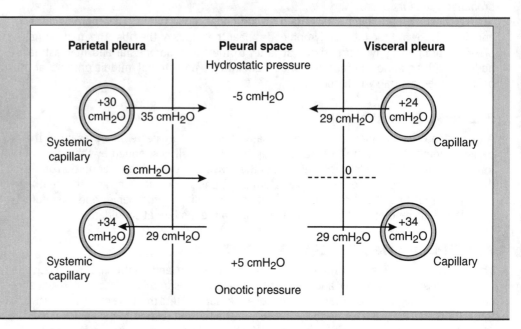

Case Study:
Continued

On physical exam, the patient has a temperature of 103.6°F, blood pressure of 84/50, a pulse of 134, and a respiratory rate of 24. She is sitting on a stretcher and appears uncomfortable. She is awake, alert, and orientated to person, place, and time. Her skin is warm and dry. Head and neck exams are unremarkable. Chest exam reveals dullness to percussion at the left base to halfway up the chest. There are decreased breath sounds accompanied by egophony. The right side is unremarkable. Heart, abdomen, and extremities are normal. On admission, her white blood cell count is 34,000 with 76% segmented cells, 18% bands, 3% lymphocytes, and 1% monocytes. An arterial blood gas on 2 liters of oxygen showed a pH of 7.44, a PCO$_2$ of 26 mmHg, and a PO$_2$ of 92 mmHg. Her hemoglobin and hematocrit are 8.0 and 24.5, respectively. Her chest x-ray reveals a large left pleural effusion associated with an infiltrate in the left lower lung.

PLEURAL EFFUSIONS

PATHOGENESIS OF PLEURAL EFFUSIONS

Accumulation of pleural fluid is caused by increased pleural fluid formation or decreased fluid resorption, or both.

The major mechanisms of pleural fluid formation include increased pleural fluid formation or decreased lymphatic clearance, or both. The major causes of pleural effusions are listed in Table 18-1. The most common cause in this study was congestive heart failure, with an annual incidence of 500,000 cases. The two next most frequent etiologies were pneumonia and malignant disease.

Clinically, patients usually present with complaints of shortness of breath or dyspnea on exertion. They may also complain of paroxysmal nocturnal dyspnea and orthopnea. In cases of infected pleural fluid, additional symptoms include fever, chills, and pleuritic chest pain on the side of the effusion. On physical exam, there is dullness to percussion on the affected side, decreased to absent breath sounds, and decreased tactile fremitus, and a pleural rub may be heard.

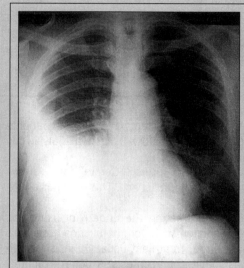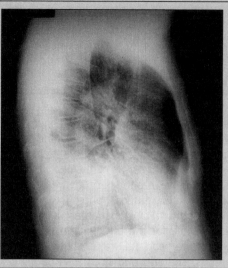

FIGURE 18-4
A posterior-anterior and lateral chest x-ray of a right-sided pleural effusion. Note the loss of the right diaphragm on the PA film. Courtesy of the Department of Diagnostic Imaging, Temple University Hospital.

Congestive heart failure	500,000
Pneumonia (bacterial)	300,000
Malignant disease	200,000
Lung	60,000
Breast	50,000
Lymphoma	40,000
Other	50,000
Pulmonary embolism	150,000
Viral disease	100,000
Cirrhosis with ascites	50,000

Table 18-1
Annual Incidence of Various Types of Pleural Disease in the United

Modified from Light RW: *Pleural Disease*. Baltimore: Williams & Wilkins, 1995.

CATEGORIES OF EFFUSIONS

Pleural effusions are defined as transudates or exudates. An exudate is defined as 1) a ratio of pleural fluid protein to serum protein greater than 0.5, 2) a ratio of pleural fluid lactate dehydrogenase (LDH) to serum LDH greater than 0.6, or 3) a total pleural fluid LDH greater than two-thirds of the upper limit of normal serum LDH. If at least one of these criteria is fulfilled, the effusion is considered to be an exudate. In the appropriate clinical setting, thoracentesis provides the cause of an effusion in approximately 75% of patients. If additional tests are performed on pleural fluid, thoracentesis has been found to significantly alter patient management in more than 90% of all cases.

An exudate is defined as pleural fluid total protein–serum total protein ratio greater than 0.5, pleural fluid LDH–serum LDH ratio greater than 0.6, or total pleural fluid LDH greater than two-thirds of the upper limit of normal serum LDH.

TRANSUDATIVE EFFUSIONS

Transudates (Table 18-2) usually result from alterations in systemic or pulmonary capillary pressure or plasma oncotic pressure. An example of elevated visceral or parietal pleura capillary hydrostatic pressures is seen in congestive heart failure, the most common cause of transudative pleural effusions. These effusions are usually bilateral, equal in size, and associated with cardiomegaly. Hypoalbuminemia is an example of pleural fluid formation resulting from decreases in plasma oncotic pressure. Pleural effusions can also result from movement of fluid from another space into the pleural space, such as from the peritoneal space (hepatic hydrothorax) or from the retroperitoneal space (urinothorax). There are also iatrogenic causes of pleural effusions, such as a hemothorax developing after a central line placement.

Hepatic hydrothorax occurs in 6% to 8% of patients with cirrhosis and ascites and is another cause of transudates. Hepatic hydrothorax is rarely seen in the absence of ascites and occur more frequently on the right side than on the left. Hepatic hydrothorax is thought to occur secondary to anatomic tears in the diaphragm.

Effusions in patients with nephrotic syndrome occur as a result of low oncotic pressure secondary to severe protein loss. Nephrotic syndrome also is associated with an

Transudates are caused by increases in capillary hydrostatic pressures (such as in congestive heart failure) or by changes in oncotic pressures (clinical conditions associated with low albumin or protein, such as nephrotic syndrome and hypoalbuminemia).

Table 18-2
Causes of Transudative Pleural Effusions

Congestive heart failure
Liver cirrhosis
Nephrotic syndrome
Peritoneal dialysis
Hypoalbuminemia
Urinothorax (urine in the pleural space)
Atelectasis

increased risk for pulmonary embolism, and this diagnosis should be ruled out in patients with new effusion on chest x-ray and a clinically relevant history. Peritoneal dialysis can cause effusions secondary to rents in the diaphragm.

Urinothorax (urine in the pleural space) occurs when rupture of Gerota's fascia allows urine to move into the peritoneum and eventually the pleural space. This fluid has a high creatine, a low glucose, and a low pH.

Treatment of transudates is usually aimed at treating the underlying condition responsible for the effusion. In conditions associated with volume overload, such as congestive heart failure, cirrhosis, and renal failure, treatment usually consists of diuretics, sodium, and fluid restriction. Occasionally, thoracentesis is done in acutely symptomatic patients to provide immediate relief.

EXUDATIVE EFFUSIONS

Exudative effusions are caused by increased permeability of the pleural space, decreased lymphatic flow from the pleural space, or increased negative pleural pressure in the pleural space.

Unlike those that cause transudates, disease processes that cause exudates usually involve the pleural space, lung inflammation (pneumonia), or impaired lymphatic drainage (malignancy). The mechanisms by which exudates form are thought to include 1) increased permeability of the pleural space, 2) decreased lymphatic flow from the pleural space, or 3) an increase in the negativity of the pleural pressure. Table 18-3 lists some of the numerous etiologies of exudates. Among those listed, the most common cause of an exudative effusion is pneumonia followed by malignancy.

Table 18-3
Causes of Exudative Pleural Effusions

Neoplastic Disease	**Drug-Induced Disease**
	Nitrofurantoin
Infectious Diseases	Dantrolene
Bacterial disease	Methysergide
Tuberculosis	Amiodarone
Fungal infections	Bromocriptine
Parasitic infections	Methotrexate
Viral infections	
	Pulmonary Embolism
Collagen Vascular Diseases	
Wegener's granulomatosis	**Hemothorax**
Rheumatoid pleuritis	
Sjögren's syndrome	**Chylothorax**
Systemic lupus erythematosus	
Drug-induced lupus	**Miscellaneous**
	Sarcoidosis
	Amyloidosis
	Radiation
	Asbestos exposure

ADDITIONAL TESTS FOR EFFUSIONS OR PLEURAL EFFUSIONS

Aside from LDH and protein, there are several other studies that are carried out on pleural fluid that aid in the diagnosis and treatment of effusions. These tests include pH, cell count, glucose, amylase, antinuclear antibody (ANA), rheumatoid factor, and lupus erythematosus (LE) cell prep. The presence of pleural fluid with a pH of less than 7.20 indicates the presence of increased lactic acid. The differential diagnosis includes parapneumonic effusions, esophageal perforation, rheumatoid arthritis, tuberculosis, malignancy, and blood. ANA levels can be attained on pleural fluid in patients for which there is suspicion of a collagen vascular disease, especially rheumatoid arthritis (RA), or systemic lupus erythematosus (SLE). A rheumatoid factor of 1:320 or higher is diagnostic for an effusion as a result of RA. Pleural fluid can be examined for the presence of SLE using an LE prep. Adenosine deaminase (ADA) elevations in effusions indicate the presence of *Mycobacterium tuberculosis* (TB). Finally, counterimmunoelectrophoresis (CIE) can be run to exclude specific bacterial pathogens such as *Staphylococcus*, *Streptococcus*, and *Haemophilus influenzae*. The pleural fluid can undergo Gram, fungal, and acid-fast bacilli (AFB) staining and culture to identify a possible bacterial, tuberculosis, or fungal pathogen.

In diseases such as tuberculosis and cancer, a sample of the pleura can be obtained in order to improve diagnostic yield. Pleural biopsy is positive in 40% of patients with cancer involving the pleura. This test is generally less sensitive than pleural fluid cytology, which is positive in 55% to 60% of patients. In 5% to 15% of patients, the pleural biopsy is positive and pleural fluid cytology is negative. In cases of granulomatous involvement of the pleura, pleural biopsy is positive in 50% to 80% of patients. Among the differential diagnosis for disease processes that can involve the pleura are fungi, sarcoidosis, TB, and RA. Pleural biopsy culture for AFB is positive in 75% of patients with TB. AFB smear accompanied by biopsy and culture is positive in 95% of patients. A second biopsy can increase the rate of positive diagnosis by 10% to 40%. In cases in which biopsies were nondiagnostic, a follow-up study over 1 to 3 years revealed that 29 of 143 patients developed cancer and 1 of 143 developed TB. The complications associated with pleural biopsy include a 1% incidence of pneumothorax and a 0.5% incidence of fatal hemorrhage.

Bronchoscopy is indicated in the presence of parenchymal disease on chest x-ray or computed tomography (CT) of the chest.

A thoracentesis is attempted under ultrasound and is unsuccessful. CT of the chest shows a large left pleural effusion that has areas of loculation along the medial left heart border. Thoracentesis done under CT guidance obtains 120 mL of purulent fluid; white blood cell count is 260,000 with 99% segmented cells, 1% lymphocytes, and 0% monocytes. Pleural fluid glucose is 6 mg/dL, pleural fluid protein is 5.2 mg/dL, and pleural fluid LDH is 18,895 U/L. The patient's serum LDH is 252 U/L (normal range, 100 to 190 U/L), and serum protein is 4.0 mg/dL. Pleural fluid Gram stain reports many white blood cells and few gram-positive cocci. Pleural fluid cultures grow group A Streptococcus sensitive to ampicillin, clindamycin, cefazolin, erythromycin, tetracycline, and vancomycin. Blood cultures are negative. Sputum cultures reveal many white blood cells, rare epithelial cells, and many gram-positive cocci, and grow Staphylococcus aureus sensitive to cefazolin, ciprofloxicin, tetracycline, clindamycin, erythromycin, oxacillin, and vancomycin.

Case Study:
Continued

■ MANAGEMENT OF PLEURAL EFFUSIONS

APPROACH TO THE PATIENT

The first test to confirm the presence of a pleural effusion is a chest x-ray (Figure 18-4). If the chest x-ray is consistent with an effusion, bilateral decubital films can be done to determine if the effusion is free flowing and of adequate size. In order for an effusion to be adequate for thoracentesis, at least 10 mm of fluid should be seen on a lateral decubital chest x-ray. If adequate fluid is present, a thoracentesis should be done and the resulting pleural fluid sent for total protein, LDH, and cell count. At this time, other studies, such as pH, cultures, glucose, and others, should be performed if warranted by the clinical setting. Further management depends on whether the effusion is a transudate or an exudate.

EFFECTS OF PLEURAL EFFUSIONS ON RESPIRATION

When pleural effusions are small, they have no significant effect on respiration; however, larger pleural effusions can lead to restrictive defects on pulmonary function tests, as noted by decreases in functional residual capacity (FRC) and total lung capacity (TLC). In large effusions, there may be an increased alveolar-arterial (A-a) oxygen gradient owing to atelectasis of the lung and subsequent ventilation-perfusion mismatching. Cases of untreated infected pleural effusions and blood in the pleural space (empyema and

Large pleural effusions can lead to a decrease in TLC and FRC. The A-a gradient may also be increased by mismatching of ventilation and perfusion in the affected lung.

FIGURE 18-5
Diagram of the initial work-up for a pleural effusion. Further work-up depends on the etiology of the pleural effusion. Modified from Light RW: *Pleural Disease.* Baltimore: Williams & Wilkins, 1995.

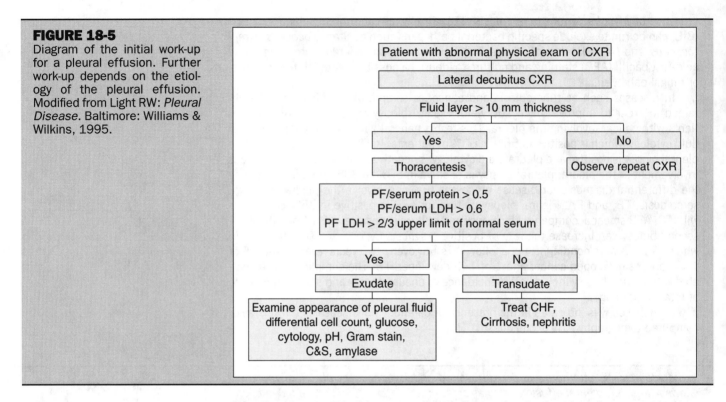

hemothorax, respectively) can result in inflammation in the pleural space and subsequent development of a thick pleural peel, which results in development of restrictive defects (trapped lung) as seen on pulmonary function tests.

PARAPNEUMONIC EFFUSIONS

Effusions resulting from pneumonia are called parapneumonic effusions. Parapneumonic effusions may also be associated with lung abscesses and bronchiectasis. The incidence of parapneumonic effusions is increased if appropriate treatment is delayed or if bacteremia is present. Parapneumonic effusions are divided into complicated and noncomplicated. A noncomplicated effusion is considered one for which the pH is greater than 7.3, glucose is higher than 60, and LDH is lower 1000. Parapneumonic effusions become complicated when pH is below 7.0, glucose is less than 40, and LDH is greater than 1000. A patient with a pleural fluid pH between 7.1 and 7.3 should be monitored closely, and if there is no improvement, a repeat thoracentesis or CT of the chest is advisable.

In patients with parapneumonic effusions, the indications for chest tube placement are as follows: pus on aspiration, a positive Gram stain for organisms, and glucose less than 50 or pH less than 7.1. If chest tube drainage has slowed and there are loculated areas that have not been drained, 250,000 units in about 100 mL of normal saline instilled through the chest tube can be used to lyse adhesions that have formed. In patients who do not improve with chest tube drainage, surgical intervention—either thorascopic debridement or open thoracotomy—may be needed.

MALIGNANT PLEURAL EFFUSIONS

Malignant effusions are caused by either spread of malignant disease to the pleural surface or decreased fluid resorption from the pleural space as a result of destruction of lymphatics by tumor. Initial work-up for pleural effusions in patients with malignancy is similar to what has been previously discussed. In this case, pleural fluid can be sent for cytology if a diagnosis is required. In the case of recurrent pleural effusions owing to malignancy, a chest tube may be placed. Once the daily fluid output has decreased to less than 100 mL per day, sclerotherapy can be attempted. Sclerotherapy is the instillation of a sterile substance such as tetracycline or doxycycline into the pleural space. These agents set up an inflammatory reaction and cause pleural surfaces to adhere to each other, thus obliterating the pleural space. Chemotherapy and radiation therapy are also used.

▌ PNEUMOTHORAX

A pneumothorax by definition is air in the pleural space. The mechanisms by which a pneumothorax develops (Figure 18-7) are as follows: 1) communication between the alveoli and the pleural space (bronchopleural fistula); 2) communication between the atmosphere and the pleural space (penetrating chest wounds or trauma); and 3) gas-producing organisms within the pleural space. Pneumothoraces are categorized as either spontaneous or traumatic. Spontaneous pneumothoraces are subdivided into primary (in the absence of known parenchymal disease) and secondary (in patients with known diseases that predispose them to pneumothoraces).

Mechanisms for formation of pneumothorax are communication between the alveoli and the pleural space, communication between the atmosphere and the pleural space (trauma), and gas-producing organisms.

CLINICAL MANIFESTATIONS

The clinical manifestations of a pneumothorax depend on the volume of the pneumothorax and on the presence or absence of underlying lung disease. About 90% of patients present with complaints of dyspnea and ipsilateral, pleuritic chest pain. These symptoms are more severe with larger pneumothoraces and in the presence of lung disease. A nonproductive cough may or may not be present. A small pneumothorax may be entirely asymptomatic and without clinical findings. However, the physical examination in significant pneumothoraces reveals decreased breath sounds, hyperresonance to percussion, and decreased tactile fremitus over the affected hemithorax. In cases of tension pneumothorax, tracheal shift away from the affected side, tachycardia, distant heart sounds, and cyanosis are present.

Categories of Pneumothorax

Spontaneous
   Primary (no underlying disease)
   Secondary (has a predisposing
      disease)
Traumatic (includes iatrogenic)

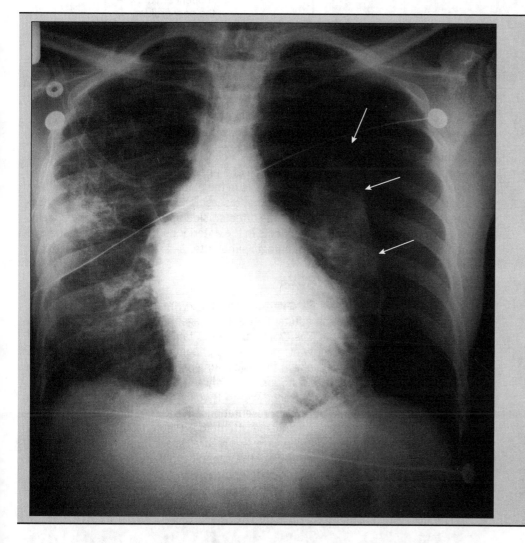

FIGURE 18-6
Chest x-ray of a left pneumothorax in a patient with carcoidosis. The arrows indicate the visible reflection of the visceral pleura. Courtesy of the Department of Diagnostic Imaging, Temple University Hospital.

PHYSIOLOGICAL EFFECTS OF PNEUMOTHORAX

Entry of air into the pleural space results in expansion of the chest wall and collapse of the lung. Vital capacity, lung volumes, and lung compliance are reduced. Arterial hypoxemia is common.

When a pneumothorax develops, the gas that enters the pleural cavity is similar in composition to atmospheric air. As PO_2 and PCO_2 equilibrate with the surrounding tissue, the volume of the pneumothorax decreases (in the absence of a continued air leak) and the PN_2 increases relative to the PN_2 of tissues. As the nitrogen is reabsorbed, the volume of gas decreases, which raises the intrapleural PO_2 and PCO_2 to favor continued reabsorption. The rate of reabsorption of a pneumothorax is about 1.25% per day. This rate can be increased by raising the inspired oxygen concentration.

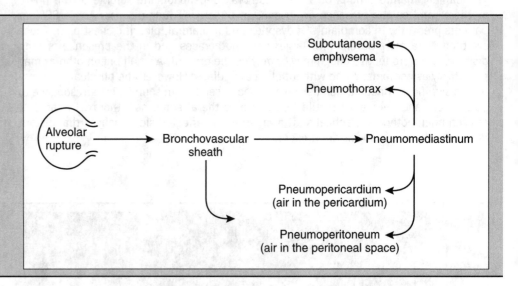

FIGURE 18-7
Depiction of the several pathways that air can follow once alveolar rupture occurs. Air tracks along the bronchovascular sheath and can present clinically in several forms. From Murray JF, Nadel JA: *Textbook of Respiratory Medicine*. Philadelphia: Saunders, 1994.

RADIOGRAPHIC APPEARANCE OF PNEUMOTHORAX

A pneumothorax is confirmed by its appearance on chest radiography. A chest x-ray taken at end-expiration can enhance the appearance of a pneumothorax.

Air within the pleural space usually collects in the apices of the lungs. However, the presence of pleural adhesions, or parenchymal disease, may result in loculated collections of air. A lateral decubitus film with the affected side up may facilitate the appearance of air. In the supine patient, air collects in the anterior portion of the chest and can present as an enhanced cardiac or diaphragm silhouette.

TYPES OF PNEUMOTHORACES

Primary Spontaneous Pneumothorax. Primary spontaneous pneumothorax usually occurs in young adults, between the ages of 20 and 40, and is more common in men than in women. The typical patient is tall and thin, and most have a history of tobacco use. The majority of spontaneous pneumothoraces are thought to be caused by rupture of subpleural blebs in the apical lung regions. Primary pneumothorax in young patients with normal lung function is usually self-limited.

There is a 40% chance of recurrence within 2 years, and the risk of recurrence increases further with subsequent repeat presentations. In the case of recurrent spontaneous pneumothorax, pleurodesis should be attempted. Pleurodesis is the procedure wherein an irritating agent is instilled into the pleural space in order to induce an inflammatory reaction and cause adhesion of the visceral and parietal pleurae. The most common agents used today include doxycycline, bleomycin, and talc.

In recent years, thoracoscopy has been used to diagnose and treat primary pneumothorax. Blebs or bullae can be ligated through various methods. Use of this therapy has a recurrence rate of about 2%.

Secondary Spontaneous Pneumothorax. There are several pulmonary processes that are associated with increased risk of pneumothorax development, some of which are listed in Table 18-4. The patients in this group tend to be older than those at risk for primary pneumothorax. One exception is cystic fibrosis, which occurs in 8% of the population with an average age of about 17. Chronic obstructive pulmonary disease (COPD) is the most common disorder predisposing to pneumothorax. Other common etiologies include pulmonary fibrosis secondary to mycobacterium tuberculosis. In recent years there has been an increase in the incidence of pneumothorax in patients with AIDS, to about 26%.

Asthma Sarcoidosis Chronic obstructive pulmonary disease Emphysema Cystic fibrosis *Pneumocystis carinii* pneumonia with AIDS Tuberculosis	**Table 18-4** **Diseases Associated with Secondary Spontaneous Pneumothorax**

Secondary pneumothorax further compromises lung function in these patients and can lead to respiratory failure. Although the rates of recurrence of primary and secondary pneumothorax are similar, a more aggressive approach is warranted for secondary pneumothorax because of its potentially life-threatening complications.

Traumatic Pneumothorax. Traumatic pneumothorax can occur secondary to penetrating or blunt chest trauma. A separate category under traumatic pneumothorax is iatrogenic pneumothorax (i.e., pneumothorax resulting from procedures). It is thought that the incidence of iatrogenic pneumothorax is almost as high as that of pneumothorax resulting from trauma. Table 18-5 lists the various procedures associated with iatrogenic pneumothorax. It should be noted that iatrogenic causes include not only central line placements and needle biopsies, but also mechanical ventilation. The risk of a pneumothorax from mechanical ventilation is substantially increased in the presence of underlying pulmonary disease such as asthma, emphysema, or COPD. Treatment of an iatrogenic pneumothorax, again, depends on the clinical status of the patient and on whether or not the patient is on mechanical ventilation.

Transthoracic needle aspiration Subclavian needle stick Thoracentesis Pleural biopsy Positive pressure ventilation Supraclavicular needle stick Nerve block Miscellaneous	**Table 18-5** **Causes of Iatrogenic Pneumothorax**

MANAGEMENT OF PNEUMOTHORAX

In cases where the pneumothorax is small (less than 15%), and the patient is asymptomatic, observation is recommended, accompanied by patient education and close follow-up. Oxygen administration aids resorption of the intrapleural air.

If the pneumothorax is large and the patient is symptomatic, simple aspiration of the air can be attempted. More than half of all patients respond to this conservative therapy. In the case of persistent air leak, or of pneumothorax in a ventilated patient, a chest tube can be inserted and negative pressure applied until the lung reexpands and the leak is sealed. This therapy is effective in about 90% of the cases. If after 7 days an air leak is still present, more aggressive treatment may be needed to close it.

Although the rates of recurrence of primary and secondary pneumothorax are similar, a more aggressive approach is warranted for secondary pneumothorax as a result of possibly life-threatening complications. Usually these patients are treated with chest tube placement and application of negative pressure in order to reexpand the lung. Once the leak is closed, sclerosis is recommended to prevent recurrence. If a bronchopleural fistula still exists, thoracoscopy may be needed to close the air leak.

| **Case Study:** *Resolution* | *A left chest tube is placed, with initial drainage of 1 liter of purulent secretions. The patient's temperature and white blood cell count decrease, but she continues to have low-grade fever accompanied by a persistent elevation in white blood cell count. Drainage by chest tube decreases, and a repeat chest x-ray shows persistent areas of loculated fluid. She is then treated with streptokinase by way of the chest tube in order to improve drainage. The chest tube output subsequently improves, and a repeat CT of the chest shows resolution of the effusion and improvement in the lung infiltrate. She becomes afebrile, the chest tube is removed, and she is discharged to home on antibiotics.* |

■ REVIEW QUESTIONS

1. Which one of the following statements is false?

   (A) The visceral pleura has no sensory innervation.
   (B) The parietal pleura is supplied by the local systemic capillaries.
   (C) Stimulation of the costal pleura over the central diaphragm refers pain to the ipsilateral shoulder.
   (D) At end-expiration (FRC), pleural pressure is positive ($+10 \, cmH_2O$).

2. Which one of the following statements is false?

   (A) Pleural effusion formation in patients with congestive heart failure is related to changes in the filtration coefficient of the pleura.
   (B) Parapneumonic effusions develop in patients with pneumonia as a result of changes in the permeability of the pleural surface.
   (C) Pleural effusions in nephrotic syndrome result from decreases in the oncotic pressure gradient.

3. An exudate is defined as

   (A) pleural fluid protein–serum protein ratio greater than 0.5
   (B) total pleural fluid LDH greater than two-thirds of the upper limit of normal serum LDH
   (C) pleural fluid LDH–serum LDH ratio greater than 0.6
   (D) pleural fluid white blood cell count greater than 10,000/mm³

4. Each of the following is associated with transudative pleural effusions except

   (A) congestive heart failure
   (B) malignancy
   (C) liver cirrhosis
   (D) nephrotic syndrome

5. Which of the following factors is not associated with an increased risk of pneumothorax?

   (A) A penetrating chest wound in a 30-year-old man
   (B) Transthoracic needle biopsy in a 50-year-old man with emphysema
   (C) Diagnosis of stage I adenocarcinoma of the lung in a 60-year-old woman with no history of tobacco use
   (D) Mechanical ventilation in a 30-year-old woman admitted for status asthmaticus

■ ANSWERS AND EXPLANATIONS

1. The answer is D. The pleura is divided into visceral and parietal surfaces. The visceral pleura overlies the lung whereas the parietal pleura lines the chest wall, diaphragm, and mediastinal structures. The visceral pleura has no sensory innervation. The costal and peripheral diaphragmatic parietal pleura receives sensory innervation from the intercostal nerves and refers pain directly to the overlying area. The central portion of the diaphragmatic pleura is supplied by the phrenic nerve, and pain is referred to the ipsilateral shoulder. The bronchial arterial system supplies the visceral pleura whereas the parietal pleura is supplied by the local systemic circulation. The superior phrenic and musculophrenic arteries supply the diaphragm, intercostal arteries supply the costal pleura, and the pericardiophrenic artery supplies the majority of the mediastinal pleura. Pleural pressure at end-expiration (FRC) and during normal quiet breathing is always negative (approximately -5 cmH$_2$O at FRC to -10 cmH$_2$O at end-inspiration).

2. The answer is A. The movement of fluid into and out of the pleural space is dependent on several factors. Starling's law of transcapillary exchange is thought to best define the relationship between pleural fluid formation and removal. In summary, fluid formation is dependent on the surface area of the membrane, its filtration coefficient, and the difference between the hydrostatic and oncotic pressure gradients between the pleural space and capillaries in the pleura. Congestive heart failure is one of the most common causes of pleural effusions. Here there is an increase in pleural fluid formation owing to increased hydrostatic pressure in the pulmonary capillaries that results in increased fluid within the interstitium and eventually in the pleural space. Parapneumonic effusions are thought to result from altered permeability of the membrane caused by inflammatory changes. Pleural effusions in patients with nephrotic syndrome develop because the decreased oncotic pressure is thought to result in increased pleural fluid formation.

3. The answer is D. Pleural effusions are separated into transudates and exudates. An exudate is defined as meeting the following criteria: pleural fluid protein–serum protein ratio greater than 0.5, pleural fluid LDH–serum LDH ratio greater than 0.6, and total pleural fluid LDH greater than two-thirds of the upper limit of normal serum LDH. Although more recent investigations have suggested other tests, such as pleural fluid cholesterol and the ratio between pleural fluid and serum bilirubin, the aforementioned criteria, initially defined by Light, remain the best way of separating transudates from exudates. Pleural fluid white blood cell count is usually less than 1000/mm^3 in transudative effusions. White blood cell counts above 10,000/mm^3 are associated with parapneumonic effusions, malignant effusions, tuberculous effusions, and effusions occurring in pulmonary embolism, postmyocardial infarction, pancreatitis, and systemic lupus erythematosus.

4. The answer is B. Transudative effusions usually result from alterations in the hydrostatic and oncotic pressure gradients between the pleural capillaries and the pleural space, and result in increased pleural fluid formation. Congestive heart failure (CHF) is the most common cause of transudative pleural effusions. Effusions caused by CHF develop in association with left ventricular failure, and are usually bilateral. Increased hydrostatic pressure results in increased fluid in the lung interstitium that subsequently migrates across the visceral pleura and into the pleural space. Malignancy is among the most common causes of exudative effusions. Malignant effusions occur either through direct invasion of the pleura by tumor or through indirect effects by lymphatic destruction or occlusion, which causes decreased fluid removal. The development of pleural effusion in liver cirrhosis is termed hepatic hydrothorax. The majority of these effusions occur in the presence of ascites. Although many theories exist, recent experiments have demonstrated that movement of ascitic fluid across the diaphragm and into the pleural space is the pathophysiologic mechanism. Approximately 20% of patients with nephrotic syndrome develop transudative pleural effusions. The decreased oncotic pressure is thought to result in increased pleural fluid formation. Like congestive heart failure, these effusions are usually bilateral.

5. The answer is C. Pneumothorax occurs when there is communication between the alveoli and the pleural space or between the atmosphere and the pleural space. Primary pneumothoraces occur in healthy individuals without a history of lung disease. Secondary pneumothoraces are seen in patients with underlying lung diseases such as chronic obstructive lung disease, *Pneumocystis carinii* pneumonia in AIDS patients, tuberculosis, cystic fibrosis, and asthma. There are also iatrogenic causes of a pneumothorax. Among these are procedures such as central venous line placement, transthoracic needle aspiration, thoracentesis, pleural biopsy, and mechanical ventilation. Of the choices above, only malignancy has not been associated with an increased risk for pneumothorax. The patient in option A has a penetrating chest wound that can result in pneumothorax as a result of communication between the atmosphere and the pleural space. The patient in B is at increased risk because of his emphysema, and also because of the transthoracic needle biopsy procedure he is undergoing. The patient in D has severe airflow obstruction owing to her asthma exacerbation, and mechanical ventilation may result in air trapping and lead to alveolar rupture and pneumothorax.

∎ SUGGESTED READING

Clausen JL: Pneumothorax. *In* Bordlow RA, Moser KM, eds.: *Manual of Clinical Problems in Pulmonary Medicine*, 3rd ed. Boston: Little, Brown, 1991.

Light RW: *Pleural Disease*. Baltimore: Williams & Wilkins, 1995.

Moser KM: Pleural effusion. *In* Bordlow RA, Moser KM, eds.: *Manual of Clinical Problems in Pulmonary Medicine*, 3rd ed. Boston: Little, Brown, 1991.

Pleural diseases. *Sem Resp Crit Care Med* 16(4):1995.

Chapter 19

OCCUPATIONAL LUNG DISEASES

Francis C. Cordova, M.D.

Daniel Shade, Jr., M.D.

▊ CHAPTER OUTLINE

Learning Objectives
Case Study: Introduction
Overview of Occupational Lung Diseases
Silicosis
Case Study: Continued
Case Study: Continued
Asbestos-Related Pulmonary Disorders
Case Study: Continued
Coal Worker's Pneumoconiosis
Occupational Asthma
Effects of Air Pollution
Case Study: Resolution
Review Questions

▊ LEARNING OBJECTIVES

At the completion of this chapter, the reader should:

- Be familiar with the clinical features, pathologic changes, work-up, and therapy of selected occupational lung diseases.
- Understand the pathophysiology and recognize the three types of silicosis, and be able to identify the common complications associated with silicosis.
- Be able to identify the different forms of asbestos-related lung injury.
- Be able to recognize the clinical features, pathology, and management of coal worker's pneumoconiosis.
- Be able to differentiate occupational asthma from intrinsic asthma.
- Be able to identify the most common air pollutants and their effects on lung function.

Case Study:
Introduction

J. R., a 62-year-old white man, is admitted to the hospital for an elective surgical repair of inguinal hernia. He is referred to you because routine preoperative chest x-ray is abnormal. Review of his pertinent history shows that he has been having intermittent cough for 6 months, but he denies any history of dyspnea, hemoptysis, or weight loss. He started smoking as a teenager and continued to smoke one pack per day. He worked at an automobile brake repair shop for 5 years, then worked in a South African quarry for 25 years as a truck driver before coming back to the United States. His father died of lung cancer at 55 years of age.

On physical exam, he appears well nourished and is not in respiratory distress. Auscultation of the chest reveals scattered expiratory rhonchi. Chest excursion is normal. No clubbing is noted.

Laboratory data reveal normal CBC and chemistry. Antinuclear antibody (ANA) and rheumatoid factor are positive. Chest x-ray shows bilateral interstitial lung nodules involving predominantly the upper lung zones and bilateral hilar adenopathy. Purified protein derivative (PPD) skin test is negative. Acid-fast bacilli (AFB) smear of the sputum is negative. Arterial blood gas (ABG) while inspiring room air shows a pH of 7.38, a P_aO_2 of 83 mmHg, and a PCO_2 of 42 mmHg. Spirometry results were forced expiratory volume in 1 second (FEV_1), 2.3 liters (70% of predicted); forced vital capacity (FVC), 3.4 liters (82%); FEV_1/FVC, 68%; total lung capacity (TLC), 5.4 liters (75% of predicted); and residual volume (RV), 1.9 liters (71% of predicted).

■ OVERVIEW OF OCCUPATIONAL LUNG DISEASES

The lung's extensive alveolar surface area and constant contact with ambient air to fulfill its gas-exchange function make it extremely vulnerable to toxic environmental exposures. Occupational lung diseases encompass a diverse group of pulmonary disorders resulting from dusts, fumes, and chemical exposures from the workplace and living environment. Pneumoconiosis, derived from the term "pneumonokoniosis," which means "dusty lung," refers to the fibrotic reaction of the lung resulting from inhalation of mineral or inorganic dusts. The three main types of pneumoconiosis are silicosis, asbestosis and other asbestos-related lung diseases, and coal worker's pneumoconiosis. Other less common types of pneumoconiosis include aluminosis (aluminum), berylliosis (beryllium), and siderosis (iron), to name a few.

The pathologic changes associated with the different occupational lung diseases are quite varied. Depending on the nature of the toxic exposure (physicochemical properties) and the host reaction (rate of ciliary clearance, humoral antibody formation, and hereditary defects), the major site of injury to the respiratory system may be in the upper airways (rhinitis, septal perforation, or nasal cancer), lower airways (bronchospasm or bronchitis), alveolar parenchyma (diffuse alveolar damage, interstitial fibrosis, nodular fibrosis, macule formation, or focal emphysema), or pleura (pleural effusion or pleural fibrosis). In pneumoconiosis, the dust particles that escape the filtering mechanism of the upper airways are deposited in the alveoli. The dust particles either induce alveolitis or are engulfed by alveolar macrophages, which then migrate into the interstitial and lymphatic tissues. The end results of these two host reactions are interstitial fibrosis and nodular fibrosis, respectively. The types of pathologic reactions in different regions of the respiratory system are shown in Table 19-1.

Table 19-1
Typical pathological reactions of the different compartments of the lung due to exposure to various toxic materials. (Reproduced with permission from Gibbs AR: Pathological Reactions of the Lung to Dust. In Morgan WKC, Seaton A, eds.: *Occupational Lung Disease,* 3rd ed. p 127, Philadelphia: WB Saunders, 1995.)

SITE OF INJURY	TYPE OF REACTION	EXAMPLES OF OFFENDING AGENTS
Airways	Asthma	Isocyanates, metals
	Bronchiolitis	Nitrogen dioxide
Airways-parenchyma	Centrilobular fibrosis	Coal, kaolin, talc, silica
	Diffuse interstitial fibrosis	Asbestos
	Extrinsic allergic alveolitis	Farmer's lung
	Sarcoid-like	Beryllium
Parenchyma	Diffuse alveolar damage	Toxic fumes, asbestos, silica
	Giant interstitial pneumonitis	Hard metal
	Pulmonary alveolar proteinosis	Silica
	Emphysema	Coal, cadmium
Diffuse/random	Progressive massive fibrosis	Coal, kaolin, talc
	Carcinoma	Asbestos, nickel, arsenic
Pleura	Benign effusion	Asbestos
	Plaques	Asbestos, talc
	Diffuse fibrosis	Asbestos
	Mesothelioma	Asbestos

The clinical presentations of the different occupational lung diseases are similarly diverse. In pneumoconiosis, for example, patients may be asymptomatic and present with only an abnormal chest x-ray ordered for routine presurgery clearance. In more advanced disease states, the most common symptom is dyspnea, which may occur at rest or only during exercise. In addition, the duration of symptoms can be acute (occupational asthma and acute silicosis), subacute (hypersensitivity pneumonitis), or chronic (silicosis, coal worker's pneumoconiosis, and asbestosis). Some diseases are self-limiting (occupational asthma and hypersensitivity pneumonitis) if no further exposures occur, whereas other diseases are progressive (accelerated silicosis and asbestosis).

The diagnosis of occupational lung disease requires high clinical suspicion. In most cases, a detailed clinical history and physical examination, in addition to a few diagnostic tests, are all that are required to make the correct diagnosis. A detailed employment history, including a knowledge of the total period of employment, the pattern of daily work activity, and the characteristics of exposure (e.g., sandblasting in an enclosed space without protective mask), will provide information about the extent and magnitude of the occupational exposure. Because many occupational lung diseases, such as the pneumoconioses, have long latency periods before the onset of symptoms, job descriptions should include in detail actual daily periods of exposure. The nature of various pulmonary toxins (fumes, dusts, and chemicals) should be obtained. In addition, an attempt should be made to establish the temporal relationship of symptoms to the work environment (occupational asthma, byssinosis, and hypersensitivity pneumonitis).

Early in the course of the disease, patients with occupational lung disease may have a relative paucity of physical signs. None of these physical signs is specific for any of the occupational lung diseases, but they are useful aids in determining the severity of the underlying disorder. Nevertheless, certain physical findings are helpful in the diagnostic process. For example, clubbing of the fingers can be seen in asbestosis but is not usually found in other pneumoconioses or in hypersensitivity pneumonitis. On auscultation, adventitial sounds such as crepitations occurring during late inspiration are heard in pulmonary fibrosis (asbestosis) and chronic allergic alveolitis but not in silicosis or coal worker's pneumoconiosis. Wheezing temporally associated with the work environment may indicate the presence of occupational asthma, hypersensitivity pneumonitis, or reactive airways disease syndrome.

One essential aid in the evaluation of patients suspected of having work-related respiratory illness is the chest x-ray. In fact, the radiographic patterns of some of these diseases (silicosis, asbestosis, and coal worker's pneumoconiosis) are characteristic of the disorders. Radiographic findings may include increased interstitial markings (asbestosis and hypersensitivity pneumonitis) (Figure 19-1), nodular densities (silicosis and coal worker's pneumoconiosis) (Figure 19-2), pleural effusions or pleural plaques (asbestosis) (Figure 19-3), and hyperinflation (occupational asthma). In the pneumoconioses, radiographic opacities are graded according to size, shape, and location within the different lung zones, and to the extent of the changes. Moreover, radiographic abnormalities may be the only findings that suggest a significant dust load in the lung.

Pulmonary function tests usually reveal restrictive, obstructive, or mixed ventilatory disorders in patients with occupational lung diseases. Table 19-2 lists the ventilatory defects observed on spirometry of the different occupational lung diseases. Diseases with fixed airflow obstruction, such as emphysema and chronic byssinosis, are best evaluated with simple spirometry. In patients with variable obstruction, such as occupational asthma, serial peak flow measurements conducted by the patients both at home and at work may be useful in diagnosis and management. Diseases causing pulmonary fibrosis are best evaluated by spirometry (FVC, FEV_1, and FEV_1/FVC), lung volumes, and diffusion capacity. Arterial blood-gas examination is useful in detecting and assessing the severity of hypercapneic and hypoxemic respiratory failure in patients with advanced occupational lung disease. Cardiopulmonary reserve can be assessed by cardiopulmonary exercise testing and followed serially by a simpler test such as a 6-minute walk test (i.e., total distance the patient can walk in 6 minutes).

Physical Findings in Occupational Lung Diseases

- Clubbing (asbestosis)
- Crepitations (asbestosis and hypersensitivity pneumonitis)
- Wheezing (occupational asthma and reactive airways disease syndrome)

Radiographic Patterns in Occupational Lung Diseases

- Increased interstitial markings (asbestosis and hypersensitivity pneumonitis)
- Nodular densities (silicosis and coal worker's pneumoconiosis)
- Pleural effusions or plaques (asbestosis)
- Hyperinflation (occupational asthma)

Disorders Revealed by Pulmonary Function Tests

- Restrictive disorders
- Obstructive disorders
- Mixed disorders

OBSTRUCTIVE VENTILATORY	RESTRICTIVE VENTILATORY DEFECT	MIXED RESTRICTIVE/ OBSTRUCTIVE DEFECT
Occupational asthma	Silicosis	Silicosis
Industrial bronchitis	Asbestosis	Asbestosis
Progressive massive fibrosis	Asbestos associated pleural diseases	Progressive massive fibrosis
Reactive airways dysfunction syndrome	Hypersensitivity pneumonitis	
Byssinosis		

Table 19-2
Different Patterns of Abnormal Spirometry in Different Occupational Lung Diseases.

Tissue confirmation often is not required in the diagnosis of occupational lung disease when the proper clinical setting and typical radiographic features are present. If a lung biopsy is required to rule out other disease entities, or if the diagnosis is in doubt, an open-lung biopsy is the preferred procedure because of a higher diagnostic yield compared with transbronchial biopsy. Pleural biopsy, in conjunction with thoracentesis, is

FIGURE 19-1
Chest x-ray showing increased interstitial lung markings at both lung bases in a patient with asbestosis for more than 20 years. Reproduced with permission from Parkes WR: Silicates and Lung Disease. In *Occupational Lung Disorders*, 2nd ed. London: Butterworths, 1982, p 266.

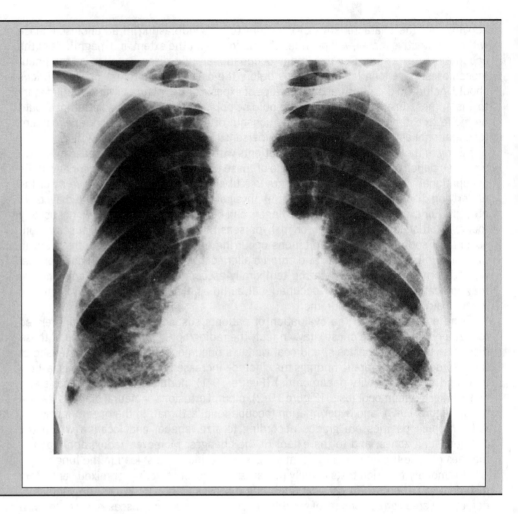

useful in ruling out tuberculosis in patients with pleural effusions and a history of asbestos exposure.

Once the diagnosis of occupational lung disease has been established, management includes avoidance to further exposure of the offending toxins, general supportive care (supplemental oxygen and bronchodilators), and detailed evaluation of the extent of pulmonary disability, if present. Steroids are often used in occupational asthma and hypersensitivity pneumonitis. In patients with functional limitations, a pulmonary rehabilitation program may be helpful in maintaining exercise capacity.

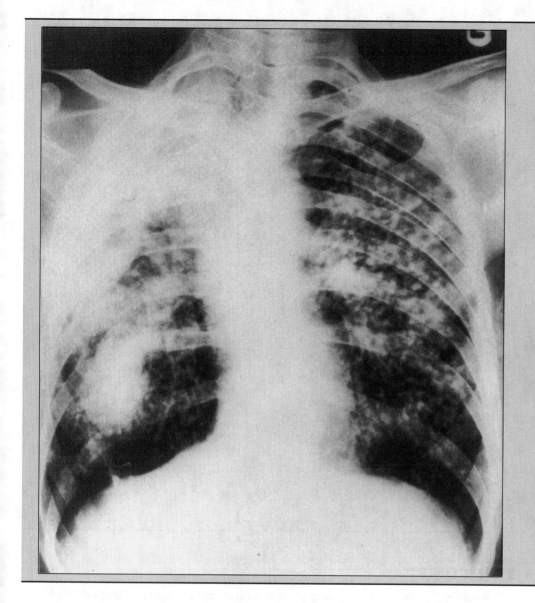

FIGURE 19-2
Chest x-ray showing nodular opacity in left upper lung field and extensive fibrosis in the right upper lobe in a patient with complicated silicosis. Reproduced with permission from Seaton A: Silicosis. In Morgan WKC, Seaton A, eds: *Occupational Lung Diseases*, 3rd ed. Philadelphia: WB Saunders, 1995, p 246.

FIGURE 19-3
Chest x-ray showing bilateral pleural plaques on the chest wall and diaphragm (rim calcification along the left hemidiaphragm). Reproduced with permission from Parkes WR. Silicates and Lung Disease. In *Occupational Lung Disorders*, 2nd ed. London: Butterworths, 1982, p 247.

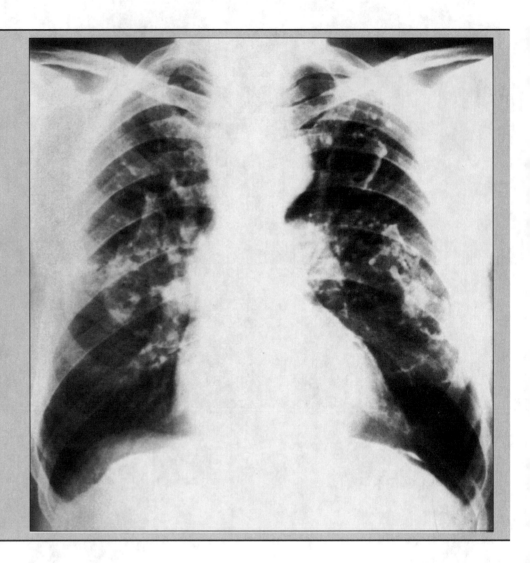

■ SILICOSIS

Silicosis is a chronic fibrotic lung disease resulting from inhalation of dusts containing crystalline silicon dioxide. The clinical presentation varies depending on the duration and intensity of exposure, the nature of the quartz crystals (tridymite or cristobalite) inhaled, and the presence of other organic and inorganic dusts. In addition, the presence of chronic obstructive pulmonary disease (COPD) and pulmonary tuberculosis often complicates the disease process. Although the incidence of silicosis is declining with improved industrial hygiene, it has been estimated that more than a million workers are exposed to quartz crystals. It has been estimated that as many as 1500 cases of silicosis could be diagnosed annually.

TYPES OF SILICOSIS

Chronic silicosis, the most common form of silicosis, is caused by many years of low-level quartz exposure. Patients are usually asymptomatic early in the course of the disease but may complain of cough and dyspnea on exertion. In advanced cases, progressive shortness of breath may occur with a paucity of physical findings. Finger clubbing and bibasilar crackles may be present, but are not commonly found.

Accelerated silicosis is a rapidly progressive disease caused by high concentrations of quartz exposure over periods as short as 5 years. This disease is marked by progressive shortness of breath and may eventually culminate in respiratory failure.

Acute silicosis is an acute form of silicosis that results from exposure to very high quartz concentrations. The duration of exposure can be as short as a few weeks. Patients usually present with fever, cough, and progressive dyspnea, including weight loss. Physical findings such as tachypnea, accessory muscle use, nasal flaring, and cyanosis are indicative of severe hypoxemic respiratory failure as a complication of progressive silicosis.

PATHOGENESIS

Quartz is the most common form of crystalline silica. Other crystalline forms are cristobalite and tridymite, which are thought to be more fibrogenic than quartz crystals. Silica combined with other minerals is called silicate crystals. Quartz is the most common form of silica exposure found in the workplace. Occupations where exposure to high concentrations of quartz crystals are reported are listed in Table 19-3.

Mining, quarrying, and tunneling Stonecutting, dressing, polishing, and cleaning monumental masonry Abrasives and abrasive blasting Glass manufacture Foundry work Pottery, porcelain, lining bricks Boiler scaling Vitreous enameling	**Table 19-3** **List of Industries with High** **Risk for Silica Exposure**

In vitro and in vivo evidence has shown that the type of quartz and the presence of other dust particles are important in modulating the lung's fibrogenic response. Inhaled quartz particles less than 10 μm in size are deposited in the alveoli, where they are engulfed by macrophages or deposited in the interstitial spaces. Phagocytosis of the quartz crystals by macrophages leads to cell lysis as a result of peroxidation of the lipid cell membrane. It has been suggested recently that silicate inhalation can lead to oxidant generation as a result of the formation of silicate-iron complexes. Inflammatory mediators are then released following cell lysis, which initiates a cascade of events leading to an alteration in macrophage function and activation of humoral and cellular immunity, thus leading to collagen deposition and lung fibrosis. The fibrosis appears as discrete nodules usually surrounded by normal lung tissue. Although a portion of the quartz crystals may eventually drain to regional lymph nodes, some of the inhaled material remains in the lung and contributes to progressive disease long after exposure has occurred.

CLINICAL FEATURES

In general, clinical symptoms and radiographic changes related to silicosis first appear 15 to 20 years after the onset of exposure to silica dust. Patients who are exposed to high concentrations of quartz may present soon after exposure and progress rapidly to acute hypoxemic respiratory failure. In contrast, patients who are exposed to low levels of quartz may be asymptomatic for long periods before presenting with mild symptoms of dyspnea on exertion or dry cough.

In chronic silicosis, the latency period between exposure and onset of signs and symptoms is very long.

PULMONARY FUNCTION TESTS

Changes in lung function are nonspecific in silicosis because of concomitant exposures to other dusts and cigarette smoking. Lung functions are usually normal in simple silicosis, but complicated silicosis, mild reductions in diffusion capacity, lung volumes, and compliance are found. An obstructive ventilatory pattern is frequently superimposed on an underlying restrictive defect. In advanced cases, exercise-induced hypoxemia is usually evident. In patients with simple silicosis, it has been estimated that the annual declines in FVC and FEV_1 are 59 mL and 64 mL, respectively. With implementation of current dust control standards, the reported annual decline in pulmonary function is much less than previously estimated.

Pulmonary Function Changes in Advanced Silicosis

- Decreased diffusion capacity
- Decreased lung volumes
- Decreased lung compliance
- Obstructive ventilatory pattern

RADIOGRAPHIC EVALUATIONS

The characteristic radiographic findings in silicosis are rounded (nodular) densities distributed predominantly in the upper lobes. Cavitation is unusual and always suggests the possibility of tuberculosis. Pulmonary nodule calcification is uncommon and usually is observed only in patients with rheumatoid arthritis (Caplan's syndrome). Eggshell calcification of hilar nodes (Figure 19-4) is almost pathognomonic of quartz exposure but

Radiographic Findings in Silicosis

- Nodular densities predominantly in upper lobes
- Eggshell calcification of hilar nodes
- Pulmonary nodule calcification is uncommon

FIGURE 19-4
Hilar lymphadenopathy with eggshell calcification in a patient with silicosis. Reproduced with permission from Parkes WR. Diseases of Free Silica. In *Occupational Lung Disorders*, 2nd ed. London: Butterworths, 1982, p 150.

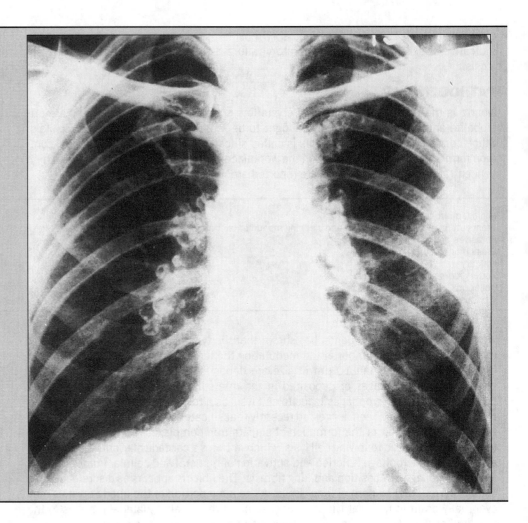

in rare cases may be seen in sarcoidosis and in lymphoma after radiotherapy. Coalescence of small nodular densities may lead to contraction of the upper lobes and the development of emphysematous changes in the lung bases. Pleural fibrosis is usually associated with massive fibrosis. In accelerated silicosis, the radiographic features are similar to those of chronic silicosis but the changes occur earlier and progress more rapidly.

In acute silicosis, diffuse bilateral alveolar and interstitial infiltrates are often present and are indistinguishable from pulmonary edema. Nodular densities are observed unless the disease is superimposed on chronic silicosis. The presence of pleural effusions often suggests another disease entity such as tuberculosis, malignancy, or congestive heart failure. A computed tomography (CT) scan of the chest is more sensitive than the plain chest x-ray in detecting as well as defining the silicotic nodules, especially when there is early conglomeration.

Case Study:
Continued

Based on the paucity of clinical symptoms, significant occupational history, and chest radiographic findings, the most likely diagnosis is chronic silicosis. Although the patient also has a history of asbestos exposure in the brake repair shop, the exposure period was too short for asbestosis. Likewise, the chest x-ray is not typical of asbestosis. His arterial blood gas is normal. Pulmonary function tests show a mixed obstructive and restrictive lung pattern that is common in any of the pneumoconioses, especially in smokers.

Tuberculin skin test and sputum AFB are negative. The patient is advised to stop smoking 2 weeks prior to surgery and is started on inhaled albuterol. He subsequently undergoes uneventful hernia repair.

THERAPY FOR SILICOSIS

Once simple silicosis develops, the fibrotic process of lung repair becomes irreversible. Management of individual cases is directed toward preventing progression and warding off complications. Continued exposure in the workplace may lead to progressive disease, except in foundry work, where progression to progressive massive fibrosis is infrequent. In advanced cases, treatment consists of supplemental oxygen, beta agonists, anticholinergics, theophylline if chronic airflow obstruction is present, and diuretics as well as inotropic drugs in the presence of cor pulmonale. To date, no specific drugs have been proven to be of benefit in the treatment of silicosis. Recent reports have suggested that short courses of corticosteroids in simple and complicated silicosis may improve lung function. However, the effect of long-term use of corticosteroids in preventing the progression of silicosis is unclear.

> Treatment of silicosis is supportive.

PROGNOSIS

Simple silicosis is not associated with increased mortality. The major causes of death are respiratory complications. Among the predictors of mortality are an age less than 45 years, advanced silicosis, and the occurrence of tuberculosis.

Six months after the inguinal hernia repair, the patient returns to your office for follow-up. He complains of night sweats, low-grade fever, and cough productive of light yellow, bloodstreaked sputum. He also reports losing 30 lb in 1 month. He lives in a nursing home. On physical exam, he is mildly tachypneic with a respiratory rate of 24 breaths per minute. His temperature is 100.1°F. Auscultation of the chest reveals bronchial breath sounds in the right upper lung field with egophony. Laboratory data include a white blood cell count of 14,000 per cubic millimeter, with 75% neutrophils and 25% lymphocytes. PPD shows 7-mm induration. Sputum is positive for acid-fast organisms. Chest x-ray shows two new 2.5-cm cavitary lesions in the apicoposterior segment of the left upper lobe. The patient is immediately started on quadruple antituberculous drug therapy (isoniazid, rifampin, ethambutol, and pyrazinamide).

Case Study:
Continued

COMPLICATIONS OF SILICOSIS

Tuberculosis is the major complication of silicosis. Diligent efforts should be undertaken to rule out active tuberculosis. In Third World countries during the 1960s, the incidence of active tuberculosis was 20%. In the same period in the United States, the incidence of tuberculosis in metal miners with silicosis was 5.3%, compared with 0.6% in those without silicosis. Infections with atypical mycobacteria (*Mycobacterium kansasii* and *Mycobacterium avium-intracellulare*) have also been reported. Pneumothorax may result from rupture of bullous emphysema secondary to massive fibrosis. Rheumatoid nodules may appear in patients with silicosis. Epidemiologic and experimental studies suggest an association between silica exposure and increased risk of pulmonary malignancy. However, a cause-and-effect relationship cannot be established in most of the studies linking silicosis and lung cancer because of the presence of confounding variables (smoking and exposure to cocarcinogens).

Complications of Silicosis

- Tuberculosis
- Pneumothorax
- Rheumatoid nodules

■ ASBESTOS-RELATED PULMONARY DISORDERS

Asbestos is a collective term for fibrous mineral silicates of the serpentine and amphibole groups. These minerals are valued for their durability and fire-resistant qualities. Inhalation of asbestos fibers can lead to different pulmonary disorders such as asbestosis, lung cancer, malignant mesothelioma, asbestos pleural effusions, and pleural plaques or circumscribed pleural thickening.

TYPES OF ASBESTOS-RELATED PULMONARY DISORDERS

Asbestosis is diffuse interstitial fibrosis of the lung parenchyma caused by exposure to asbestos fibers. Asbestos exposure can lead to both benign and malignant pleural diseases. Benign pleural diseases can present as pleural plaques, pleural effusions, or diffuse pleural thickening that on occasion leads to fibrothorax.

Asbestos bodies are asbestos fibers coated with iron-protein complex.

PATHOGENESIS

Deposition of asbestos fibers in the alveoli results in macrophage-induced alveolitis and, depending on the dust load, may lead to increased oxidant and fibronectin production, cytokine release, and recruitment of inflammatory cells, eventually leading to chronic interstitial lung disease. Pulmonary fibrosis associated with asbestosis tends to be most prominent in the lower lobes at the subpleural regions. Microscopic examination may reveal asbestos bodies or uncoated asbestos fibers (Figure 19-5), which are considered pathognomonic for asbestos exposure. Asbestos bodies are asbestos fibers coated by iron-containing protein, which have a golden yellow or brown color. They can also be detected in sputum specimens dissolved in sodium hydroxide. It is important to remember that the presence of asbestos bodies indicates only past exposure to asbestos fibers, not asbestosis or other asbestos-related diseases.

On postmortem examination or open thoracotomy, pleural plaques appear as shiny, white, and slightly raised areas (Figure 19-6). Pleural plaques are most commonly found in the inferolateral chest wall and over the central portion of the diaphragm, although the anterior or posterior chest wall may be initially involved. Histologically, pleural plaques consist of hyaline fibrous tissue that is almost completely acellular and avascular (Figure 19-7). Calcifications are commonly observed, especially in the parietal pleura. Pleural plaques are believed to develop as a result of the release of short asbestos fibers into the pleural space by way of subpleural and parietal pleural lymphatics. Pleural fibrosis commonly involves the visceral and parietal pleurae of both lower lobes. On gross inspection, the lung is encased by a white peel. Occasionally, the pleural reaction may fold on itself, trapping the underlying parenchyma and causing atelectasis of the trapped lung. This process leads to the development of pleuroparenchymal lesions known as rounded atelectasis (Figure 19-8).

FIGURE 19-5
An example of an asbestos body identified in a sputum specimen. Reproduced with permission from Morgan WKC, Gee JBL: Asbestos-related diseases. In Morgan WKC, Seaton A, eds.: *Occupational Lung Diseases*, 3rd ed. Philadelphia: WB Saunders, 1995, p 327.

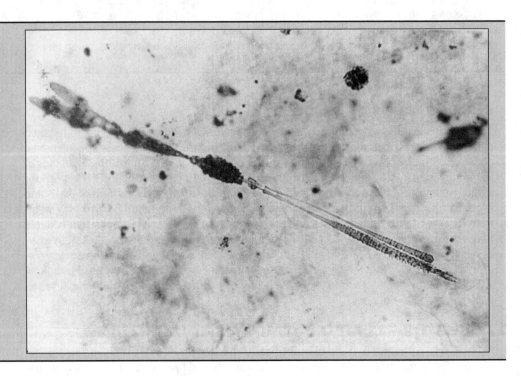

CLINICAL FEATURES

The onset is often insidious. The most common presenting complaint is initial shortness of breath on exertion, which progresses to breathlessness at rest as the disease advances. Persistent cough and sputum are also commonly reported. Chest pain is not unusual but suggests pleural involvement. The earliest physical examination findings are the presence of basilar end-inspiratory crackles. Finger clubbing is seen in 15% to 20% of cases and portends a poorer prognosis.

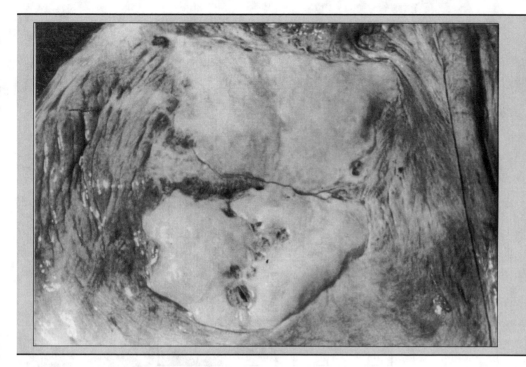

FIGURE 19-6
Gross appearance of pleural plaques. Reproduced with permission from Morgan WKC, Gee JBL: Asbestos-related diseases. In Morgan WKC, Seaton A, eds.: *Occupational Lung Diseases*, 3rd ed. Philadelphia: WB Saunders, 1995, p 338.

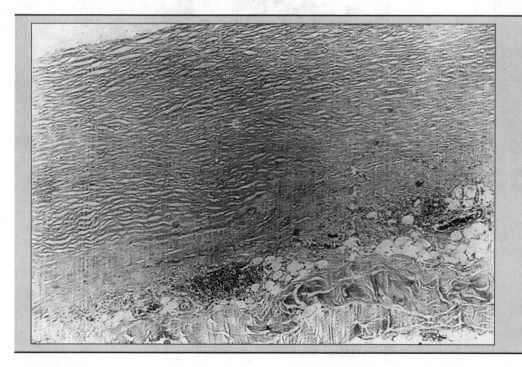

FIGURE 19-7
Histologic section of pleural plaques. Note the whorls of collagen fibers around the plaques. Reproduced with permission from Morgan WKC, Gee JBL: Asbestos-related diseases. In Morgan WKC, Seaton A, eds.: *Occupational Lung Diseases*, 3rd ed. Philadelphia: WB Saunders, 1995, p 338.

In the absence of parenchymal disease, patients usually demonstrate no symptoms. The diagnosis of pleural plaques is usually made as an incidental finding on chest x-ray. Shortness of breath and pleuritic chest pain are the usual presenting complaints; however, some patients may be asymptomatic. A pleural rub may be heard on occasion. In patients with extensive pleural involvement, the most common complaint is dyspnea on exertion.

It usually requires 20 years from the first asbestos exposure for pleural plaques to become radiographically apparent. Only 5% of pleural plaques are calcified, and most

FIGURE 19-8
(A) Rounded atelectasis in the left upper lobe. Note the pulmonary vessel passing through the inferior aspect of the opacity. (B) CT scan showing an elongated mass in the lingula. Note the pleural thickening, curvilinear path of the vessels, and subpleural fat. Reproduced with permission from Fraser RG, Peter Paré JA, Paré PD, et al: Roentgenologic signs in the diagnosis of chest disease. In Fraser RG, Peter Paré JA, Paré PD, et al., eds: *Diagnosis of Diseases of the Chest*, 3rd ed. Philadelphia: WB Saunders, 1988, p 488.

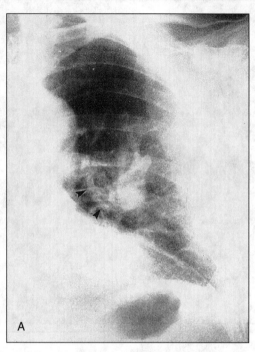

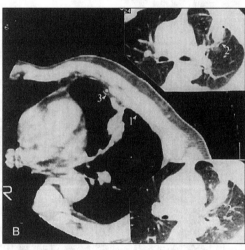

present as irregular shadows on the lateral margins of the chest x-ray without clear margins. In addition to occupational exposure, domestic and residential exposures have been implicated in the production of pleural plaques. As many as 50% of patients with pleural plaques have concomitant asbestos-related parenchymal lung disease.

PULMONARY FUNCTION TESTS

Pulmonary function testing usually reveals either restrictive or combined restrictive (reduction in FVC and TLC) and obstructive (FEV$_1$ and FEF$_{25-75}$) ventilatory defects. The restrictive defects in asbestosis are caused by a decrease in lung compliance. Obstructive defects are present at lower lung volumes as a result of the development of peribronchiolar fibrosis. In advanced cases, an impairment in gas exchange manifested by hypoxemia is observed, with decreased diffusion capacity and arterial oxygen on blood-gas analysis. Isolated pleural plaques are not usually associated with clinically detectable restrictive defects on pulmonary function testing. A reduction in vital capacity may be seen in selected patients with rare presentations of extensive pleural plaques or moderate to large pleural effusions.

RADIOGRAPHIC EVALUATION

The posteroanterior chest radiograph remains a useful initial test in the diagnosis of asbestosis and in the health surveillance of exposed workers. Typically, small irregular opacities are seen in the lower lung zones between the rib shadows. As the opacities coalesce, the heart borders may become obscured. Rounded opacities caused by asbestos are unusual unless concomitant exposures to silica dusts occur. In contrast to silicosis, hilar adenopathies are not seen in asbestosis. Early fibrotic changes of asbestosis are better visualized by chest CT scan than by chest x-ray, especially in the presence of pleural fibrosis. In addition, chest CT scanning is helpful in characterizing localized pleuropulmonary lesions, such as rounded atelectasis, which must be differentiated from lung cancer.

Pleural plaques are usually seen as bilateral localized pleural thickenings on the anterolateral or diaphragmatic parietal pleura on chest x-ray. Rounded atelectasis may also be observed on the chest x-ray. This type of pleural thickening is distinguished from circumscribed pleural thickening by obliteration of the costophrenic angle, and a loss of lung volumes. Chest CT scanning is helpful in evaluating the extent of pleural fibrosis and defining the nature of pleural-based masses such as rounded atelectasis. Pathognomonic chest CT appearances of rounded atelectasis have been described, including a peripheral lesion located adjacent to a broadly based pleural thickening with a "comet tail" of bronchovascular structures radiating from the lesion to the hilum.

> Calcified pleural plaques may be the only abnormal radiographic findings in asbestosis.

Radiographic Abnormalities in Asbestos-Related Lung Diseases

- Increased interstitial markings predominantly at lung bases
- Rounded atelectasis
- Pleural thickening

THERAPY FOR ASBESTOS-RELATED PULMONARY DISORDERS

There is no effective treatment once pulmonary fibrosis has been established. The usefulness of steroids and other anti-inflammatory agents or cytotoxic agents in the presence of active alveolitis is unclear. The avoidance of further asbestos exposure and smoking cessation are helpful. Because of the increased incidence of lung fibrosis in patients with pleural plaques, avoidance of further exposure to asbestos is advised. The role of surgery in diffuse pleural fibrosis is unclear; however, pleurectomy may be effective in providing symptomatic relief from pleuritic chest pain resulting from benign asbestos pleural disease. Smoking cessation programs should be offered to decrease the risk of lung cancer.

After 8 weeks, a sputum culture grows Mycobacterium kansasii *that is sensitive to all antituberculous drugs. Pyrazinamide is discontinued, and the patient is treated with isoniazid, rifampin, and ethambutol. His symptoms improve after 2 months of therapy, and repeat sputum AFB and culture after 6 months of therapy are negative. He also has gained 25 lb in the last 6 months. He is given pneumococcal vaccine and yearly influenza vaccination. He continues the medications for 18 months and is then lost to follow-up.*

Ten years later, he is admitted to the hospital for progressive shortness of breath, dry cough, nonpleuritic chest pain, low-grade fever, and weight loss of 2 months' duration. A chest x-ray reveals a moderate left pleural effusion. Repeat tuberculin skin test is negative, with a positive anergy panel. Sputum AFB staining is negative. A diagnostic thoracentesis is performed and 200 mL of bloody fluid is obtained. Analysis of the pleural fluid reveals a protein of 4.5 gm/dL and a pleural fluid LDH of 1200 IU/dL. All bacterial and mycobacterial cultures are negative. Thoracoscopic biopsy of the pleura reveals sheets of poorly differentiated mesenchymal cells forming cordlike patterns.

Case Study:
Continued

COMPLICATIONS

Epidemiologic evidence has shown that there is a tenfold increase in the risk for lung cancer in patients with asbestosis. This increased risk is dependent on the duration and intensity of asbestos exposure. Smoking enhances the carcinogenicity of asbestos. Individuals with histories of exposure to asbestos have an increased risk of developing mesothelioma. Malignant mesothelioma is thought to arise from pleural mesothelial cells. Unlike other asbestos-related lung diseases, no close relationship exists between the duration and intensity of asbestos exposure and the development of mesothelioma. The majority of patients present with an insidious onset of chest pain, dry cough, and

Complications of Asbestosis

- Lung cancer
- Mesothelioma

shortness of breath. The most common radiographic finding is a large pleural effusion. Pleural plaques may also be seen on the contralateral side in one-third of the cases. A diagnosis of mesothelioma often requires an open pleural biopsy.

COAL WORKER'S PNEUMOCONIOSIS

Coal worker's pneumoconiosis is a pulmonary disease resulting from the deposition of coal dusts in the lungs. Depending on the radiographic appearance, the disease may be classified as simple pneumoconiosis, if the lesion is less than 1 cm in diameter, or complicated pneumoconiosis (progressive massive fibrosis), if the cumulative size of the lesions is greater than 1 cm. The severity of the disease is related to the worker's cumulative exposure to coal mine dusts and concomitant exposure to silica. Inhalation of coal mine dust can also lead to silicosis, industrial bronchitis, and chronic airflow obstruction independent of smoking.

PATHOGENESIS

The primary lesion in coal worker's pneumoconiosis is the coal macule (Figure 19-9), distributed mainly in both upper lobes, although the lower lobes may eventually become involved. On histologic examination, the lesions consist of aggregates of dusts, dust-laden macrophages, and fibroblasts in the respiratory bronchioles and alveoli. The coal macules may eventually enlarge to form nodules that eventually weaken the bronchioles, leading to focal emphysema. Coalescence of the perivascularly located coal nodules leads to bulky, rubbery masses located mainly in the posterior segments of the upper lobes. This pattern is termed progressive massive fibrosis (PMF). As in the other pneumoconioses, the initial pathogenic mechanism involves the deposition of coal dusts in the distal airways, followed by macrophage-triggered alveolitis leading eventually to fibrosis. The development of focal and centriacinar emphysema is thought to result from release of inflammatory mediators by inflammatory cells, causing alveolar and epithelial cell damage. The exact pathogenetic events triggering PMF are speculative but are thought to be attributable mainly to dust load and, by inference, to the degree of immunologic response.

CLINICAL FEATURES

In simple pneumoconiosis, there are usually no symptoms. The diagnosis is made on the basis of the chest x-ray in patients who have histories of coal exposure. The presence of cough and sputum early in the disease process is probably the result of chronic bronchitis from dust inhalation. As the disease progresses to PMF, dyspnea on exertion becomes the predominant symptom. Occasionally, coughing of black sputum (melanoptysis) may occur as a result of rupture of the cavitating PMF lesions into the airway. Blue-black discoloration of the skin on the hands, forearms, and face by coal tattoo marks may indicate past coal exposure. Finger clubbing is not a feature of this disease, and if present should prompt a search for alternative diagnoses.

PULMONARY FUNCTION TESTS

There are no identifiable patterns of impairment on lung function testing in simple pneumoconiosis. In more advanced diseases, such as in PMF, reductions in FVC and FEV_1 are usually seen even after allowing for the effects of smoking. Residual volume may increase, reflecting air trapping from emphysema and small airways disease. In addition, reductions in diffusion capacity and increases in dead space ventilation (V_D/V_T) are also noted.

RADIOGRAPHIC EVALUATIONS

A hallmark chest radiographic finding in simple pneumoconiosis is the presence of small, rounded opacities in the lung parenchyma. The upper lung zones are initially involved, and cavitation and calcification of the lesions may occur. Hilar adenopathy may occur, but eggshell calcifications are unusual. Progressive massive fibrosis lesions usually are observed in the upper lobes. Bullous lesions may develop around the PMF lesions as they shrink toward the apices. High-resolution CT scanning usually reveals the presence of nodules before they become visible on the chest x-ray.

Types of Coal Worker's Pneumoconiosis

- Simple (lesion smaller than 1 cm)
- Complicated (lesion larger than 1 cm)

Coalescence of coal macules results in progressive massive fibrosis (PMF).

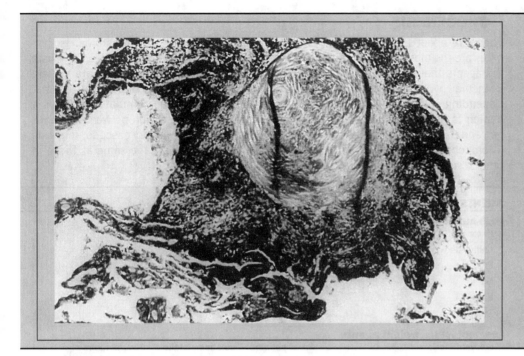

FIGURE 19-9
Histologic picture of a coal macule. Reproduced with permission from Seaton A: Coal workers' pneumoconiosis. In Morgan WKC, Seaton A, eds.: *Occupational Lung Diseases*, 3rd ed. Philadelphia: WB Saunders, 1995, p 397.

THERAPY FOR COAL WORKER'S PNEUMOCONIOSIS

Management is directed at the prevention, early diagnosis, and treatment of complications. The principles of management is the same as in silicosis. Retraining of younger patients with extensive exposure is advised to prevent the development of progressive massive fibrosis. Patients with significant airflow obstruction or PMF should receive appropriate immunizations with influenza and pneumococcal vaccines.

COMPLICATIONS

Both *Mycobacterium tuberculosis* and atypical mycobacteriosis can complicate coal worker's pneumoconiosis, although they occur much less frequently than in silicosis. Nevertheless, continued surveillance and treatment of tuberculosis is of paramount importance. Caplan's syndrome (rheumatoid pneumoconiosis) is a syndrome that describes the association between coal worker's pneumoconiosis and rheumatoid arthritis. The chest x-ray typically shows rounded densities less than 5 cm in diameter that appear in crops over short periods of time. The lesions may cavitate, calcify, or develop air-fluid levels, or may even disappear occasionally. Radiographic abnormalities may precede the onset of rheumatoid arthritis by 5 to 10 years. There is an association between the rheumatoid nodules found in the elbows and over the Achilles tendon and those that appear in the lungs.

Caplan's syndrome is the association between rheumatoid arthritis and coal worker's pneumoconiosis.

■ OCCUPATIONAL ASTHMA

Occupational asthma is characterized by the presence of variable airflow obstruction or bronchial hyperresponsiveness, or both, as a result of exposure to airborne dusts, gases, vapors, and fumes in the workplace. Occupational asthma has an estimated prevalence of 2% to 15% and is becoming the most prevalent occupational respiratory disease, surpassing even silicosis and asbestosis.

TYPES OF OCCUPATIONAL ASTHMA

Occupational asthma can be divided into allergic and nonallergic varieties. Allergic occupational asthma is caused by exposure to a specific sensitizing agent present in the workplace, and is characterized by a preceding latency period before the onset of symptoms. Nonallergic occupational asthma results from exposure to inhaled irritants, and is notable for absence of latency period and persistent, nonspecific bronchial hyperreactivity. Reactive airways dysfunction syndrome is classically a result of exposure to high levels of extremely irritating agents, resulting in a persistent asthma-like illness. This illness is in contradistinction to preexisting asthma aggravated by irritants in the workplace.

Types of Occupational Asthma

- Allergic (immunologically mediated; latency period before onset of symptoms)
- Nonallergic (exposure to irritating gases; absence of latency period)

PATHOGENESIS

There are about 250 agents that can potentially cause occupational asthma. Isocyanates are the most common causative agents that have been identified. Table 19-4 lists the agents that cause occupational asthma and the types of workers who are at risk. Bronchial hyperresponsiveness is the characteristic feature of occupational asthma. Depending on the nature of the offending agent, it can directly stimulate, or act as a hapten to produce, IgE-specific antibodies. The specific interaction between the antigen and the IgE antibody complex can then initiate the inflammatory cascade, resulting in bronchial edema and hyperreactivity. Pathologic changes are the same as those in other forms of asthma.

Table 19-4
Agents Implicated in Occupational Asthma and Workers Who Are Potentially Exposed to These Sensitizing Agents.

AGENTS	WORKERS AT RISK
High-molecular weight agents	
Cereals	Bakers, millers
Animal-derived allergens	Animal handlers
Enzymes	Detergents users, pharmaceutical workers, bakers
Gums	Carpet makers, pharmaceutical workers
Latex	Health professionals
Seafoods	Seafood processors
Low-molecular weight agents	
Isocyanates	Spray painters; insulation installers; manufacturers of plastics, rubbers, foams
Wood dusts	Forest workers, carpenters, cabinet makers
Anhydrides	Users of plastics, epoxy resins
Amines	Shellac and lacquer handlers, solderers
Fluxes	Electronic workers
Chloramine-T	Janitors, cleaners
Dyes	Textile workers
Persulfate	Hairdressers
Formaldehyde glutaraldehyde	Hospital staffs
Acrylate	Adhesive handlers
Drugs	Pharmaceutical workers, health professionals
Metals	Solderers, refiners

Reproduced with permission from Chan-Yeung M, Malo JL. Current concepts: occupational asthma. *N Engl J Med* 333:107-112, 1995.

CLINICAL FEATURES

Symptoms of occupational asthma improve on weekends and holidays and worsen on return to work.

The onset of symptoms may be immediate, or it may have a prolonged latency of a few weeks to several years from the time of initial exposure. Symptoms such as dyspnea, cough, and wheezing usually improve on weekends and holidays and worsen on return to work. However, symptoms may be prolonged and persistent if the disease is not recognized and treated early. Allergic symptoms such as rhinitis, itchy eyes, and sneezing often accompany respiratory symptoms. Symptoms may first appear at night or late in the day, because of the late response of asthma following an exposure encountered at work.

PULMONARY FUNCTION TESTS

Normal pulmonary function tests do not rule out occupational asthma. Bronchoprovocation tests and serial spirometric tests may be helpful if initial spirometry is normal.

Because occupational asthma is a reversible airflow limitation, normal spirometry does not exclude the diagnosis. Pulmonary function measured on a day away from work may be normal in up to 50% of patients with occupational asthma. Bronchoprovocation testing is helpful if the symptoms are atypical, such as cough and chest tightness, or if initial spirometry shows no evidence of airflow limitation. A negative study does not rule out occupational asthma if the patient has not been exposed for an extended period of time. However, the absence of bronchial hyperresponsiveness after the individual has worked for 2 weeks virtually rules out asthma. Other indications for testing include the need to provide safe guidelines for specific bronchial challenge testing, in following the recovery of the patient after cessation of exposure and quantitation of bronchial hyperresponsiveness.

Serial measurements of peak expiratory flow rates done every 2 hours while the patient is awake both at work (for 2 weeks) and at home (for 2 weeks), in conjunction with a diary of symptoms, help examine the relationship between asthma and the work environment. These tests are sensitive but not specific and are limited by patient effort.

SKIN TESTING

If appropriate allergens are available, a skin test or blood test for IgE antibodies may be helpful in identifying the specific offending agent. A positive test, however, indicates only prior sensitization and not disease causation.

THERAPY FOR OCCUPATIONAL ASTHMA

For occupational asthma with a latency period, the ideal treatment is avoidance of further exposure to the offending agent. In the ideal situation, the worker is reassigned to a different workplace so as to avoid exposure to sensitizing agents. If occupational asthma is a result of toxic irritation of the airways, an emphasis should be placed on improving the workplace. The pharmacologic treatment of occupational asthma is similar to treatment of other types of asthma.

■ EFFECTS OF AIR POLLUTION

The adverse effects of dust, fumes, and toxic chemicals from certain industries are not limited to the workplace environment but also afflict the surrounding communities. Since the advent of the industrial revolution, the detrimental effects of low-level exposure to air pollutants on human health have been increasingly recognized. Excessive mortality owing to cardiopulmonary diseases was recorded in highly industrialized countries such as Belgium, England, and the United States during the 1930s to 1950s. Although there are individual differences in sensitivity to air pollutants, patients with underlying chronic pulmonary disorders are especially susceptible to the adverse effects of air pollution.

In general, air pollutants are defined as concentrations of gases or particles to levels above normal. Alternatively, they can be defined as gases or particles present in ambient air that cause ill effects on human health. Some of the major pollutants and their adverse effects on the lung are listed in Table 19-5. Because many air pollutants are present in the atmosphere at the same time, it is not clear from epidemiologic data which agents cause the most toxicity. Nevertheless, three major pollutants—namely, sulfur dioxide, ozone, and nitrogen dioxide—have been well studied and will be discussed further.

POLLUTANTS	SOURCES	ADVERSE EFFECTS
Sulfur oxides	Power plants, oil refineries Kerosene space heaters	Bronchoconstriction
Oxides of Nitrogen	Automobile exhaust, oil refineries Gas stoves and furnaces	Airway injury, pulmonary edema, bronchiolitis
Ozone	Automobile exhaust, aircraft cabin, electrical appliances	Airway injury, pulmonary edema, bronchiolitis
Polycyclic hydrocarbons	Diesel exhaust, cigarette smoke	Lung cancer
Asbestos	Insulation, building materials Workers' clothing	Mesothelioma, pulmonary fibrosis
Ionizing radiation	Building materials	Lung cancer
Arsenic	Smelters	Lung cancer
Allergens	Pollen	Exacerbation of asthma

Table 19-5
Examples of Major Pollutants and Its Associated Adverse Pulmonary Effects

Adapted from Boushey, et al: Air Pollution. In Murray JF, Nadel JA, ed. *Textbook of Respiratory Medicine*, 2nd ed. p. 2033, Philadelphia: W.B. Saunders, 1994.

LUNG DEFENSE MECHANISMS

The lung has several defense mechanisms to guard it against air pollutants. Because air pollutants exist in the form of either gas or particulate matter, the upper airway, particularly the nose, acts as an efficient filter to remove air pollutants. The turbulent flow of air in the nose induced by the turbinates traps large particles and removes harmful gases

Lung Defense Mechanisms

- Nose acts as an efficient filter system
- Mucociliary escalator
- Alveolar macrophages

through adsorption. For example, the concentration of sulfur dioxide that reaches the lung is less than 2% of the concentration inspired at the nose. The mouth is less efficient than the nose in filtering noxious gases. Thus, mouth breathing during high ventilatory demands such as strenuous exercise increases the concentration of soluble pollutants reaching the lower airway and lung parenchyma. Smaller particles (less than 10 μm in diameter) that escape the initial filtering function of the nose are removed by the mucociliary escalator and subsequently swallowed. Still smaller particles (0.5 to 3.0 μm in diameter) that reach the alveoli are engulfed by the alveolar macrophages. Individuals with congenital defects such as the immotile cilia syndrome are especially susceptible to inhaled polluted air.

EFFECTS OF SPECIFIC POLLUTANTS

Factors Affecting Toxicity of Air Pollutants

- Physicochemical properties
- Concentration
- Duration of exposure
- Individual susceptibility

The site of injury in the respiratory system depends on the physicochemical properties of the air pollutant, its concentration, the duration of exposure, and individual susceptibility. Highly soluble gases such as sulfur dioxide usually cause immediate irritation of the upper airway. Less water soluble gases, such as oxides of nitrogen and ozone, cause delayed cellular injury in the distal airways and alveoli. Large particles, because of aerodynamic drag and turbulent flow, impact in the upper airway and result in less airway injury. Small particles (smaller than 5 μm) that pass through the upper airway cause distal and alveolar injury.

Sulfur dioxide is produced by burning of fossil fuels such as coal and crude oil. The major sources of sulfur dioxide are power plants, oil refineries, smelters, paper pulp mills, and wineries. Sulfur dioxide is a clear, highly water-soluble gas that can easily react with other air pollutants and form particulate aerosols of sulfuric acids and various metallic, acidic, and ammonium sulfates. Inhalation of sulfur dioxide in concentrations greater than 5 ppm causes an increase in airway resistance in normal human volunteers. Patients with bronchial asthma are especially susceptible to the bronchoconstrictor effect of sulfur dioxide. Epidemiologic studies show that approximately 90% of people who complain of respiratory symptoms and who have been exposed to polluted air with high concentrations of sulfur dioxide have asthma. Exercise increases the bronchoconstrictor effect of sulfur dioxide by virtue of high minute ventilation and mouth breathing. Apart from its bronchoconstrictor effect, sulfur dioxide also decreases the clearance of inhaled particles. In animal studies, short-term exposure to sulfur dioxide stimulates submucosal gland secretion as well as hypertrophy of airway submucosal glands.

Nitrogen dioxide and ozone are both by-products of internal combustion engines. Nitrogen dioxide may be present in indoor air in concentrations higher than in outdoor air in homes that use natural gas for heating and cooking. On the other hand, ozone levels three times higher than permitted have been measured in high-flying commercial aircraft. Both nitrogen dioxide and ozone exist as relatively insoluble gases, and thus cause injury in the distal airway and alveoli. High ozone concentrations have been linked to a higher incidence of exacerbations of airflow obstruction in patients with chronic obstructive pulmonary disease (COPD) and asthma. In healthy subjects, ozone causes cough, substernal chest pain, and transient decreases in airflow and lung compliance. These effects become more marked during prolonged exposure or strenuous exercise. Similar changes in lung function can result from nitrogen dioxide exposure. In addition, extremely high concentrations of nitric oxide commonly found in silos can cause pulmonary edema and acute respiratory failure.

Case Study:
Resolution

It is important to remember that mixed pneumoconiosis can occur because silica is quite ubiquitous. For example, coal workers may also develop silicosis. In this case, the patient develops mesothelioma as a result of prior asbestos exposure. Overall, about 50% of all cases of mesothelioma have documented histories of asbestos exposure.

■ REVIEW QUESTIONS

1. A 55-year-old man who has been working in a local coal mine for 10 years is concerned about his health after learning that one of his coworkers was recently admitted to a hospital for respiratory failure. He complains of intermittent cough productive of scanty whitish sputum but otherwise is in fairly good health. He has smoked one pack of cigarettes per day for the last 30 years. Physical examination is normal. The most appropriate next step in this patient's evaluation is

   (A) chest x-ray
   (B) arterial blood gas
   (C) sputum Gram stain and culture
   (D) pulmonary function test

2. A 55-year-old pottery worker comes to your office complaining of worsening shortness of breath, productive cough, and low-grade temperature, especially in the late afternoon, for the last 2 months. He was told 5 years ago by the company physician after routine chest x-ray that he had silicosis. He denies a significant smoking history. A repeat chest x-ray a day after the office visit shows bilateral nodular densities on both upper lobes that are slightly worse than they were on the chest x-ray 5 years ago. The most appropriate next diagnostic test is

   (A) tuberculin skin test and sputum AFB
   (B) CT scan of the chest
   (C) referral to a pulmonary specialist for transbronchial lung biopsy
   (D) serum rheumatoid factor

3. The presence of asbestos bodies in respiratory secretions

   (A) indicates previous asbestos exposure
   (B) is an early marker for asbestosis
   (C) is associated with an increased risk of lung cancer
   (D) is associated with late development of malignant mesothelioma, especially in the presence of pleural plaques

4. Spirometry in patients with pneumoconiosis may show

   (A) a restrictive lung defect
   (B) an obstructive lung defect
   (C) a mixed restrictive and obstructive lung defect
   (D) all of the above

5. A 32-year-old first-year medical student complains of cough, shortness of breath, and intermittent wheezing, especially on exertion, for the past 2 months. He has no fever. He denies any history of asthma. After meticulous questioning, he recalls being exposed to formalin after it was accidentally spilled on the floor during anatomy class. Which one of the following statements about this disorder is false?

   (A) The respiratory symptoms result from the irritant nature of the offending gas.
   (B) The symptoms occur immediately after exposure and may persist for several months.
   (C) The airway edema and hyperreactivity observed in this syndrome are caused by IgE-mediated release of inflammatory mediators such as histamine and leukotriene.
   (D) Upper airway mucosal injury may also occur in this syndrome.

6. Which of the following air pollutants may cause an exacerbation of bronchial asthma?

   (A) Sulfur dioxide
   (B) Ozone
   (C) Nitrogen dioxide
   (D) All of the above

■ ANSWERS AND EXPLANATIONS

1. The answer is A. Chest x-ray, in addition to clinical history and physical examination, is the best initial screening test for detection of significant dust load in the lung. In the presence of simple pneumoconiosis, avoidance of further exposure to prevent progressive disease may be helpful. Significant radiographic abnormalities may be seen in the absence of symptoms. On the other hand, chronic cough in a smoker may be not be a result of simple pneumoconiosis. Pulmonary function tests (spirometry, lung volumes, diffusion capacity, and arterial blood gases) are helpful in disability evaluation but are otherwise nonspecific. Sputum Gram stain and culture are important in ruling out concomitant bacterial infection, but they are unlikely to be helpful in this patient with purulent sputum and fever.

2. The answer is A. The incidence of both typical and atypical pulmonary tuberculosis is high in patients with silicosis. In patients with symptoms of productive cough, weight loss, and low-grade fever, pulmonary tuberculosis should be ruled out. Tuberculin skin test and sputum examination for acid-fast organisms should be part of the diagnostic evaluation. If malignancy is a consideration, chest CT scan may be helpful in further defining the parenchymal lesions and in evaluating the hilum and mediastinum for malignancy. Tissue diagnosis is seldom required in the diagnosis of pneumoconiosis if significant exposure history is obtained and malignancy is not highly suspected. A positive serum rheumatoid factor is present in patients with Caplan's syndrome.

3. The answer is A. Asbestos bodies are asbestos fibers coated with iron complex with protein. The presence of asbestos bodies in sputum indicates only prior exposure to asbestos. It does not indicate progressive asbestos lung disease or a higher risk for lung cancer. Asbestosis increases the risk of lung cancer, and the effects of asbestosis and smoking on the risk of lung cancer are addictive. The association between malignant mesothelioma and asbestos exposure was recognized in the early 1960s. The risk of mesothelioma is highest with crocidolite, which has a high length-diameter ratio. Chrysolite, which is widely used commercially, has relatively low potential in causing malignant mesothelioma. There is no association between smoking and malignant mesothelioma. The latency period between asbestos exposure and the diagnosis of the tumor is very long—30 to 40 years on average.

4. The answer is D. Any of the ventilatory defect patterns on spirometry may be observed in patients with pneumoconiosis. Mixed restrictive and obstructive ventilatory defects are often present as a result of pulmonary fibrosis and of traction emphysema on the surrounding area. Moreover, most patients with pneumoconiosis are smokers and may have concomitant chronic airflow obstruction.

5. The answer is C. This patient has reactive airways dysfunction syndrome, which occurs after significant exposure to an irritating gas. The clinical presentation may be difficult to differentiate from asthma, especially if a history of exposure to irritant gas is not obtained. Unlike asthma, the airway injury is not immunologically mediated.

6. The answer is D. All of the pollutants listed not only cause bronchitis but also can exacerbate airflow obstruction such as asthma or COPD. Epidemiologic data have shown that patients with underlying airflow obstruction are especially susceptible to the effects of air pollutants.

■ SUGGESTED READING

Chan-Yeung M, Malo JL: Occupational asthma. *N Engl J Med* 333:107, 1995, pp. 107–112.

Gibbs AR: Pathological reactions of the lung to dust. In Morgan WKC, Seaton A, eds.: *Occupational Lung Diseases*, 3rd ed. Philadelphia: WB Saunders, 1995, pp. 127–157.

Gong H Jr.: Health effects of air pollution: a review of clinical studies. *Clin Chest Med* 13(2):201, 1992, pp. 201–214.

Graham WGB: Silicosis. *Clin Chest Med* 13(2):253, 1992, pp. 253–267.

LeRoy Lapp N, Parker JE: Coal worker's pneumoconiosis. *Clin Chest Med* 13(2):243, 1992, pp. 243–252.

Morgan WKC: The deposition and clearance of dust from the lungs—their role in etiology of occupational lung disease. In Morgan WKC, Seaton A, eds.: *Occupational Lung Diseases*, 3rd ed. Philadelphia: WB Saunders, 1995, pp. 111–126.

Morgan WKC, Gee JBL: Asbestos-related diseases. In Morgan WKC, Seaton A, eds.: *Occupational Lung Diseases*, 3rd ed. Philadelphia: WB Saunders, 1995, pp. 308–373.

Seaton A: The clinical approach. In Morgan WKC, Seaton A, eds.: *Occupational Lung Diseases*. Philadelphia: WB Saunders, 1995, pp. 17–26.

INDEX

NOTE: An f after a page number denotes a figure; a t after a page number denotes a table.

A

A-aDO$_2$. *See* Alveolar-arterial oxygen gradient (A-aDO$_2$)
A1AT (alpha$_1$-antitrypsin) deficiency, chronic obstructive pulmonary disease due to, 237–238
Abdomen, in respiratory mechanics, 12
Abdominal muscles, 16
ABPA (allergic bronchopulmonary aspergillosis), 228
Accessory muscles, 16
ACE (angiotensin converting enzyme), in sarcoidosis, 252, 252t
Acetylcholine (ACh), in regulation of airway caliber, 120f
Acid-base disturbances, 81–85
    metabolic acidosis, 83, 83t
    metabolic alkalosis, 84, 84t
    mixed, 84, 85f
    respiratory acidosis, 81–82, 82t
    respiratory alkalosis, 83, 83t
Acid-base status, 79–81, 81f
Acidemia, 81
Acidosis
    metabolic, 82t, 83, 83t
    respiratory, 81–82, 81f, 82t
Acinus, 20f, 23
Acquired immunodeficiency syndrome (AIDS). *See* Human immunodeficiency virus (HIV)
ACTH (adrenocorticotropic hormone), excess, with lung cancer, 308t, 310
Acute lung injury (ALI), 135–147
    cellular response to, 140–141, 142f
    cytokines in, 140, 140t
    defined, 138
    diagnosis of, 138–139
    exudative phase of, 139f, 139–143, 140t, 141f, 142f
    fibrotic phase of, 144f, 144–145, 145t
    gas-exchange abnormalities in, 145
    humoral response to, 140, 140t, 141f
    due to inhalation, 137–138
    lung function in, 145–146, 146f
    macrophages in, 140
    proliferative phase of, 143, 143f
    pulmonary capillary injury in, 141–143
    pulmonary hypertension with, 146
    therapy and outcome of, 146–147
    ventilation in, 145–146, 146f
Acute phase response (APR) proteins, 140
Adenocarcinoma, 305
Adenosine deaminase (ADA), in pleural effusions, 373
Adenosine triphosphate (ATP), during exercise, 193
Adhesion molecules, in asthma, 215–216
β-Adrenergic receptor agonists, for asthma, 223, 225, 227
β-Adrenergic receptor system, in airway smooth muscle contraction, 122–123, 123f
Adrenocorticotropic hormone (ACTH), excess, with lung cancer, 308t, 310
Adult respiratory distress syndrome (ARDS), lung compliance in, 24
Aerobic capacity, during exercise, 109, 109f, 111–112
Aerobic training, effect in healthy adults of, 111–112
Aging, respiratory system with, 7, 7t
AIDS. *See* Human immunodeficiency virus (HIV)
Airflow obstruction, 115–129
    airway conductance in, 124, 124f
    airway resistance in, 116–117, 123

due to airway smooth muscle contraction, 122t, 122–123, 123f
    and cardiac function, 129
    in chronic obstructive pulmonary disease, 238, 238f
    defined, 115
    diffusion capacity for carbon monoxide with, 128
    diseases causing, 115t, 115–116
    effect of effort on airflow rate in, 118–119, 119f
    exercise physiology in, 203–204
    expiratory airflow rates in, 123
    flow-volume curve with, 124–125, 125f
    forced expiration and equal pressure point in, 117f, 117–118, 118f
    gas-exchange abnormalities with, 129
    due to lung cancer, 308t, 309, 309f
    lung compliance with, 127, 127f
    lung volumes with, 127–128, 128f
    mechanisms of, 121f, 121–123, 122t, 123f
    pulmonary function in, 123–129
    regulation of airway caliber in, 119–120, 120f
    during sleep, 358–361, 358–361f
    spirometry with, 124, 124t
    static lung volumes with, 125–127, 128f
    due to structural abnormalities, 121, 121f, 122t
    work of breathing with, 128
Airflow rate, effort effect on, 118–119, 119f
Air pollution, 399t, 399–400
Airway(s), 20f, 20–22, 21f, 22t
    narrowing of, in asthma, 212t, 212–213, 213f
    premature closure of, 45
    smooth muscle of, 20–21, 21f
    upper and lower, 115
Airway caliber, regulation of, 119–120, 120f
Airway conductance, in obstructive airways diseases, 124, 124f
Airway resistance, 25, 116–117
    in obstructive airways diseases, 123
Albuterol, for asthma, 223, 227
ALI. *See* Acute lung injury (ALI)
Alkalemia, 81
Alkalosis
    metabolic, 82t, 84, 84t
    respiratory, 81f, 83, 83t
        in pulmonary hypertension, 165
Allergic bronchopulmonary aspergillosis (ABPA), 228
Alpha$_1$-antitrypsin (A1AT) deficiency, chronic obstructive pulmonary disease due to, 237–238
Alveolar-arterial oxygen gradient (A-aDO$_2$), 92, 99–101, 101f
    during exercise, 107, 109f
    in hypoventilation, 92–93
    in interstitial lung disease, 266, 267f
    with pulmonary embolism, 289
    in respiratory failure, 181–182
    with shunt, 100
    with ventilation-perfusion inequality, 100–101, 101f
Alveolar-capillary exchange units, 22f, 22–23, 23f, 26, 27f
Alveolar damage, diffuse, in interstitial lung disease, 276
Alveolar dead space, 39–42, 40f, 41f
Alveolar ducts, 20f
Alveolar gas equation, 41–42
    in respiratory failure, 178, 179f
Alveolar hemorrhage syndromes, 274t, 274–275
Alveolar hyperventilation, 83

Alveolar hypoventilation, 363
Alveolar hypoxia, 52, 52f
    and pulmonary vascular resistance, 63, 64f
Alveolar macrophage growth factor (AMDGF), in acute lung
        injury, 145t
Alveolar minute ventilation, 38
Alveolar PCO_2, 89–92, 90f, 91f
Alveolar plateau, 46
Alveolar PO_2, 89–92, 90f, 91f
Alveolar pores of Kohn, 23
Alveolar sacs, 20f
Alveolar ventilation, 37
    during exercise, 107, 108f
    in respiratory failure, 178, 179f
Alveolar vessels, 27, 28f
    resistance in, 61–62, 63f
Alveolar volume, 37
Alveolitis, in interstitial lung disease, 268
Alveolus(i), 136
    development of, 1t, 2, 2t, 3
    structure of, 22–23, 23f
AMDGF (alveolar macrophage growth factor), in acute lung
        injury, 145t
Amine precursor uptake and decarboxylation (APUD)
        system, 32
Amiodarone, interstitial lung disease due to, 272
Amphotericin B, for cryptococcosis, 339
ANA (antinuclear antibody), in pleural effusions, 373
Anaerobic glycolysis, 105–106, 111
Anaerobic threshold (AT), during exercise, 107, 108f, 111–
        112, 193, 197, 197f, 198f
Anatomic dead space, 37, 38, 39f
Anemia, carboxyhemoglobin, 74
Angina
    exercise-related, 195
    in pulmonary hypertension, 164, 165
Angiography, pulmonary
    of pulmonary embolism, 294
    of pulmonary hypertension, 161, 163f
Angiotensin converting enzyme (ACE), in sarcoidosis, 252,
        252t
Anterior intercostal membrane, 16
Anti-basement membrane antibody disease, 275–276
Anticholinergics, for asthma, 223, 226
Anticoagulation, for pulmonary hypertension, 167
Antidiuretic hormone, syndrome of inappropriate, with lung
        cancer, 308t, 310
Anti-inflammatory agents, for asthma, 222, 222t, 223–
        224, 225f, 227
Antinuclear antibody (ANA), in pleural effusions, 373
Antipneumococcal vaccination, with chronic obstructive
        pulmonary disease, 240
α_1-Antitrypsin (A1AT) deficiency, chronic obstructive
        pulmonary disease due to, 237–238
Apnea, 358
    central sleep, 362–363
    obstructive sleep, 358–361, 358–361f
APR (acute phase response) proteins, 140
APUD (amine precursor uptake and decarboxylation)
        system, 32
Arachidonic acid, in acute lung injury, 140, 141f
ARDS (adult respiratory distress syndrome), lung
        compliance in, 24
Arrhythmias, during exercise, 202–203
Arterial blood gas(es), 99
    in chronic obstructive pulmonary disease, 234t
    in pulmonary embolism, 289
Arterial blood gas analysis
    in pulmonary hypertension, 159
    in respiratory failure, 180–182, 181t, 182f, 182t
Arterial oxygen tension (P_aO_2), with pulmonary embolism,
        289
Arterial PCO_2
    shunt and, 95, 98f
    ventilation-perfusion inequality and, 94, 95f

Arterial pH, in respiratory failure, 182, 182f, 182t
Arterial PO_2
    shunt and, 95–97, 98f, 99f
    ventilation-perfusion inequality and, 94f, 94–95, 96f,
        97f
Arthritis, rheumatoid, with interstitial lung disease, 273
Asbestos bodies, 392, 392f
Asbestos exposure, lung cancer due to, 303, 303t
Asbestos-related pulmonary disorders, 391–396, 392–
        394f
    clinical features of, 392–394
    complications of, 395–396
    pathogenesis of, 392–394f
    pulmonary function tests with, 394
    radiographic evaluation of, 386f, 395
    therapy for, 395
    types of, 391
Aspergillosis
    allergic bronchopulmonary, 228
    with human immunodeficiency virus, 341
Aspirin, asthma due to, 221
Asthma, 116, 211–228
    acute
        complications of, 228
        diagnosis of, 217–218, 218f
        management of, 225t, 225–226
        pulmonary function in, 219
        signs and symptoms of, 212
    adhesion molecules in, 215–216
    airway hyperresponsiveness in, 216–217
    airway inflammation and inflammatory mediators in,
        213–216
    airway narrowing in, 212t, 212–213, 213f
    airway resistance and expiratory airflow rates in, 123
    anticholinergics for, 223, 226
    anti-inflammatory agents for, 222, 222t, 223–224,
        225f, 227
    aspirin-induced, 221
    beta-adrenergic receptor agonists for, 223, 225, 227
    bronchodilators for, 222, 222t, 223
    cardiac function in, 220
    case study of, 211, 217, 222
    chronic
        complications of, 228
        management of, 226t, 226–228, 227t
        pulmonary function in, 219
    in Churg-Strauss vasculitis, 277
    clinical features of, 212
    complications of, 228
    constitutive cells in, 216
    cytokines in, 214–215, 215t
    defined, 212
    diagnosis and laboratory evaluation of, 217f, 217–219,
        218f, 218t, 219t
    differential diagnosis of, 219, 219t
    early and late responses in, 214
    eosinophils in, 215
    epidemiology of, 212
    exercise-induced, 221
    gas-exchange abnormalities in, 129, 220–221
    hyperinflation in, 219
    lung compliance in, 127, 127f
    lung volumes in, 127–128
    lymphocytes in, 213, 214–215
    mast cells in, 214
    mechanical ventilation for, 226
    migration of leukocytes in, 215–216
    occupational, 221, 397–399, 398t
    oxygen therapy for, 226
    pathology of, 212t, 212–213, 213f
    peak expiratory flow in, 217, 217f
    pulmonary function changes in, 219–220
    pulsus paradoxus in, 220
    severity of, 222, 226, 226t
    special categories of, 221

theophylline for, 223, 224t, 226
    therapy for, 222t, 222–228, 224–227t, 225f
    triggers for, 217, 218t, 227
AT (anaerobic threshold), during exercise, 107, 108f, 111–
        112, 193, 197, 197f, 198f
Atelectasis
    in acute lung injury, 146
    with pulmonary embolism, 290
    rounded, in asbestos-related pulmonary disorders, 392,
        394f
ATP (adenosine triphosphate), during exercise, 193
Azygos lobe, 7

B

Bacille-Calmette-Guérin (BCG) vaccination, 323
Bacterial infections, with human immunodeficiency virus,
        333–335, 334t
BAL. See Bronchoalveolar lavage (BAL)
BALT (bronchial-associated lymphoid tissue), 22
Basal cells, 20, 21f
Basement membrane, 21f
Beta-adrenergic receptor agonists, for asthma, 223, 225,
        227
Beta-adrenergic receptor system, in airway smooth muscle
        contraction, 122–123, 123f
Bicarbonate (HCO$_3$)
    in acid-base balance, 79, 80, 80f, 81f
    in carbon dioxide transport, 77, 77f
    in metabolic acidosis, 83
Biopsy
    lung, in pulmonary hypertension, 164
    pleural, 373
    transbronchial, in interstitial lung disease, 268, 268t
Birbeck's granules, 278
Bird's nest filter, 295f
Blastomyces dermatitidis, with human immunodeficiency
        virus, 340–341
Blastomycosis, with human immunodeficiency virus, 340–
        341
Blood flow, during exercise, 111
Blood oxygen-carbon dioxide diagram, 90, 90f
Blood pressure (BP)
    during exercise, 111, 201–202
    during sleep, 360
Blood supply. See Circulation
    to pleura, 368–369
Bochdalek's hernia, 8
Body plethysmography, 126
Bohr effect, 73
    during exercise, 197, 197f
Bohr's method, 40
Bony thorax, 12, 13f
BOOP (bronchiolitis obliterans with organizing pneumonia),
        279
BP. See Blood pressure (BP)
Breathing, control of
    normal, 354–356, 354–356f
    during sleep, 357–358
Breathing pattern, during exercise, 199, 199f
Breathing reserve, during exercise, 198–199
Bronchi, 20, 21f
    abnormalities of, 8
Bronchial-associated lymphoid tissue (BALT), 22
Bronchial circulation, 30, 30f
Bronchiectasis, 116
Bronchioles, 20, 20f, 21f
Bronchiolitis obliterans with organizing pneumonia (BOOP),
        279
Bronchitis, chronic, 116, 233–242
    airway resistance and expiratory airflow rates in, 123
    causes of, 237–238
    characteristics of bronchial wall in, 235f
    clinical history of, 239
    defined, 233

diagnosis of, 235t, 239
    epidemiology of, 239
    gas-exchange abnormalities in, 129
    lung volumes in, 127–128
    obstruction in, 238, 238f
    physical examination of, 239
    treatment of, 239–240
Bronchoalveolar lavage (BAL)
    with human immunodeficiency virus, 346
    in interstitial lung disease, 268
    in sarcoidosis, 245, 245t
Bronchoconstriction, 21–22
Bronchodilators
    for asthma, 222, 222t, 223
    for chronic obstructive pulmonary disease, 239
    for pulmonary hypertension, 166
Bronchoprovocation tests, 219
Bronchoscopy
    with human immunodeficiency virus, 346
    of interstitial lung disease, 268
    of lung cancer, 304f, 305
    of pleural effusions, 373
Buffering systems, 79

C

Calcium channel antagonists, for pulmonary hypertension,
        167
Canalicular period, 1t, 2
Cancer. See Lung cancer
Capillaries, injury of, in acute lung injury, 141–143
Capillaritis, 274–275
Capillary endothelial cells, 136
Caplan's syndrome, 397
Carbamino compounds
    in carbon dioxide transport, 77, 77f
    and oxyhemoglobin dissociation curve, 74
Carbon dioxide (CO$_2$)
    fractional concentration of, 39, 40f
    and oxyhemoglobin dissociation curve, 74
    partial pressure of. See PCO$_2$
        and acid-base status, 80, 81f
    production and removal of, 79, 80f
Carbon dioxide (CO$_2$) diffusion, 54, 55f
Carbon dioxide-hemoglobin dissociation curve, 76, 76f
Carbon dioxide (CO$_2$) transport, 76–78, 76f, 77f
Carbonic acid
    in acid-base balance, 79–81
    in carbon dioxide transport, 77
Carbon monoxide (CO), bound to hemoglobin, 74
Carbon monoxide (CO) diffusion capacity, 50, 51f, 53f, 53–
        54, 128
Carboxyhemoglobin, 74
Carboxyhemoglobin dissociation curve, in respiratory
        failure, 175, 176f
Carcinoma. See Lung cancer
Cardiac arrhythmia, during exercise, 202–203
Cardiac function
    airflow obstruction effect on, 129
    in asthma, 220
Cardiac index (CI), 67t
Cardiac lobe, 7
Cardiac output (CO)
    during exercise, 109, 110f, 193, 202, 202f
    and oxygen consumption, 75–76
    during sleep, 360
    thermodilution technique for, 66
Cardiovascular responses, to exercise, 193
Carotid bodies, in control of breathing, 355
CD4+ cells, in human immunodeficiency virus, 332
Cellular response, to acute lung injury, 140–141, 142f
Central sleep apnea, 362–363
C fibers, 31, 32t
    in control of breathing, 356
Chemoreceptors, in control of breathing, 354–355

Chemotherapeutic agents
  interstitial lung disease due to, 271
  for lung cancer, 307
Chest radiography
  in asbestos-related pulmonary disorders, 386f, 395
  of chronic obstructive pulmonary disease, 236f
  in coal worker's pneumoconiosis, 396
  with human immunodeficiency virus, 34t, 345
  of interstitial lung disease, 260f, 262–263, 263t
  of lung cancer, 304, 304t
  of occupational lung disease, 385, 386–388f
  of pleural effusions, 374
  of pneumothorax, 376f, 377
  of pulmonary embolism, 288–289, 289t
  of pulmonary hypertension, 156f, 159, 165
  of respiratory failure, 181t, 183
  of sarcoidosis, 249
  in silicosis, 387f, 389–390, 390f
  of tuberculosis, 320
Chest tube
  for pleural effusions, 375
  for pneumothorax, 378
Chest wall, 12, 14f
  static volume-pressure curves of, 12, 14f
Chest wall compliance
  with aging, 7
  in newborns, 6
Cheyne-Stokes respiration (CSR), in congestive heart
       failure, 361f, 362–363
CHF (congestive heart failure), Cheyne-Stokes respiration,
       361f, 362–363
Chloride shift, in carbon dioxide transport, 77
Cholinergic nervous system, in regulation of airway caliber,
       119, 120f
Chronic obstructive pulmonary disease (COPD), 115t, 115–
       116, 233–242
  arterial blood-gas determination in, 234t
  case study of, 234
  causes of, 237–238
  characteristics of, 233–234
  chest x-ray of, 236f
  clinical history of, 239
  CT scans of, 237f
  defined, 233
  diagnosis of, 234, 234t, 235t, 235–237f, 239
  diaphragm in, 16
  epidemiology of, 239
  histology of, 236f
  lung volumes in, 127–128
  obstruction in, 238, 238f
  physical examination of, 239
  pulmonary function in, 123–129, 234t
  sleep-related breathing disorders in, 363, 363f
  treatment of, 239–240
Churg-Strauss vasculitis, interstitial lung disease due to,
       277
CI (cardiac index), 67t
CIE (counterimmunoelectrophoresis), of pleural effusions,
       373
Cigarette smoking
  chronic obstructive pulmonary disease due to, 237
  lung cancer due to, 302–303, 303t
Cilia, 20, 21f
Ciliated cells, development of, 3
Ciliated columnar epithelial cell, 21f
Circulation
  bronchial, 30, 30f
  distention and recruitment of, 59, 60f
  during exercise, 59, 60t, 109f, 109–111, 110f
  fetal, 4f, 4–5
  function of, 59–67
  hemodynamic monitoring of, 66, 66t, 67t
  hemodynamics of, 59, 60t
  lung zones of, 64–65, 65f
  pleural, 368–369

and pulmonary vascular resistance, 60–63, 61–64f
  at rest, 59, 60t
  structure of, 26–30, 27–29f, 30t, 30f
Circulatory time delay, 362
Clara cells, 20, 21f
Claudication, exercise-related, 195
Closing volume, 45f, 45–46
Clubbing
  with lung cancer, 308t, 310
  with occupational lung disease, 385, 385f
CMV (cytomegalovirus), with human immunodeficiency
       virus, 341
CO. See Carbon monoxide (CO); Cardiac output (CO)
CO$_2$. See Carbon dioxide (CO$_2$)
Coal macule, 396, 397f
Coal-worker's pneumoconiosis, 396–397, 397f
Coccidioidomycosis, with human immunodeficiency virus, 340
Collagen vascular disorders
  with interstitial lung disease, 272–274, 273t
  with pulmonary hypertension, 153
Collateral ventilation, 23
Complement, in acute lung injury, 140
Compliance. See Lung compliance
Compliance curves, in obstructive airways diseases, 127,
       127f
Computed tomography (CT)
  of chronic obstructive pulmonary disease, 237f
  with human immunodeficiency virus, 345
  of interstitial lung disease, 263, 265f
  of lung cancer, 308f
  of pleural effusions, 373
  of respiratory failure, 183–184
Conducting airways, 20
Congenital defects, 7–8
Congestive heart failure (CHF), Cheyne-Stokes respiration,
       361f, 362–363
Connective tissue disorders, with interstitial lung disease,
       272–274, 273t
Constitutive cells, in asthma, 216
Continuous positive airway pressure (CPAP), nasal, 361,
       362–363
COPD. See Chronic obstructive pulmonary disease (COPD)
Corticosteroids
  for asthma, 224, 226, 227, 228
  for *Mycobacterium avium* complex, 338, 339t
  for sarcoidosis, 254–255
Counterimmunoelectrophoresis (CIE), of pleural effusions,
       373
CPAP (continuous positive airway pressure), nasal, 361,
       362–363
Cromolyn sodium, for asthma, 223–224, 227
Cryptococcosis, with human immunodeficiency virus, 339
Cryptococcus neoformans, with human immunodeficiency
       virus, 339
CSR (Cheyne-Stokes respiration), in congestive heart
       failure, 361f, 362–363
CT. See Computed tomography (CT)
Cutaneous anergy, in sarcoidosis, 246
Cyanosis, in pulmonary hypertension, 165
Cystic fibrosis, 116
Cytokines
  in acute lung injury, 140, 140t, 144–145, 145t
  in asthma, 214–215, 215t
  in sarcoidosis, 245, 246, 246t
Cytomegalovirus (CMV), with human immunodeficiency
       virus, 341
Cytotoxic T cells, in human immunodeficiency virus, 332

D

Davenport diagram, 80–81, 81f
Dead space
  alveolar, 39–42, 40f, 41f
  anatomic, 37, 38, 39f
  physiologic, 38, 39f

Dead space minute ventilation, 38
Dead space to tidal volume ratio (V_D/V_T), during exercise, 107, 200–201
Deep venous thrombosis (DVT)
    diagnosis of, 292, 292f, 293f
    incidence of, 285
    management of, 296t, 296–297, 297t
    in pathophysiology of pulmonary embolism, 286
    prophylaxis for, 296t
    risk factors for, 286t
Development, 1–8
    abnormalities of, 7–8
    with aging, 7, 7t
    at birth, 5–6, 6f
    case study of, 1, 5, 8
    of diaphragm and pleura, 3
    of lungs, 1t, 1–3, 2t
    of lung vasculature, 3–5, 4f
    postnatal, childhood, and adult, 6–7
    surfactant in, 5–6, 6f
    in utero, 1t, 1–5, 2t, 4f
Diaphragm, 14–16, 15f
    congenital defects of, 8
    in COPD, 16
    costal, 14–15
    crural, 15
    development of, 3
    eventration of, 8
Diaphragmatic hernias, 8
Diffusion, 49
    carbon dioxide, 54, 55f
    factors affecting, 49, 50f
    impairment in, 93
    limitations on, 50–52, 51f, 52f
Diffusion abnormality, respiratory failure due to, 174
Diffusion capacity, 49–55
    for carbon monoxide, 50, 51f, 53f, 53–54, 128
    of helium, 53–54
    measurement of, 53–54
Diffusion limited gas transfer, 50, 51f
Digital clubbing
    with lung cancer, 308t, 310
    with occupational lung disease, 385, 385f
Digitalis, for pulmonary hypertension, 166–167
2, 3-Diphosphoglycerate (2, 3-DPG), and oxyhemoglobin dissociation curve, 73, 74
Directly observed therapy (DOT), for tuberculosis, 322
Distention, 26
    pulmonary vascular, 59, 60f
Diuretics, for pulmonary hypertension, 167
$D_L CO$ (diffusion capacity for carbon monoxide), 50, 51f, 53f, 53–54, 128
Doppler ultrasound, for pulmonary embolism, 292, 292f
Dorsal respiratory group (DRG), 354
DOT (directly observed therapy), for tuberculosis, 322
2, 3-DPG (2, 3-diphosphoglycerate), and oxyhemoglobin dissociation curve, 73, 74
Drug-induced interstitial lung disease, 271–272, 272t
Ductus arteriosus, 3, 4, 4f, 5
Ductus venosus, 5
DVT. See Deep venous thrombosis (DVT)
Dyspnea
    exercise-related, 195
    in pulmonary hypertension, 159, 164, 165
    in respiratory failure, 179

E

Eaton-Lambert syndrome, with lung cancer, 308t, 310
Echocardiography, of pulmonary hypertension, 159–160, 160f, 165
Effort, and airflow rate, 118–119, 119f
Effusions. See Pleural effusions
EIA (exercise-induced asthma), 221
Elastic recoil, 24, 25f

Electrocardiography
    of pulmonary embolism, 288f, 289, 289t
    of pulmonary hypertension, 155f, 159
Embolectomy, 297
Embolism. See Pulmonary embolism (PE)
Embryonic period, 1t, 2
Emphysema, 116, 233–242
    airway resistance and expiratory airflow rates in, 123
    arterial blood gases in, 234t
    case study of, 234
    causes of, 237–238
    chest x-ray of, 236f
    clinical history of, 239
    CT scans of, 237f
    defined, 233
    diagnosis of, 235t, 239
    epidemiology of, 239
    gas-exchange abnormalities in, 129
    with human immunodeficiency virus, 344
    lung compliance in, 24, 25f, 127, 127f
    lung volumes in, 127–128
    obstruction in, 238, 238f
    physical exam in, 239
    pulmonary function tests in, 234t
    pulmonary histology of, 236f
    treatment of, 239–240
E-NANC (excitatory nonadrenergic, noncholinergic) nervous system, in regulation of airway caliber, 120, 120f
End-capillary PCO_2, 92
End-capillary PO_2, 92, 98, 101
Endothelial cells, in asthma, 216
Endotracheal intubation, for respiratory failure, 186
Energetics, 105–107, 106f, 107t
Eosinophil(s), in asthma, 215
Eosinophilic granuloma, interstitial lung disease due to, 278–279
Eosinophilic pneumonia, chronic, 279
Epithelial cells, in asthma, 216
Equal pressure point, 118, 118f
ERV (expiratory reserve volume), 126, 126f
Erythema nodosum, in sarcoidosis, 250
Ethambutol, for tuberculosis, 332
    in HIV patients, 336, 336t
Excitatory nonadrenergic, noncholinergic (E-NANC) nervous system, in regulation of airway caliber, 120, 120f
Exercise, 191–206
    blood flow and vascular pressures during, 111
    blood pressure during, 201–202
    breathing pattern during, 199, 199f
    breathing reserve during, 198–199
    cardiac arrhythmia during, 202–203
    cardiac output during, 193, 202, 202f
    case studies of, 203, 204, 205, 206
    circulation during, 109f, 109–111, 110f
    effect on healthy adults of, 111–112
    energetics of, 105–107, 106f, 107t
    gas exchange during, 107, 108f, 109f
    hemodynamics during, 60t
    hypoxemia during, 200
    maximum minute ventilation during, 198–199
    myocardial ischemia during, 202–203
    oxygenation during, 200
    oxygen pulse during, 201, 201f
    physiology of, 105–112
    in pulmonary hypertension, 165
    ventilation-perfusion mismatch during, 200f, 200–201
Exercise capacity, 195–196
Exercise endurance, 192
Exercise-induced asthma (EIA), 221
Exercise limitation
    cardiac parameters in, 201f, 201–203, 202f
    clinical signs of, 195
    diseases associated with, 191, 192t

Exercise limitation (*continued*)
early symptoms of, 192
functional classification of, 192, 193t
pulmonary parameters in, 198–201, 199f, 200f
Exercise physiology
normal, 193–194
in obstructive lung diseases, 203–204
in pulmonary vascular diseases, 206
in restrictive lung diseases, 205
Exercise testing, 194
complications of, 194
contraindications to, 194, 194t
indications for, 194
measurements during, 195–197–198f
Exercise time, total, 196
Expiratory airflow rates, in obstructive airways diseases, 123
Expiratory reserve volume (ERV), 126, 126f
Extra-alveolar vessels, 26–27, 28f
resistance in, 62, 63f
Exudative effusions, 371, 372t, 372–373
Exudative phase, of acute lung injury, 139f, 139–143, 140t, 141f, 142f

F

Fatigue, exercise-related, 195
FCO_2 (fractional concentration of carbon dioxide), 39, 40f
Fetal circulation, 4f, 4–5
Fetal development
of diaphragm and pleura, 3
of lungs, 1t, 1–3, 2t
of lung vasculature, 3–5, 4f
surfactant in, 5–6, 6f
Fetal hemoglobin, 74
FEV_1. *See* Forced expiratory volume in one second (FEV_1)
Fiberoptic bronchoscopy. *See* Bronchoscopy
Fibroblasts
in acute lung injury, 143–144
in asthma, 216
Fibrosis. *See* Pulmonary fibrosis
Fibrotic phase, of acute lung injury, 144f, 144–145, 145t
Fick principle, 75–76
Fick's law, 22, 22f, 49
FIO_2 (inspired oxygen fraction)
and shunt, 97, 99f
and ventilation-perfusion inequality, 95, 97f
Flow-volume curve, in obstructive airways diseases, 124–125, 125f
Flow-volume loops, in lung cancer, 302f, 309, 309f
Fluconazole, for cryptococcosis, 339
Foramen of Bochdalek, 15
Foramen of Morgagni, 15
Foramen ovale, 4, 5
patent, with pulmonary embolism, 290
Forced expiration, 117f, 117–118, 118f
Forced expiratory volume in one second (FEV_1)
with aging, 7
in obstructive airways diseases, 124, 124t, 125f
in respiratory failure, 183
Forced expiratory volume in one second to forced vital capacity ratio (FEV_1/FEV), in obstructive airways diseases, 124, 124t, 125f
Forced vital capacity (FVC), in obstructive airways diseases, 124, 124t, 125f
Force-frequency relationship, 18–19, 19f
Force-length relationship, 17–18, 18f
Force-velocity relationship, 18, 19f
Fractional concentration of carbon dioxide (FCO_2), 39, 40f
Functional residual capacity (FRC), 126–127, 126f
in obstructive airways diseases, 127, 128f
Fungal infections, with human immunodeficiency virus, 339–341
Fusion frequency, 18

FVC (forced vital capacity), in obstructive airways diseases, 124, 124t, 125f

G

Ganciclovir, for cytomegalovirus, 341
Gas diffusion. *See* Diffusion
Gas dilution technique, 126
Gas exchange, 22f, 22–23, 23f
abnormal, 92–99
due to diffusion impairment, 93
due to hypoventilation, 92–93
due to nonpulmonary factors, 97–99, 100f
due to shunt, 95–97, 98f, 99f
due to ventilation-perfusion inequality, 93–95, 94f, 96f, 97f
in acute lung injury, 145
with airflow obstruction, 129
assessing efficiency of, 99–102, 101f, 102f
in asthma, 220–221
during exercise, 107, 108f, 109f, 193
in interstitial lung disease, 265t, 266–267, 267f
in pulmonary embolism, 289–290
in pulmonary hypertension, 165
Glomus cells, in control of breathing, 355
Glycogen, muscle, 106
Glycolysis, anaerobic, 105–106, 111
Goblet cells, 20, 21f
development of, 3
Goodpasture's syndrome, 275–276
Granulomas
eosinophilic, interstitial lung disease due to, 278–279
in sarcoidosis, 246, 247f, 248f, 248t
in tuberculosis, 318, 319f
Granulomatosis
lymphomatoid, interstitial lung disease due to, 277
Wegener's, interstitial lung disease due to, 276
Greenfield filter, 295, 295f
Group B streptococcal infection, with human immunodeficiency virus, 334
Growth and development, 1–8
abnormalities of, 7–8
with aging, 7, 7t
at birth, 5–6, 6f
case study of, 1, 5, 8
of diaphragm and pleura, 3
of lungs, 1t, 1–3, 2t
of lung vasculature, 3–5, 4f
postnatal, childhood, and adult, 6–7
surfactant in, 5–6, 6f
in utero, 1t, 1–5, 2t, 4f
Growth factors, in acute lung injury, 144–145, 145t

H

Haemophilus influenzae, with human immunodeficiency virus, 334, 335
Haldane effect, 77, 78, 78f
Hampton's hump, 288–289
HCO_3. *See* Bicarbonate (HCO_3)
Heart catheterization, in pulmonary hypertension, 161–162
Heart rate
during exercise, 109, 110f, 111, 193, 202, 202f
during sleep, 360
Heart rate reserve, conditions associated with high, 195t
Heat production, during exercise, 111
Helium diffusion capacity, 53–54
Hemodynamic monitoring, 66, 66t, 67t
Hemodynamics
in pulmonary embolism, 290
at rest and during exercise, 60t
Hemoglobin, oxygen capacity and, 71–72
Hemoglobin S, 74
Hemolysis, during exercise, 111
Henderson-Hasselbalch equation, 80, 182, 182t

Heparin, for pulmonary embolism and deep venous thrombosis, 296–297, 297t
Hepatic hydrothorax, 372
Hernias, diaphragmatic, 8
Herpes simplex virus, with human immunodeficiency virus, 341
Histiocytosis X, interstitial lung disease due to, 278–279
Histology, of lung development, 2–3
Histoplasma capsulatum, with human immunodeficiency virus, 339–340
Histoplasmosis, with human immunodeficiency virus, 339–340
HIV. *See* Human immunodeficiency virus (HIV)
Hoarseness, in pulmonary hypertension, 165
Horner's syndrome, 309
Human immunodeficiency virus (HIV)
  bacterial infections with, 333–335, 334t
  emphysema with, 344
  fungal infections with, 339–341
  interstitial pneumonitis with, 343
  Kaposi's sarcoma with, 342
  lymphoma with, 342
  mycobacterial infections with, 335–337, 336t
  pleural effusions with, 344
  Pneumocystis carinii pneumonia with, 337–338, 339t
  pneumothorax with, 343–344
  pulmonary complication(s) of, 331–349
    case study of, 332, 333, 335, 337, 343
    diagnostic approach to, 344–347, 345t, 347–349f
    incidence of, 331
    pathogenesis of, 332f, 332–333
    pulmonary hypertension with, 344
    quasispecies of, 332
    tuberculosis with, 320, 323–324
    viral infections with, 341
Humoral response, to acute lung injury, 140, 140t, 141f
Hyaline membrane disease, 6, 23
Hydrogen ion
  in carbon dioxide transport, 77
  and oxyhemoglobin dissociation curve, 73
  production and removal of, 79, 80f
Hydrothorax, hepatic, 372
Hypercalcemia, with lung cancer, 308t, 310
Hypercapnia
  in asthma, 220
  in respiratory failure, 182
  ventilatory response to, 355, 355f
Hyperinflation, in asthma, 219
Hyperresponsiveness, in asthma, 216–217
Hypersensitivity pneumonitis, 269–271, 270t
Hypertension, pulmonary. *See* Pulmonary hypertension (PH)
Hypertrophic pulmonary osteoarthropathy, with lung cancer, 308t, 310
Hyperventilation, alveolar, 83
Hypocapnia, in asthma, 220
Hypopnea, 358, 359f
Hypotension, during exercise, 201–202
Hypoventilation, 92–93
  respiratory failure due to, 176–178, 179f
Hypoxemia
  in acute lung injury, 145
  in asthma, 220
  during exercise, 200
  in interstitial lung disease, 266–267
  in pulmonary hypertension, 159, 165
  in respiratory failure, 180–182
  ventilatory response to, 355, 356f
Hypoxia
  alveolar, 52, 52f
    and pulmonary vascular resistance, 63, 64f
  vasoconstriction in, 29–30
Hysteresis, 24, 24f

I
IC (inspiratory capacity), 126, 126f
Idiopathic pulmonary fibrosis (IPF), interstitial lung disease due to, 277–278
IGF (insulin-like growth factor), in acute lung injury, 144, 145t
Immune response, in sarcoidosis, 245t, 245–246, 246t
I-NANC (inhibitory nonadrenergic, noncholinergic) nervous system, in regulation of airway caliber, 120, 120f
Increased controller gain, 362
Infant respiratory distress syndrome, 6, 23
Infectious agents, in sarcoidosis, 244–245, 245t
Inferior vena cava (IVC) filter, 295, 295f
Inferior vena cava (IVC) interruption, 297, 297t
Infiltrative lung diseases, 204
Inflammation, in asthma, 213–216
Inflammatory mediators, in asthma, 213–216
INH (isoniazid), for tuberculosis, 322
  in HIV patients, 336, 336t
Inhalation injury, 137–138
Inhibitory nonadrenergic, noncholinergic (I-NANC) nervous system, in regulation of airway caliber, 120, 120f
Inspiratory capacity (IC), 126, 126f
Inspiratory reserve volume (IRV), 126, 126f
Inspired oxygen fraction (FIO$_2$)
  and shunt, 97, 99f
  and ventilation-perfusion inequality, 95, 97f
Insulin-like growth factor (IGF), in acute lung injury, 144, 145t
Intercostal muscles, 16
Interferon gamma, in acute lung injury, 140t
Interleukins, in acute lung injury, 140t, 145t
Interstitial lung disease(s), 259–283
  alveolar hemorrhage syndromes with, 274t, 274–275
  alveolitis in, 268
  assessment of disease activity in, 268
  due to bronchiolitis obliterans with organizing pneumonia, 279
  case study of, 259–260, 264, 267–268, 269
  chest x-ray of, 260f, 262–263, 263t
  due to chronic eosinophilic pneumonia, 279
  due to Churg-Strauss vasculitis, 277
  classification of, 261t
  clinical features of, 261–267
  connective tissue/collagen vascular disorders with, 272–274, 273t
  CT scan of, 263, 265f
  defined, 260
  diagnosis of, 268, 268t
  diffuse alveolar damage in, 276
  drug-induced, 271–272, 272t
  due to eosinophilic granuloma, 278–279
  etiology of, 260
  examples of, 269–279
  gas exchange in, 265t, 266–267, 267f
  in Goodpasture's syndrome, 275–276
  history of, 261–262, 262t
  hypersensitivity pneumonitis as, 269–271, 270t
  idiopathic causes of, 276–279
  due to idiopathic pulmonary fibrosis, 277–278
  lung compliance in, 264–265, 265t, 266f
  due to lymphomatoid granulomatosis, 277
  mixed connective tissue disease with, 274
  physical examination of, 262, 262t
  physiologic alterations in, 263–267, 265t
  pressure-volume curve in, 265, 266f
  progressive systemic sclerosis with, 273
  pulmonary fibrosis in, 268
  pulmonary function tests in, 264f, 265t, 266
  pulmonary hypertension in, 265t, 267
  with pulmonary involvement only, 277–279
  rheumatoid arthritis with, 273
  symptoms of, 261–262, 262t
  systemic lupus erythematosus with, 274

Interstitial lung disease(s) (*continued*)
    systemic necrotizing vasculitis with, 275
    therapy for, 269, 269t
    due to vasculitides, 276–277
    ventilation in, 264–265, 265t, 266f
    due to Wegener's granulomatosis, 276
Interstitial pneumonitis, with human immunodeficiency
        virus, 343
Interstitial space, between alveoli, 136, 137f
Intrapulmonary shunt, respiratory failure due to, 176, 177f
In utero development
    of diaphragm and pleura, 3
    of lungs, 1t, 1–3, 2t
    of lung vasculature, 3–5, 4f
    surfactant in, 5–6, 6f
Ion channels, in airway smooth muscle contraction, 122,
        123f
IPF (idiopathic pulmonary fibrosis), interstitial lung disease
        due to, 277–278
Ipratropium bromide, for asthma, 223, 226
Irritant receptors, in control of breathing, 355–356
IRV (inspiratory reserve volume), 126, 126f
Isoniazid (INH), for tuberculosis, 322
    in HIV patients, 336, 336t
IVC (inferior vena cava) filter, 295, 295f
IVC (inferior vena cava) interruption, 297, 297t

J

J receptors, in control of breathing, 356
Jugular vein waves, in pulmonary hypertension, 153, 154f

K

Kaposi's sarcoma (KS), with human immunodeficiency
        virus, 342
Krogh's constant, 54
Kulchitsky (K) cells, 20
    development of, 3
Kyphoscoliosis, 82

L

Lactic acid, 105–106, 111
Lactic acidosis, during exercise, 197
Laminar flow, 117
Langerhans' granules, 278
Left atrial pressure (LAP), 60
Left ventricular stroke work index (LVSWI), 67t
Legionella pneumophila, with human immunodeficiency
        virus, 334
Leukocytes, in asthma, 215–216
Leukotriene(s), in acute lung injury, 140
Leukotriene modifiers, for asthma, 224, 225f, 227
LIP (lymphocytic interstitial pneumonitis), with human
        immunodeficiency virus, 343
Lobes, abnormal formation of, 7
Lower airways, 115
Lung(s)
    agenesis of, 7
    defense mechanisms of, 399–400
    development of, 1t, 1–3, 2t
    sequestration of, 8
    simplified diagram of, 38f
    static volume-pressure curves of, 12, 14f
    structure of, 11–32
        airway resistance and, 25
        airways in, 20f, 20–22, 21f, 22t
        alveolar-capillary exchange units in, 22f, 22–23,
            23f
        bony thorax and chest wall in, 12, 13f, 14f
        case study of, 12, 30, 32
        circulation in, 25–30, 27–29f, 30t, 30f
        lung compliance and, 23–24, 24f, 25f
        lymphatics in, 31

    nervous system in, 31–32, 32t
    respiratory muscles in, 14–19, 15f, 18f, 19f
Lung biopsy
    open-, with human immunodeficiency virus, 346–347
    in pulmonary hypertension, 164
Lung cancer, 301–313
    adenocarcinoma type of, 305
    with asbestos-related pulmonary disorders, 395–396
    bronchoscopy of, 304f, 305
    case study of, 301, 303, 308, 310
    chest x-rays of, 304, 304t
    clinical presentation of, 303, 305
    complications of, 308t, 308–310, 309f
    CT scan of, 308f
    diagnostic workup for, 304–305
    epidemiology of, 302
    etiology of, 302–303, 303t
    flow-volume loops in, 302f, 309, 309f
    histologic types of, 305, 306f
    large cell, 305
    non-small cell, 305, 306f, 307, 307t
    paraneoplastic syndromes in, 308t, 309–310
    prognosis in, 311
    pulmonary function tests in, 302t
    small cell, 305, 306f, 307, 307t
    with solitary pulmonary nodule, 307
    squamous cell, 305, 306f
    staging of, 306–307, 307t
    therapy for, 307, 307t
Lung capacity, 126–127, 126f
Lung compliance, 23–24, 24f, 25f
    in acute lung injury, 145–146
    in interstitial lung disease, 264–265, 265t, 266f
    in obstructive airway diseases, 127, 127f
Lung diffusion capacity. *See* Diffusion capacity
Lung failure, 172, 172f, 173f
Lung function, 35–114
    in acute lung injury, 145–146, 146f
    case study of
    diffusion capacity in, 49–57
    during exercise, 105–114
    gas transport and acid-base balance in, 71–87
    pulmonary circulation in, 59–69
    ventilation in, 37–48
    ventilation-perfusion relationships in, 89–104
Lung function tests. *See* Pulmonary function tests (PFTs)
Lung perfusion, topographical differences in, 28, 29f
Lung scanning
    in pulmonary hypertension, 160f,162f, 160–161
    in respiratory failure, 184
Lung size, at various ages, 2, 2t
Lung transplantation
    for pulmonary hypertension, 168
    for respiratory failure, 187
    for sarcoidosis, 255
Lung volumes
    in chronic obstructive pulmonary disease, 234t
    in obstructive airway diseases, 127–128, 128f
    and pulmonary vascular resistance, 61–62, 63f
    static, in obstructive airway diseases, 125–127, 128f
    and ventilation distribution, 42–45, 44f
Lung zones, 64–65, 65f
Lupus erythematosus, systemic, with interstitial lung
        disease, 274
Lupus pernio, in sarcoidosis, 250
LVSWI (left ventricular stroke work index), 67t
Lymphatics, 31
    pleural, 369
Lymphocytes, 22
    in asthma, 213, 214–215
Lymphocytic interstitial pneumonitis (LIP), with human
        immunodeficiency virus, 343
Lymphoma, with human immunodeficiency virus, 342
Lymphomatoid granulomatosis, interstitial lung disease due
        to, 277

M

MAC (*Mycobacterium avium* complex), 324
  with human immunodeficiency virus, 336–338, 339t
Macrophages
  in acute lung injury, 140
  in sarcoidosis, 245
Malignancy. *See* Lung cancer
Malignant pleural effusions, 375
Mantoux tuberculin test, 319, 320t
Mast cells, in asthma, 214
Maximal midexpiratory flow ($MMEF_{25\%-75\%}$), in
    obstructive airways diseases, 124, 124t
Maximal oxygen uptake (VO_{2max}), during exercise testing,
    195–196, 196f
Maximum exercise ventilation ($V_{E}max$), 198–199
Maximum minute ventilation, during exercise, 198–199
Maximum oxygen consumption, during exercise, 109, 109f,
    110f, 111–112
Maximum voluntary ventilation (MVV), 198
MCTD (mixed connective tissue disease), with interstitial
    lung disease, 274
MDRTB (multidrug resistant tuberculosis), 321–322
Mechanical ventilation
  for asthma, 226
  for respiratory failure, 186–187
Mechanoreceptors, in control of breathing, 355–356
Metabolic acidosis, 82t, 83, 83t
Metabolic alkalosis, 82t, 84, 84t
Methemoglobin, 74
Methemoglobinemia, 74
Methotrexate, interstitial lung disease due to, 272
Minute ventilation, 37–38, 38f
  in acute lung injury, 146
  during exercise, 107, 108f, 109f
  maximum, during exercise, 198–199
Mixed acid-base disturbances, 84, 85f
Mixed connective tissue disease (MCTD), with interstitial
    lung disease, 274
Mixed-venous PO_2, and gas exchange, 97–99, 100f
$MMEF_{25\%-75\%}$ (maximal midexpiratory flow), in obstructive
    airways diseases, 124, 124t
Morgagni's hernia, 8
Motor unit, 17
Mucociliary elevator, 20
Mucosa, 20
Mucous gland, 21f
Multidrug resistant tuberculosis (MDRTB), 321–322, 332
Muscle(s)
  energy sources for, 105–107, 106f, 107t
  force-frequency relationship of, 18–19, 19f
  force-length relationship of, 17–18, 18f
  force-velocity relationship of, 18, 19f
  respiratory, 14–19
    anatomy of, 14–16, 15f
    contractile properties of, 17–19, 18f, 19f
    functional characteristics of, 17
Muscle fibers, 17
Muscle pain, exercise-related, 195
Muscle pressures, in respiratory failure, 183
Muscle spindles, in control of breathing, 356
MVV (maximum voluntary ventilation), 198
Mycobacterial diseases, 315–329
  case study of, 317, 319, 321, 323, 325
  classification of, 316f, 316–317, 317t
  with coal worker's pneumoconiosis, 397
  with human immunodeficiency virus, 335–337, 336t
  nontuberculous (atypical), 317, 317t, 324
  with silicosis, 391
  tuberculosis, 317–324
    BCG vaccination for, 323
    with coal worker's pneumoconiosis, 397
    diagnosis of, 320–321
    epidemiology of, 317f, 317–318, 318t
    in HIV-infected patients, 323–324

  with human immunodeficiency virus, 335–336, 336t
  multidrug resistant, 321–322, 332
  pathogenesis of, 318–319, 319f
  preventative therapy for, 323, 323t
  risk factors for, 318, 318t
  screening for, 319–320, 320t
  with silicosis, 391
  transmission of, 318
  treatment for, 321–322, 322t
Mycobacterium avium complex (MAC), 324
  with human immunodeficiency virus, 336–338, 339t
Mycobacterium chelonei, 324
Mycobacterium fortuitum, 324
Mycobacterium kansasii, 324
Mycobacterium tuberculosis. See Mycobacterial diseases,
    tuberculosis
Myocardial contractility, during exercise, 111
Myocardial ischemia, during exercise, 202–203

N

NANC (nonadrenergic, noncholinergic) nervous system, in
    regulation of airway caliber, 120, 120f
Nasal continuous positive airway pressure, 361, 362–363
Nedocromil sodium, for asthma, 224, 227
Neoplasms. *See* Lung cancer
Nephrotic syndrome, effusions with, 372
Nerves, in pleura, 369
Nervous system, 31–32, 32t
Neurokinins, in regulation of airway caliber, 120f
Neutrophils, in acute lung injury, 140–141, 142f
Nitric oxide, in regulation of airway caliber, 120f
Nitrofurantoin, interstitial lung disease due to, 272
Nitrogen dioxide, 400
Nitrogen washout curve, 45f, 45–46
Nitrous oxide (N_2O), and perfusion limitations, 50, 51f
Nocardia asteroides, with human immunodeficiency virus,
    334
Nocturnal noninvasive positive pressure ventilation, for
    chronic obstructive pulmonary disease, 363
Nocturnal oxygen desaturation (NOD), 363, 363f
Nonadrenergic, noncholinergic (NANC) nervous system, in
    regulation of airway caliber, 120, 120f
Non-Hodgkin's lymphoma, with human immunodeficiency
    virus, 342
Noninvasive positive pressure ventilation (NPPV), nocturnal,
    for chronic obstructive pulmonary disease, 363
Non-rapid eye movement (NREM) sleep, 356
Non-small cell lung carcinoma (NSCLC), 305, 306f, 307,
    307t
Nonsteroidal anti-inflammatory drugs (NSAIDs), asthma due
    to, 221
Nontuberculous mycobacteria (NTM), 317, 317t, 324

O

Obesity-hypoventilation syndrome, 82
Oblique muscles, 16
Obstruction, in chronic obstructive pulmonary disease, 238,
    238f
Obstructive lung diseases, 203. *See also* Chronic
    obstructive pulmonary disease (COPD)
  exercise physiology in, 203–204
Obstructive sleep apnea syndrome (OSAS), 358–361, 358–
    361f
Occupational asthma, 221
Occupational lung disease(s), 383–403
  due to air pollution, 399t, 399–400
  asbestos-related, 391–396, 392–394f
  asthma as, 397–399, 398t
  case study of, 383, 390, 391, 395, 400
  chest x-ray of, 385, 386–388f
  clinical presentation of, 384
  coal-worker's pneumoconiosis as, 396–397, 397f
  diagnosis of, 384–387

Occupational lung disease(s) (*continued*)
  management of, 387
  overview of, 384–387
  pathological changes with, 384, 384t
  physical findings in, 385, 385f
  pulmonary function tests in, 386, 386t
  silicosis as, 388–391, 389t, 390f
  types of, 384
O_2P (oxygen pulse), during exercise, 201, 201f
Organophosphate, and oxyhemoglobin dissociation curve, 73, 74
OSAS (obstructive sleep apnea syndrome), 358–361, 358–361f
Osteoarthropathy, hypertrophic pulmonary, with lung cancer, 308t, 310
Oxygen, partial pressure of. *See* PO_2
Oxygenation, during exercise, 200
Oxygen capacity, and hemoglobin, 71–72
Oxygen-carbon dioxide diagram, 90, 90f
Oxygen consumption, 75–76
  maximum, during exercise, 109, 109f, 110f, 111–112
Oxygen delivery, 75
Oxygen demand, during exercise, 107
Oxygen desaturation, nocturnal, 363, 363f
Oxygen pulse (O_2P), during exercise, 201, 201f
Oxygen tension, arterial, with pulmonary embolism, 289
Oxygen therapy
  for asthma, 226
  for Cheyne-Stokes respiration in congestive heart failure, 362
  for chronic obstructive pulmonary disease, 363
  for pulmonary hypertension, 166
  for respiratory failure, 184–185
Oxygen transport, 75–76
Oxygen uptake (VO_2), maximal, during exercise testing, 195–196, 196f
Oxyhemoglobin dissociation curve, 72f, 72–74, 73f
  during exercise, 197, 197f
  in respiratory failure, 175, 176f
Ozone, 400

P

Pain, exercise-related, 195
Pancoast's tumor, 308t, 309
P_aO_2 (arterial oxygen tension), with pulmonary embolism, 289
PAP. *See* Pulmonary arterial pressure (PAP)
Paraneoplastic syndromes, 308t, 309–310
Parapneumonic effusions, 374–375
Parasympathetic nervous system, in regulation of airway caliber, 119, 120f
Parenchyma, structure and function of, 136–137, 136–138f
Parenchymal inflammation and injury, 135–147
  due to acute lung injury, 138–145
    exudative phase of, 139f, 139–143, 140t, 141f, 142f
    fibrotic phase of, 144f, 144–145, 145t
    proliferative phase of, 143, 143f
  case study of, 135, 137, 147
  gas-exchange abnormalities in, 145
  due to inhalation injury, 137–138
  lung function in, 145–146, 146f
  pulmonary hypertension with, 146
  therapy and outcome of, 146–147
  ventilation in, 145–146, 146f
Partial pressure of carbon dioxide (PCO_2). *See* PCO_2
Partial pressure of oxygen (PO_2). *See* PO_2
PCO_2, 39–42, 41f
  and acid-base status, 80, 81f
  alveolar, 39–42, 41f, 89–92, 90f, 91f
  arterial
    shunt and, 95, 98f
    ventilation-perfusion inequality and, 94, 95f
  end-capillary, 92

PCP (*Pneumocystis carinii* pneumonia), with human immunodeficiency virus, 337–338, 339t
PCR (polymerase chain reaction) test, for tuberculosis, 321
PCWP (pulmonary capillary wedge pressure), in pulmonary hypertension, 162
PDGF (platelet-derived growth factor), in acute lung injury, 144, 145t
PE. *See* Pulmonary embolism (PE)
Peak expiratory flow (PEF), in asthma, 217, 217f
Peak expiratory flow rate (PEFR)
  in obstructive airways diseases, 124, 124t
  in respiratory failure, 183
Pentamidine, for *Mycobacterium avium* complex, 338
Perfusion, limitations on, 50–52, 51f, 52f
Perfusion limited gas transfer, 50, 51f
PFTs. *See* Pulmonary function tests (PFTs)
PGI_2 (prostaglandin I_2), 165, 166, 167
PH. *See* Pulmonary hypertension (PH)
pH
  arterial, in respiratory failure, 182, 182f, 182t
  and oxyhemoglobin dissociation curve, 73
  of pleural effusions, 373
pH balance, 79–85, 80f, 82t, 83t, 84t, 85f
Phrenic nerve, 15
Physiologic dead space, 38, 39f
Physiologic dead space to tidal volume ratio (V_D/V_T), during exercise, 107, 200–201
Pickwickian syndrome, 82
PKA (protein kinase A), in airway smooth muscle contraction, 123, 123f
Plasma volume, during exercise, 111
Platelet-derived growth factor (PDGF), in acute lung injury, 144, 145t
Pleura
  development of, 3
  normal anatomy and physiology of, 368f, 368–370, 370f
Pleural biopsy, 373
Pleural disease, 367–381
  case studies of, 367, 370, 373, 378
Pleural effusions, 371–375
  categories of, 371–373
  causes of, 371t
  chest x-ray of, 371f
  diagnosis of, 373–374
  effects on respiration of, 374
  exudative, 371, 372t, 372–373
  with human immunodeficiency virus, 344
  malignant, 375
  management of, 374f, 374–375
  parapneumonic, 374–375
  pathogenesis of, 371
  transudative, 372, 372t
Pleural fluid, 369–370, 370f
Pleural plaques
  in asbestos-related pulmonary disorders, 392, 393t, 393–394, 395
  in occupational lung disease, 388f
Pleural pressure gradient, 42, 43f, 44f
Pleural space, physiology of, 369–370, 370f
PMNs (polymorphonuclear cells), in sarcoidosis, 246
Pneumococcal pneumonia, with human immunodeficiency virus, 334–335
Pneumoconiosis, 384. *See also* Occupational lung disease(s)
  coal-worker's, 396–397, 397f
Pneumocystis carinii pneumonia (PCP), with human immunodeficiency virus, 337–338, 339t
Pneumonia
  bronchiolitis obliterans with, 279
  chronic eosinophilic, 279
  pleural effusions due to, 374–375
  pneumococcal, with human immunodeficiency virus, 334–335
  Pneumocystis carinii, with human immunodeficiency virus, 337–338, 339t

Pneumonitis
  herpes simplex, 341
  hypersensitivity, 269–271, 270t
  interstitial, with human immunodeficiency virus, 343
Pneumothorax(ces), 375–378
  categories of, 375
  clinical manifestations of, 375
  defined, 375
  with human immunodeficiency virus, 343–344
  iatrogenic, 377–378, 378t
  management of, 378
  physiological effects of, 375
  primary spontaneous, 377
  radiographic appearance of, 376f, 377
  secondary spontaneous, 377, 377t
  traumatic, 377–378
  types of, 377–378
PO$_2$, 41f, 41–42
  alveolar, 41f, 41–42, 89–92, 90f, 91f
  arterial
    shunt and, 95–97, 98f, 99f
    ventilation-perfusion inequality and, 94f, 94–95, 96f, 97f
  end-capillary, 92, 98, 101
  mixed-venous, and gas exchange, 97–99, 100f
  with pulmonary embolism, 289
Pollution, air, 399t, 399–400
Polymerase chain reaction (PCR) test, for tuberculosis, 321
Polymorphonuclear cells (PMNs), in sarcoidosis, 246
Polysomnography (PSG), 360, 361f
  of pulmonary hypertension, 162–164
PPD (purified protein derivative) tuberculin test, 319, 320t
PPH (primary pulmonary hypertension), 152, 161, 161f, 164–166
Premature infants, hyaline membrane disease in, 6
Prenatal development
  of diaphragm and pleura, 3
  of lungs, 1t, 1–3, 2t
  of lung vasculature, 3–5, 4f
  surfactant in, 5–6, 6f
Pressure-volume curves
  in acute lung injury, 146, 146f
  in interstitial lung disease, 265, 266f
Primary lobule, 23
Primary pulmonary hypertension (PPH), 152, 161, 161f, 164–166
Progressive massive fibrosis (PMF), in coal worker's pneumoconiosis, 396
Progressive systemic sclerosis (PSS), with interstitial lung disease, 273
Proliferative phase, of acute lung injury, 143, 143f
Prostaglandin I$_2$ (PGI$_2$, prostacyclin), 165, 166, 167
Prostaglandins, in acute lung injury, 140
Protein kinase A (PKA), in airway smooth muscle contraction, 123, 123f
Pseudoglandular period, 1t, 2
PSG (polysomnography), 360, 361f
  of pulmonary hypertension, 162–164
PSS (progressive systemic sclerosis), with interstitial lung disease, 273
Pulmonary angiography
  of pulmonary embolism, 294
  of pulmonary hypertension, 161, 163f
Pulmonary arterial pressure (PAP), 60
  and pulmonary vascular resistance, 61, 62f
  during sleep, 360
Pulmonary arteries, 26
  development of, 3–4
Pulmonary artery catheter
  hemodynamic measurements using, 66t, 67t
  in pulmonary hypertension, 161
Pulmonary capillary wedge pressure (PCWP), in pulmonary hypertension, 162
Pulmonary circulation. See Circulation

Pulmonary embolism (PE), 285–299
  arterial blood gases in, 289
  case study of, 286, 288, 291, 295
  chest radiography of, 288–289, 289t
  clinical features of, 287–289
  diagnostic tests for, 292–295, 293f, 294f
  Doppler ultrasound of, 292, 292f
  electrocardiogram of, 288f, 289, 289t
  gas-exchange abnormalities in, 289–290
  hemodynamics in, 290
  incidence of, 285
  management of, 295f, 296–297, 297t
  pathophysiology of, 286
  prophylaxis for, 296t
  pulmonary angiography of, 294
  pulmonary infarction due to, 290–291
  risk factors for, 286, 286t, 296t
  signs and symptoms of, 287, 287t, 288t
  venography of, 292
  ventilation-perfusion lung scan of, 291f, 294–295, 295f
Pulmonary fibrosis
  idiopathic, interstitial lung disease due to, 277–278
  in interstitial lung disease, 268
  lung compliance in, 24, 25f, 127, 127f
  in sarcoidosis, 248, 249f
Pulmonary function tests (PFTs)
  in asbestos-related pulmonary disorders, 394
  in asthma, 219–220
  in chronic obstructive pulmonary disease, 234t
  in coal worker's pneumoconiosis, 396
  with human immunodeficiency virus, 346
  in interstitial lung disease, 264f, 265t, 266
  in lung cancer, 302t
  in obstructive airways diseases, 123–129
  in occupational asthma, 398–399
  in occupational lung disease, 386, 386t
  in pulmonary hypertension, 157f, 159, 165
  in respiratory failure, 181t, 183
  in sarcoidosis, 252, 253t, 254t, 255f
  in silicosis, 389
Pulmonary hypertension (PH), 151–168
  in acute lung injury, 146
  arterial blood gas testing in, 159
  case study of, 153, 154, 159, 164, 166
  chest radiography of, 156f, 159, 165
  classification of, 151–153, 152t
  collagen vascular diseases with, 153
  defined, 151
  diagnostic evaluation of, 157–164, 158f
  echocardiography of, 159–160, 160f, 165
  electrocardiography of, 155f, 159
  exercise in, 165
  with human immunodeficiency virus, 344
  hyperkinetic, 152t
  in interstitial lung disease, 265t, 267
  lung biopsy in, 164
  management of, 166–168
  mixed capillary (precapillary), 152, 152t
  with normal or near-normal lungs, 152, 152t
  obliterative, 152t
  obstructive, 152t
  passive, 152t
  physical examination for, 153, 153t, 154f, 157f
  polygenic, 152t
  polysomnography of, 162–164
  postcapillary, 151–152, 152t
  primary (unexplained, idiopathic), 152, 161, 161f, 164–166
  pulmonary angiography of, 161, 163f
  pulmonary capillary wedge pressure in, 162
  pulmonary function testing in, 157f, 159, 165
  right heart catheterization in, 161–162
  thromboembolic, 161, 162f, 163f
  vasoconstrictive, 152t

Pulmonary hypertension (PH) (*continued*)
  ventilation-perfusion lung scanning in, 160f,162f, 160–161
  waves in jugular vein in, 153, 154f
Pulmonary infarction, due to pulmonary embolism, 290–291
Pulmonary nodule, solitary, 307
Pulmonary parenchyma, structure and function of, 136–137, 136–138f
Pulmonary sequestration, 8
Pulmonary trunk, 26
Pulmonary vascular bed
  active influences on, 62–63, 64f
  passive influences on, 61–62, 62f, 63f
  unique characteristics of, 59, 60f, 60t
Pulmonary vascular diseases, exercise physiology in, 206
Pulmonary vascular distention, 59, 60f
Pulmonary vascular recruitment, 59, 60f
Pulmonary vascular resistance (PVR), 26, 27–29f, 60–63, 61–64f, 67t
Pulmonary veins, 26
  development of, 4
Pulsus paradoxus, in asthma, 220
Pump failure, 172, 172f, 173f
Purified protein derivative (PPD) tuberculin test, 319, 320t
Pyrazinamide (PZA), for tuberculosis, 332
  in HIV patients, 336, 336t

R

R (respiratory exchange ratio), 41
RA (rheumatoid arthritis), with interstitial lung disease, 273
Radiography, chest. *See* Chest radiography
Radon, lung cancer due to, 303
Rapid eye movement (REM) sleep, 356
Rapidly adapting pulmonary stretch receptors (RARs), 31, 32t
Raynaud's phenomenon, in pulmonary hypertension, 164
Recruitment, 26
  pulmonary vascular, 59, 60f
Rectus abdominis muscles, 16
Reid index, 3
Residual volume (RV), 126, 126f
  in obstructive airways diseases, 127, 128f
Resistance
  airway, 25, 116–117
    in obstructive airways diseases, 123
  to gas flow, 52
  tissue, 116
Respiration, pleural effusion effect on, 374
Respiratory acidosis, 81–82, 81f, 82t
Respiratory alkalosis, 81f, 83, 83t
  in pulmonary hypertension, 165
Respiratory control center
  central, 354, 354f
  normal, 354–356, 354–356f
  during sleep, 357–358
Respiratory exchange ratio (R), 41
Respiratory failure, 171–188
  acute *vs.* chronic, 173f, 173–174
  anatomic components of, 172, 173f
  arterial blood-gas analysis in, 180–182, 181t, 182f, 182t
  arterial pH in, 182, 182f, 182t
  case study of, 171, 174, 184, 188
  chest imaging in, 181t, 183–184
  defined, 172–174
  diagnosis of, 179–182t, 179–184, 182f
  due to diffusion abnormality, 174
  hypercapnia in, 182
  due to hypoventilation, 176–178, 179f
  hypoxemia in, 180–182
  due to intrapulmonary shunt, 176, 177f
  laboratory diagnosis of, 180–184, 181t, 182f, 182t
  lung failure in, 172, 172f, 173f

  lung function testing in, 181t, 183
  medications for, 185
  oxygen therapy for, 184–185
  pathophysiology of, 174–178, 175–177f, 179f
  physical examination of, 180, 180t
  pump failure in, 172, 172f, 173f
  reducing ventilatory work load for, 186–187
  supportive therapy for, 185–186
  symptoms of, 179, 179t
  treatment of, 184–187, 185f
  due to ventilation-perfusion inequality, 174f, 174–175, 175f
Respiratory mechanics, in respiratory failure, 181t, 183
Respiratory muscles. *See* Muscles
Respiratory quotient (RQ), 41
  during exercise, 106
Respiratory rate, during exercise, 107, 108f
Restrictive lung diseases, 204
  exercise physiology in, 205
Rheumatoid arthritis (RA), with interstitial lung disease, 273
Rhodococcus equi, with human immunodeficiency virus, 334
Rib cage, 12, 13f
Rifampin, for tuberculosis, 322
  in HIV patients, 336, 336t
Right heart catheterization, in pulmonary hypertension, 161–162
Right-to-left shunting, with pulmonary embolism, 289–290
Right ventricular hypertrophy, in pulmonary hypertension, 153, 155f, 159, 160f
Right ventricular stroke work index (RVSWI), 67t
Rounded atelectasis, in asbestos-related pulmonary disorders, 392, 394f
RQ (respiratory quotient), 41
  during exercise, 106
Runyon classification, 317, 317t
RV (residual volume), 126, 126f
  in obstructive airways diseases, 127, 128f

S

Saccular period, 1t, 2
Salmeterol, for asthma, 223
Sarcoidosis, 243–258
  angiotensin converting enzyme in, 252, 252t
  assessment of disease activity in, 253
  case study of, 243, 244f, 253–254, 254f, 255, 255f
  clinical manifestations of, 249–250, 250f, 251f, 251t
  cutaneous anergy in, 246
  defined, 244
  diagnosis of, 252t, 252–254, 253f, 254f
  erythema nodosum in, 250
  etiology of, 244–248, 245t, 246t, 247–249f, 248t
  granulomas in, 246, 247f, 248f, 248t
  immune response in, 245t, 245–246, 246t
  incidence of, 244
  infectious agents associated with, 244–245, 245t
  lupus pernio in, 250
  myocardial, 249
  ocular, 250
  pathophysiology of, 244–248, 245t, 246t, 247–249f, 248t
  prognosis in, 254, 254t
  pulmonary fibrosis in, 248, 249f
  pulmonary function tests in, 252, 253t, 254t, 255f
  stages of, 251t
  treatment of, 254–255, 255f, 255t
SARs (slowly adapting pulmonary stretch receptors), 31, 32t
Scalenus muscles, 16
SCLC (small cell lung carcinoma), 305, 306f, 307, 307t
Sclerosis, progressive systemic, with interstitial lung disease, 273
Sclerotherapy, for malignant pleural effusions, 375

Sensors, in control of breathing, 354–356
Sequestration, pulmonary, 8
Shunt, 95–97, 98f, 99f
    alveolar-arterial oxygen gradient with, 100
    with pulmonary embolism, 289–290
    respiratory failure due to, 176, 177f
SIADH (syndrome of inappropriate antidiuretic hormone),
        with lung cancer, 308t, 310
Sickle cell disease, 74
Signal transduction, in airway smooth muscle contraction,
        122, 123f
Silicosis, 387f, 388–391, 389t, 390f
Single-breath nitrogen washout test, 45f, 45–46
Skeletal muscle, energy sources for, 105–107, 106f, 107t
Skin testing, in occupational asthma, 399
SLE (systemic lupus erythematosus), with interstitial lung
        disease, 274
Sleep, normal, 356–357, 357f
Sleep apnea
    central, 362–363
    obstructive, 358–361, 358–361f
Sleep-related breathing disorders, 162–164, 353–365
    case study of, 353, 356, 357, 358, 362, 363, 364
    due to central sleep apnea, 362–363
    due to chronic obstructive pulmonary disease, 363, 363f
    control of breathing and
        normal, 354–356, 354–356f
        during sleep, 357–358
    normal sleep and, 356–357, 357f
    due to obstructive sleep apnea syndrome, 358–361,
        358–361f
Slowly adapting pulmonary stretch receptors (SARs), 31,
        32t
Slow-wave sleep (SWS), 356
Small cell lung carcinoma (SCLC), 305, 306f, 307, 307t
Smoke inhalation, 137–138
Smoking. See Cigarette smoking
Smooth muscle, airway, 20–21, 21f
Smooth muscle contraction, 122t, 122–123, 123f
Solitary pulmonary nodule, 307
Specific compliance, 24
Spirometry
    in obstructive airways diseases, 124, 124t
    in occupation lung diseases, 386, 386t
Sputum analysis
    with human immunodeficiency virus, 346
    in tuberculosis, 320–321
Squamous cell carcinoma, 305, 306f
Staphylococcus aureus, with human immunodeficiency
        virus, 334
Starling's law, 369
Static lung volumes, in obstructive airways diseases, 125–
        127, 128f
Static volume-pressure curves, 12, 14f
Sternocleidomastoid muscles, 16
Streptococcus pneumonia, with human immunodeficiency
        virus, 334–335
Stretch receptors, 31, 32t
    in control of breathing, 355–356
Stroke volume, during exercise, 109, 110f
Stroke volume index (SVI), 67t
Submucosa, 20
Substance P, in regulation of airway caliber, 120f
Sulfur dioxide, 400
Superior vena cava (SVC) syndrome, 308t, 309
Surfactant, 3, 5–6, 6f, 23, 24
    in acute lung injury, 139
Surfactants, 136
SVI (stroke volume index), 67t
SVR (systemic vascular resistance), 67t
Swan-Ganz catheterization, 30, 30f, 66
SWS (slow-wave sleep), 356
Sympathetic nervous system, in regulation of airway caliber,
        119–120, 120f
Symptom-limited cardiopulmonary exercise test, 192

Syncope, in pulmonary hypertension, 164, 165
Syndrome of inappropriate antidiuretic hormone (SIADH),
        with lung cancer, 308t, 310
Systemic lupus erythematosus (SLE), with interstitial lung
        disease, 274
Systemic necrotizing vasculitis, with interstitial lung
        disease, 275
Systemic vascular resistance (SVR), 67t

T

Tachykinins, in regulation of airway caliber, 120f
TB. See Tuberculosis (TB)
T cells
    in human immunodeficiency virus, 332
    in sarcoidosis, 245, 246
Terminal respiratory unit, 136, 136f
TGFs (transforming growth factors), in acute lung injury,
        144, 145, 145t
Theophylline
    for asthma, 223, 224t, 226
    for chronic obstructive pulmonary disease, 239
Thermodilution technique, for cardiac output, 66
Thoracic cage, 12
Thoracocentesis, of pleural effusions, 371, 373
Thoracotomy, in interstitial lung disease, 268
Thorax, 12, 13f
Thromboembolic pulmonary hypertension, 161, 162f, 163f
Thromboembolism. See Pulmonary embolism (PE)
Thrombolytic therapy, for pulmonary embolism and deep
        venous thrombosis, 297
Thromboxane, 165
Tidal volume (TV), 37, 126, 126f
    during exercise, 107, 108f, 109f
Timed distance test, 192
Tissue resistance, 116
TMP/SMX (trimethoprim-sulfamethoxazole), for
        Mycobacterium avium complex, 338
TNF (tumor necrosis factor), in acute lung injury, 140t
Total lung capacity (TLC), 126, 126f
    in acute lung injury, 146f
    in obstructive airways diseases, 127, 128f
Total pressure of respiratory system, 12, 14f
Total sleep time (TST), 357
Trachea, 20, 21f
    abnormalities of, 8
Tracheobronchial glands, development of, 3
Tracheostomy, for obstructive sleep apnea, 361
Training, effect in healthy adults of, 111–112
Transbronchial biopsy, in interstitial lung disease, 268,
        268t
Transcapillary exchange, Starling's law of, 369
Transforming growth factors (TGFs), in acute lung injury,
        144, 145, 145t
Transplantation
    for pulmonary hypertension, 168
    for respiratory failure, 187
    for sarcoidosis, 255
Transpulmonary pressure, 42
Transudative effusions, 372, 372t
Transverse septum, 3
Transversus abdominis muscle, 16
Trauma, pneumothorax due to, 377–378
Tricuspid regurgitation, in pulmonary hypertension, 153,
        154f
Trimethoprim-sulfamethoxazole (TMP/SMX), for
        Mycobacterium avium complex, 338
TST (total sleep time), 357
Tuberculin skin test, 319, 320t
Tuberculosis (TB), 317–324
    BCG vaccination for, 323
    with coal worker's pneumoconiosis, 397
    diagnosis of, 320–321
    epidemiology of, 317f, 317–318, 318t
    in HIV-infected patients, 320, 323–324

Tuberculosis (TB) (*continued*)
  with human immunodeficiency virus, 335–336, 336t
  multidrug resistant, 321–322, 332
  pathogenesis of, 318–319, 319f
  preventative therapy for, 323, 323t
  risk factors for, 318, 318t
  screening for, 319–320, 320t
  with silicosis, 391
  transmission of, 318
  treatment for, 321–322, 322t
Tumor necrosis factor (TNF), in acute lung injury, 140t
Turbulent flow, 116–117
TV. *See* Tidal volume (TV)
Type I pneumocytes, 3, 23, 23f, 136, 137f
  in acute lung injury, 139, 139t
Type II pneumocytes, 3, 23, 23f, 136
  in acute lung injury, 139

U

Ultrasound, Doppler, for pulmonary embolism, 292, 292f
Underdamping, 362
Upper airway(s), 115
Upper airway receptors, in control of breathing, 356
Urinothorax, 372
Uvulopalatalpharyngoplasty (UPPP), for obstructive sleep
         apnea, 361

V

Vaccination, antipneumococcal, 240
Vascular pressures, during exercise, 111
Vascular resistance, 26, 27–29f, 60–63, 61–64f, 67t
Vascular system. *See* Circulation
Vascular tone, 30, 30t
Vasculature. *See* Circulation
Vasculitis(ides)
  Churg-Strauss, 277
  interstitial lung disease due to, 275, 276–277
  systemic necrotizing, 275
Vasoactive intestinal peptide (VIP), in regulation of airway
         caliber, 120f
Vasoactive substances, 30, 30t
Vasoconstriction, 29–30
  during exercise, 111
Vasodilation, during exercise, 111
Vasodilator therapy, for pulmonary hypertension, 165, 166,
         167–168
VC (vital capacity), 126, 126f
  in respiratory failure, 183
V_D/V_T (physiologic dead space to tidal volume ratio), during
         exercise, 107, 200–201
V_{Emax} (maximum exercise ventilation), 198–199
Vena cava. *See* Inferior vena cava (IVC); Superior vena cava
         (SVC)
Venography, for pulmonary embolism, 292
Venous admixture, 101–102, 102f
Venous thromboembolism. *See* Pulmonary embolism (PE)
Ventilation, 23, 37–46
  in acute lung injury, 145–146, 146f
  alveolar, 37
  alveolar dead space in, 39–42, 40f, 41f
  closing volume in, 45f, 45–46
  defined, 37
  during exercise, 107, 108f, 109f
  in interstitial lung disease, 264–265, 265t, 266f

  lung volume and, 42–45
  minute, 37–38, 38f
  regional differences in, 42–46, 43–45f
  in simplified lung, 37–38, 38f, 39f
Ventilation-perfusion (V/Q) inequality, 93–95, 94f, 96f,
         97f
  alveolar-arterial oxygen gradient with, 100–101, 101f
  respiratory failure due to, 174–175, 175f, 176f
Ventilation-perfusion (V/Q) lung scan
  for pulmonary embolism, 291f, 294–295, 295f
  for pulmonary hypertension, 160f,162f, 160–161
  for respiratory failure, 184
Ventilation-perfusion (V/Q) mismatch, during exercise,
         200f, 200–201
Ventilation-perfusion (V/Q) ratio, 93
Ventilation-perfusion (V/Q) relationships, 89–102
  alveolar-arterial oxygen difference, 92
  and alveolar PO_2 and PCO_2, 89–92, 90f, 91f
  diffusion impairment, 93
  gas exchange
    abnormal, 92–99
      nonpulmonary factors in, 97–99, 100f
      assessing efficiency of, 99–102, 101f, 102f
  hypoventilation, 92–93
  regional variations in, 90–92, 91f
  shunt, 95–97, 98f, 99f
  ventilation-perfusion inequality, 93–95, 94f, 96f, 97f
Ventilator equivalence method, 197, 198f
Ventilatory response
  to exercise, 193
  to hypercapnia, 355, 355f
  to hypoxemia, 355, 356f
Ventral respiratory group (VRG), 354
VIP (vasoactive intestinal peptide), in regulation of airway
         caliber, 120f
Viral infections, with human immunodeficiency virus, 341
Vital capacity (VC), 126, 126f
  in respiratory failure, 183
VO_2 (oxygen uptake), maximal, during exercise testing,
         195–196, 196f
Volume-pressure curves, in acute lung injury, 146, 146f
VO_{2max} (maximal oxygen uptake), during exercise testing,
         195–196, 196f
V/Q. *See under* Ventilation-perfusion (V/Q)
VRG (ventral respiratory group), 354
V slope method, 197, 198f

W

Warfarin
  for pulmonary embolism and deep venous thrombosis,
         297, 297t
  for pulmonary hypertension, 167
Wegener's granulomatosis, interstitial lung disease due to,
         276
Work of breathing
  in acute lung injury, 146
  in airflow obstruction, 128

X

X-ray, chest. *See* Chest radiography

Z

Zone of apposition, 12, 13f, 15–16